D1560864

Principles and Practice of Radiation Therapy

Practical Applications

Edited by

Charles M. Washington, BS, RT(T)

Director, Radiation Therapy Program
M.D. Anderson Cancer Center
The University of Texas
Houston, Texas

Dennis T. Leaver, MS, RT(R)(T)

Director, Radiation Therapy Program
Southern Maine Technical College
South Portland, Maine

with 301 illustrations

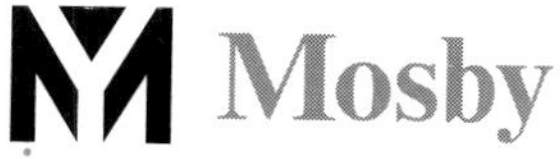

St. Louis Baltimore Boston Carlsbad Chicago Naples New York Philadelphia Portland
London Madrid Mexico City Singapore Sydney Tokyo Toronto Wiesbaden

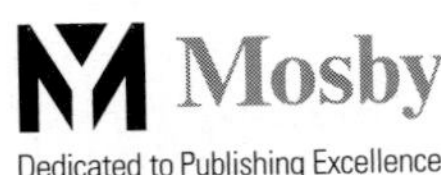

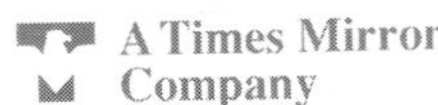

Vice President and Publisher: Don Ladig
Senior Editor: Jeanne Rowland
Senior Developmental Editor: Lisa Potts
Project Manager: Linda McKinley
Production Editor: Paul Stoecklein
Designer: Elizabeth Young
Electronic Production Coordinator: Joan Herron
Manufacturing Supervisor: Linda Ierardi

Printed in the United States of America

Composition by Mosby Electronic Production—St. Louis
Lithography by Top Graphics
Printing/binding by Maple Vail Book Manufacturing Group

Mosby–Year Book, Inc.
11830 Westline Industrial Drive
St. Louis, Missouri 63146

Library of Congress Cataloging in Publication Data
Principles and practice of radiation therapy / edited by Charles M.
Washington, Dennis T. Leaver.
p. cm.
Includes bibliographical references and index.
Contents: v. 3. Practical applications.
ISBN 0-8151-9137-5 (hardback)
1. Cancer--Radiotherapy. I. Washington, Charles M. II. Leaver,
Dennis T.
[DNLM: 1. Radiation Oncology--methods. WN 250 P957 1997]
RC271.R3P734 1997
616.99' 442--dc20
DNLM/DLC
for Library of Congress 96—4954
CIP

97 98 99 00 01 / 9 8 7 6 5 4 3 2 1

Contributors

Susan Barber-Derus, BA, RT(R)(T)
Director, Department of Radiation Oncology,
Froedtert Memorial Lutheran Hospital,
Milwaukee, Wisconsin

James D. Becht, MD
Radiation Oncologist,
Department of Radiation Oncology,
Elliot Regional Cancer Center,
Manchester, New Hampshire

Susan Belinsky, MPA, RT(R)(T)
Director, Radiation Therapy Program,
Labore College,
Boston, Massachusetts

Todd Blobe, BA, RT(T)
Program Director,
School of Radiation Therapy,
Baptist/St. Vincent's Health Systems,
Jacksonville, Florida

Leila A. Bussman, BS, RT(R)(T)
Director, Radiation Therapy Program,
Mayo Clinic/Mayo Foundation,
Rochester, Minnesota

Timothy Dziuk, MD
Director, Department of Radiation Oncology,
Texoma Regional Cancer Center,
Sherman, Texas

Russell L. Gerber, MS
Instructor in Radiology,
Mallinckrodt Institute of Technology,
Washington University Medical School,
St. Louis, Missouri

Cheryl Glisch, BS, RT(R)(T)
Director of Quality Management,
Department of Radiation Oncology,
Medical College of Wisconsin,
Milwaukee, Wisconsin

Theresa Grady, BS, RT(T)
Chief Therapist,
Department of Radiation Oncology,
New England Medical Center,
Boston, Massachusetts

Sally V. Green, BS, RT(T)
Clinical Coordinator, Radiation Therapy Program,
Bellevue Community College,
Bellevue, Washington

J. Michael Kerley, MD
Director, Department of Radiation Oncology,
Paris Regional Cancer Center and
St. Joseph's Radiation Oncology Center,
Paris, Texas

Linda Langlin, RT(R)(T)
Clinical Supervisor,
Department of Radiation Oncology,
Central Maine Medical Center,
Lewiston, Maine

Janice M. Manolis, RT(T), CMD
Certified Medical Dosimetrist,
Department of Radiation Therapy,
St. Mary's Hospital,
St. Louis, Missouri

James A. Martenson, MD
Radiation Therapy Program,
Mayo Clinic/Mayo Foundation,
Rochester, Minnesota

Tammy Newell, RT(T)
Radiation Therapist,
Department of Radiation Oncology,
Elliot Regional Cancer Center,
Manchester, New Hampshire

Carlos Perez, MD
Director, Radiation Oncology Center,
Mallinckrodt Institute of Radiology,
Washington University Medical Center,
St. Louis, Missouri

Jean Roane, RT(R)(T)
Radiation Therapist,
Department of Radiation Oncology,
Maine Medical Center,
Portland, Maine

Cheryl Sanders, MPA, RT(R)(T)
Director, Radiation Therapy Program,
The University of Nebraska,
Omaha, Nebraska

Donna Stinson, MPA, RT(R)(T)
Director, Radiation Therapy Program,
Cooper Hospital/University Medical Center,
Camden, New Jersey

Dan Strahan, BS, RT(T)
Director, Radiation Therapy Program,
Methodist Hospital of Indiana,
Indianapolis, Indiana

Cathy Turley, MS, RT(R)(T)
Assistant Professor of Radiology,
School of Medicine and Health Sciences,
The George Washington University,
Washington, DC

Paul Wallner, DO, FACR
Radiation Oncologist,
Cooper Hospital/University Medical Center,
Camden, New Jersey

Jeffrey Young, MD
Clinical Assistant Professor,
Department of Radiation Oncology,
Maine Medical Center,
Portland, Maine

Reviewers

Eric Anderson, PhD
Assistant Professor of Physics,
Avila College,
Kansas City, Missouri

Sucha Asbell, MD
Chairman, Radiation Oncology,
Albert Einstein Medical Center,
Philadelphia, Pennsylvania

Joseph Baranowsky, BS
Field Service Engineer,
Dornier Medical Systems,
Kennesaw, Georgia

Cecelia Bouchard, MS, RT(R)(T)
Clinical Coordinator, Radiation Therapy,
Southern Maine Technical College,
South Portland, Maine

Andrew P. Brown, MD
Radiation Oncologist,
Elliott Regional Cancer Center,
Manchester, New Hampshire

Cynthia P. Burns, AS, RT(R)(T)
Radiation Therapist,
Cynthia A. Rydholm Cancer Treatment Center,
Central Maine Medical Center,
Lewiston, Maine

Shaun T. Caldwell, BS, RT(R)(T)
Educational Director, Radiation Therapy,
College of Health Professions,
Weber State University,
Ogden, Utah

Anne T. Campbell, BHS, RT(R)(T)
Program Director, Radiation Therapy Technology Program,
Chandler Medical Center,
University of Kentucky,
Lexington, Kentucky

Sandra Bouquet Carslick, RT(R)(T)
Senior Radiation Therapist,
Costal Cancer Treatment Center,
Maine Medical Center,
Bath, Maine

Peter Y. Chen, MD
Associate Director of Education,
Department of Radiation Oncology,
William Beaumont Hospital,
Royal Oak, Michigan

Melvin C. Cheney, MS, RT(T)
Director of Patient Services,
Northwest Arkansas Radiation Therapy Institute;
Program Director, Radiation Therapist Program,
Northwest Arkansas Community College,
Springdale, Arkansas

Annette Coleman, MA, RT(T)
Director, Radiation Therapy Program,
Harvard Joint Center for Radiation Therapy,
Massachusetts College of Pharmacy and Allied Health Sciences,
Boston, Massachusetts

Joseph Digel, RT(R)(T)
Chief Therapist, Radiation Oncology,
Program Director, Radiation Therapy Program,
The Johns Hopkins Hospital,
Baltimore, Maryland

Barbara Flexner, BS, RT(T)
Educational Coordinator, Program Director,
Allied Health and Radiation Therapy Technology,
Vanderbilt University Medical Center,
Nashville, Tennessee

Diana Freeman, BS, RT(T)
Program Director, Certified Medical Dosimetrist,
Parkland College,
Decatur Memorial Hospital,
Decatur, Illinois

Tilly Gibbs, BA, RT(T)
Chief Therapist, Director,
Radiation Therapy Program,
University of Utah Hospital,
Salt Lake City, Utah

Patricia Giordano, MS, RT(T)
Program Director, Assistant Professor,
Gwynedd-Mercy College,
Gwynedd Valley, Pennsylvania

Charleen Gombert, BS, RT(T)
Professor, Program Director,
Radiation Therapy Technology Program,
Community College of Allegheny County,
Pittsburgh, Pennsylvania

Mark Graniero, BS, RT(T)
Chief Radiation Therapist,
Four County Radiation Medicine,
Utica, New York

Roslyn Ham, AS, RT(T)
Radiation Therapist,
Florida East Coast Cancer Center,
Ft. Pierce, Florida

Robert Holihan, BS, RT(R)
Instructor, Radiography Program,
Ferris State University,
Big Rapids, Michigan

Edna Holmes, MPA, RT(R)
Director, Radiography Program,
Lake Michigan College,
Benton Harbor, Michigan

Kathleen Kienstra, BS, RT(R)(T)
Program Director,
Barnes Hospital School of Radiation Therapy,
St. Louis, Missouri

Julianne Kinsman, MEd, RT(T)
Department Chairperson, Radiation Therapy Technology,
Springfield Technical Community College,
Springfield, Massachusetts

Druellen Kolker, BS, RT(T)
Program Director, Radiation Therapy Technology,
University of Chicago Hospitals,
Roosevelt University,
Chicago, Illinois

Sue M. Merkel, BS, RT(R)(T)
Program Director, Radiation Oncology,
University of Michigan Medical Center,
Ann Arbor, Michigan

Carmen Mesina, MS
Clinical Radiation Therapy Physicist,
Harper Hospital,
Wayne State University,
Detroit, Michigan

Roy A. Miller, BS, RT(T)
Coordinator, Radiation Therapy Program,
Owens Community College,
Toledo, Ohio

Sharon J. Morretti, RT(T)
Supervisor, Radiation Therapy Program,
North Shore Cancer Center,
Peabody, Massachusetts

Cindy Mueller, BS, RT(R)(T)
Program Director, School of Radiation Therapy,
St. Joseph's Hospital,
Milwaukee, Wisconsin

Diane Mulkhey, AS, RT(T)
Manager, Radiation Therapy Department,
Central Maine Medical Center,
Lewiston, Maine

Joann M. Murray, BS, RT(R)(T)
Program Director, School of Radiation Therapy,
Welborn Cancer Center,
Evansville, Indiana

Larry Oliver, RT(T)
Program Director, Radiation Therapy Technology,
University of Kansas Medical Center,
Kansas City, Kansas

Brad Owen, RT(T)
Radiation Therapist,
Glens Falls, New York

Christina M. Paugh, BA, RT(R)(T)
Program Director, Educational Coordinator,
Radiation Oncology,
West Virginia University Hospital,
Morgantown, West Virginia

Joan Pierson, RT(R)(T)
Program Coordinator,
School of Radiation Therapy,
Henry Ford Hospital,
Detroit, Michigan

Nancy Quinn-Fagan, MEd, RT(R)(T)
Director of Education,
M.D. Anderson-Moncrief Cancer Center,
Ft. Worth, Texas

Marie L.A. Racine, BS, RT(R)(T)
Program Director, Radiation Therapy Technology,
Galveston College/University of Texas School of Allied Health Sciences,
Galveston, Texas

Mary Jo Repasky, MHSA, RT(R)(T)
Program Director, Radiation Therapy Technology,
College of Health Professions,
Medical University of South Carolina,
Charleston, South Carolina

Pamela J. Ross, RT(T)
Coordinator of Technology,
Clinical Coordinator,
School of Radiation Therapy,
New York Methodist Hospital,
Brooklyn, New York

David Schatanoff, MD
Radiation Oncologist,
Radiation Oncology Department,
Mercy Regional Health System,
Altoona, Pennsylvania

Deborah Semanchik, RT(R)(T)
Radiation Therapist,
Radiation Oncology Department,
Mercy Regional Health System,
Altoona, Pennsylvania

Diane Skog, BS, RT(T)
Senior Radiation Therapist,
Maine Medical Center,
Portland, Maine

Shirley N. Smith, MPA, RT(R)(T)
Associate Dean of Radiation Therapy,
Baker College,
Owosso, Michigan

Carole A. Sullivan, PhD, RT(R)(T), FASRT
Dean, College of Allied Health,
Health Sciences Center,
University of Oklahoma,
Oklahoma City, Oklahoma

Larry Swafford, BS, RT(T)
Program Director, Radiation Therapy Technology,
Virginia Commonwealth University/Medical College of Virginia,
Richmond, Virginia

Wanda Teasley, MHSA, RT(R)(T), FASRT
Chairperson, Associate Professor,
Clinical Services Department,
College of Health Professions,
Medical University of South Carolina,
Charleston, South Carolina

Giles Toole, MS, RT(R)(T)
Program Director, Radiation Therapy Technology,
Thomas Technical Institute,
Thomasville, Georgia

George M. Ushold, EdD, RT(T)
Director of Education, School of Radiation Therapy,
University of Rochester Cancer Center,
Rochester, New York

Ann Marie Vann, MEd, RT(R)(T)
Program Director, Radiation Therapy,
Medical College of Georgia,
Augusta, Georgia

David G. Ward, BS, Ed, RT(R)(T)
Program Director, Radiation Therapy Technology,
University Hospital of Cleveland,
Cleveland, Ohio

To those who have run and continue to run the race against cancer.
We sincerely hope those who read this work will grow in the knowledge
and understanding necessary to provide direction and compassion to their patients.
Let us not grow tired in running our own race,
but instead encourage those around us.

Preface

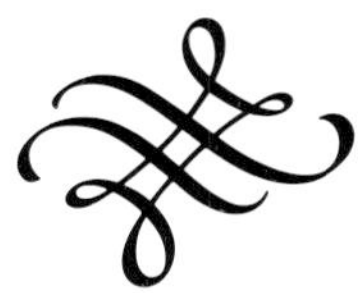

Cancer is the second leading cause of death in the United States. According to estimates of the American Cancer Society, over 1.3 million new cases of cancer were diagnosed in 1996. The problem of controlling the disease and the important role of those involved in clinical and research activities is evident by the vast amount of money spent on cancer research each year and the immeasurable cost in compromised quality and loss of human life. Radiation therapy, a vital resource involved in cancer management, is used in well over half the diagnosed cases.

Practical Applications is one of three texts in the *Principles and Practice of Radiation Therapy* series designed to contribute to a comprehensive understanding of cancer management, improve techniques involved in delivering a prescribed dose of radiation therapy, and apply knowledge and complex concepts associated with radiation therapy treatment. Each text is designed to stand on its own and at the same time provide a continuum of information in the series to the student, therapist, dosimetrist, oncologist, nurse, and others involved in radiation oncology.

This first-ever text offers a comprehensive overview of radiation therapy. Different types of cancer are discussed, such as skin and melanoma cancer, soft tissue sarcomas, bone tumors, leukemia, and pediatric tumors. Also covered are the specific body systems that are often the recipients of cancer, including the lymphoreticular system, endocrine system, respiratory system, head and neck region, central nervous system, digestive system, breast, gynecological system, and male reproductive and genitourinary systems.

Pedagogical features designed to enhance comprehension and high-level learning are incorporated into each chapter. Elements include chapter outlines, key terms, and a complete glossary. Other notable features are the review questions and questions to ponder at the end of each chapter. The review questions reiterate the cognitive information presented in the chapter to help the reader incorporate the information into the basic understanding of radiation therapy concepts. The questions to ponder are open-ended, divergent questions intended to stimulate critical thinking and analytical judgment during information processing. Each chapter offers a reference list, thus providing the reader with additional sources. Again, the focus on each chapter is the comprehensive needs of the radiation therapy management team.

Creating a series of this magnitude has been a collaborative effort by numerous individuals. Although the idea for such a work began several years ago as one comprehensive text, the impossibility of the task was soon realized, considering the complexity and vast amount of information. Instead, three texts were proposed: *Introduction to Radiation Therapy; Radiation Therapy Physics, Simulation, and Treatment Planning;* and *Practical Applications.* A survey of nearly all radiation therapy, dosimetry, and radiation oncology resident program directors and a smaller number of oncology nurses revealed a strong need for such a work with a notable percentage of the respondents recommending a multivolume approach. Survey results not only were encouraging, but also provided us with various individuals interested in lending their expertise as contributing authors, consultants, and reviewers. The result is a truly collaborative effort from the oncology community. This has been especially helpful because a great deal of individuality exists among treatment centers, hospitals, and universities in the techniques of irradiation.

Our hope is that the *Principles and Practice of Radiation Therapy* series will add to the body of knowledge specific to the profession. In addition, we sincerely hope the expanded knowledge and progress gained in administering a prescribed dose of radiation will ultimately enrich the quality of life of the patient and reduce suffering from cancer.

Charles M. Washington
Dennis T. Leaver

Acknowledgments

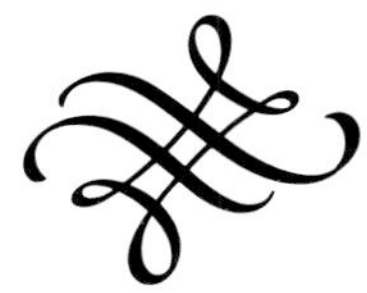

This book is the result of a tremendous team effort involving 61 contributing authors, more than 50 reviewers, our illustrators, and the dedicated professionals at Mosby–Year Book, Inc. All of us have had individuals who believed in and encouraged us when we encountered obstacles. We would like to acknowledge and thank those professionals who were instrumental in helping us build our professional foundation: Diane Chadwell and Adam Kempa from Wayne State University in Detroit, Michigan, and Dr. Banice Webber and Beverly Raymond from Radiation Oncology Associates in Providence, Rhode Island. Without their guidance and support, we could not have addressed the need for this work.

We would like to give special thanks to our students and reviewers who provided suggestions and comments that improved the manuscript. The continued support and encouragement of our colleagues at The University of Texas M.D. Anderson Cancer Center and Southern Maine Technical College are greatly appreciated. We are also grateful to Deborah Nickson and Jeanne Leaver for their dedicated service, secretarial assistance, and help with the glossary.

Above all, we gratefully acknowledge our families because they are the silent force behind this book. The idea for this project began at a conference in 1992. The idea was developed by many colleagues, friends, and the challenge to add to the body of knowledge in radiation oncology. We are grateful for the love, support, and encouragement from our wives, Connie Washington and Jeanne Leaver. They are also extremely important to this project. Finally, a special thanks goes to our heavenly Father, who sustains us and makes things grow.

Contents

Principles and Practice of Radiation Therapy

Practical Applications

CHAPTER

1

Skin and Melanoma

Todd Blobe

Outline

Key terms

Actinic (solar) keratoses
Basal cell carcinoma
Dermis
Desquamation
Epidermis
Erythema
Keratin
Keratinocytes
Keratoacanthoma
Malignant melanoma
Melanin
Melanocytes
Mohs' surgery
Mycosis fungoides
Nevus
Squamous cell carcinoma
Subcutaneous layer
Telangiectases
Xeroderma pigmentosum

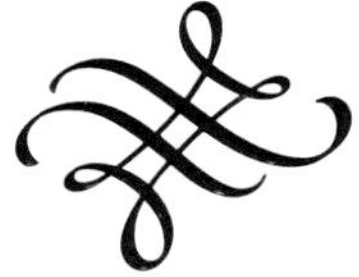

During a lifetime the skin, one of the most visible and vulnerable organs of the body, is subjected to many external influences, including cold, heat, friction, ultraviolet (UV) light, pressure, and chemicals. As a result, the skin is especially susceptible to trauma, infection, and disease.

This chapter focuses on the three main types of skin cancer: basal cell carcinoma, squamous cell carcinoma, and malignant melanoma. Basal cell and squamous cell carcinomas are commonly referred to as *nonmelanoma cancers of the skin.*

SKIN AND MELANOMA

Epidemiology

Cancer of the skin is the most common type of malignancy. Approximately 50% of all people who live to age 65 will develop at least one skin cancer during their lifetime.[6] In 1996 the incidence of basal cell and squamous cell skin cancer is estimated to be more than 800,000 new cases (basal cell cancers outnumber squamous cell cancers of the skin approximately five to one), whereas **malignant melanoma** was expected to account for 38,300 new cases.[4] The reason such a large range for nonmelanoma skin cancer estimates exists is that many early skin cancer lesions are easily treated by primary physicians and dermatologists and are not reported to the various cancer-tracking agencies.

Unfortunately, the incidence of skin cancers and melanomas is rising. "During the past decade, the annual increase in malignant melanoma was approximately 7 percent *per year,* the most rapidly increasing rate for any cancer in the United States."[63] For adults between the ages of 25 and 29 and men aged 30 to 40, melanoma now displaces other cancers in occurrence. In women between the ages of 30 and 40, only breast cancer outnumbers the cases of melanoma. The number of basal cell and squamous cell skin cancers have also increased by as much as 65% since 1983,[53] and more young people are being affected. A few theories that might account for this trend are as follows:

1. The "healthy tan" has become fashionable in recent years. Crowded beaches and the proliferation of tanning salons seem to indicate people are interested in that look.
2. Clothing trends have changed in recent years. Everyday fashions and swimwear have become more liberal, allowing for more skin to be exposed to the sun's rays.
3. The depletion of the ozone layer has diminished the atmosphere's ability to protect the earth and its inhabitants from the sun's harmful UV rays. Rays that were formerly filtered by the ozone layer now reach the earth's surface and its inhabitants. "According to the latest projections, a one percent decrease in ozone heralds a 2.6 percent increase in basal and squamous cell cancers."[58]

In addition to increasing rates of incidence, death rates as a result of skin cancer have also changed over the years. Between 1958 and 1960 the death rate for melanomas per 100,000 people was 1.4 in males and 1.0 in females. Between 1988 and 1990 the death rate was 3.0 in males and 1.5 in females, a 120% and 48% increase, respectively, over the past 30 years.[4]

Nonmelanomas, however, have experienced a decreased death rate over the same period. From 1958 to 1960 the death rate for nonmelanoma skin cancer per 100,000 people was 1.7 for males and 0.8 for females. From 1988 to 1990 the death rate was 1.3 for males and 0.4 for females, a decrease of 25% and 56%, respectively.[4] The fact that death rates are so low and declining for nonmelanoma skin cancer is good news, but the comparatively higher and rising death rates for melanomas are alarming.

Melanomas are much more lethal than their nonmelanoma counterparts. About 7300 people (4600 males and 2700 females) will die from melanoma in 1996. This number accounts for 1.3% of all cancer deaths. An additional 2100 people are expected to die from nonmelanoma skin cancers in 1994 (75% from squamous cell carcinoma), accounting for only 0.4% of all cancer deaths.[4] Although nonmelanomas outnumber melanomas approximately 30 to 1, three times as many people die each year from melanoma than from nonmelanoma skin cancers.

Some individuals are more prone to skin cancer than others. Tendencies for people to develop skin cancers and melanomas can be grouped into four main categories: geographical location, skin type, multiplicity, and gender.

Geographical location. People who live near the equator have a high chance of developing skin cancer because the sun's rays are intense and direct. At latitudes away from the equator, the sun's rays are angled and are not as intense. This angulation causes the rays to travel through more of the atmosphere, allowing it to absorb more harmful rays in areas away from the equator than those at the equator itself (Fig. 1-1). Table 1-1 shows annual UV levels in selected cities, with Anchorage's level as an arbitrary baseline. On average,

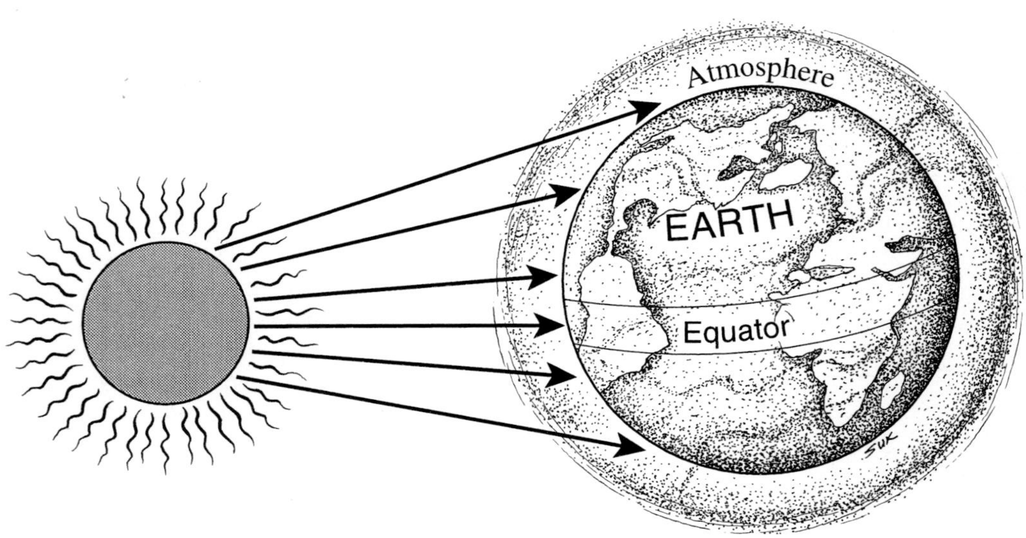

Fig. 1-1 Areas near the equator receive more direct sunlight than areas closer to the poles. Notice the way the angled rays near the poles are filtered through larger amounts of the atmosphere before they reach the earth.

the closer a city is to the equator, the higher the UV exposure. The higher the UV exposure, the higher the rates for skin cancer. For example, melanoma rates in Honolulu are twice those in Detroit. This difference corresponds roughly with that in the UV index. Similarly, people living at high altitudes are more prone to develop skin cancer because high levels have less atmosphere to filter the sun's rays. Each 1000-foot climb in elevation is accompanied by a 4% to 5% increase in UV radiation exposure.[58]

Skin type. Individuals with fair complexions are 10 times more likely to develop skin cancer than those with dark skin. Especially susceptible are albinos, people with freckles or light-colored eyes, and people who suffer from **xeroderma pigmentosum** (a genetic condition caused by a defect in mechanisms that repair deoxyribunucleic acid [DNA] damage caused by UV light, characterized by the development of pigment abnormalities and multiple skin cancers in body areas exposed to the sun). These people tend to tan poorly and burn easily.

People with dark skin have greater quantities of melanin in their skin, giving them more protection from the UV rays of the sun. This does not mean that dark-skinned individuals are free of skin cancers, but they get them less often and in more unusual places, such as on the palm of the hand, on the sole of the foot, or in the mucous membranes. Among African-Americans, squamous cell carcinoma is more common than basal cell carcinoma. Squamous cell carcinoma tends to occur in sites not exposed to the sun and is often aggressive.[53]

Multiplicity. Prior skin cancer occurrence increases the odds that a second primary skin cancer will develop. Reasons for this may include the following: (1) Other areas of the skin may have been exposed to the same carcinogens that caused the initial skin cancer, and (2) the individual may have a weakness in the immune system that hinders the ability to fight off skin cancers naturally.

A previous melanoma of the skin increases the risk of another primary melanoma by five to nine times. The rate of second primary melanomas is higher in persons under age 40 at the original time of diagnosis compared with persons diagnosed at age 40 or older. The risk is highest in the first year after the original diagnosis but remains highly elevated long afterward.[57]

For individuals with at least one nonmelanoma cancer occurrence, the chances of developing a second malignancy are 17% within 1 year and 50% within 5 years.[32] Because of these elevated risks, any patient diagnosed with skin cancer should be closely monitored for signs of recurrence or new primaries.

Gender. Rates for melanoma skin cancers are slightly more for men than women, but men are three times more likely than women to develop nonmelanomas, except on the legs, where women have higher rates of nonmelanoma skin cancers.[47] This trend seems to be related to skin care habit differences between the genders rather than genetics. Men tend to work outside more often and do not wear sunscreens as often (50% less) as women. Also, men have a more nonchalant attitude about sun exposure and its effects. In general, women seem to pay more attention to their skin than men.[34]

Table 1-1 Comparison of latitude on ultraviolet exposure

City	Degrees of latitude	Elevation (ft)	Ultraviolet index
Anchorage	61	118	100
Seattle	47	10	477
Detroit	42	585	630
Philadelphia	40	100	656
Boise*	43	2704	715
Phoenix	33	1090	889
Denver*	39	5280	951
Houston	29	40	999
Miami	25	10	1028
Honolulu	21	21	1147

Modified from Roach M, Hastings J, Finch S: Sun Struck: here's the hole story about the ozone and your chances of getting skin cancer, *Health* 11:40, May-June, 1992.

*UV readings for Boise and Denver seem to be out of place, but in comparing the elevations of those two cities, a significant difference is evident. High elevations also contribute to higher UV exposures.

Etiology

Many factors are directly and indirectly responsible for the development of the various forms of skin cancer, but the major cause is exposure to UV light.

UV light. The American Cancer Society estimates that approximately 90% of all skin cancers would be prevented if people protected their skin from the sun's rays.[6] The risk of developing melanoma increases four to five times after three or more blistering sunburns during adolescence.[7] The time between the initial stimulus (sunburn) and the appearance of a melanoma is believed to be between 10 and 20 years.[64] At greatest risk for developing a malignant melanoma is the person who primarily stays indoors and receives occasional sun exposure. In contrast, people who spend a majority of the time in the sun (e.g., farmers, construction workers) are most apt to develop basal cell or squamous cell carcinomas.

Sunlight contains two types of UV rays that are harmful to the skin: ultraviolet A (UVA) and ultraviolet B (UVB). Their wavelengths are between 290 and 320 nanometers (UVA) and between 320 and 400 nanometers (UVB).[63]

UVB is thought to cause cancer by damaging DNA and its repair systems, resulting in mutations that may lead to cancer. It is also thought to play a role in cellular immunity by impairing T-cell* function and increasing suppressor T-cell† numbers.[53]

*T cells are cells that normally help protect against cancer.

†Suppressor T cells are cells that aid in shutting down the immune response.

UVA rays have long been considered relatively harmless compared with UVB rays. In fact, "most tanning equipment emits ultraviolet A light."[53] Recent studies have shown that the stratum corneum absorbs UVB (see anatomy and physiology section in this chapter), whereas 50% of UVA radiation is able to penetrate to the highly mitotic basal layer of the skin, where the potential for malignant changes and premature aging of the skin exists. Evidence also suggests that UVA acts to promote tumors initiated by UVB.[64]

Like many other cancers, skin cancer is a disease of aging. Most skin cancers appear after age 50, but the damaging effects of the sun's rays are accumulated over a lifetime. However, skin cancers can develop in infants, children, and young adults, especially those with high-risk factors (e.g., xeroderma pigmentosum, giant hairy nevi).

Other factors associated with nonmelanoma skin cancers. Other factors that contribute to nonmelanoma skin cancers include exposure to arsenic (an element used in medicines and poisons) and therapeutic or occupational exposure to radiation. After irradiation the risk to the exposed individual is up to 20%, and latent periods may extend up to 50 years beyond the initial exposure. Squamous cell carcinomas account for two thirds of these radiation-induced lesions, which tend to be aggressive and result in a 10% mortality rate.[16]

Besides xeroderma pigmentosum, another genetic condition associated with the formation of basal cell carcinomas is called *basal cell nevus syndrome* (a genetically linked condition that appears during the late teen years). Symptoms include multiple basal cell carcinomas of the skin, cysts of the jaw bones, pitting of the palms and soles, and skeletal anomalies (particularly of the ribs).[6]

Squamous cell carcinomas of the skin have also been associated with the following[69]:

- Human papilloma virus infection
- Immunosuppression as a result of organ transplant, lymphoma, or leukemia
- Thermal or electrical burns and chronic heat exposure
- Scars or chronic inflammatory conditions
- Hydrocarbons derived from coal and petroleum
- Areas of chronic drainage (e.g., fistulas, sinuses)

Smoking is a proven cause of squamous cell carcinoma of the lip. It has also been linked to the development of squamous cell skin cancer in other anatomical areas. However, it is not known whether cigarette smoke acts directly as a skin carcinogen or has an adverse effect on the immune system, inhibiting the body's ability to defend itself from cancer.[32]

Other factors associated with melanoma skin cancers. Melanomas tend to develop from **melanocytes,** which grow in clusters to form a mole, or **nevus**. Moles can be broadly classified according to when they are acquired: congenital melanocytic nevi (those present at birth) and common acquired nevi (those that develop later in life).

Congenital melanocytic nevi can be classified into three sizes: small (less than 1.5 cm in diameter), medium (1.5 cm to 19.9 cm in diameter), and large (20 cm or more in diameter). Large nevi (Fig. 1-2) are accompanied by an approximate 6% to 8% risk of developing melanoma compared with a 1% risk in the general population. Accordingly, some surgeons feel these moles should be removed prophylactically before malignant changes can occur. Prophylactic removal of small and medium lesions should be made individually because the chance of malignant change in them is small.[25]

Melanocytic nevi can be grouped into three main categories: junctional, compound, and intradermal. Junctional nevi tend to be small (usually less than 6 mm), well-circumscribed, flat lesions with smooth surfaces that are uniformly brown or black and circular. The melanocyte clusters in junctional nevi are found above the basement layer. Compound nevi contain melanocyte clusters in the dermis and epidermis. They appear as small, well-circumscribed, slightly raised papules that often contain excess hair. The surface is rough and color ranges from tan to brown throughout. Over time, these lesions may take on a nodular appear-

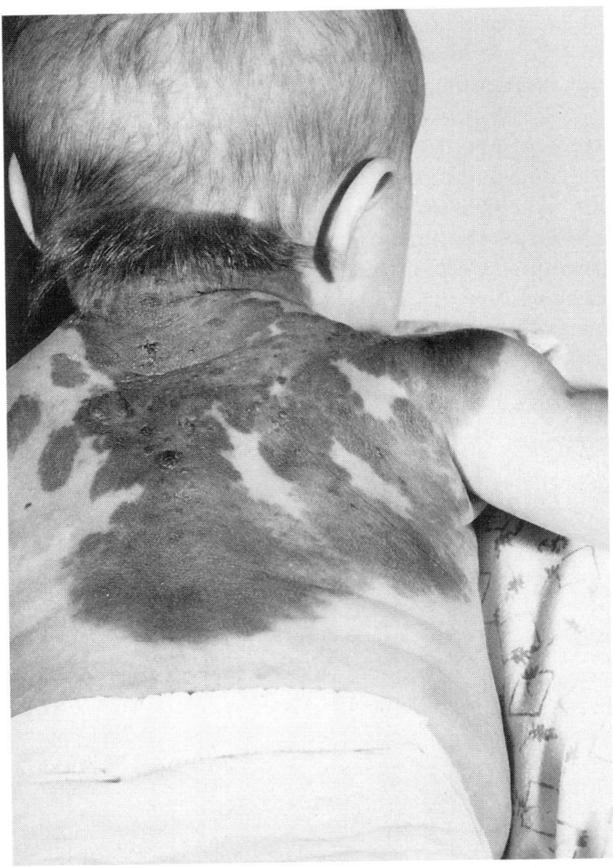

Fig. 1-2 This child with a giant hairy nevus has approximately an 8% chance of developing a melanoma within the first 15 years of life. Because of the high risk, this lesion will be removed in a series of prophylactic surgical procedures. (Photo and information courtesy R. Dean Glassman, M.D.)

ance. Intradermal nevi are small, well-circumscribed, dome-shaped lesions that range from flesh to brown. They too may contain excess hair. Melanocytic clusters are found only in the dermal layer in these moles.[25]

The propensity of a mole to develop into a melanoma is related to the location of the melanocytic clusters found in the moles. Intradermal nevi rarely transform into melanomas; the likelihood of junctional and compound nevi transforming into melanomas is far greater. One theory for this pattern is that melanocytes located in the dermis do not receive as much UV exposure because they are located deep in the skin. Melanocytes in junctional and compound nevi are closer to the skin's surface and therefore receive higher amounts of melanoma-inducing UV radiation.[15]

Dysplastic nevi, also known as *B-K* or *atypical moles,* are acquired pigmented lesions of the skin that have one or more of the clinical features of melanoma-asymmetry, border irregularity, color variation, or a diameter greater than 6 mm.[25] "The presence of dysplastic moles marks an individual as having a seven-fold to seventy-fold increased risk of melanoma. Even a single dysplastic mole appears to be a significant risk factor for melanoma."[57]

The number of moles a person has also influences the chances of acquiring melanoma. One study showed that "persons who have twelve moles at least 5 mm in diameter have an estimated 41-fold increased risk of melanoma while those who have fifty or more moles at least 2 mm in diameter have a 64-fold increased risk of melanoma."[57]

People with a family history of melanoma have an eight fold increase in their chances of acquiring the disease.[57] Several studies have pinpointed a region on the short arm of chromosome 9 (9p) as one involved in the early stage development of melanoma tumors.[14] Genetic material from this area is thought to play a vital role in the suppression of tumor formation. Without this material a person may be more susceptible to tumor formation because one of the normal defense mechanisms may be missing. Other chromosomal abnormalities associated with melanomas can be found on chromosomes 1, 6, 7, 11, and 19.[30]

"Some families are affected with an inherited familial atypical mole and melanoma (FAM-M) syndrome, also known as B-K mole syndrome or dysplastic nevus syndrome (DNS). The syndrome is defined by: 1.) occurrence of melanoma in one or more first- or second-degree relatives, 2.) large numbers of moles (often 50+), some of which are atypical and often variable in size, and 3.) moles that demonstrate certain distinct histological features. Persons with this syndrome have a markedly increased risk of developing melanoma. Their lifetime risk may be as much as 100%."[48] These patients require close monitoring because of the high risks involved. This syndrome has also been described in the nonfamilial setting.[25]

"Hormones, pregnancy, birth control pills, and certain environmental exposures have also been linked to the development of malignant melanoma, but these factors need further study."[5]

Anatomy and physiology

The skin is the largest organ of the body, covering about 22 square feet and weighing 10 to 12 pounds on the average person. The skin provides many functions, including the following:

- Regulates body temperature through perspiration (as perspiration evaporates, it carries heat away from the body) and blood flow through vessels located in the skin (the skin allows heat carried by the blood to radiate off its surface)
- Acts as a barrier between the external environment and the body, offering protection against factors such as trauma, UV light, and bacterial invasion
- Participates in the production of vitamin D, which is vital to the process enabling the body to absorb and use calcium in the gastrointestinal tract
- Provides receptors for external stimuli such as heat, cold, pressure, and touch, allowing the body to be aware of its environment

The skin is an example of an epithelial membrane, a connective tissue covered by a layer of epithelial tissue. The connective tissue layer in the skin is called the **dermis;** the epithelial layer is called the **epidermis** (Fig. 1-3). These layers are held together by an intermediate layer called the *basement membrane.*[67]

The dermis is the deeper layer of the skin composed of connective tissue that contains blood and lymphatic vessels, nerves and nerve endings, sweat glands, and hair follicles. It contains mainly elastic and collagen fibers that allow for the flexibility and strength of the skin. The upper 20% of the dermis is referred to as the *papillary region* and contains dermal papillae, ridges that are responsible for the formation of fingerprints. The lower 80% of the dermis is the reticular region and contains many accessory structures of the skin, such as the following: hair follicles, sebaceous (oil) and sudoriferous (sweat) glands and their ducts, nerve endings, and blood vessels.[67]

A **subcutaneous layer** containing nerves, blood vessels, adipose (fat) tissue, and areolar connective tissue lies beneath the dermis. Because the epidermis is avascular, the blood vessels of the dermis and subcutaneous layer are responsible for the nutritional status of the epidermis.

The epidermis is the extremely thin outer layer of the skin, composed of four to five layers (depending on its location). These layers are as follows, from deepest to most superficial.[67]

1. Stratum basale (stratum germinativum)—This is the basal layer containing stem cells capable of producing **keratinocytes** (which comprise 90% of the epidermal cells of the skin) and cells that give rise to glands and hair follicles. This layer also contains melanocytes (which comprise 8% of the epidermal cells of the skin), cells with branching processes that produce the pigment melanin. In hairless skin a third type of cell, Merkel's cell, can also be found. Together with a

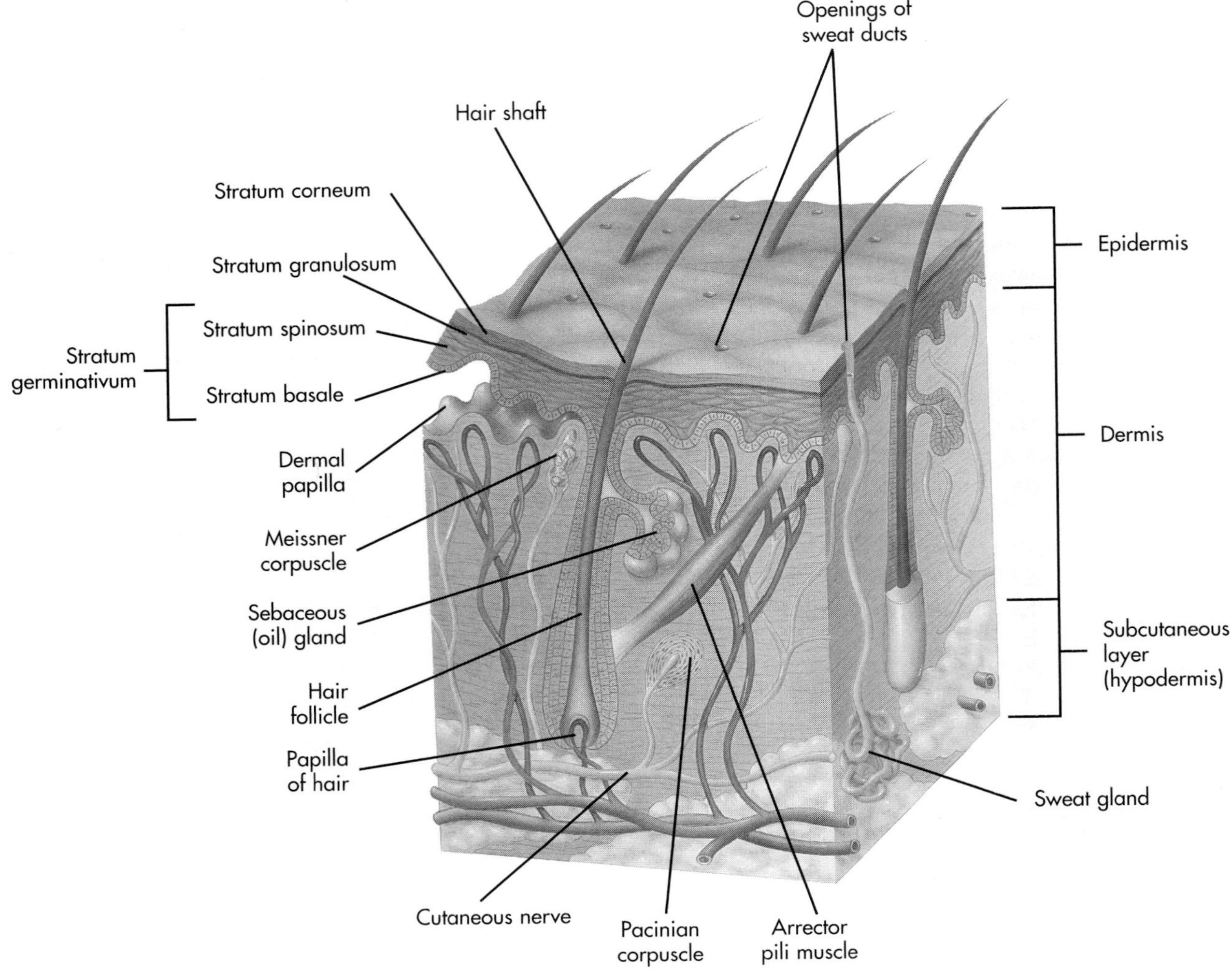

Fig. 1-3 This cross section of the skin shows the relationship between the epidermis, dermis, and subcutaneous layers. Notice how thick the dermis is compared with the epidermis. Also shown are the various accessory structures of the skin and their location. (From Thibodeau GA, Patton KT: *Anatomy & physiology,* ed 3, St Louis, 1996, Mosby.)

flattened portion of a neuron called a *tactile* (Merkel's disc), Merkel's cells function in the sensation of touch.

2. Stratum spinosum—This layer contains 8 to 10 rows of keratinocytes, which have a spiny appearance microscopically. Branches from the melanocytes reach into this layer, allowing the keratinocytes to absorb the protective pigment melanin via exocytosis.
3. Stratum granulosum—This layer contains three to five rows of somewhat flattened cells. The keratinocytes begin to produce a substance called *keratohyalin,* which is a precursor to a waterproof protein called **keratin.**
4. Stratum lucidum—This layer is normally found only in areas in which thick skin is present (soles and palms) and contains three to five rows of clear, flat cells that contain eleidin, another keratin precursor.
5. Stratum corneum—This layer forms the skin surface and contains 25 to 30 rows of flat, dead, scaly (squamous) cells that are completely filled with keratin and have lost all their internal organelles, including nuclei. The lower layers of cells are closely packed and adhere to each other, whereas the upper layers of cells are loosely packed and continually flake away from the surface.

Basically, the outer, protective layer of the skin is composed of dead cells filled with keratin. Each day, millions of these cells are sloughed off and continually replaced by cells from the lower layers of the epidermis. Germ cells in the stratum basale give rise to keratinocytes, which go through a process called *keratinization* as they are pushed toward the surface by new cells. As the cells are relocated, they accumulate keratin to the point that the cell can no longer function and dies. The mature keratinocytes serve their protective function and are eventually shed from the surface of the skin. The time necessary for the cell to travel from the germ layer to the surface is approximately 2 to 4 weeks. This cycle continually repeats itself.

Melanin is a pigment that serves a protective function of the skin. It is produced by the melanocytes and absorbed by the keratinocytes in the stratum spinosum layer of the epidermis. UV light damages the keratinocytes by inhibiting synthesis of DNA and ribonucleic acid (RNA) (genetic material in the cell), leading to cell dysfunction or death. The melanin absorbed by the keratinocytes is placed in the cell so that it lies between the skin surface and nucleus of the cell, thus protecting it from the sun's rays like an umbrella (Fig. 1-4).

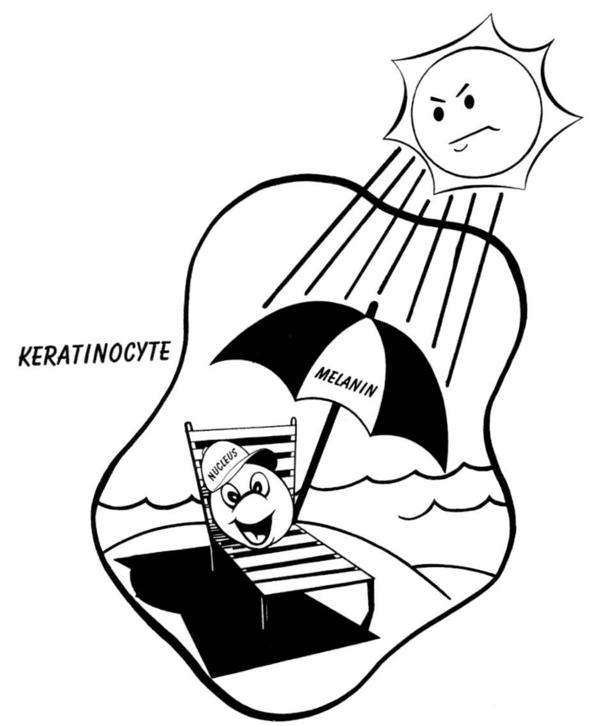

Fig. 1-4 This cartoon depicts the way melanin is strategically placed inside the keratinocyte between the nucleus and sun's rays, protecting it from ultraviolet radiation.

Melanin is one of the pigments responsible for differences in skin color among individuals. The more melanin a person's skin contains, the darker the skin. The number of melanocytes is about the same in all races. Differences in skin darkness are attributed to the amount of melanin the melanocytes produce. The systemic release of melanocyte-stimulating hormone (MSH) from the anterior pituitary gland controls overall skin darkness. The more MSH released by the pituitary, the more melanin the melanocytes produce and the darker the person's skin. Variations in skin darkness can occur in localized areas of the body as a result of exposure to UV light. Brief exposure to UV light causes melanin already present in the epidermis to darken considerably, whereas long-term exposure causes melanocytes to increase melanin production. Both processes result in darker or tanned skin. A tan is actually a response by the body to damage caused by UV light.[58] In the absence of UV stimulation, melanocytes decrease melanin production to normal levels and the skin returns to normal color.[71]

Skin cancers can be classified according to the cell of the skin from which they originate. Malignant melanoma, the most lethal form of skin cancer, arises from the melanocytes located in the stratum basale. The most common sites for melanoma are the legs of women and the trunk and face of men. Melanomas can also arise in other areas of the body, such as the choroid or ciliary body of the eye, the eyelids, the mucosa of the oral cavity, the genitalia, and the anus.

Basal cell carcinoma, a slow-growing form of skin cancer that does not tend to metastasize, arises from the stem cells of the stratum basale. It is the most prevalent cancer in humans and, if left untreated, can cause extensive damage.

Squamous cell carcinoma, a faster-growing cancer than the basal cell type with a higher propensity for metastasis, arises from the more mature keratinocytes of the upper layers of the epidermis. This type of nonmelanoma skin cancer can arise anywhere on the body but is especially common on sun-exposed areas such as the head, neck, face, arms, and hands.

Other types of cancers can arise in the skin but are not covered in detail in this chapter. These include, but are not limited to, the following[49]:

1. Adenocarcinoma of the sebaceous and sudoriferous glands—This type of cancer arises in the dermal layer of the skin and is a slow-growing lesion capable of metastasis. It tends to be radioresistant; therefore surgery is the treatment of choice.
2. Cutaneous T-cell lymphoma, including **mycosis fungoides**—This is a disease of the T lymphocytes. It resembles eczema or other inflammatory conditions and tends to remain localized to the skin for long periods. Total-body irradiation with electrons and topical nitrogen mustard has been used to control early stages of the disease.
3. Kaposi's sarcoma—This is a slow-growing, temperate tumor thought to arise from vascular tissue. The associated nodular purple lesions are often multifocal and common in individuals affected with acquired immunodeficiency syndrome (AIDS) and those living in the Mediterranean region. Surgical excision is indicated for individual lesions and radiation therapy for multiple lesions.

The AIDS epidemic has introduced an aggressive variant of this disease. Although associated lesions are radiosensitive, AIDS patients who acquire this disease have a poor prognosis and are best treated systemically with chemotherapy. Radiation therapy is used to palliate local areas.

4. Merkel's cell carcinoma—This is a rare tumor thought to arise from Merkel's (tactile) cells. It is known for high rates of recurrence after surgical excision, frequent involvement of regional lymph nodes, and distant metastatic failure. These tumors are structurally similar to small cell carcinomas and appear as firm, nontender, pink-red nodular lesions with an intact epidermis.[51] These types of cancers are often treated with a combination of chemotherapy and radiation therapy or surgery.

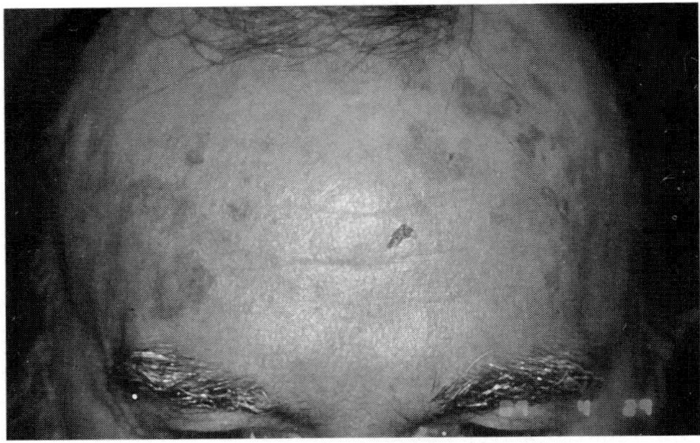

Fig. 1-5 Actinic keratosis. (Courtesy Mark McLaughlin, M.D.)

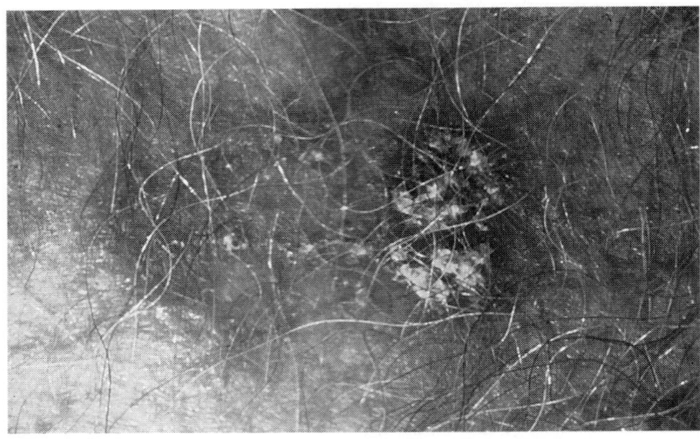

Fig. 1-6 Bowen's disease. (Courtesy Mark McLaughlin, M.D.)

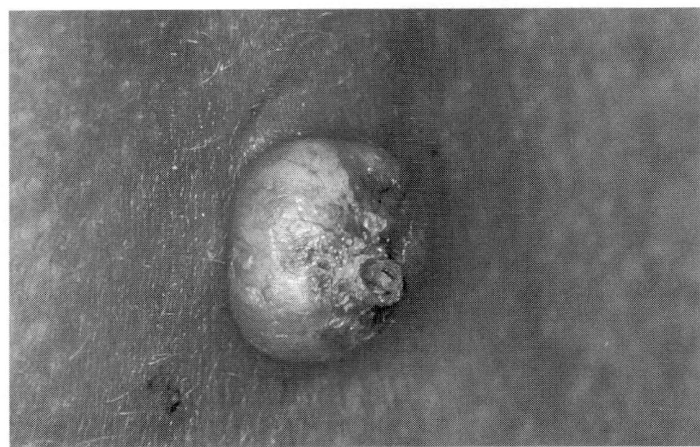

Fig. 1-7 Keratoacanthoma. (Courtesy Mark McLaughlin, M.D.)

Clinical presentation

Although skin cancers and melanomas occur in a wide variety of shapes, sizes, and appearances, similarities exist that facilitate lesion classification. Following is a discussion concerning the tumors seen most often and premalignant growths that may precede them.

Nonmelanoma precursors and characteristics. Premalignant lesions are those that, if left untreated or not closely monitored, can develop into cancer. Squamous cell carcinomas tend to arise more often from precursor lesions compared with basal cell carcinomas.[70] The American Cancer Society classifies some of the precancerous lesions for nonmelanomas as follows[6]:

1. **Actinic (solar) keratoses**—These are warty lesions or areas of red, scaly patches occurring on the sun-exposed skin of the face or hands of older, light-skinned individuals (Fig. 1-5). Because actinic keratoses have a 5% to 10% chance[33] of degrading into squamous cell carcinoma, some physicians remove them surgically or treat them with 5-fluorouracil (5-FU), liquid nitrogen, or electrodesiccation to destroy them and eliminate the possibility of cancerous change.[16]
2. Arsenical keratoses—These are multiple, hard, cornlike masses on the palms of hands or soles of feet resulting from long-term arsenic ingestion.
3. Bowen's disease—This is a precancerous dermatosis or carcinoma in situ characterized by the development of pink or brown papules covered with a thickened, horny layer (Fig. 1-6).
4. Keratoacanthoma—This is a rapid-growing lesion that can appear suddenly as a dome-shaped mass on a sun-exposed area (Fig. 1-7). Microscopically, the nodules are composed of well-differentiated squamous epithelia with a necrotic center or central keratin mass. They can be difficult to distinguish from squamous cell cancer and usually resolve themselves if left untreated.

Nonmelanoma skin cancers have a multitude of appearances (Figs. 1-8 and 1-9). Basal cell carcinomas tend to arise as smooth, red, or milky lumps and have a pearly border and multiple **telangiectases** (tiny blood vessels visible on the skin's surface). Basal cell carcinomas can be shiny or pale. About 80% of basal cell carcinomas occur on the head and

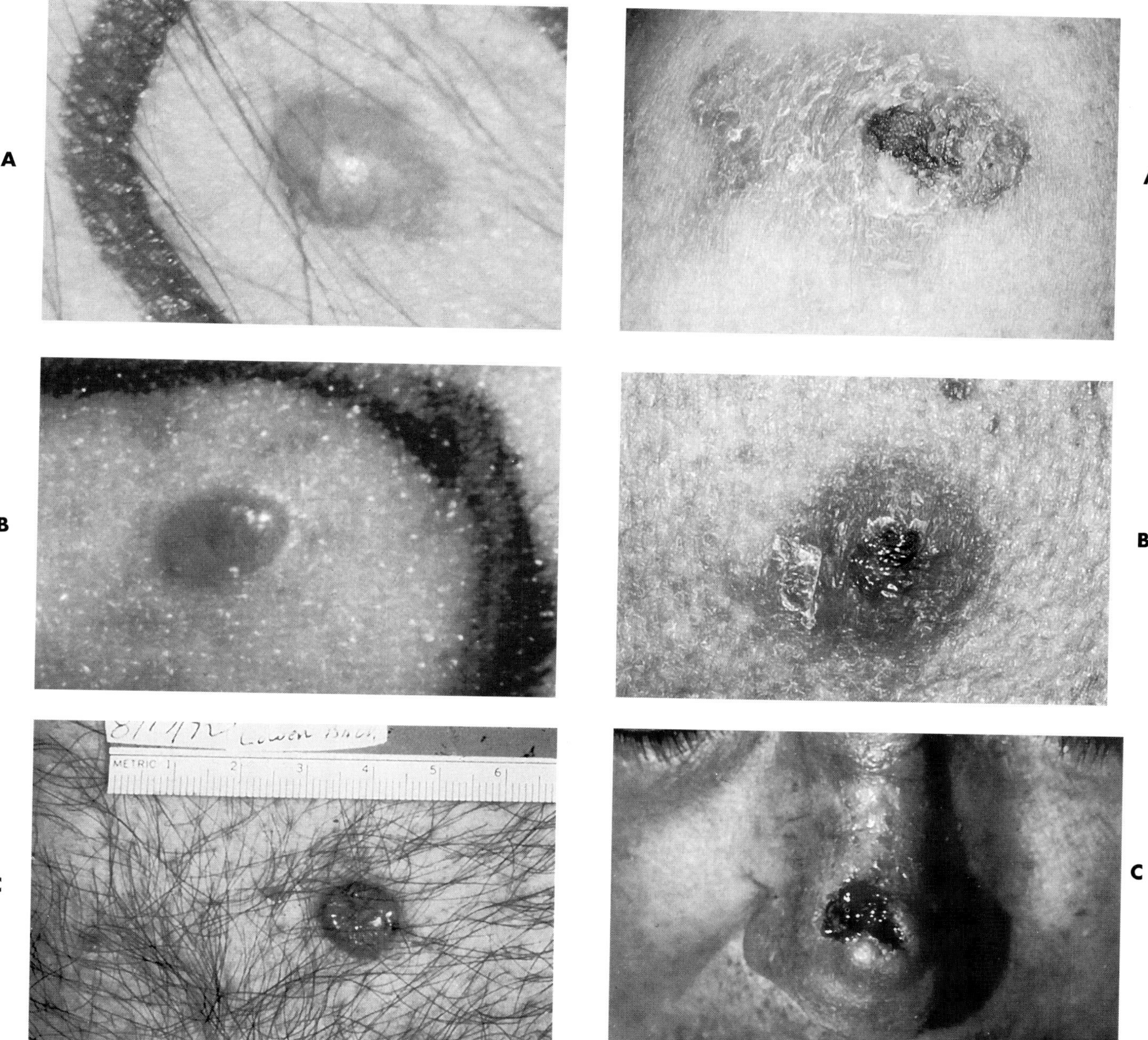

Fig. 1-8 **A, B,** and **C:** Examples of basal cell carcinomas. (**A, B,** and **C,** courtesy the National Cancer Institute.)

Fig. 1-9 **A, B,** and **C:** Examples of squamous cell carcinomas. (**A, B,** and **C,** courtesy the National Cancer Institute.)

neck. Squamous cell carcinomas tend to have a scaly, crusty, slightly elevated lesion that may have a cutaneous horn. Approximately 80% of UV-induced squamous cell carcinomas develop on the arms, head, and neck.[53] Other symptoms possibly indicating a basal cell or squamous cell carcinoma include a sore that takes longer than 3 weeks to heal, a recurrent red patch that may itch or be tender, and a wart that bleeds or scabs. Some basal cell carcinomas may contain melanin, causing the lesion to appear black and resemble a melanoma. In general, any new growths that persist or change in appearance should be reported to a physician.

Melanoma precursors and characteristics. Approximately 70% of melanomas occur as the result of a change in a preexisting nevus. The other 30% arise from de novo melanomas, growths not associated with previously observed nevi.[16] The American Cancer Society[7] has released the ABCD rules for early detection of melanoma (Fig. 1-10). These are as follows:

A

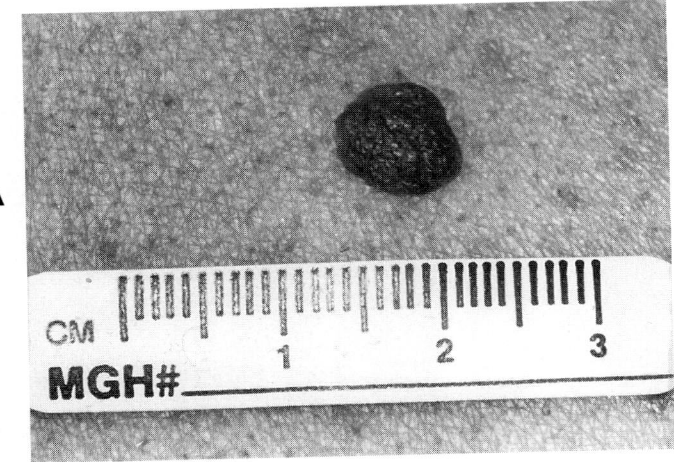

C

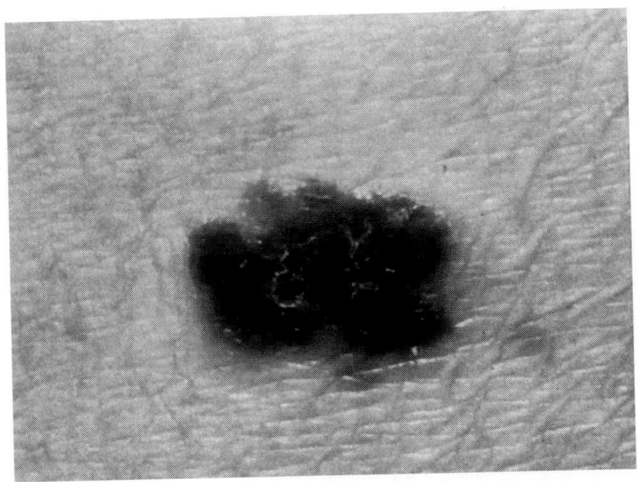

B

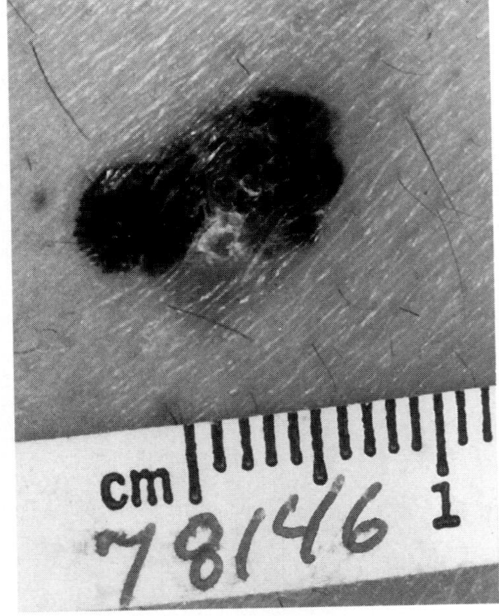

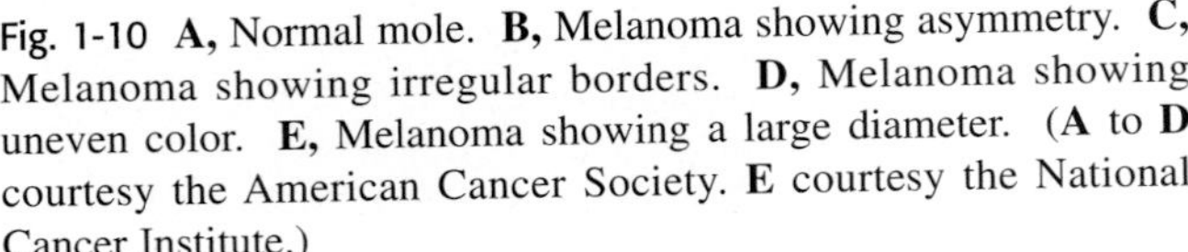

D

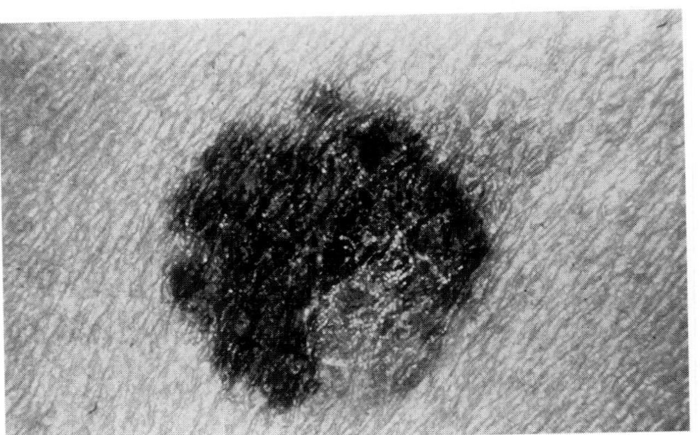

E

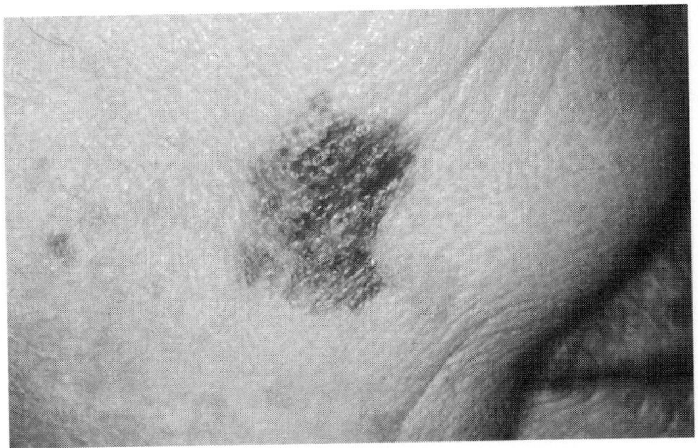

Fig. 1-10 **A,** Normal mole. **B,** Melanoma showing asymmetry. **C,** Melanoma showing irregular borders. **D,** Melanoma showing uneven color. **E,** Melanoma showing a large diameter. (**A** to **D** courtesy the American Cancer Society. **E** courtesy the National Cancer Institute.)

A, *A*symmetry—Melanomas tend to be asymmetrical; most benign moles tend to be symmetrical.

B, *B*order—Melanomas tend to have notched, uneven borders; most benign moles tend to possess clearly defined, smooth borders.

C, *C*olor—Melanomas can contain different shades of black, brown, or tan; benign moles tend to be uniformly tan or brown.

D, *D*iameter—Most melanomas have a diameter greater than 6 mm; most benign moles tend to be less than 6 mm in diameter.

In addition to the ABCD rules, the following changes in the appearance of a mole should be monitored as possible signs of melanoma[46]:

1. Change in color—Red, white, and/or blue areas in addition to black and tan
2. Change in surface—Scaly, flaky, bleeding, or oozing moles or a sore that does not heal
3. Change in texture—Hard, lumpy, or elevated moles

4. Change in surrounding skin—Spread of pigmentation, swelling, or redness to surrounding skin
5. Change in sensation—Unusual pain or tenderness in a mole
6. Change in previously normal skin—Pigmented areas that arise in previously normal skin

A few pigmented lesions of the skin are benign, but these can be difficult to distinguish from melanoma.[25] They are as follows:

1. Simple lentigo—This is a small (1 to 5 mm), brown to black macule. It is round with sharply defined edges, and the surface is flat, similar to a freckle. Thought to be the precursor to the common mole, some simple lentigines are clinically indistinguishable from junctional nevi.
2. Solar lentigo—This is a small to medium, flat, lightly pigmented macule better known as a *liver spot.* It is especially common in older caucasians on areas of the skin chronically exposed to the sun.
3. Seborrheic keratoses—These are round or ovoid, wartlike papules ranging from a few to several millimeters. These growths tend to be raised (often with a warty, "stuck-on" appearance) and composed of proliferating epidermal cells, especially of the basal type.
4. Others—Some common moles may be difficult to distinguish from melanoma. For a description of common moles, see the Etiology Section.

Although all these above lesions tend to be benign, they should be watched for signs of malignant change. Questionable lesions should be biopsied and analyzed to rule out malignancy.

Detection and diagnosis

Theoretically, no one should die from skin cancer because the skin lends itself easily to self-inspection and cancer detection. If the public were educated on the way to detect skin cancer and actually took the time to inspect themselves, cancer should be found at an early stage and therefore be easily treatable. Following are some of the methods used to detect and diagnose skin cancer.

Everyone should inspect the total surface area of the skin monthly for signs of cancer. High-risk individuals should have photographs of the skin taken to document existing moles to which they can refer when questions arise concerning factors such as the size, color, and shape of moles. Body charts indicating the location and size of moles may also be useful.

Inspections should take place in well-lighted areas. Familiarity with existing moles, freckles, and blemishes is important so that newly pigmented areas or blemishes can be distinguished from older ones. When surveying the skin, individuals should remember the ABCD rules. In addition, people should watch for sores that do not heal or other areas of unexplained changes in the skin. (See the box below for recommended steps to follow when inspecting skin.)

Any unusual changes should be brought to the attention of a physician. The earlier skin cancer is detected, the better the chance it will be cured. People who find unusual lesions must not let their fears of pain, cost, and disfigurement get in the way of seeking a proper diagnosis and treatment. Skin cancer is obviously not something that will go away by itself.

A routine physical examination should include a thorough inspection of the skin's surface by the physician. Physicians must be knowledgable in distinguishing between benign and malignant conditions. Also, regional lymph nodes should be inspected for signs or symptoms of metastasis.

A family history should be taken to determine whether a person is at a higher risk for developing melanoma because a family member previously had the disease. Patients with a family history of melanoma should be monitored closely.

Individuals should have a biopsy performed for unusual or suspicious lesions. Depending on the size and location of the lesion, the biopsy may be incisional (only a portion of the lesion is removed for tissue diagnosis—usually reserved for large lesions) or excisional (entire lesion is removed). Excisional biopsies (including punch, saucerization, or elliptical incision) may be indicated for suspected squamous cell carcinomas or melanomas to ascertain the depth of the tumor's penetration and should include a portion of the underlying sub-

The National Cancer Institute Recommendations for Inspecting the Skin

STEP 1—Using a full-length mirror, inspect the front and back of the trunk of the body. A hand-held mirror may be used with the full-length mirror for inspecting the posterior areas of the body.
STEP 2—Inspect the arms, forearms (including the undersides) and upper arms. Hands, including the palms and fingernails, should also be inspected.
STEP 3—Using the full-length mirror, examine the back, front, and sides of the legs, including areas around the buttocks and genitals. (A hand-held mirror may be needed for these areas.)
STEP 4—Sit and closely examine the feet, including the toenails, soles, and spaces between the toes.
STEP 5—Inspect the face, neck, ears, and scalp. Again, the combination of full-length and hand-held mirrors may be helpful. A comb or blow dryer may be used to part the hair in different ways until the scalp is better exposed. Also, a friend or relative can aid in inspecting the scalp or other difficult areas of the body.

Modified from the National Cancer Institute: *What you need to know about melanoma,* National Institutes of Health publication number 93-1563, Bethesda, Maryland, April 1993, The Institute.

cutaneous fat for accurate microstaging. A shave or curettage may be adequate to diagnose basal cell carcinoma but is not recommended for lesions suspected to be melanoma.[48]

To the naked eye, some lesions are difficult to define as malignant or nonmalignant without a biopsy. A relatively new technique in diagnosing melanomas is in vivo (in tissue) epiluminescence microscopy (ELM), or dermoscopy. ELM is a noninvasive procedure that allows physicians to differentiate between benign and malignant lesions while they are in the early phases of development and have not yet begun to exhibit the features displayed by later melanomatous lesions. The procedure uses a dermatoscope (R), which looks similar to a ophthalmoscope. Mineral oil is placed on the surface of the lesion, causing the stratum corneum to become almost invisible and facilitating the examination of the epidermis, particularly the dermal-epidermal junction. ELM images can be digitized by primary care physicians and sent to ELM experts by telephone for quick analysis.[38] Digitized ELM images can also be fed into computers run by specially designed software. These programs evaluate lesions based on factors such as shape, size, color, and border and attempt to make an objective analysis on a previously subjective science.[25]

A dermatologist should be able to identify a type of lesion just by its appearance. Based on this information, the dermatologist should also have a good idea concerning the metastatic potential of the lesion. Again, basal cell carcinomas have an extremely small chance of metastases, squamous cell carcinomas have a slightly higher chance, and malignant melanomas have the highest chance of all the major skin cancers.

If the physician suspects that a patient may have an advanced squamous cell carcinoma or melanoma, an evaluation for metastasis should be conducted. This evaluation should include the following:

- Physical examination of the patient to find evidence of lymphadenopathy, secondary lesions of the skin, or second primaries
- Evaluation of motor skills to detect possible brain involvement
- Chest x-ray examination to rule out lung metastasis
- Liver function tests to rule out liver involvement
- Evaluation of alkaline phosphatase levels and bone scan if patient complains of bone pain
- CBCs to detect anemias that may be the result of gastrointestinal bleeding caused by metastasis
- Biopsy of regional lymph nodes to compare the number of positive lymph nodes with the total number in the biopsy

Computed tomography (CT) and magnetic resonance imaging (MRI) examinations, because of their cost, are often done only when signs and symptoms point to metastatic disease. Because melanoma can spread to virtually any part of the body, CT scans of the head, chest, abdomen, and pelvis may be ordered to rule out involvement of the brain, lung, liver, bowel, adrenals, and subcutaneous skin. MRI is mainly used as an adjuvant to CT or in instances in which central nervous system involvement is suspected.[27]

Pathology and staging

Melanoma. After it has been removed, the biopsy specimen is sent to a pathologist, who examines it microscopically and provides much useful information that is used to diagnose, stage, and develop a prognosis for the patient. Essential to a pathology report for melanoma are the diagnosis (whether the biopsy specimen indicates cancer), thickness of the tumor, and status of the margins (whether tumor cells are present on the edges of the biopsy specimen). If cancer is diagnosed, additional information may include the following:

- Specific cancer subtype
- Depth of tumor penetration
- Degree of mitotic activity (reproductive rate of cells)
- Growth pattern (radial versus lateral)
- Level of host response (number of lymphocytes present in and/or around the tumor)
- Presence, if any, of tumor ulceration, tumor regression, or satellitosis (lymphatic extensions of the tumor that result in small lesions adjacent to the primary)[48]

Melanomas can be classified according to their growth patterns, and histological appearances can be grouped into the following four major categories[16,18,49]:

1. Superficial spreading melanomas (SSMs), also called *radial spreading melanomas,* are the most common melanoma subtype, accounting for approximately 70% of all lesions. They generally arise on any anatomical site as preexisting lesions that evolve over several years and have a radial (horizontal) growth pattern. The periphery of these deeply pigmented lesions is often notched or irregular and colors in the tumors can vary from brown, black, red, pink, or white. Partial regression of the tumor is common. As time passes, the tumor tends to grow more vertically, resulting in a more elevated, irregular surface.
2. Nodular melanomas (NMs) account for approximately 15% of all lesions and can also occur on any anatomical site. They are twice as common in men than women. Lesions tend to be raised throughout and vary in color from dark brown, blue, or blue-black. Some lesions may not contain any pigment at all (amelanotic). These tumors are particularly lethal because they lack a radial growth phase, making an early diagnosis difficult. They tend

to invade early and frequently show ulceration when advanced.

3. Lentigo maligna melanomas (LMMs), also called *Hutchinson's freckles,* account for approximately 5% of all lesions and tend to occur in chronically sun-exposed skin of older caucasians, especially females. LMM begins with a relatively benign radial growth phase that may last for decades before it enters its vertical growth phase. The appearance of an LMM is similar to that of an SMM but lacks the red hues and has minimal elevation during its vertical growth phase.
4. Acral lentiginous melanomas (ALMs) account for approximately 10% of all lesions and are found mainly on the palms, soles, nail beds, or mucous membranes. The ALM is the most common form of melanoma in black and oriental people and has a tan or brown flat stain on the palms or soles. An ALM can also appear as a brown to black discoloration under the nail bed and is often mistaken for a fungal infection.

Because melanocytes are found in the basal layer of the epidermis, melanoma formation takes place in this area. Most melanomas begin their development with a radial (horizontal) growth phase (Fig. 1-11), during which abnormal melanocytes form nests along the basal layer. Later, some of the melanocytes begin to migrate into and form nests in the upper layers of the epidermis. The horizontal phase can last as long as 15 years in instances of SSM, 5 years in instances of LMM, or an extremely short (or nonexistent) period in instances of NM.

The second phase of development is the vertical growth phase. During this phase melanocytes descend across the basal lamina and into the dermis. Also during this phase nodules can become raised on the skin's surface. After invasion into the dermis has taken place, inflammatory cells arrive to defend the body from foreign invaders. If these cells are successful, a spontaneous regression takes place. If they are not successful, the melanoma grows deeper into the dermis and may involve the blood and lymphatic vessels, thus possibly helping the melanoma spread to regional lymph nodes and/or virtually any organ of the body.[1]

Dr. Wallace Clark and Dr. Alexander Breslow developed the main microstaging systems for melanomas. Both systems are basically indirect measures of tumor volume. Clark's system categorizes melanomas based on their level of invasion through the epidermis and layers of the dermis. Clark's levels (Fig. 1-12) may indicate the potential for metastasis because the access of tumor cells to lymphatic and vascular structures are assessable. Also, the extent of invasion may indicate the tumor's progression from relatively harmless radial growth to more aggressive vertical growth.[43] Clark's levels are as follows:

- Level 1—Confinement to the epidermis above the basement membrane

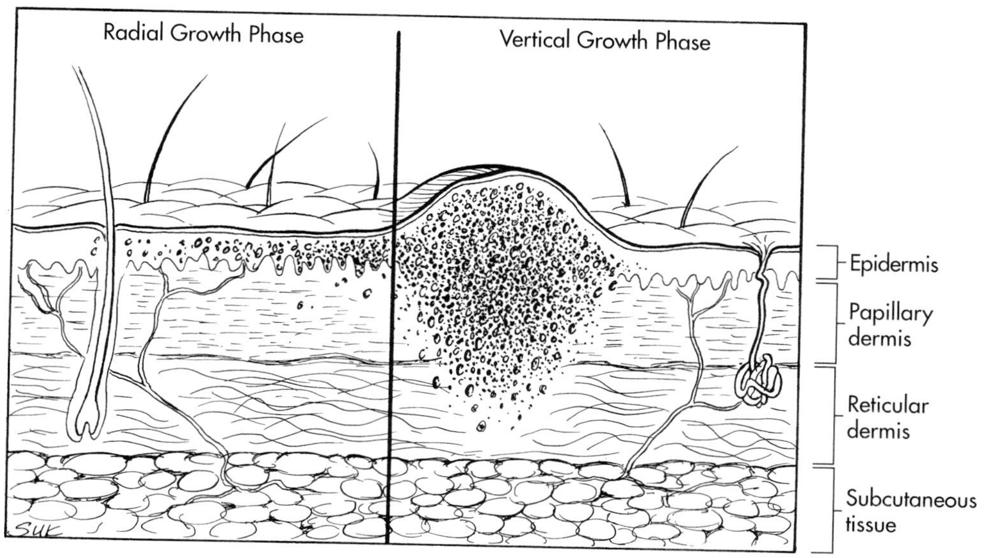

Fig. 1-11 A cross section of a superficial spreading melanoma showing the radial growth phases indicative of most early melanomas *(left)*, and the vertical phase indicative of most late melanomas *(right)*.

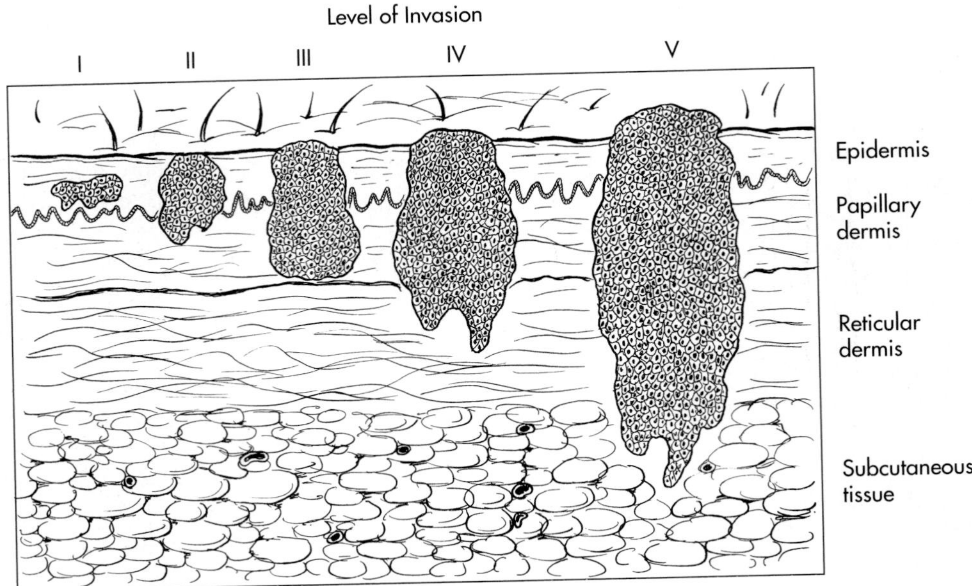

Fig. 1-12 A schematic relating Clark's levels to the layer of the skin through which the tumor has penetrated.

- Level 2—Invasion through the basement membrane to the papillary dermis
- Level 3—Presence of tumor cells at the papillary-reticular junction of the dermis
- Level 4—Invasion into the reticular dermis
- Level 5—Invasion into subcutaneous fat

Breslow's system categorizes melanomas based on tumor thickness from the top of the granular layer of the epidermis or, if the primary tumor is ulcerated, from the ulcer surface to the deepest identifiable melanoma cell as measured by an ocular micrometer.[13] Breslow's levels are as follows:

- Level 1—Melanoma in situ, limited to the epidermis
- Level 2—Less than 0.75 mm
- Level 3—0.76 mm to 1.5 mm
- Level 4—1.51 mm to 4 mm
- Level 5—Greater than 4 mm

Because Breslow's system has more to do with tumor bulk than penetration, some experts feel this system is more reproducible and correlates more accurately with the risk of metastatic disease and prognosis than Clark's system. One problem that Clark's system does not address is the variation in skin thickness throughout the body. In contrasting the extremely thin skin of the eyelids with the extremely thick skin of the soles of the feet, a 0.75-mm lesion would be far more penetrating in the eyelid than on the sole of the foot, yet the size of the tumor is the same in both instances. Other problems pathologists may encounter with Clark's system occur when specimens are taken from areas of the body where the papillary-reticular junction of the dermis (an important demarcation point) is not well defined or when the integrity of the tissue layers in the surgical specimen is compromised.[26] Using both the Clark and Breslow methods, physicians at the John Wayne Cancer Institute in Santa Monica, California, have calculated 5-year survival rates based on microstaging data (Table 1-2). The researchers who compiled the data concluded that Breslow's measurement of thickness is a more powerful prognostic factor because it remains highly significant in every subset of Clark's levels.[43]

The American Joint Committee on Cancer (AJCC)[8] has developed a macrostaging system for malignant melanoma of the skin, taking into account Clark's levels of invasion, Breslow's measurements of thickness, and known patterns of metastasis (see the box at the bottom of p. 15).

After it has been arranged according to the TNM system, the tumor can be further classified into a specific stage. Stage groupings allow health care workers to assemble patients with similar disease patterns to aid physicians in treatment planning, facilitate information exchange, indicate prognosis, and help evaluate treatment results. (See the top box on p. 15 for the stage groupings for melanomas.)

The 5-year survival rates based on the AJCC stage are as follows: Stage I = 95%, Stage II = 78%, Stage III = 51%, and Stage IV = 13%.[4,8]

Prognostic factors for malignant melanoma include the following[59]:

1. Tumor thickness—Thicker tumors yield a poorer prognosis.
2. Depth of invasion—The deeper the level of penetration, the poorer the prognosis.

3. Ulceration—Ulcerated tumors have a worse prognosis than nonulcerated tumors, especially if the area of ulceration exceeds 6 mm in diameter.
4. Lymph node status—A positive lymph status equals a poorer prognosis.
5. Metastatic status—The prognosis for metastatic patients is grim.
6. Gender—All things being equal, women have a 22% survival advantage over men when the disease is found before it has metastasized.[66]
7. Location of primary tumor—Tumors located on the extremities, excluding the feet, have a better prognosis than tumors on the head and neck, which have a better prognosis than a tumor found on the trunk.[18]

Table 1-2 5-year survival rates

Level	Clark survival rate	Breslow survival rate
Level I	100%	100%
Level II	95%	95%
Level III	81%	85%
Level IV	68%	66%
Level V	47%	46%

Courtesy John Wayne Cancer Institute, Santa Monica, California.

Stage Groupings for Melanomas

Stage IA—Melanoma ≤ 0.75 mm in thickness that invades the papillary dermis with no lymph node involvement (T_1, N_0, M_0)
Stage IB—Melanoma 0.76 mm to 1.5 mm in thickness and/or invasion to the papillary-reticular dermal junction; no lymph node involvement (T_2, N_0, M_0)
Stage IIA—Melanoma 1.51 mm to 4.0 mm and/or invasion of the reticular dermis; no lymph node involvement (T_3, N_0, M_0)
Stage IIB—Melanoma greater than 4.0 mm and/or invasion of the subcutaneous tissue and/or metastasis to the skin or subcutaneous tissue within 2 cm of the primary tumor; no lymph node involvement (T_4, N_0, M_0)
Stage IIIA—Melanoma of any size that has metastasized to regional lymph node(s), none of which is greater than 3 cm in greatest dimension (any T, N_1, M_0)
Stage IIIB—Melanoma of any size that has metastasized to regional lymph node(s), some of which may be larger than 3 cm in greatest dimension and/or evidence of in-transit metastasis (any T, N_2, M_0).
Stage IV—Melanoma that has spread beyond regional lymph nodes (any T, Any N, M_1)
Note: In-transit metastasis involves skin or subcutaneous tissue more than 2 cm from the primary tumor not beyond the regional lymph nodes.

TNM System for Staging Malignant Melanomas

T = Primary tumor status

TX = Primary not assessable
T_0 = No evidence of primary tumor
Tis = Melanoma in situ, lesions that have not invaded the basement membrane
T_1 = Tumor ≤ 0.75 mm in thickness and invades the papillary dermis
T_2 = Tumor >0.75 mm but ≤ 1.5 mm in thickness and/or invades to the papillary-reticular dermal junction
T_3 = Tumor >1.5 mm but ≤ 4 mm in thickness and/or invades the reticular dermis
- T_{3a} = Tumor >1.5 mm but ≤ 3 mm in thickness
- T_{3b} = Tumor >3 mm but ≤4 mm in thickness

T_4 = Tumor >4 mm in thickness and/or invades the subcutaneous tissue and/or contains satellite(s) within 2 cm of the primary tumor
- T_{4a} = Tumor >4 mm in thickness and/or invades the subcutaneous tissue
- T_{4b} = Satellite(s) within 2 cm of the primary tumor

N = Lymph node status

NX = Lymph nodes not assessable
N_0 = No evidence of disease in nodes
N_1 = Metastasis ≤ 3 cm in greatest dimension in any regional lymph node(s)
N_2 = Metastasis >3 cm in greatest dimension in any regional lymph node(s) and/or in-transit metastasis
- N_{2a} = Metastasis >3 cm in greatest dimension in any regional lymph nodes
- N_{2b} = In-transit metastasis
- N_{2c} = Both (N_{2a} and N_{2b})

M = Metastatic disease status

MX = Presence of metastatic disease not assessable
M_0 = No evidence of metastatic disease
M_1 = Distant metastasis
- M_{1a} = Metastatic disease found in distant skin or lymph nodes
- M_{1b} = Metastatic disease found in other distant sites

Note: When the thickness and level of invasion do not coincide, the less favorable finding should prevail.

Modified from Beahrs OH et al: *AJCC manual for staging of cancer,* ed 4, Philadelphia, 1992, JB Lippincott.

8. Age—The prognosis for older patients is worse than that for younger patients.[62]

The clinical-histological subtype does not appear to provide additional prognostic information when the depth of invasion is taken into consideration.[48]

Because the epidermis does not contain any blood vessels or lymphatics, skin cancers confined to that area have virtually no chance of spreading other than via direct extension. After a tumor invades the superficial lymphatic plexus of the dermis (which is devoid of valves characteristic of deeper lymphatic vessels),[40] it can spread in any direction to and from the tumor. Because melanomas can occur on a multitude of different locations throughout the body, physicians must be aware of the lymphatic drainage patterns of the specific area where the melanoma is found. Obviously, a melanoma found on the shoulder will affect different regional nodes than a melanoma found on the leg. Approximately 5% of patients have metastatic melanoma from an unknown primary site.[16] Following are areas of the body and the regional nodes that may be affected if a melanoma developed there[8]:

- Ipsilateral preauricular, submandibular, cervical, and head and neck—Supraclavicular nodes
- Thorax—Ipsilateral axillary lymph nodes
- Arm—Ipsilateral epitrochlear and axillary lymph nodes
- Abdomen, loins, and buttocks—Ipsilateral inguinal lymph nodes
- Leg—Ipsilateral popliteal and inguinal lymph nodes
- Anal margin and perianal skin—Ipsilateral inguinal lymph nodes

Some melanomas do not fit into specific drainage categories, but rather between drainage areas. In such instances, regions on both sides of the area containing the tumor must be considered potential drainage sites. Procedures have been developed to aid physicians in determining the actual lymphatic flow patterns from the primary melanoma site. A study called *lymphoscintigraphy* uses a radioactive isotope that is injected into the primary melanoma site. The isotope then filters through the lymphatic channels that drain the tumor, and the patient is scanned to determine which lymph node stations could potentially harbor malignant cells. Another procedure, called *intraoperative lymphatic mapping,* uses special dyes that are injected into the primary tumor. As these dyes are transported through the lymphatic channels, they stain the tissues they contact. During surgery the physician can identify the draining lymphatics and follow them to the lymph node closest to the tumor, or the sentinel node. The most likely site of early metastases, the sentinel node is removed and analyzed to determine whether it contains malignant cells.[43]

Melanomas can spread to virtually any organ of the body. Melanomas tend to spread in the following order: (1) direct extension of the primary, including invasion into the subcutaneous tissues; (2) regional lymphatics; (3) distant skin and subcutaneous tissues; (4) lung; and (5) liver, bone, and brain.

Nonmelanoma. After a biopsy is taken (incisional or excisional) the cell type of the carcinoma must be determined.

The four main subtypes of basal cell carcinoma (BCC) are as follows[18]:

1. Nodular-ulcerated basal cell carcinoma is the most common type and is found mainly on the head and neck. Lesions are generally smooth, shiny, and translucent and accompanied by telangiectasis, an abnormal dilation of capillaries and arterioles that may be visible on the skin's surface. Ulceration is common and lesions may be pigmented. Pigmented lesions may sometimes be mistaken for melanoma.
2. Superficial basal cell carcinoma is found mainly on the trunk and appears as a red plaque, which may develop areas of translucent papules as it spreads over the skin's surface. These lesions may also develop areas of pigmentation.
3. Morphea-form, or sclerosing, basal cell carcinoma often appears as a scarlike lesion, often with indistinct margins. This type of lesion is uncommon, is found mainly on the head and neck, and has a rather high propensity for invasion and recurrence after treatment.
4. Cystic basal cell carcinoma is an uncommon cancer that "undergoes central degeneration to form a cystic lesion."[16]

Although basal cell carcinoma do not have a propensity to metastasize, they are capable of extensive local invasion and destruction. They tend to follow the path of least resistance, although they have been known to destroy bone and cartilage if left untreated.

However, rare cases of metastatic basal cell carcinoma have been reported. The rate of metastasis is less than 1 per 4000 cases, and the condition is often detected 10 or more years after treatment of the primary. Tumors most likely to metastasize are large, ulcerated, resistant tumors found on the head or neck of middle-aged men.[53] Regional lymph nodes are usually involved, but the involvement of liver, lung, and bone has been reported.

Squamous cell carcinomas can take on a variety of appearances. As mentioned earlier, they can be scaly, slightly ulcerated, or nodular. Occasionally, tumors contain characteristics of basal cell *and* squamous cell cancers.

A verrucous variety of squamous cell carcinoma has been described as a low grade, warty neoplasm with a greasy, foul discharge. These lesions are most commonly found on the sole of the foot.[23]

Squamous cell carcinomas have a higher propensity to metastasize than basal cell carcinomas. This tendency is based on a variety of factors, including the following[53]:

1. Differentiation—Poorly differentiated lesions have a higher propensity to metastasize than well-differentiated lesions.

2. Etiology—Tumors developing in immunosuppressed patients or in areas of chronic inflammation, scar tissue, and radiation dermatitis have higher rates of metastasis compared with tumors that develop in sun-exposed areas.
3. Size and invasion—Tumors greater than 1 cm in size and more than 4 mm deep have a higher propensity for metastasis, even in sun-exposed areas.

Most studies report a 3% to 10% rate of metastasis from squamous cell skin cancer, but patients with high-risk factors can have up to a 30% chance of developing metastasis. Regional lymph nodes are affected 85% of the time in metastatic patients, with possible involvement of liver, bone, brain, and especially lung.[53]

Because nonmelanoma skin cancers can occur anywhere on the skin's surface, multiple lymphatic regions may be affected. Lymphatic drainage patterns for nonmelanomas are the same as those for melanomas. (See the box at right for the staging of nonmelanomas, according to the AJCC.)

Basal cell and squamous cell cancers of the skin are not reportable diseases. In other words, physicians are not responsible for keeping accurate records concerning factors such as incidence and survival. Therefore a strong database does not exist for calculating survival rates stage by stage. Although the overall survival rate is not known, early nonmelanoma lesions are almost 100% curable.[45]

TNM System for Staging Nonmelanomas

T = Primary tumor status

TX	=	Primary tumor not assessable
T_0	=	No evidence of primary tumor
Tis	=	Carcinoma in situ
T_1	=	Tumor ≤ 2 cm in greatest dimension
T_2	=	Tumor >2 cm but ≤5 cm in greatest dimension
T_3	=	Tumor >5 cm in greatest dimension
T_4	=	Tumor invasion of deep extradermal structures (cartilage, skeletal muscle, or bone)

N = Lymph node status

NX	=	Regional lymph nodes not assessable
N_0	=	No regional lymph node metastasis
N_1	=	Regional lymph node metastasis

Metastatic disease status

MX	=	Presence of distant metastases not assessable
M_0	=	No distant metastasis
M_1	=	Distant metastasis

Stage grouping

Stage I—Tumor ≤ 2 cm, with no lymph node involvement (T_1, N_0, M_0)
Stage IIA—Tumor >2 cm but ≤ 5 cm, with no lymph node involvement (T_2, N_0, M_0)
Stage IIB—Tumor > 5 cm with no lymph node involvement (T_3, N_0, M_0)
Stage IIIA: Any tumor that invades internal structures such as cartilage, bone, muscle, with no lymph node involvement (T_4, N_0, M_0)
Stage IIIB—Any tumor in which the regional lymph nodes are involved (T_4, N_1, M_0)
Stage IV—Any tumor in which distant metastases are present

Modified from Beahrs OH et al: *AJCC manual for staging of cancer,* ed 4, Philadelphia, 1992, JB Lippincott.

Treatment techniques

Melanoma. The treatment of primary melanoma of the skin for cure is limited to surgical resection. Chemotherapy and immunotherapy are used to keep diagnosed malignant melanomas from metastasizing and as a treatment for melanomas that have metastasized. The role of radiation therapy is limited primarily to the palliative treatment of metastatic disease sites. Melanoma has a reputation for being a radioresistant tumor, but radiation therapy has been successfully used as an adjuvant to surgery and as the primary treatment modality in selected tumors and tumor sites.

Although there is no doubt that surgery is currently the only form of curative therapy for malignant melanoma, controversy exists concerning surgical margins and the use of prophylactic lymph node removal to help prevent the occurrence of metastasis.

Before the 1970s, wide local excisions with 5-cm margins of normal skin surrounding the tumor were routine, sometimes creating large defects closeable only with skin grafts. Recent studies, however, indicate that wide margins are not always required. The thickness of the tumor, site of the tumor, and potential morbidity of the operation should determine the margin size around the primary. The decision to use wider margins should be based on the chance of local recurrence because no clear evidence exists to prove that creating larger margins increases the likelihood of survival.[66]

Although firm guidelines for surgical margins in the treatment of melanoma have not been established, some recommendations are as follows: (1) Melanoma in situ can be excised with a 0.5-cm margin and considered cured because the chance of metastases is small, and (2) 1-cm margins are adequate for tumors less than 1 mm in thickness.[48] Tumors with a thickness of 1 to 2 mm can be treated with a 1-cm or 3-cm margin. Studies have shown both to be similar in effectiveness. A possible deciding factor is the site on which the lesion was found. For example, a patient may opt for the aggressive therapy if the tumor is on the trunk and the conservative approach if it is on the face. A melanoma greater than 2 mm in thickness should be excised with a 3-cm margin if possible.[62] However, the recurrence of melanomas more than 2 mm thick seems to be related more to tumor thickness than to the size of excisional margins. Although 3-cm margins are more effective in tumor control versus 1-cm margins in treating these lesions, even large margins of 5 cm are no guarântee against local recurrence.[66] For all excisions, surgical margins should include subcutaneous tissue down to the fascia and should show no involvement of the tumor.

Biopsies of questionable lesions often encompass a 0.5-cm margin around the tumor. If at the time of the pathological examination the lesion is found to be a malignant melanoma beyond the in-situ stage, the surgeon must go back and create the proper margins dictated by the thickness of the lesion. In the case of subungual lesions (found beneath the nail beds), all but the earliest lesions are treated by the amputation of the complete digit.[15]

The elective prophylactic removal of regional lymph nodes in clinically negative (nonpalpable) lymph nodes is questionable. A prophylactic lymphadenectomy in a patient with a tumor less than 1 cm thick is most likely overkill because of the low metastatic risk of the tumor. Patients with tumors greater than 4 mm in thickness have a high risk of distant disease and do not benefit much from the removal of regional disease as a form of curative therapy. The persons who most likely benefit from this procedure are those with tumors between 1 mm and 4 mm in thickness, provided the lymphatic removal was carried out early in the course of the disease. The results of studies concerning prophylactic lymph node removal are inconclusive but may be beneficial to well-selected patients if the surgical technique does not cause significant complications.[23]

The key to melanoma treatment is the eradication of the tumor before it has a chance to metastasize. Although a tumor may be removed with clear margins, a few stray cells that can lead to recurrence or metastasis may be left behind. This is the area in which chemotherapy and immunotherapy play a role. These agents will hopefully cause the destruction of stray cells before they can reseed. (Specifics concerning chemotherapy and immunotherapy are discussed in the section concerning metastatic disease.)

Patients with proven lymph node metastasis should undergo a radical excision of regional lymph nodes, removing as much of the soft tissue and its associated lymphatics as possible between the tumor site and the regional lymph nodes. Even with such treatment the risk of distant metastasis is high (85%).[23]

Patients who have melanomas on an extremity are treatable with isolated limb perfusion, which combines chemotherapy with hyperthermia. With this technique the extremity is isolated with a tourniquet while the blood in the limb circulates through a machine that pumps, oxygenates, and heats it. Because this blood is cut off from the rest of the body, large doses of chemotherapy can be introduced and circulated through the limb. Melphalan (L-PAM) is the agent of choice in most instances, although cisplatin (DDP) has been used successfully.[30] Because melanoma cells cannot survive above 105.8° F, the heating action provides an extra mode of cell killing to the process. After about 1 hour of treatment the treated blood is completely drained and the tourniquet is removed, allowing the normal blood supply to return to the limb.[58]

For patients who have developed distant metastasis, no successful curative treatment options are available. The options available are for symptomatic relief and the prolongation of life.

Surgery can be used to remove local recurrences and localized metastatic areas such as nonregional lymph nodes, distant skin lesions, and subcutaneous metastases. Because surgery of this type is palliative, it should only be done on patients whose quality of life would be enhanced with low morbidity (side effects).

Radiation therapy can also be used for palliation. It can be used to relieve symptoms caused by skin, soft tissue, or bone metastasis, as well as those found in the brain and spinal cord. Dosage and fractionation are important and will be discussed later in the chapter.

Chemotherapy has been successful in producing remissions in some patients, but its use in the treatment of malignant melanoma is largely palliative. Dacarbazine (DTIC) as a single agent is the drug of choice, although nitrosoureas and Vinca alkaloids have also been used. "Tumors of the skin, lymph nodes, and soft tissues respond better to drugs than do visceral metastasis."[36] Unfortunately, the response rate is only about 15% to 18%,[17] and responses only last an average of 4 to 6 months.[23] The problem with cytoxic regimens is their lack of tumor specificity. They affect the surrounding tissue as much as they do the tumor, causing serious complications in large doses. Through the study of the biochemical properties and behavior of melanomas, hopes are that an agent can be found or incorporated into molecules that will selectively seek out and bind with melanoma cells to destroy them. Potential vehicles that may be used are molecules that normally bind to melanocytes, such as growth factors, MSHs, and monoclonal antibodies.

Studies have shown that some melanomas contain estrogen (hormones affecting the secondary sex characteristics as well as systematic effects such as the growth and maturity of long bones) receptors, allowing for responses to antiestrogen therapy. Antiestrogens block receptor sites for estrogen, denying the cell the effect that estrogen would have had on the cell. Research has shown that dacarbazine plus tamoxifen (TAM), an antiestrogen, is more effective than dacarbazine alone in terms of response rate and median survival. The effects of tamoxifen-aided treatment are more pronounced in women and in men and postmenopausal women with higher than normal body mass indexes (weight divided by height).[17] Tamoxifen also has a synergistic effect on cisplatin.[36]

A recent study by McClay and McClay concentrated on the overall effectiveness of various chemotherapeutic regimens and concluded that a combination of dacarbazine, carmustine (BCNU), cisplatin, and tamoxifen (overall regimen code = DBDT) may be the chemotherapeutic treatment of choice for metastatic melanoma. Combined data using this regimen have reported response rates of 47% with relatively modest toxicity.[35]

A bone marrow transplant using high-dose chemotherapy and autologous (self-donated) marrow can also improve the response to chemotherapy treatment. Although improvements in short-term survival have been seen, long-term survival has not been affected.[36]

Immunotherapy also plays a role in metastatic melanoma treatments. Melanomas have a history of spontaneous regression in which the body is somehow able to fend off the disease using its own natural defenses. Basically, immunotherapy attempts to take advantage of this phenomenon and bolster the body's immune system so that it is able to fight off the melanoma on its own.

Immunotherapy can be divided into the following five major types[41]:

1. Active—Stimulation of the body's natural defenses
   - Nonspecific—Use of microbial or chemical adjuvants to activate macrophages, natural killer cells, and other nonspecific defenses; stimulation of the immune system in general
   - Specific—Use of tumor cells or tumor-associated antigens sometimes mixed with haptens, viruses, or enzymes to activate T cells, macrophages, or other cells the body uses to fight specific tumor cells; stimulation of particular areas of the immune system
2. Adoptive—Transfer of cells with antitumor properties into the tumor-bearing host to directly or indirectly cause tumor regression
3. Restorative—Replacement of depleted immunological subpopulations, such as T cells, or inhibition of the body's natural suppressor mechanisms (suppressor T cells or suppressor macrophages) to allow the body to replace the depleted subpopulations on its own
4. Passive—Transfer of antibodies or other short-lived antitumor factors into the tumor-bearing host to control tumor growth
5. Cytomodularitive—Enhancement of tumor-associated antigens and histocompatibility (HLA) antigens on the surface of tumor cells to make them more recognizable as foreign invaders by the body's immune system

Nonspecific active immunotherapy has been used to bolster the immune system in general and therefore raise the body's ability to fight the melanoma cells. One such stimulant is Bacillus Calmette and Guerin (BCG), a weakened strain of Mycobacterium bovis. Through the introduction of BCG into the body, the hope is that the body perceives that it is under attack and defends itself against all invaders, including melanoma cells.

Other agents used to promote a general immune response are interferons and interleukins.

Interferons are special proteins that activate and enhance the tumor-killing ability of monocytes and produce chemicals toxic to cells. Studies have shown that response rates are in the 15% to 20% range and usually brief. Interferons tend to be toxic to the patient and are not often used in single-agent therapy.[30]

Interleukins are substances that act as costimulators and intensifiers of immune responses. Malcolm Mitchell et al. administered cyclophosphamide (CY), a chemotherapeutic agent, to patients and then gave a dose of interleukin-2 (IL-2). Because IL-2 stimulates all subsets of T cells (helpers, killers, and suppressors), CY was given to decrease the number of suppressor T cells so the IL-2 could stimulate the helper and killer T cells that ultimately combat the tumor. Approximately 26% (10 of 39) patients responded to the therapy, with most patients having moderate symptoms of toxicity.[41]

David Berd et al. has used an autologous tumor cell vaccine to produce a specific, active immune response in patients with metastatic melanoma. The vaccine was a mixture of BCG and tumor cells removed from the patients and irradiated to keep the cells from reproducing. The patients were injected with low-dose CY 3 days before the introduction of the vaccine to depress the natural mechanisms in the body that suppress immune reactions. The theory behind this treatment is that the body does not recognize the melanoma cells as foreign. Through the mixing of the tumor cells with BCG, the body recognizes tumor cells as foreign as a result of their association with the BCG and responds to them accordingly. Of the 40 patients treated with this regimen, 5 (12.5%) showed a response; 4 of those responses were complete. Side effects of treatment included nausea and vomiting, which were controlled with medication.[12]

Mitchell and his group used a different approach to get a similar response via a generic (allogenic) vaccine. Mitchell reasoned that autologous vaccines do not allow large groups of patients to be treated with the same vaccine because each vaccine contains tumor cells from a different patient. Another problem is that not every patient has an accessible tumor from which cells can be drawn to be made into a vaccine. Mitchell's vaccine uses two melanoma cell lines drawn from two female patients chosen for their complementary characteristics. The cells are grown in culture to obtain a large cell population from which the vaccine can be made. After mechanical disruption the cell lysates (cellular debris and fluid caused by the destruction of the cell) are combined and mixed with an immunological adjuvant called *DETOX**. Of the 106 patients who received this therapy, 20 (19%) had objective clinical responses and 5 (5%) had complete responses.[42]

Steven Rosenberg and his colleagues at the National Cancer Institute have used adoptive immunotherapy in the treatment of melanoma. In one study, lymphocytes removed from the peripheral blood of the patient through multiple leukapheresis were incubated with IL-2 to generate lym-

*DETOX is made by Ribi Immunochem Research, Inc., Hamilton, Montana.

phoid cells capable of destroying tumor cells that are normally resistant to the activity of killer T cells. These resulting lymphoid cells are referred to as *lymphokine-activated killer (LAK) cells.* The major problem with this type of therapy is generating enough LAK cells for systemic therapy. After the appropriate number of LAK cells were produced, they were infused into the patient; then doses of recombinant IL-2 were given. The LAK cells released into the patient's body were in most instances more effective than the body's normal killer T cells in fighting the resistant melanoma cells.[60] About 21% of patients have complete or partial responses to this type of therapy, although severe toxicity can result.[61] Because results of this therapy are similar to therapy using IL-2 alone, questions are raised about the necessity of adding LAK cells to the regimen.

Rosenberg et al. also did a similar study in which the LAK cells were replaced with tumor-infiltrating lymphocytes (TIL). TILS are lymphocytes formed by the body in response to the melanoma that can be found in freshly resected melanomas. After the TILs were removed from the resected tumor, they were expanded in culture for 4 to 8 weeks. Before the reinfusion of the TILs the immune system of the patient was suppressed with CY or whole-body irradiation. After the administration of the TILs, IL-2 was also given. The main side effect of this therapy was "intravascular volume and accumulation of fluid in visceral organs and soft tissues" from the IL-2.[60,61] Tumor models have shown that TILs are 50 to 100 times more effective than LAK cells in eliminating tumor cells. Preliminary response rates of 40% to 60% have been reported with the TIL adoptive immunotherapy. The problem with this and other types of immunotherapy is that responses are often brief and do not have a significant effect on overall survival rates.[61]

Rosenberg has also inserted a gene for tumor necrosis factor (TNF)* into TILs. The problem with TNF is that it is toxic in large doses, so the special TILs are used to transport the TNF to the tumor, where it is then released. Because it theoretically does not come into contact with normal tissue, the TNF's toxicity to the patient is greatly diminished.[22]

Rosenberg also believes he has isolated the gene for a protein present on melanoma cells. He hopes to someday develop a vaccine that will help the body recognize these proteins and destroy melanomas before they have a chance to gain a stronghold.[22]

Although the results of immunotherapy are rather dismal thus far, the fact that the body is able to cause tumor regression at all gives researchers hope that someday immunology will play a bigger role in the fight against melanoma and other cancers.

Nonmelanoma. Patients with basal cell or squamous cell carcinomas of the skin have several treatment options. The technique selected depends on factors such as previous methods of treatment (if any), the location on the body, the risk of recurrence and metastasis, and the volume of tissue invasion. The number one goal of treatment is eradication of the tumor, followed by good cosmetic results. In instances in which cure rates are similar but the cosmetic results will differ, the modality offering the better cosmesis should prevail. If control rates are similar and cosmetic results are similar or unimportant, the most cost-effective and/or quickest treatment method is preferred.[44]

Surgery can be performed to remove nonmelanoma skin cancers from areas where scarring is acceptable and patients want expedient results. Often, the original excisional biopsy contains all the tumor with acceptable margins, and no further treatment is needed. Otherwise, the surgeon may have to operate on the site a second time to ensure that safe margins around the tumor have been created. No uniform recommendation exists concerning the size of margins, but many surgeons use 3- to 5-mm margins for small, well-defined lesions and at least 1-cm margins for larger or more aggressive tumors.[53]

For large, salvageable, eroding tumors, extensive surgery may be needed to remove not only the tumor but also additional tissue that may have been invaded, such as bone or muscle tissue. Such intervention may include the use of skin grafts and/or prosthetic devices.[16]

A more precise type of surgery, referred to as **Mohs' surgery** (developed by Dr. Fredric Mohs at the University of Wisconsin), is used in areas where normal tissue sparing is important, areas of known or high risk of cancer recurrence, areas where the extent of the cancer is unknown, or in instances of aggressive, rapidly growing tumors.[29]

Mohs' surgery, or microscopic surgery, is different from conventional surgery in that the tumor is completely mapped out through the examination of each piece of removed tissue to determine the presence and extent of any tumor. Through the removal of only tissue containing a tumor a major amount of tissue is preserved versus conventional surgery. Mohs' surgery is indicated for recurrent basal and squamous cell carcinomas, those in known high-risk sites for recurrence, and those with aggressive histological subtypes.[55]

This surgery is performed on an outpatient basis with a local anesthetic. The tumor is removed one layer at a time and examined under a microscope. From the microscopic sample the surgeon knows where to obtain the next sample. This process repeats itself until the tumor is excised completely. The wound is then stitched or allowed to heal on its own.[29] Of all therapeutic modalities, Mohs' surgery has the highest success rate (96%).[16]

One reason Mohs' surgery has not replaced conventional surgery in the treatment of nonmelanoma skin cancers is that it is a time-consuming process, thus making it expensive. Cancers that are not viewed as problematic are treated almost as effectively and more inexpensively with conventional surgery.

Curettage and electrodesiccation are often used to treat basal cell carcinoma and early squamous cell carcinoma.

*TNF is a body protein that dramatically reduces tumors in mice.

With the patient under local anesthesia, the cancer is scooped out with a curette, an instrument in the form of a loop, ring, or scoop with sharpened edges. The destruction of any remaining tumor cells and stoppage of bleeding is carried out through a process called *electrodesiccation,* which entails the use of a probe emitting a high-frequency electric current to destroy tissue and cauterize blood vessels. The advantage of this method, also known as *electrosurgery,* is that it often leaves a white scar, which is less noticeable on people with fair skin.[47]

Another method of treating early nonmelanoma skin lesions is cryosurgery, in which liquid nitrogen or carbon dioxide is applied to a lesion, lowering its temperature to around -50° Celsius and thereby freezing and killing the abnormal cells. This procedure may have to be repeated once or twice to completely eliminate the tumor. Again, a white scar is generally formed as a result. Cryosurgery is not recommended for lesions of the scalp or lower legs because of poor healing in those areas.[23]

Lasers (light amplification by stimulated emission of radiation) can also be used to treat early basal cell carcinomas and in-situ squamous cell carcinomas. Lasers use highly focused beams of light that are able to destroy areas of a tumor with pinpoint accuracy while preserving the surrounding normal tissue. Advantages of laser surgery include little blood loss or pain because the blood vessels and nerves are instantly sealed. In addition, laser surgery provides faster healing than conventional surgery. Disadvantages include the high cost of obtaining the necessary equipment and the reluctance of physicians to use it because it is a relatively new technology.

Radiation therapy is used on basal cell and squamous cell carcinomas located in places of cosmetic significance, such as the eyelids, lips, nose, face, and ears. It is also used on tumors in which surgical removal is difficult or in areas of recurrence. The major advantage of radiation therapy is normal tissue sparing. Disadvantages include its relatively high cost, multiple treatments, and late skin changes in the treatment area. Doses and fractionation schedules should be carefully planned (especially in young people) to avoid these late changes, which could include scarring, necrosis, and chronic radiation dermatitis.[23]

Finally, early nonmelanoma skin cancers can be treated with 5-FU in the form of a solution or cream. Applying 5-FU to the affected area daily for several weeks causes the area to become inflamed and irritated during treatment, but scarring does not usually result.[47]

A few investigational therapies are being researched that may someday be used to treat nonmelanoma skin cancers. In photodynamic therapy (PDT), a photosensitizing agent is injected into the body and absorbed by all cells. The agent is quickly discharged from normal cells but is retained longer by cancer cells. Light from a laser is directed on the tumor area, causing a reaction within the cells containing the photosensitizing agent that destroys the cell.[47]

As with melanomas, immunotherapy is also being researched for use against nonmelanoma cancers. Intralesional interferon alpha has been used experimentally in nodular and superficial basal cell carcinomas as well as in squamous cell carcinomas. Cosmetic results with this method are good, but cure rates are lower and recurrence rates are higher compared with conventional therapies. Because of side effects such as local pain, skin necrosis, and an influenza-type syndrome, interferon alpha is not expected to be a major player in the treatment of skin cancer.[53]

Radiation therapy

Nonmelanoma. Radiation therapy is effective in the treatment of nonmelanoma skin cancers, especially in the treatment of small tumors in which cosmetic results are important or in areas of extensive disease where the primary tumor and affected lymph nodes can be included in the radiation field. Because most skin lesions tend to be superficially located, electrons and kilovoltage x-rays are often used in their treatment. Megavoltage x-rays are rarely used in the treatment of skin cancers but may be used with or without electrons for special circumstances such as scalp lesions or tumors that are deeply infiltrating.[39]

Brachytherapy, including temporary implants or superficial molds using iridium 192 or cesium 137 sources as well as permanent implants using gold seeds, has produced good curative and cosmetic results. However, brachytherapy does not possess any significant advantages over external beam radiation therapy. Disadvantages of brachytherapy for skin cancer include the cost, trauma, and length of stay required for the procedure; radiation exposure to personnel; uncertain dose distribution; and risk associated with anesthesia.[44]

Radiation therapy is often used to treat lesions on the lips, nose, eyelids, face, and ears because they are highly visible and cosmetic results are important. The choice between treatment with kilovoltage x-rays and electrons comes down to the size of the treatment volume, depth of the lesion, underlying anatomical structures, and physician preference. The availability of equipment may be a factor, considering that most radiation therapy departments are acquiring linear accelerators capable of producing electrons with energies from 4 MeV to over 20 MeV, whereas kilovoltage machines dedicated to therapy are becoming scarce.

Each modality has advantages and disadvantages that can be compared by using the following four main categories[3]:

1. Field size—For the treatment of next-to-critical structures such as the eye, kilovoltage x-rays allow the target volume to be covered with a smaller field size compared with that of a field producing similar effects near the skin surface through the use of electrons. Fig. 1-13 *A* and *B* shows the isodose distributions of a 250-kVp x-ray using surface collimation compared with a 6-MeV electron beam using no surface collimation. The 95% isodose line is approximately

twice as wide with the x-rays versus the electrons. The electron field must be opened considerably to produce the same effect at the 95% line as that produced by the x-rays. One solution to help minimize this problem with electrons is to increase the field size and use tertiary collimation on the skin's surface. In so doing the width of the 95% isodose area is increased 46% without the exposure of any extra tissue. Even with this method the area that the 95% isodose line covers is about a third smaller than that covered with the x-rays (Fig. 1-13 *C*).

Electrons tend to lose energy as field size decreases, especially in lower energy beams blocked to a width less than half the beam energy. This decrease in small fields is the result of the loss of lateral scatter when the field size is less than the lateral range of the scattered photons.[52] In general, electron doses are not reliable toward the edges of the field; therefore judicious use of margins is indicated.

2. Depth of maximum dose (D_{max})—A surface dose less than 90% to 95% is generally unacceptable in the treatment of skin cancer.[52] The characteristics of the beam to be used must be known for each specific setup to ensure that the skin surface is receiving the correct dose. This is relatively easy with low-energy x-rays because D_{max} is always at the surface regardless of field size or collimation technique. The D_{max} of electrons, in contrast, is a function of field size, location of secondary collimation, and surface contour. Because the D_{max} of electron beams is a function of energy and is usually found at a depth beneath the skin's surface, bolus material of appropriate thickness should be used to bring the dose toward the surface. To obtain exact information concerning D_{max} via electrons with or without bolus, dosimetric measurements should be taken through the use of phantom material to determine the characteristics of the beam on each patient—a potentially time-consuming process.
3. Deep-tissue dose—A characteristic of electrons is their rapid falloff; they penetrate the tissue to a certain point and dissipate, allowing for the sparing of some of the underlying tissues. Kilovoltage x-rays penetrate much deeper, however, and affect a greater volume of underlying tissue. As long as no deep tumor extensions are present, the treatment of choice is electron therapy.
4. Differential bone absorption—Gram for gram, the absorbed dose is higher in bone and cartilage than in soft tissue with the use of kilovoltage x-rays. This can result in underlying bone and cartilage receiving higher doses than the dose at D_{max}. No significant difference exists between bone and soft-tissue doses for electrons used in clinical practice.
5. Cosmesis and control rates—A study by Perez, Lovett, and Gerber,[52] indicated excellent or good cosmesis in 95% of patients treated with kilovoltage x-rays, compared with 80% of patients treated with electrons. Also, cosmetic results were superior for patients in whom less than 50% of the dose was delivered with bolus. Patients treated with electrons seem to have slightly lower control rates, although the differences are not statistically significant.

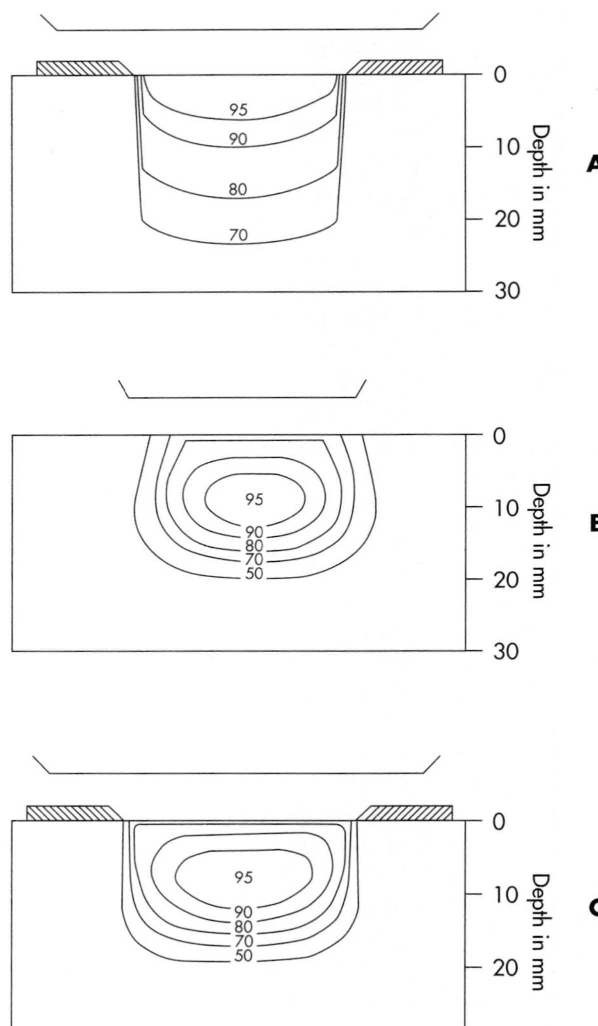

Fig. 1-13 Isodose distributions were measured through the center of a 3 × 3 cm square field defined on the surface of a water phantom. **A,** 250-kVp x-rays (HVL 1.4 mm Cu) with secondary collimation on the phantom surface. SSD = 50 cm. **B,** 6-MeV electron beam with secondary collimation 5 cm above the phantom surface (at the level of the electron cone). Source to collimator distance (SCD) = 95 cm. SSD = 100 cm. **C,** 6-MeV electron beam with tertiary collimation on the phantom surface. SSD = SCD = 100 cm. (Redrawn from Amdur RJ et al: RT for skin cancer near the eye, *Int J Radiat Oncol Biol Phys* 23:775, 1992.)

A few technical differences are involved in setting up a patient for a treatment with electrons produced by a linear accelerator versus x-rays produced by an orthovoltage machine (capable of producing x-rays with potentials ranging from 150 to 500 kVp).[31] Both types of equipment use cones to delineate the beam. Cones for electrons generally range from 4 × 4 cm to 25 × 25 cm and from 1 to 4 cm for orthovoltage machines (Figs. 1-14 and 1-15). The use of cones is not required with orthovoltage equipment because the field may be defined via primary collimators. Interchangeable filters (Fig. 1-16) are necessary to "harden" the beam during orthovoltage therapy. Aluminum, copper, or combination filters may be used, depending on the energy of the beam. An example of a combination filter is the Thoraeus filter, which is composed of tin, copper, and aluminum; the tin side faces the target, whereas the aluminum side faces the patient. Linear accelerators use special scattering foils to take electrons that are concentrated in a pencil-thin beam and disperse them over the desired treatment field. Shorter source-skin distances (SSDs) are used with orthovoltage equipment (generally 30 to 50 cm, compared with 100 cm SSDs used with linear accelerators).

Cutouts for each type of beam are manufactured by different means. In electron therapy most departments manufacture their own custom cutouts by using an alloy with a low melting point (70° C) called *Lipowitz metal* (brand name, *Cerrobend*).[31] These cutouts outline the field and protect normal tissues as the radiation oncologist dictates. The cutouts are inserted into a special housing located at the distal end of the electron cone before each treatment (Fig. 1-17) During treatment the bottom of the cutout normally rests about 5 cm from the skin's surface (Fig. 1-18). Depending on the type of linear accelerator used, cutouts may be substituted with a series of lead strips layered to produce the desired outline. These strips rest on the lower rungs of the cone and are taped into position.

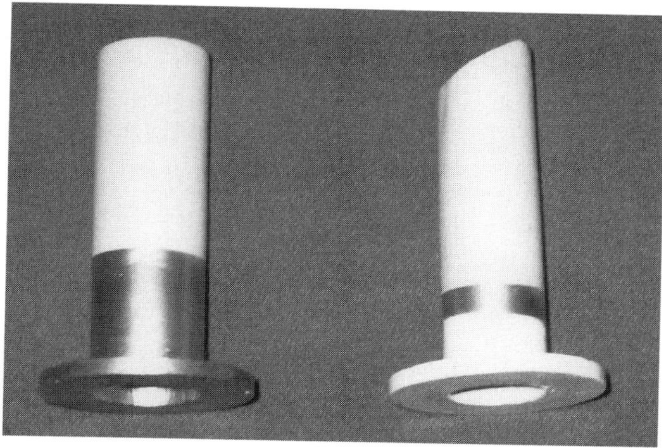

Fig. 1-14 Typical cones used with orthovoltage equipment. (Courtesy Shands Radiation Therapy Department, Gainesville, Florida.)

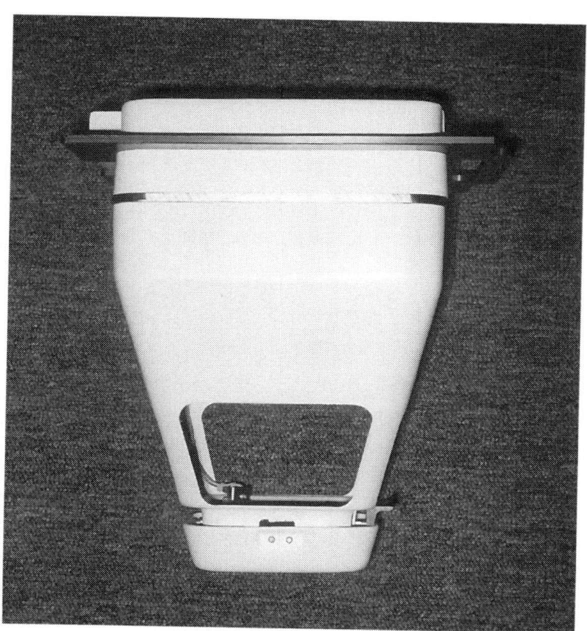

Fig. 1-15 Typical cone used with electrons produced by a linear accelerator. (Courtesy St. Vincent's Medical Center, Department of Radiation Therapy, Jacksonville, Florida.)

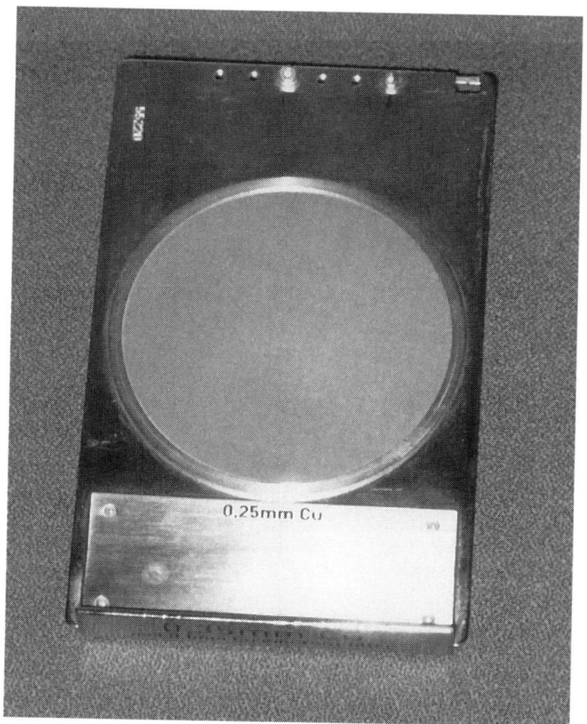

Fig. 1-16 An orthovoltage filter composed of 0.25 mm of copper that is used to filter low-energy x-rays.

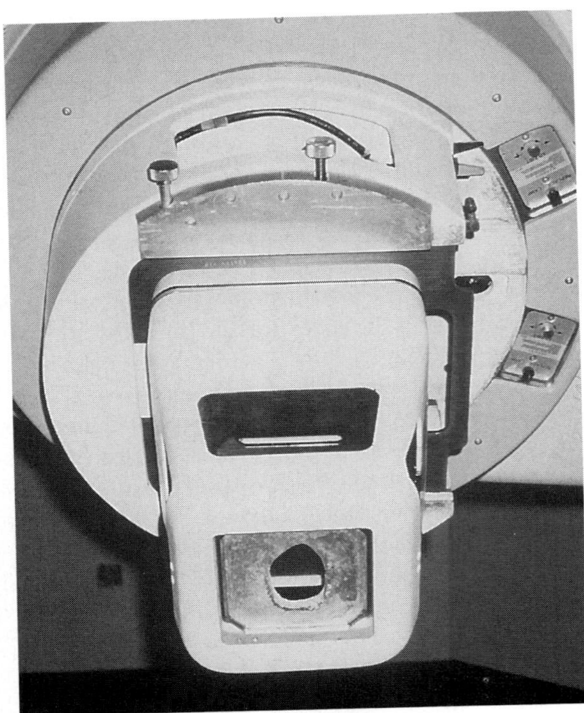

Fig. 1-17 An electron cone with a cutout in place. (Courtesy St. Vincent's Medical Center, Department of Radiation Therapy, Jacksonville, Florida.)

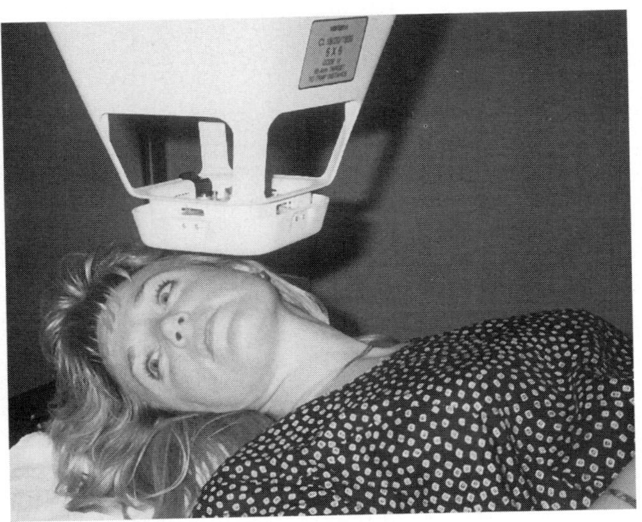

Fig. 1-18 A simulated electron setup showing the normal distance of the cone from the patient. (Courtesy St. Vincent's Medical Center, Department of Radiation Therapy, Jacksonville, Florida.)

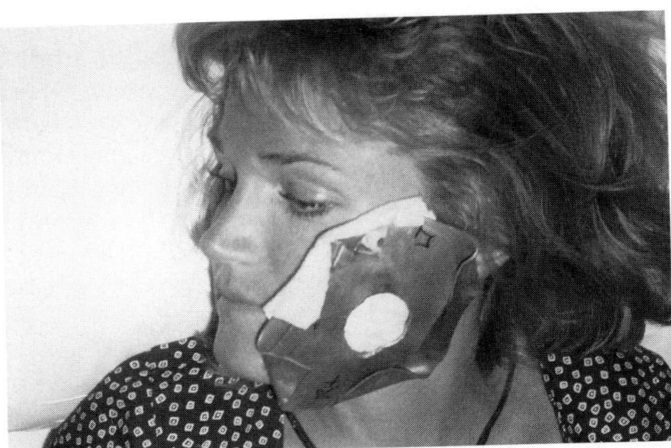

Fig. 1-19 Blocking material for orthovoltage equipment often consists of a thin strip of lead shielding that rests directly on the patient's skin.

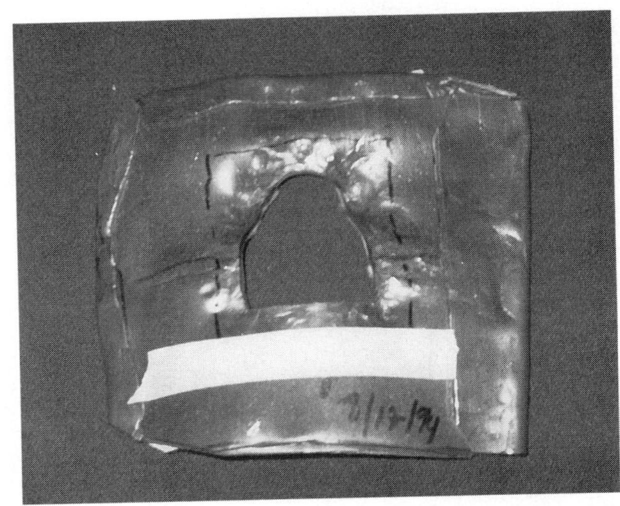

Fig. 1-20 A typical lead mask used during orthovoltage treatment. The radiation passes through the hole cut into the central part of the mask. (Courtesy Shands Radiation Therapy Department, Gainesville, Florida.)

Orthovoltage treatment requires a different type of blocking scheme. Instead of being attached to the machine, the blocking material rests on the patient (Fig. 1-19). Because lead is a soft metal, it can be formed into thin sheets that are somewhat pliable. These sheets can be contoured to the patient's anatomy, and holes can be cut into the sheets, creating the field through which the radiation passes (Fig. 1-20). The cones used are larger than and actually come into contact with the resulting cutout (Fig. 1-21), thus allowing the lead shielding to define the field. This type of blocking scheme can also be used as tertiary shielding in electron beam therapy. Regardless of the type of radiation used, the transmission factor for the blocking material should not exceed 5%.[31]

Radiation fields as a general rule should include a 2-cm margin completely surrounding the tumor to cover possible microscopic extension.[2] A 1-cm margin may be adequate for small, superficial basal cell carcinomas. Tumors and their

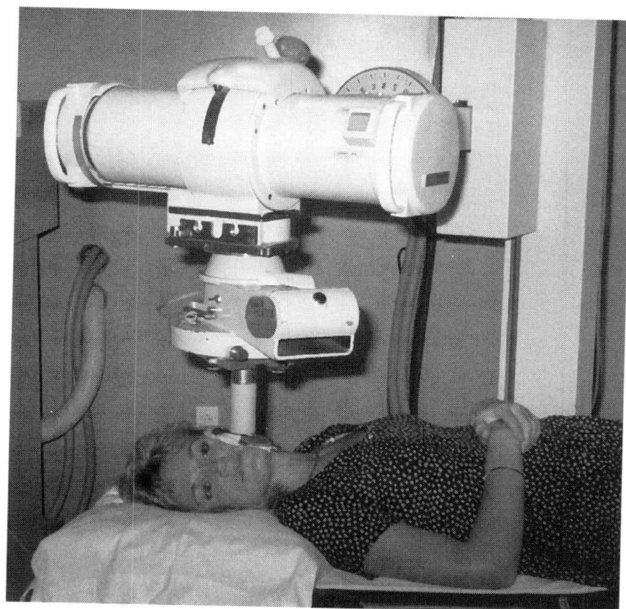

Fig. 1-21 A simulated setup on an orthovoltage machine showing the way the cone actually comes into contact with the lead mask that rests on the patient's skin. (Courtesy Shands Radiation Therapy Department, Gainesville, Florida.)

full margins should receive between 67% and 75% of the total dose, with a boost field encompassing the clinical tumor to deliver the full dose to the tumor itself. In doing so the amount of normal tissue treated is reduced, and the cosmetic effect is improved.[24]

Doses vary according to the size and penetration of the tumor and may differ from institution to institution. At the Mallinckrodt Institute of Radiology, doses ranged from 3,500 to 4,000 cGy for small basal cell carcinomas and from 5,000 to 6,000 cGy for basal cell tumors >5 cm and squamous cell carcinomas. Daily fractions were 250 to 300 cGy × 4 days a week for fields <20 square cm or 200 cGy × 5 days a week for larger lesions.[52]

At the University of Florida in Gainesville, doses for nonmelanoma tumors were as follows[39]:

6000 cGy/7 weeks	Large, untreated lesions with minimal bone or cartilage invasion
5000 cGy/4 weeks	Small, thin lesions (<5 cm around the ears, nose, or eyes)
4500 cGy/3 weeks	Moderate-sized lesions not involving the ears, nose, or eyes
4000 cGy/2 weeks or 3000 cGy/1 week	Small lesions (≤1 cm) not involving the ears, nose, or eyes

Figs. 1-22 and 1-23 show the results of patients who received radiation therapy to treat their nonmelanoma skin cancer.

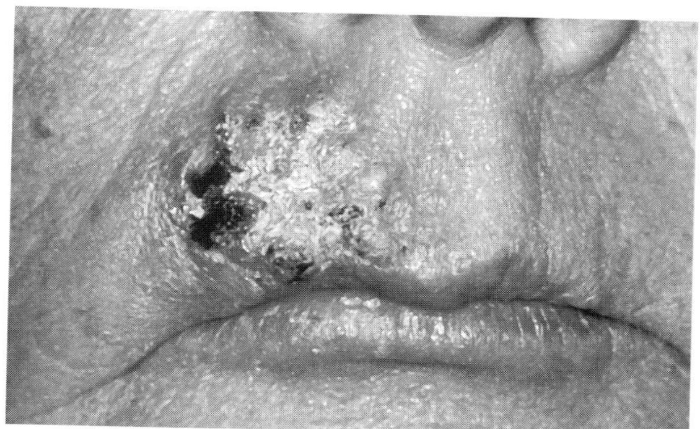

A

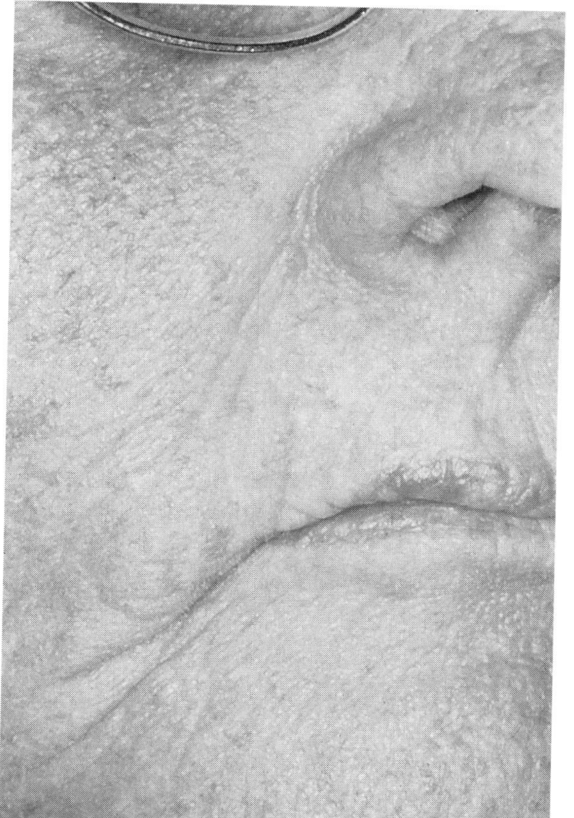

B

Fig. 1-22 A patient with squamous cell skin cancer before **(A)** and after **(B)** radiation therapy. (**A** and **B** courtesy Mark McLaughlin, M.D.)

Rapid fractionation schemes may be used in areas where late cosmetic results are not important or in instances in which transportation to and from the treatment site is difficult for the patient. Fraction size is the dominant factor in producing adverse reactions in late-responding normal tissue (the higher the daily dose, the greater the likelihood of adverse late effects).[68]

The radiation oncologist can determine the extent of the tumor through CT scans, through palpation, or by casting a

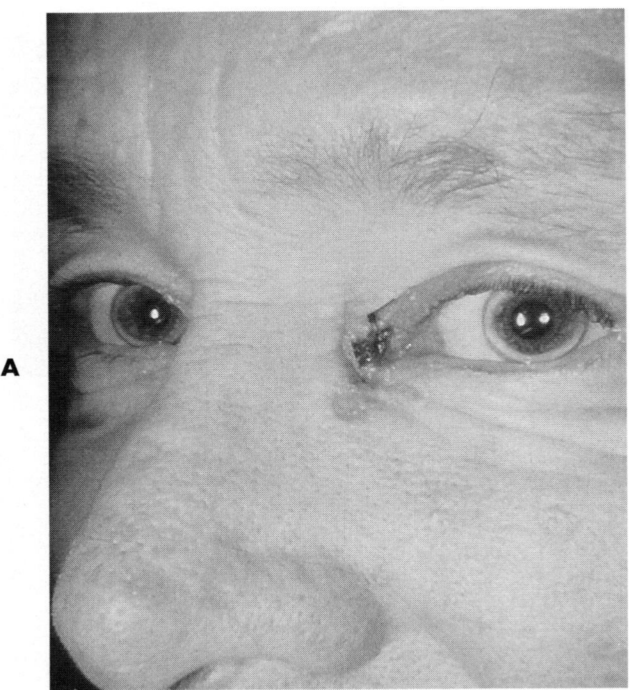

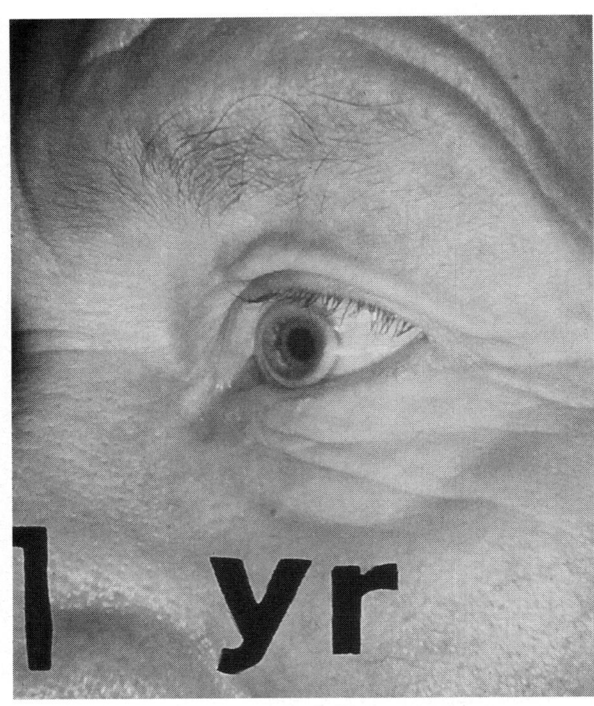

Fig. 1-23 A patient with basal cell cancer of the inner canthus of the eye before (**A**) and after (**B**) radiation therapy. (**A** and **B** courtesy Shands Radiation Therapy Department, Gainesville, Florida.)

light on the lesion from different angles, possibly allowing the detection of changes not visible from the surface.[44] Fields are designed according to the extent of the tumor and its projected growth pattern.

Depending on the area to be treated and type of radiation used, special considerations exist, including the following:

- Carcinomas of the skin overlying the pinna of the ear or nasal cartilages require special care in dose fractionation. Poorly designed treatment regimens can result in painful chondritis, which may require excision.[44]
- Bolus may be used with electron therapy to fill in gaps on uneven surfaces, maximize the surface dose, or reduce the underlying tissue dose.
- Lip—Cancers that cross the vermilion border of the lip have a higher risk of nodal metastasis, possibly indicating the need for prophylactic neck irradiation.[2] In the designing of a radiation field for the lip, a lead shield should be created to protect the teeth and gums. Paraffin wax on the outside of the shield helps prevent electron backscatter, reducing the dose to the buccal mucosa.
- Nose—Radiation treatments for skin cancers involving the nose should also include a wax-coated lead strip in the nostril to help protect the nasal septum. For more invasive lesions, tissue-equivalent material should be inserted into the nostril to remove the air gap and create a more uniform dose to the deeper tissues.
- Eye—For the treatment of carcinomas of the eyelid with radiation, the lens of the eye should be protected with an appropriately sized eye shield. These shields are usually composed of lead ranging in thickness from 1.7 to 7 mm. Sizes range from 2 to 3.4 cm in diameter. Small-to-medium shields can be placed between the eyelid and eye, while larger shields can be used to cover the eyelid. A thin film of antibacterial ointment can be applied to the inside of the shield before insertion to aid in the prevention of infection and help protect against scratching of the lens. Concern about the increase in lid dose from backscatter is avoidable by coating the outer surface of the shield with a low-atomic-number material such as wax or dental acrylic.[31] The lens of the eye is one of the most radiosensitive structures. A single dose of 200 cGy may cause the development of cataracts, (a loss of transparency in the lens of the eye).[11] Larger doses are required for cataractogenesis in fractionated regimens. The latent period between irradiation and the appearance of cataracts is also dose related. The latency is about 8 years after exposure to a dose in the range of 250 to 650 cGy.[28]

- Ear—In the treatment of skin cancers of the ear with radiation, treatment planning should be done so that doses to the inner ear do not exceed 1000 cGy.[24] Because of the unique and varied shape of the external ear and depending on the location and extent of the tumor, bolus material may be necessary to "flatten" the surface of the ear or get rid of the air gap behind the external ear in tumors involving the base of the auricle.

Malignant melanoma. Traditionally, malignant melanoma has been considered a radioresistant tumor; radiation therapy was reserved mainly for the treatment of metastases. Recently, however, the role of radiation therapy has expanded to that of an adjuvant and, in some instances, the primary treatment modality.

Researchers have discovered that treatment results improve with the use of larger fractions. Because of the initial shoulder of the cell survival curve of melanoma cells exposed to radiation, standard fraction sizes of 180 to 200 cGy are not effective. Larger doses per fraction are needed to overcome the apparent repair processes that melanoma cells seem to possess.[10,54]

Radiation therapy as the primary treatment modality is limited to large facial lentigo maligna melanomas for which wide surgical resection requires extensive reconstruction. Most of these lesions are controllable with proper fractionation, but up to 24 months may be necessary for the lesion to regress completely.[10]

One of the problems physicians face in the treatment of melanoma patients with bad prognostic features (i.e., lesions >1.5 mm thick or positive nodes) is local recurrence or regional relapse after wide local excision with or without limited neck dissection. Physicians at the M.D. Anderson Cancer Center in Houston are studying the use of radiation therapy as an adjuvant to surgery. Their aim is to reduce the morbidity associated with local-regional recurrences such as ulceration, disfigurement, and pressure symptoms and possibly improve the survival rate of a small subgroup of patients by helping to contain the disease before it has a chance to spread to distant sites. Patients were treated with five fractions of 600 cGy delivered twice per week via electron beams of appropriate energies when possible. The overall 5-year actuarial local-regional control (LRC) rate for the group receiving radiation was 88%, compared with historical rates of 50% for those who had surgery alone. Further research is needed to clarify the role of radiation therapy as an adjuvant in the treatment of malignant melanoma.[9]

The role of radiation therapy is greatest in the treatment of metastatic or recurrent disease. The role of megavoltage x-rays is also increased as deeper levels of tissue become involved or major organs become affected. Fractions of at least 500 cGy should be used to treat cutaneous, subcutaneous, lymph node, or visceral metastases in small treatment volumes or in areas in which late effects are irrelevant. When affected lymphatics or organs require large treatment volumes or if late effects may be detrimental, lower daily doses of 200 to 400 cGy may be used up to normal tissue tolerance or hyperfractionation may be used (115 cGy × 2 per day to a total dose of 3500 to 4000 cGy). The therapeutic outcome is based on the tumor size and dose per fraction.[18,54]

Bone metastases respond to radiation differently than metastases found in soft tissue. The former are more sensitive to total dose than to the fractionation scheme used. Fraction size should be determined by the sensitivity of the surrounding tissue, but response rates are better when total doses exceed 3000 cGy.[18]

The treatment of brain metastases of malignant melanoma also involves the use of a higher-than-normal dose per fraction. Studies have compared protocols by using twice-daily fractions of 300 to 375 cGy to total doses of 3000 to 3750 cGy in 1 week versus 190 to 240 cGy per fraction to total doses of 3750 to 4800 cGy in 2 weeks. The median survival time was drastically improved in the patients treated in 1 week. However, whether the difference was attributable to the time difference or fraction size was unclear. The incidence of acute edema and late brain atrophy was low in both regimens.[37]

Side effects. A major difference between megavoltage x-ray treatment of internal structures and kilovoltage x-ray or megavoltage-electron treatment of skin lesions is the location of the D_{max}. For the treatment of internal structures, having the D_{max} at least 0.5 cm beneath the skin surface is preferable for maintaining the skin-sparing effect. That is, if the maximum dosage of radiation is absorbed beneath the skin, the epidermal layer receives a much smaller percentage of radiation and produces fewer side effects as a result. For the treatment of skin cancers, just the opposite should occur. Maximum doses should be applied at or near the skin surface where tumors are located, whereas underlying tissues are spared. As a result, skin reactions can be expected to be worse during the treatment of primary skin cancers than during the properly planned treatment of internal structures.

Radiation reactions can be divided into acute (early) or chronic (late) changes. The severity of the reaction depends on the volume, dose, and protraction of the treatment. High doses to large volumes in short amounts of time result in more severe reactions than low doses to small volumes over long periods of time.

Early reactions that can be expected during the course of radiation treatment for skin cancers include the following:

- **Erythema** (inflammatory redness of the skin) is usually the first sign of the effects of irradiation. This condition is caused by the swelling of the capillaries of the dermal layer, increasing the blood flow to the skin.[44]
- Pigmentation is caused by the increased production of melanin by the melanocytes, causing the skin to become darker. The melanocytes respond to x-rays and

electrons the same way they do to UV rays and try to protect the young epithelial cells in the same fashion.

- Dry **desquamation,*** or shedding of the epidermis, appears at intermediate doses of radiation. The radiation affects the sensitive basal cells, and although not all are killed, enough are compromised that the basal layer has a hard time replacing the cells naturally sloughed off. The result is an abnormal thinning of the epithelial layer.[44]
- Moist desquamation* appears at the high-dose levels necessary to control skin cancer. As a result of these high doses, nearly all the cells of the basal layer are destroyed. After the cells of the epidermis have gone through their normal cycle, no cells from the germinal layer exist to replace them. The dermis then becomes exposed and begins producing a serous oozing from its surface. The epidermis is thought to be ultimately repopulated from more radioresistant cells surrounding hair follicles or sweat glands.[51]
- Temporary hair loss* appears after moderate doses of radiation. Higher doses may result in permanent hair loss.
- Sebaceous (oil) and sudoriferous (sweat) glands may show decreased or absent function when subjected to curative doses for skin cancer.[51]

Late reactions that can be expected after a curative course of radiation therapy include the following[51]:

- The skin never returns to its previous state. Damage to the dermal layer results in fibrosis, giving the skin a firmer, rougher appearance. Capillaries are dilated and fewer, resulting in telangiectasia. Also, the epithelial layer is thin and more susceptible to injury. Damage to melanocytes results in hypopigmentation and increased sensitivity to the sun.
- Necrosis is a common effect in patients who receive large doses in short amounts of time. The incidence of necrosis in carefully planned treatment regimens should not exceed 3%.

Prevention

Skin cancer is one of the few malignancies in which the causes are readily identifiable and preventable. About 90% of skin cancers can be avoided if people take proper precautions against the sun's rays.[6] If people take the time to educate themselves concerning skin cancer prevention and detection and follow through on that knowledge, the trend of rising skin cancer incidence could be reversed.

Exposure to UV light is the main triggering mechanism for skin cancer, so any type of preventive measures will stress ways to avoid UV exposure. Sun exposure also causes photoaging of the skin, including processes such as premature freckling, fine wrinkling, and dilation of the capillaries. Irregular pigmentation, commonly referred to as *liver spots,* often develops during later years in photodamaged skin.

The ozone layer is the portion of the atmosphere that protects the earth from harmful UV rays. In recent years this natural defense mechanism has been under attack by man-made substances such as chloroflourocarbons, automobile exhaust, and other agents. NASA estimates a 2% increase in UV radiation for every 1% loss of the ozone layer.[56] Efforts are under way by many governments throughout the world to limit the release of these destructive agents into the atmosphere. Through the preservation of the ozone layer the amount of UV light that reaches the earth's surface can be limited.

With or without a healthy ozone layer, plenty of UV light reaches the planet's surface and is a potential cause of skin cancer. Not all sun exposure is bad, however. The human body needs sunlight to aid in the production of vitamin D, which is essential for calcium absorption in the intestines and may help protect against certain types of cancer. Not much sun exposure is needed; only about 5 minutes a day is required to produce sufficient amounts of vitamin D. Also, a little time in the sun after an extended period of cloudy days can often give a person a psychological boost.[56]

Following are some potential UV light sources about which people should be aware[58]:

- Strong sun—Avoid exposure to the sun between 10 AM and 2 PM because the rays are directly overhead and considered strongest during this time. In the continental United States, the UV intensity is reduced by half at 3 hours before and 3 hours after peak exposure time. The peak exposure time is 12:00 noon during standard time and 1:00 PM during daylight saving time.[19] One way to judge the amount of UV exposure is by looking at a person's shadow. The longer the shadow, the lower the intensity of the UV rays. The shorter the shadow, the higher the intensity.[21]
- Reflected light—Snow, sand, water, and cement are capable of reflecting UV light. Added to the direct rays of the sun, the reflective rays can increase overall exposure rates up to 180%. Even people who wear hats or sit under umbrellas must be aware of the exposure risks of reflected light.
- Cloudy skies—UV rays can penetrate through clouds. Depending on cloud conditions, between 20% and

*Usually a 2-week delay exists between the start of radiation and the onset of desquamation and/or hair loss. On the first day of radiation the skin and hair follicles contain roughly a 2-week supply of reserve cells located between the basal layer and stratum corneum. As these cells progress toward the surface of the epidermis, they become more mature and differentiated and therefore more resistant to radiation. After the 2-week reserve supply is used up, the skin becomes red and irritated and the hair begins to fall out because the layers of cells that normally replace the reserve supply have been compromised by the effects of the radiation.

80% of UV rays still reach the ground. Proper precautions are needed even on cloudy days.

- Fluorescent lights—Fluorescent lights emit small amounts of UVA radiation, potentially boosting a desk worker's annual exposure by approximately 6%.
- Tanning lamps—Although most tanning salons and tanning equipment manufacturers would like the public to believe that tanning beds are safe, most emit UVA rays capable of skin injury, including skin cancer, premature skin aging, blood vessel damage, and immune system effects. A tan is the body's natural response to damage caused by UV light, whether that light is made by humans or nature.

If avoiding sources of UV light is impossible, certain protective measures must be undertaken. Slacks, long-sleeved shirts, hats, and visors offer excellent protection from UV light. Still, care must be taken to protect areas of the skin not directly covered by the various articles. These areas include the ears, tops of the feet, and backs of the knees.

Sunscreens are effective in protecting against UV exposure. The blocking ability of sunscreens is indicated by its sun-protection factor (SPF), which tells the number of times a person can stay in the sun with protection versus without protection before a sunburn develops. For example, a sunscreen with an SPF of 15 enables a person wearing it to stay in the sun 15 times longer than if the person was wearing no sunscreen.

Sunscreens contain different ingredients to protect against UVA and UVB rays. Agents that can block both types of rays are referred to as *broad-spectrum* sunscreens.

The use of sunscreens and their role in the prevention of skin cancers is controversial. Some experts feel that although the protective capacity of sunscreens against UVB is good, the protective capacity against UVA is lacking.

Some people feel the use of sunscreens may be counterproductive. They theorize that people using sunscreens are able to stay out in the sun for longer periods than without sunscreen because the UVB rays are being effectively blocked. With a minimum number of UVB rays available to cause the skin to feel burned, people are able to stay in the sun for longer periods. Because sunscreens are not as effective in blocking UVA, people are being exposed to higher levels of UVA than before sunscreens were developed. Increased UVA exposure can promote previous UVB damage or cause other types of damage on its own.

The American Academy of Dermatology, the Australian College of Dermatology, and the Canadian Dermatology Association strongly disagree with these views, stating, "One of the most powerful weapons in our fight against (skin cancers) is sun avoidance through the combination of protective clothing and sunscreens."[64] In fact, the Australians have initiated the "Slip, Slap, Slop" program, encouraging individuals to slip on protective clothing, slap on a hat, and slop on some sunscreen.

A statistical study at Harvard University concluded that "regular use of a SPF-15 sunscreen during the first 15 years of life would reduce a person's risk of developing the most common skin cancers by 78 percent...because people receive 80 percent of their lifetime sun exposure before the age of 20."[72] Babies are also included in this category. They are also susceptible to sunburn and can acquire damage that may lie dormant for decades.

A sunscreen with an SPF of at least 15 is the best choice.* Sunscreen should be applied at least 15 minutes before going outside to allow the skin to absorb it. Also, sunscreen should be reapplied every 2 hours and after swimming or heavy physical activity. Because the lips do not contain melanin and are a prime site for skin cancer, they should be protected with a lip balm or block having an SPF of 15.

Certain types of medications, such as antibiotics and diuretics, can increase a person's sensitivity to the sun. Before taking any medications, people should always consult drug labels, the physician, or the pharmacist regarding possible side effects, including those caused by UV exposure.

In 1994 the National Weather Service (NWS), the United States Environmental Protection Agency (EPA), and the Centers for Disease Control and Prevention (CDC) introduced the Experimental UV Index to inform the public about the type of UV conditions to expect so that proper precautions can be taken. The Index is a next-day forecast of the likely exposure to UV radiation for a specific location during the peak hour of sunlight around noon.

The Index uses a set of four skin-phototype categories into which the public is divided based on the normal color of a person's skin and its propensity for sunburn. These categories are shown in Table 1-3.

The UV Index ranges from 0 to 15; the higher the number, the shorter the amount of time the skin takes to burn. Index values, however, are based on the sensitivity level of fair-skinned individuals and are only estimates. Cloud cover, a major factor in forecasting UV exposure, can be higher or lower than projected, and therefore the actual UV intensity can be higher or lower than the day's forecast. If the actual weather is drastically different from the UV Index forecast (i.e., if the forecast calls for cloudy skies, but the sky is actually clear), common sense should prevail and proper precautions should be taken. In addition, in areas where rays are being reflected, exposure may be higher than the forecast and extra protection may be warranted. Table 1-4 shows the UV Index and the amount of time it takes for the most susceptible and least susceptible skin types to burn. Skin type is a big factor in determining the length of time a person can stay in the sun without burning.[20]

In addition to analyzing primary protection against UV rays, the National Cancer Institute is researching chemoprevention of nonmelanoma skin cancer. Chemoprevention is

*The Food and Drug Administration is researching whether a higher SPF is advantageous.

Table 1-3 The four skin phototypes

Skin phototypes	Skin color in unexposed area	Tanning history
Never tans, always burns	Pale or milky white; alabaster	Develops red sunburn; painful swelling occurs; skin peels
Sometimes tans, usually burns	Very light brown; sometimes freckles	Usually burns; pink or red coloring appears; can gradually develop light brown tan
Usually tans, sometimes burns	Light tan, brown, or olive; distinctly pigmented	Infrequently burns; shows moderately rapid tanning response
Always tans, rarely burns	Brown, dark brown, or black	Rarely burns; shows very rapid tanning response

Modified from Environmental Protection Agency: *Experimental UV Index, EPA 430-F-94-019,* Washington, DC, June, 1994, The Agency.

Table 1-4 UV Index and burn-exposure times

Exposure categories and Index values		Minutes to burn for "never tans" skin phototype (most susceptible)	Minutes to burn for "rarely burns" skin phototype (least susceptible)
Minimal	0-2	30 min	>120 min
Low	3	20 min	90 min
	4	15 min	75 min
Moderate	5	12 min	60 min
	6	10 min	50 min
High	7	8.5 min	40 min
	8	7.5 min	35 min
	9	7.0 min	33 min
Extremely high	10	6.0 min	30 min
	11	5.5 min	27 min
	12	5.0 min	25 min
	13	<5.0 min	23 min
	14	4.0 min	21 min
	15	<4.0 min	20 min

Modified from Environmental Protection Agency: *Experimental UV Index, EPA 430-F-94-019,* Washington, DC, June, 1994, The Agency.

the use of natural and man-made substances to prevent cancer. Studies indicate that high doses of vitamin A, beta-carotene, and isotretinoin, (a synthetic form of vitamin A) may help individuals who lack natural defenses (persons with albinism and xeroderma pigmentosum) to fight skin cancer.

Studies are taking place at Duke University concerning a topical solution that delivers large quantities (more than twenty times the normal amount) of vitamin C into the skin. Investigators believe that vitamin C protects the skin by controlling the body's inflammatory response to UV exposure (sunburn) and serving as an antioxidant to counteract the oxidative damage (caused by UV exposure) to collagen, elastin, and the cell membrane. By limiting the effects of UV damage, researchers hope to slow the effects of UV exposure, including skin cancer, premature wrinkling, and aging.[50]

Helping people to realize the dangers of overexposure to the sun and the importance of early detection remains a major hurdle in skin cancer prevention. Young people especially feel invulnerable to the damaging and aging effects of the sun. To many, the short-term gratification a tan provides outweighs the seemingly small risks of the sun exposure that provides it. They feel that skin cancer is for old people. In a way they are correct, because skin cancer usually shows up as people grow older. However, they do not realize that the cause of skin cancer is overexposure to the sun during a person's younger years.

Currently, mass media campaigns, educational posters, and brochures are aimed at educating the public concerning the dangers of sun exposure and the importance of early screening and detection. Health care institutions are trying to help by providing skin cancer screenings as a part of public health care fairs. Again, rising skin cancer rates can be reversed if people become educated on the prevention and detection of skin cancers and follow through on the recommendations.

Case Study

A 29-year-old white male had a 3-year history of a nonhealing ulceration just above the vermilion border of the right lip. He saw a physician, who gave the patient a prescription for Zovirax in case the ulceration was a fever blister, but the condition never resolved. He was referred to a dermatologist but never kept his appointment. Finally, his primary physician performed a biopsy, which revealed a basal cell carcinoma.

The biopsy report described the lesion as an incompletely excised basal cell carcinoma, so further treatment was necessary. Because of the location of the lesion, the physician referred the patient to a radiation oncologist for definitive treatment. Radiation therapy offered a high probability for cure and a good chance of excellent cosmetic results.

A physical examination revealed a healthy, white male without supraclavicular, cervical, or preauricular adenopathy. A 12-mm lesion without discrete edges but with some central ulceration was found on the upper lip. No other lesions were seen on the face or neck.

The patient's history was unremarkable for specific sun exposure or other skin problems. He did not smoke and was an occasional drinker. His medical history included eye surgery as a child and trauma to the lip as a youth. His family history was significant because a grandmother had breast cancer.

The patient was simulated in the supine position with a B headrest and an Aquaplast mask. A 3 × 3.5 cm electron field with a 4 × 4 cone was mapped out and encompassed the right half of the right upper lip and the surrounding tissue. He was to receive a 240-cGy D_{max} dose each day, 5 days per week for a total dose of 6000 cGy, with a 0.5-cm bolus every other day. A mouth shield was constructed to protect the teeth and gums.

The course of therapy was unremarkable until the patient was at the 3840-cGy level. The outside of the lip became red and dry; the patient was given 4 days of rest for a skiing vacation and was instructed to use Vaseline on the area to keep it moist.

After the vacation, the treatment was resumed and carried to the 6000-cGy level. At the completion of treatment a scab was present externally and moist desquamation internally in the treatment area. The patient reported little pain and good function in spite of the treatment.

The patient was seen for a follow-up visit 1 month after the completion of the radiation regimen. The skin over the lip was completely reepithelialized and flat, and no ulceration was visible around the upper lip internally or externally. He had no submental, preauricular, or cervical adenopathy and was declared clinically disease free.

About 3 months after the completion of the radiation therapy, the patient visited the radiation oncologist unexpectedly, complaining of a 2-week history of thickening in the treatment area. An examination showed a 2-mm area of swelling just above the vermilion border. The patient admitted he had been picking at the area and was encouraged to stop. He was also instructed to use Vaseline on the treated area 3 times a day for 3 weeks. If this condition were to persist or enlarge, a biopsy might determine the presence or absence of a recurrent tumor.

The patient was seen 4 weeks later, and no irritation, thickening, or irregularity was found to suggest recurrence. The patient was told to continue to use lotion in the treatment area and return for a follow-up visit in 6 months. He is expected to be fully cured.

Because of the young age at which this patient developed his skin cancer, he will be at high risk for developing future lesions. He was encouraged to contact a dermatologist to begin baseline skin screenings. The use of sunscreens and protective lip balms was also stressed.

Despite a 3-year history of skin cancer, this patient was lucky and has an excellent chance of cure. If the skin cancer had been a squamous cell carcinoma or melanoma, the patient may not have been so fortunate. Again, any suspicious lesions that do not resolve over a few weeks should be checked by a physician.

Review Questions

Multiple Choice

1. Which layer of the epidermis contains cells most sensitive to radiation?
   a. Stratum basale
   b. Stratum granulosum
   c. Stratum lucidum
   d. Stratum corneum
2. Which of following diseases is occasionally treated by total skin irradiation with electrons?
   a. Kaposi's sarcoma
   b. Malignant melanoma
   c. Mycosis fungoides
   d. Glandular adenocarcinoma
3. What are the layers of the skin, starting with the most superficial to the deepest?
   I. Subcutaneous layer
   II. Epidermis
   III. Dermis
   IV. Basement layer
   a. I, III, IV, II
   b. II, IV, III, I
   c. II, III, I, IV
   d. IV, I, III, II
4. Melanocytes are found in which layer of the skin?
   a. Stratum basale
   b. Stratum granulosum
   c. Stratum spinosum
   d. Stratum corneum

5. What is the treatment of choice for most melanoma skin cancers?
   a. Surgery
   b. Isolated limb perfusion
   c. Chemotherapy
   d. Radiation therapy
6. What is the technique in which the tumor is removed and examined one layer at a time?
   a. Curettage and electrodesiccation
   b. Mohs' surgery
   c. Cryosurgery
   d. Laser surgery
7. Tanning of the skin in the treated area after a course of radiation therapy is caused by which of the following?
   a. Damage to the basal layer
   b. Increased vascularity of the epidermis
   c. Stimulation of the melanocytes
   d. Inflammation of the dermis
8. With the use of shielding to protect the eye during irradiation, backscatter can be minimized by which of the following?
   a. Using a shield composed of Cerrobend
   b. Using a shield at least 1.7 mm in thickness
   c. Using a larger diameter shield
   d. Coating the outer surface of the shield with a low-atomic-number material such as wax

True or False

9. African-Americans have darker skin than white people because their skin contains more melanocytes.
   True _______ False _______
10. The use of kilovoltage x-rays allows the target volume to be covered with a smaller field size compared with a field that would produce similar effects near the skin through the use of electrons.
   True _______ False _______

Questions to Ponder

1. Describe the latest trends in the rates of incidence and rates of death in nonmelanoma and melanoma skin cancers.
2. Analyze circumstances that would render individuals more susceptible to developing skin cancer.
3. Contrast the microstaging systems for melanoma developed by Dr. Wallace Clark and Dr. Alexander Breslow.
4. Describe the controversy surrounding surgical margins for melanoma tumors.
5. Compare the advantages and disadvantages of electron beam therapy versus kilovoltage x-rays in the treatment of nonmelanoma skin cancer.

REFERENCES

1. Ackerman AB: Malignant melanoma: a unifying concept, *Hum pathol* 11(6): 591-595, 1980.
2. Ackerman S: Interview, August, 1994.
3. Amdur RJ et al: Radiation therapy for skin cancer near the eye: kilovoltage x-rays versus electrons, *Int J Radiat Oncol Biol Phys* 23:769, 1992.
4. American Cancer Society: *Cancer facts and figures,* Atlanta, 1996, The Society.
5. American Cancer Society: *Cancer response system: malignant melanoma, #448257*, Atlanta, The Society.
6. American Cancer Society: *Cancer response system: skin cancer, #473157*, Atlanta, The Society.
7. American Cancer Society: *Prevention and early detection of malignant melanoma, #3029-PE,* Atlanta, 1990, The Society.
8. American Joint Committee on Cancer: *Manual for staging of cancer,* ed 4, Philadelphia, 1992, JB Lippincott.
9. Ang KK et al: Postoperative radiotherapy for cutaneous melanoma of the head and neck region, *Int J Radiat Oncol Biol Phys*, 30(4):795, 1994.
10. Ang KK et al: Regional radiotherapy as adjuvant treatment for head and neck malignant melanoma, *Arch Otolaryngol Head Neck Surg* 116(4):169, February, 1990.
11. Bentel GC: *Treatment planning and dose calculation in radiation oncology,* ed 4, New York, 1989, Pergamon Press.
12. Berd D et al: Treatment of metastatic melanoma with an autologous tumor-cell vaccine: clinical and immunologic results in 64 patients, *J Clin Oncol*, 8:1858, November, 1990.
13. Breslow A: Cross-sectional areas and depth of invasion in the prognosis of cutaneous melanoma, *Ann Surg* 172:902, 1970.
14. Cannon-Albright LA: Assignment of a locus for familial melanoma, mlm, to chromosome 9p13-p22, *Science* 258:1148, November 13, 1992.
15. Cantrell BB: Interview, July, 1994.
16. Casciato DA, Lowitz BB: *Manual of clinical oncology,* ed 2, Boston, 1988, Little, Brown.
17. Cocconi G et al: Treatment of metastatic malignant melanoma with dacarbazine plus tamoxifen, *Eng J Med,* 327:516, August 20, 1992.
18. De Vita VT, Hellman S, Rosenberg SA, editors: *Cancer: principles and practice of oncology,* ed 2, Philadelphia, 1985, JB Lippincott.
19. Environmental Protection Agency: *Experimental UV Index, EPA 430-F-94-017,* Washington, DC, June, 1994, The Agency.
20. Environmental Protection Agency: *Experimental UV Index, EPA 430-F-94-019,* Washington, DC, June, 1994, The Agency.
21. Environmental Protection Agency: *The federal experimental ultraviolet index: what you need to know, EPA 430-F-94-016,* Washington, DC, June, 1994, The Agency.
22. Ezzell C: Scientists seek to fight cancer with cancer, *Science News,* 139:326, May 25, 1991.
23. Fink DJ, Holleb AI, Murphy GP: *American cancer society textbook of clinical oncology,* Atlanta, 1991, American Cancer Society.

24. Fletcher GH: *Textbook of radiotherapy,* ed 3, Philadelphia, 1980, Lea & Febiger.
25. Friedman RJ et al: Malignant melanoma in the 1990's: the continued importance of early detection and the role of physician examination and self-examination of the skin, *CA Cancer J Clin,* 41(4):201, 1991.
26. Glassman RD: Interview, June, 1994.
27. Gordon PO: Interview, December, 1994.
28. Hall EJ: *Radiobiology for the radiologist,* ed 4, Philadelphia, 1994, JB Lippincott.
29. *Healthcare update,* Roswell, Georgia, May, 1994, Publications.
30. Hunger K, McClay EF: Melanoma: new biology, new therapy, *Crit Rev Oncol Hematol* 2:299, 1991
31. Kahn F: *The physics of radiation therapy,* Baltimore, 1984, Williams & Wilkins.
32. Karagas MR et al: Risk of subsequent basal cell carcinoma of the skin among patients with prior skin cancer, T*J Am Med Associ,* 267:3305, June 24, 1992.
33. Kartsonis J: Lecture, August, 1994.
34. Katarzyna W: Safe sun, *Forbes,* 212, July 19, 1993.
35. McClay EF, McClay ME: Tamoxifen: is it useful in the treatment of patients with metastatic melanoma? *J Clini Oncol* 12:617, March, 1994.
36. Malignant melanoma. Report of a meeting of physicians and scientists, University College London Medical School, *Lancet,* 948, October 17, 1992.
37. Mauch PM, Loeffler JS, editors: *Radiation oncology: technology and biology,* Philadelphia, 1994, WB Saunders.
38. Melanoma detection: a new, improved method, *Patient Care,* 13, May 30, 1992.
39. Mendenhall WM et al: T2-T4 carcinoma of the skin of the head and neck treated with radical irradiation, *Int J Radiat Oncol Biol Phys,* 13:975, February 4, 1987.
40. Million RR, Cassisi NJ, editors: *Management of head and neck cancer,* ed 2, Philadelphia, 1994, JB Lippincott.
41. Mitchell MS: Chemotherapy in combination with biomodulation: a 5-year experience with cyclophosphamide and interleukin-2, *Semin Oncology,* 19(2 suppl 4):80-87, April, 1992.
42. Mitchell MS et al: Active specific immunotherapy of melanoma with allogenic cell lysates, *Ann NY Acad of Sci,* p 153, August 12, 1993.
43. Morton DL et al: Multivariate analysis of the relationship between survival and the microstage of primary melanoma by clark level and breslow thickness, *Cancer* 71(11):3737, June 1, 1993.
44. Moss WT, Cox JD: *Radiation oncology rationale, technique, results,* ed 6, St Louis, 1989, Mosby.
45. National Cancer Institute: *Physician's data query state of the art cancer treatment information,* Bethesda, Maryland, 1993, The Institute.
46. National Cancer Institute: *Research report: melanoma,* National Institutes of Health Publication Number 92-3020, Bethesda, Maryland, February, 1992, The Institute.
47. National Cancer Institute: *Research report: skin cancers: basal cell and squamous cell carcinomas,* National Institutes of Health Publication Number 91-2977, Bethesda, Maryland, September, 1990, The Institute.
48. NIH consensus development panel on early melanoma, *J Am Med Assoc,* 268:1314, September 9, 1992.
49. Osteen RT, editor: *Cancer manual,* ed 8, Boston, 1990, American Cancer Society, Massachusetts Division.
50. Does vitamin C protect against UVA and UVB, *Patient Care,* p14, May 30, 1992.
51. Perez CA, Brady LW: *Principles and practice of radiation oncology,* ed 2, Philadelphia, 1992, JB Lippincott.
52. Perez CA, Lovett RD, Gerber R: Electron beam and x-rays in the treatment of epithelial skin cancer: dosimetric considerations and clinical results, *Front Radiat Ther Oncol,* 25:90, 1992.
53. Preston DS, Stern RS: Nonmelanoma cancers of the skin, *N Eng J Med,* 327:1649, December 3, 1992.
54. Pyrhonen SO, Kajanti MJ: The use of large fractions in radiotherapy for malignant melanoma, *Radiother Oncol,* 24:195, 1992.
55. Randle HW: *Management of basal and squamous cell carcinomas,* Mayo Clinic lecture material, Jacksonville, Florida, The Clinic.
56. Reid K, Vikhanski L: The sun's ominous side: skin cancer, *Medical World News,* 33:18, February, 1992.
57. Rhodes AR et al: Risk factors for cutaneous melanoma: a practical method of recognizing predisposed individuals, *J Am Med Assoc,* 258:3146, December 4, 1987.
58. Roach M, Hastings J, Finch S: Sun struck: here's the hole story about the ozone and your chances of getting skin cancer, *Health,* p 40, May-June, 1992.
59. Ronan SG, Han MC, Das Gupta TK: Histologic prognostic indicators in cutaneous malignant melanoma, *Semin oncol,* 15:558, December, 1988.
60. Rosenberg SA et al: Observations on the systemic administration of autologous lymphokine-activated killer cells and recombinant interleukin-2 to patients with metastatic cancer, *N Eng J Med,* 313:1485, December 5, 1985.
61. Rosenberg SA et al: Use of tumor-infiltrating lymphocytes and interleukin-2 in the immunotherapy of patients with metastatic melanoma, *N Eng Jour Med,* 319:1676, December 22, 1988.
62. Shaw KE: Management of malignant melanoma, *Jacksonville Medicine,* p 200, May, 1991.
63. Skolnick AA: Melanoma epidemic yields grim statistics, *J Am Med Assoc,* 265:3217, June 26, 1991.
64. Skolnick AA: Sunscreen protection controversy heats up, *J Am Med Assoc,* 265:3218, June 26, 1991.
65. Stidham KR, Johnson JL, Seigler HF: Survival superiority of females with melanoma, *Arch Surgery,* 129:316, March, 1994.
66. Timmons MJ: Malignant melanoma excisions: making a choice, *Lancet* 340:1393, December 5, 1992.
67. Tortora GJ, Grabowski SR: Principles of anatomy and physiology, ed 7, New York, 1993, Harper Collins.
68. Travis EL: *Primer of medical radiobiology,* ed 2, St Louis, 1989, Year Book Medical Publishers.
69. Weinstock MA: The epidemic of squamous cell carcinoma, *J Am Med Assoc,* 262:2138, October 20, 1989.
70. White JW: *Epidemiology of skin cancer,* Mayo Clinic lecture, Jacksonville, Florida, The Clinic.
71. Williams PL, Warwick R, editors: *Gray's anatomy,* ed 36, Philadelphia, 1980, WB Saunders.
72. Zarrow S: Young skin under the sun: sun-blocking tips and new skin cancer 'cures' spell a bright future for outdoor enthusiasts, *Prevention* 40:16, May, 1988.

BIBLIOGRAPHY

Marx JL: Cancer vaccines show promise at last, *Science* 245:813, August 25, 1989.

Mitchell MS et al: Effectiveness and tolerability of low-dose cyclophosphamide and low-dose intravenous interleukin-2 disseminated melanoma, J Clin Conol 6:409, March, 1988.

Showers V: *World facts and figures,* ed 3, New York, 1989, John Wiley & Sons.

Wandycz W: Safe sun, *Forbes* 152:212, July 19, 1993.

C H A P T E R

2

Soft Tissue Sarcomas

Cheryl Sanders

Outline

Soft tissue sarcomas
- Epidemiology
- Etiology
- Prognostic indicators
- Pertinent anatomy and natural history of disease
- Clinical presentation
- Detection and diagnosis
- Pathology and staging
- Routes of spread
- Treatment techniques
- Role of radiation therapist

Key terms

ADCZ
American Joint Committee on Cancer (AJCC)
CYVADIC
iM
Limb salvage surgery (LSS)
MAID
Musculoskeletal Tumor Society (MTS)
Primary site compartment
Pseudocapsule
Radical resections
Shelling
Soft tissue sarcoma (STS)
Wide resection

SOFT TISSUE SARCOMAS

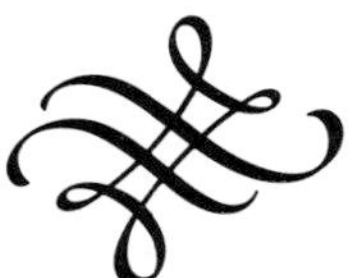

A **soft tissue sarcoma** (STS)* is a tumor occurring in the extraskeletal connective tissue. These tissues include all those that provide connection, support, and locomotion. They are grouped together because they share similarities in appearance pathologically, as well as in clinical presentation and behaviors.

The derivation of this complex and fascinating group of sarcomas is primarily from mesodermal structures and connective tissue cells. However, some of the soft tissues in this category arise from ectodermal structures and some from the epithelium. The muscles in the adult human comprise about 40% of the total body weight. The somatic soft tissues comprise about 50% of the total body weight. These structures are found throughout the entire anatomy. Therefore an STS can arise anywhere in the body. Tumors arising in connective layers of visceral organs are not considered in this section. The most common site at first presentation involves the extremities. Of the 1071 patients with an STS admitted to Memorial Sloan Kettering Cancer Center between 1982 and 1987, half (49.8%) had primaries in the upper or lower extremities. The incidence rate of the lower extremity primary was 38.9%, with most primaries located in the proximal thigh and 10.9% in the upper limbs. Other primary sites included the retroperitoneum, trunk, visceral, and head and neck[23] (Table 2-1).

This chapter presents fundamental information critical to understanding the nature of this disease, including its etiol-

*Soft tissue sarcomas are a class of malignant tumors arising primarily but not exclusively from mesenchymal connective tissues.

Table 2-1 Incidence of soft tissue sarcoma by site

Site	Percentage
Lower extremity	38.9
Retroperitonea and intraabdominal	15.2
Trunk	12.9
Upper extremity	10.9
Genitourinary	7.2
Visceral	4.8
Head and neck	5.4
Other	4.6

Modified from Holleb AI, Fink DJ, Murphy GP, editors: *ACS textbook of clinical oncology,* ed 1, Atlanta, 1991, The American Cancer Society.

ogy, tissue derivation, histology, staging, grading, and patterns of spread. Factors affecting treatment decision making and options in radiation therapy treatment planning and modalities are addressed.

Epidemiology

STS is rare. Rates of incidence range from 0.57% to 0.7% of all cancers. The incidence in the United States may now be in excess of 5700 new cases per year (the original estimate for 1990).[20,27] The American Cancer Society's estimate for 1996 was 6400 new cases, with 3700 deaths resulting from the disease.[1]

STS is more common in children than adults, comprising 6.5% of all tumors in pediatric age groups; they are the fifth highest ranked cause of death for children younger than 15 years of age.[28] A slight predilection in incidence exists for males compared with females (45% to 46%).[1,23] The literature does not indicate significant incidence by geographical location or distribution.

The most common subtypes of STS are liposarcomas (STS arising from fat), leiomyosarcomas (STS arising from smooth muscle), rhabdomyosarcomas (STS arising from striated muscle), malignant fibrous histiocytomas (deep STS showing partial fibroblastic and histiocytic differentiation with a variable storiform pattern, myxoid areas, and giant cells), fibrosarcomas (STS derived from collagen-producing fibroblasts), and a group of unclassified sarcomas. However, because of differences in the histopathological classification of criteria, precise estimates of incidence by type is difficult.[24] Because of altered identification methods and evolving classification criteria, tumors previously known as *fibrosarcomas,* or *spindle cell sarcomas,* have come to be classified as *malignant fibrous histiocytomas.* Therefore the apparent increase in malignant fibrous histiocytomas is an artificial one resulting from reclassification of other types of STS.

As new technologies emerge, further classification of histogenesis is possible. Electron microscopy, immunohistochemical staining for proteins unique to mesenchymal neoplasms, flow cytometry, and molecular biological techniques are promising adjuncts in decreasing pathological disagreements for the determination of histogenesis and tumor grade.[9]

Etiology

The etiology of STS is not known. A variety of genetic and environmental factors have been implicated. Historically, intensive radiation for benign conditions such as tuberculosis and thyroid disease gave rise to sarcomas. More recently, STS appears as a second primary resulting from high-dose irradiation for other cancers after a 5- to 15-year interval. Von Recklinghausen's disease (neurofibromatosis) involves small, discrete, pigmented skin lesions (café au lait spots and/or pigmented nevi) that develop into multiple neurofibromas along the course of peripheral nerves and may undergo malignant transformation. This disease is a familial disorder with a predisposition for malignant peripheral nerve tumors or malignant schwannomas (nonencapsulated tumors resulting from a disorderly proliferation of Schwann cells that includes portions of nerve fibers and typically undergoes a transformation to malignant schwannomas). A lymphedema of long-standing duration is occasionally followed by a lymphangiosarcoma, especially after a radical mastectomy.[23,25] Wijnmaalen et al.[30] concluded that the future incidence of angiosarcomas in previously irradiated breasts may increase because the number of patients with a long-term follow-up after conservation surgery and radiation therapy is growing rapidly.

Certain ground troops of the Vietnam War who had increased exposure to defoliant chemicals such as Agent Orange may have a higher incidence rate of STS than other soldiers serving in that war at the time.[16] Occupational exposure to vinyl chloride has been reported in association with hepatic angiosarcoma.[7] Other causes, including trauma, have also been implicated as an etiological factor giving rise to these tumors.

Prognostic indicators

Probably the most important prognostic factor in an STS diagnosis is histological grade, followed by site, size, resectability, presence or absence of metastasis, local invasion of a **pseudocapsule,*** regional lymph node involvement, and local recurrence. After an accurate histological type is determined, grading of the tumor is essential for predicting metastasis and the general outcome.

In a study of 163 patients treated at the National Cancer Institute, Costa et al.[6] graded the most common types of STS. The study indicated that the amount of necrosis present was the best predictor of the time to recurrence and overall survival.

*Pseudocapsules are STS tumors surrounded by compressed normal tissue, reactive inflammation, and fibrosis that give the gross anatomical appearance of a capsule.

In general, younger patients (less than 53 years of age) with small, low-grade primaries (less than 5 cm) in distal extremity sites who undergo a **wide resection** with an intact pseudocapsule and no regional lymph node involvement or distant metastasis will probably fare better in local control and overall survival.[14,19,21,33,35,36] Posner and Brennan[24] relate favorable signs influencing prognosis with a correlation of those prognostic signs in the stage of the disease. Combinations of one to three signs identified as favorable or unfavorable are correlated with the tumor stage and give credence to the importance of size (small versus large), site (superficial versus deep), and histological grade (low versus high). Advanced stages include increasing numbers of unfavorable signs (Table 2-2).

Table 2-2 Correlation of prognostic signs and stage

Stage	Favorable signs*	Unfavorable signs†
0	3	0
I	2	1
II	3	2
III	0	3
IV	0	Evidence of mets

Modified from Holleb AI, Fink DJ, Murphy GP, editors: *ACS textbook of clinical oncology*, ed 1, Atlanta, 1991, The American Cancer Society.
*Favorable signs include (1) small size, (2) superficial site, and (3) low histological grade.
†Unfavorable signs include (1) large size, (2) deep site, and (3) high histological grade.

Pertinent anatomy and natural history of disease

Embryologically, as the blastoderm gives rise to the endodermal, mesodermal, and ectodermal layers, the basic tissue derivations for anatomical structures and their corresponding malignancies are established. The embryonic ancestry of STS begins in the primitive mesoderm. The loosely formed network of cells in the mesoderm, the primitive mesenchyme, and/or the ectoderm give rise to the most common connective tissues, such as the pleura, peritoneum, pericardium, walls and endothelium of blood vessels, bone, cartilage, muscles, and soft connective tissue. Visceral connective tissue, similar muscle organs, and smooth muscle organs (e.g., the kidney, ureters, uterus, gonads, heart, and a variety of hematopoietic tissues) all derive from the remainder of the primitive mesoderm.

Malignant tumors are usually categorized as carcinomas or sarcomas based on whether they derive from epithelial or connective tissue. Because *epithelium* is a morphological and not an embryological term, the classification of many tumors is not precise. The endothelial lining of blood vessels, lymphatics, and the mesothelial lining of body cavities in visceral organs are epithelial in type but arise from the mesoderm germ layer of the embryo. Other deviations in derivation include Kaposi's sarcoma, which is believed to arise from endothelial cells and occurs as pigmented skin lesions. Neurofibrosarcomas have their origin in the Schwann cells of the neural tube of the primitive ectoderm. They occur as tumors of the neural sheath surrounding the peripheral nerves. Sometimes they are referred to as *neurogenic sarcomas, schwannomas,* or *malignant neurilemmomas,* and they are often associated with von Recklinghausen's disease (neurofibromatosis).[24] Structural support is required for endothelial organs, so sarcomas may arise in these connective tissues that provide the organ's form and therefore its ability to function. These connective tissue cells of origin for the corresponding malignancies determine the resulting designations as particular types of STS. (Fig. 2-1).

The local growth pattern of STS follows the lines of least resistance in the longitudinal axis of the **primary site compartment.** This involves the natural anatomical boundaries surrounding the STS primary and is composed of a common fascia plane(s) of muscles, bone, joint, skin, subcutaneous tissues, and major neurovascular structures.[27]

As undisturbed tumor size progresses, it pushes other structures away and forms a pseudocapsule that is made of compressed normal and fibrotic tissue. Trunk and head and neck primaries tend to invade adjacent muscle groups. Compartment boundaries of bone and fascia for these sites may act as a partial barrier to extension. Intermediate- and high-grade lesions typically undergo hematogenous metastasis, primarily to the lungs. Retroperitoneal primaries also have a high potential for lung metastasis but also spread to the liver and other abdominal structures. Lymph nodes are rarely involved. However, their involvement is considered an unfavorable prognostic indicator (Fig. 2-2).

Clinical presentation

Usually, STS is a painless mass that grows over several weeks or months. One study reports a median time of 4 months from the time of the mass' initial appearance until the consultation of a physician for an investigation and diagnostic workup.[19] Because surrounding anatomy is easily compressed, readily observed and troublesome symptoms are usually absent. The size and location are such that, unless the mass interferes with the normal functioning of vital organs, tumors often become quite large before the initial investigative workup, especially when they arise in the buttocks and thighs. Night pain may occur with larger lesions. Fixation to other structures and the presence of warmth or distended vascularity are also regarded as ominous indications. Systemic effects and symptoms are rare with extremity STS. Tumors causing paraneoplastic syndromes with weight loss, a fever, and general malaise are generally large and retroperitoneal or arise in the trunk or head and neck.[27]

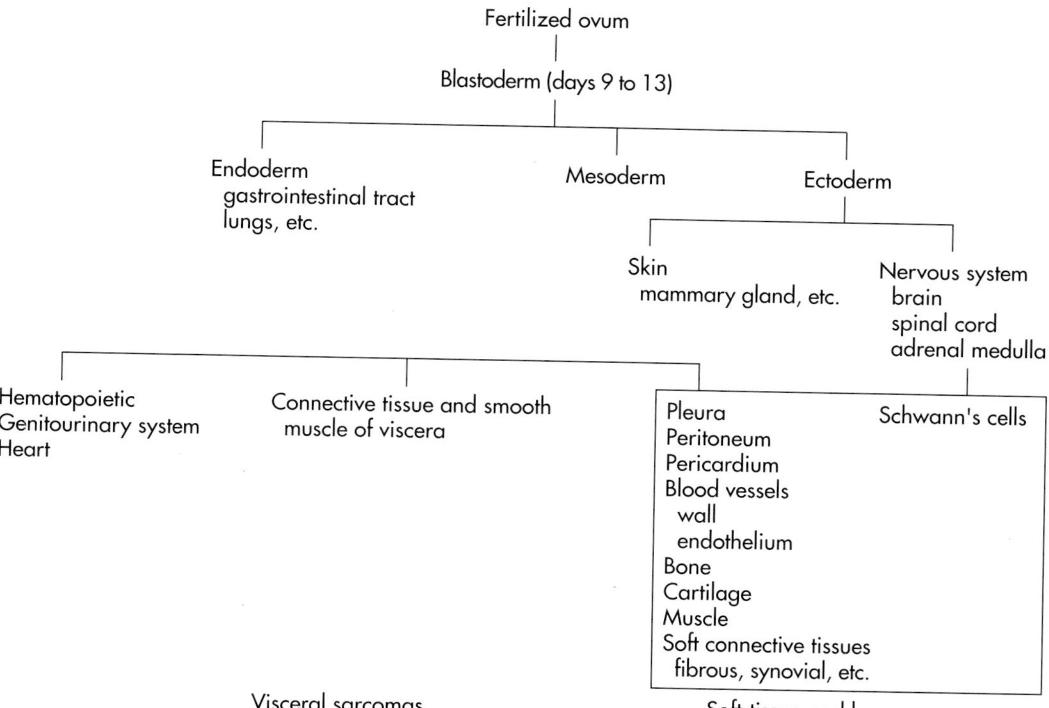

Fig. 2-1 Embryonic derivation of the soft tissue and bony sarcomas. Cells of origin determine designations as particular types of soft-tissue sarcomas. (From Rosenberg SA, Suit HA, Baker LH: Sarcomas of soft tissues. In DeVita VT, Hellman S, Rosenberg SA, editors: *Cancer: principles and practice of oncology,* vol 2, ed 2, Philadelphia, 1982, JB Lippincott.)

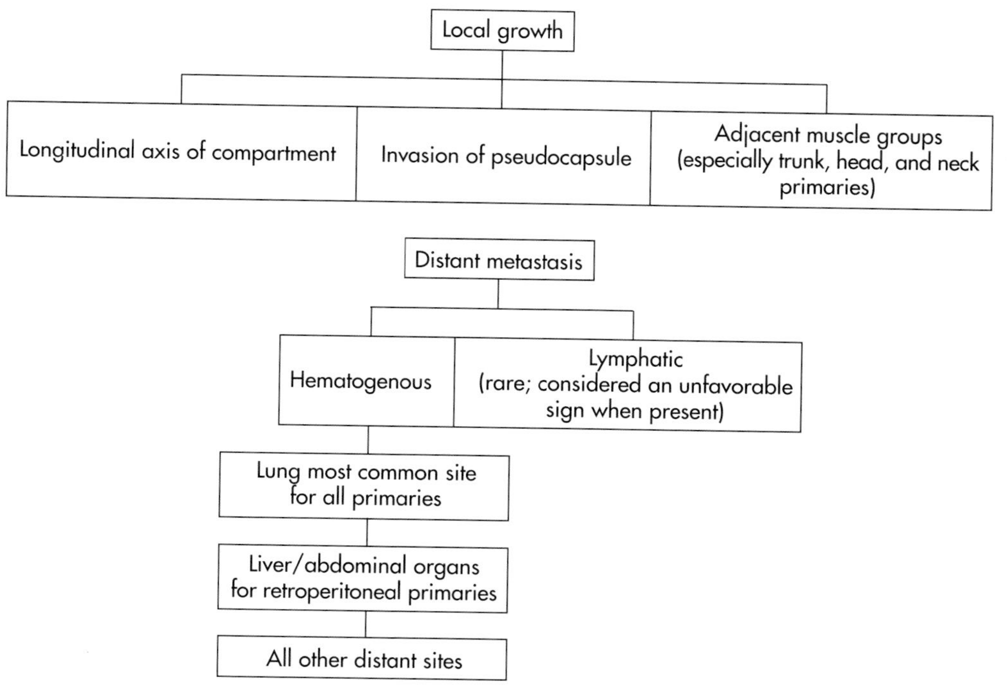

Fig. 2-2 Patterns of STS spread. STS metastatic patterns progress from local invasion to the early hematogenous extension to the lung, liver, abdominal organs, and all other distant sites. Lymphatic spread is rare.

Detection and diagnosis

After the discovery of the soft tissue mass, comprehensive diagnostic and staging procedures provide criteria that form the treatment-planning decision-making process. If the presence of a mass is apparent with inspection and palpation, suspicion demanding an accurate diagnosis should motivate the workup.

Imaging modalities include plain film radiography with soft tissue techniques and the use of contrast media studies to demonstrate subtle calcifications and the gross size, shape, and location of the primary tumor and occult or metastatic lesions, especially in the retroperitoneum. Computed tomography (CT) of the chest is useful for demonstrating additional lesions not visualized on x-ray film, especially for intermediate- and high-grade lesions.[19]

CT and magnetic resonance imaging (MRI) are essential in the localization of tumors and the relationships to blood supply, nerves, tendons, musculature, supporting fascia, and bone. MRI is considered superior to CT in differentiating normal versus abnormal tissue and in determining the anatomical extent of the tumor. However, even with enhancement agents, differentiation between malignant and benign tissue or an infection is frequently difficult. A complete history and physical examination often provides supporting information to include or rule out further suspicion of benign versus infectious possibilities in the list of probabilities.

In limited instances, arteriography may be useful in demonstrating the vasculature of the tumor. Radionuclide scans may also provide additional documentation of data accumulated with MRI. Diagnostic sonography may be useful in the initial stages to discern cystic versus solid structures. Additionally, positron emission tomography (PET) and MRI spectroscopy may provide other information regarding the metabolism and grade of a primary.

After the localization of the extent of the tumor, a biopsy to obtain viable tumor tissue is essential. This may be accomplished before the completion of the localization of all anatomical structures, but unless a team carefully manages the biopsy, future treatment options may be compromised.[8] Because of the presence of the pseudocapsule, an incisional biopsy is generally considered the preferred procedure. An excisional biopsy may be appropriate for extremely small lesions (less than 3 cm).[8,18,23,27] Control of bleeding during the procedure is necessary because hematomas provide a mechanism of spread. The longitudinal placement of the incision with avoidance of planes near neurovascular structures allows for later en bloc removal during definitive surgery with a predicted decrease in surgical contamination.

Pathology and staging

Sarcomas are classified histologically and named according to the tissues in which they arise and undergo transformation from a normal to malignant status. Because histological grade is accepted as the most critical predictor of outcomes, the importance of an accurate determination must not be underestimated.

Grading systems lack uniformity in criteria definition. Overall, however, they include the following: degree of differentiation, cellularity, amount of stroma, necrosis, vascularity, and number of mitoses. The two most commonly used classifications in staging systems are the **Musculoskeletal Tumor Society (MTS)** surgical staging system and the **American Joint Committee on Cancer (AJCC)** classifications (the classification and anatomical staging systems used for STS).

Both systems combine the anatomical stage with grade categories. The AJCC system identifies G1 as well differentiated and G2 as moderately differentiated and undifferentiated. AJCC correlates G3 and G4 with Stage IIIA and IIIB. Therefore anatomical stage is nearly synonymous with grade (see the box on p. 39). With the MTS system, G1 and G2 are simply identified as low grade or high grade.[4,12]

In the AJCC system a tumor (T) is defined by size as less than or more than 5 cm. In the MTS systems, (T) is defined by its confinement to one compartment (T1) or more than one compartment (T2). The presence of nodal involvement is equated with the presence of distant metastases.

With both systems, higher grades and an increasing anatomical extent of the disease readily correlate to an advanced stage. In all but a few specific histopathological tumors (e.g., synovial sarcomas and rhabdomyosarcomas), lymph node involvement is rare. However, when it is present, it is considered equivalent to metastasis and becomes more important than grade in determining the stage.[27]

Routes of spread

Posner and Brennan's evaluation of 1091 patients with STS at Memorial Sloan-Kettering Cancer Center from July 1, 1987 to December 13, 1987,[24] found that 22% of STS patients who had metastasis were also likely to have large (greater than 5 cm), high-grade tumors. Retroperitoneal and visceral primaries metastasized more readily than extremity lesions. Histopathologically, leiomyosarcomas spread more frequently; fibrosarcomas are less likely to have metastases at the time of the diagnosis.

STSs initially invade aggressively along local, anatomically defined planes composed of neurovascular structures, fascia, and muscle bundles. Lymphatic extension is not common. Hematological pathways are the primary route of spread; the lung is the most common site of recurrence, followed much less frequently by the bones, liver, and skin. For retroperitoneal tumors the lung is still the predominant metastatic site, but extension to the liver and other abdominal sites is also likely for recurrence. The majority of distant metastatic recurrences are likely to be reported within 2 years of the diagnosis and surgery.[18]

AJCC Staging for Soft Tissue Sarcoma

Primary tumor (T)

TX	Minimum requirements to assess primary tumor cannot be met
T_0	No demonstrable tumor
T_1	Tumor ≤5 cm in diameter
T_2	Tumor >5 cm in diameter

Nodal involvement (N)

NX	Minimum requirements to assess regional nodes cannot be met
N_0	No histologically verified metastasis to lymph nodes
N_1	Histologically verified regional lymph node metastasis

Distant metastasis (M)

MX	Minimum requirements to assess presence of distant metastasis cannot be met
M_0	No known distant metastasis
M_1	Distant metastases present (specify site)

Tumor grade

G1	Well differentiated
G2	Moderately well differentiated and undifferentiated

Stage Grouping

Stage IA	G1	T_1	N_0	M_0
Stage IB	G1	T_2	N_0	M_0
Stage IIA	G2	T_1	N_0	M_0
Stage IIB	G2	T_2	N_0	M_0
Stage IIIA	G3-4	T_1	N_0	M_0
Stage IIIB	G3-4	T_2	N_0	M_0
Stage IVA	Any G	Any T	N_1	M_0
Stage IVB	Any G	Any T	Any N	M_1

Modified from Beahrs OH et al: *AJCC manual for staging of cancer*, ed 4, Philadelphia, 1992, JB Lippincott.

Treatment techniques

Multimodality treatments. A variety of imaging procedures have resulted in the improved demonstration of tumor localization and metastatic extension. This improvement, in addition to radical wide-margin surgical techniques, sophisticated radiation therapy treatments, and effective antineoplastic agents, has helped the general management of STS to progress to a multidisciplinary team approach. This approach involves a multimodality treatment plan that may use a variety of surgical and radiation therapy techniques with or without multiagent chemotherapy. The overall treatment plan is influenced in large part by the natural history of STS and its patterns of spread and recurrence locally and systemically.

Surgery. In addition to providing tissue for a biopsy, aggressive surgery is a proven effective treatment whether used alone or with radiation therapy and/or chemotherapy. Despite the appearance of being encapsulated, an STS is surrounded by a pseudocapsule that nearly always is assumed to contain invasive foci of tumor cells. Therefore **shelling*** out these tumors surgically is inadequate. For high-grade tumors, wide or radical margins of normal tissue are required. Wide and radical margins are defined for limb-sparing and amputation techniques for extremities. **Radical resections** include all structures in every involved compartment, whereas wide resections include the tumor, its pseudocapsule, and normal tissue in the compartment. If adjuvant radiation therapy is a consideration for extremity STS, a lateral incision is best for more effective lymphatic drainage and a longitudinal incision is best with the long axis of the limb.[11,27] When used with radiation therapy, **limb salvage surgery (LSS)**† reduces the loss of function and improves local control.[10,16,29]

Radiation therapy. Based on the careful evaluation of individual patients, radiation therapy may be delivered in a variety of ways. Except for a few extremely small superficial tumors or when surgery is not medically recommended, radiation therapy is combined with surgery.

Doosenbury, Thompson, and Levitt[8] recommend preoperative radiation for extremities in the following two situations:

1. When the tumor is large enough to require extensive surgery or amputation, radiation may allow future limb-sparing surgery with adequate margins. It may also significantly reduce the amount of viable tumor at the time of surgery.
2. For patients who have had a previous biopsy, this approach has led to increased local control (37% versus 13%) at the University of Minnesota.

Reports of other experiences in the literature also support the use of preoperative radiation therapy.[2,3,18,27,28]

Generally accepted advantages include the following:

1. A smaller treatment volume will likely be possible because no surgical manipulation or disruption has taken place. The treatment volume will be planned from images demonstrating the extent of the tumor.
2. Because of tumor regression, less aggressive surgery may be possible.
3. The likelihood of surgical contamination caused by the release of viable tumor cells into the tumor bed or blood is reduced.
4. No delay in starting treatment is required.
5. The biological effect of radiation is better in terms of tumoricidal activity because hypoxia associated with postoperative scarring is absent.

*Shelling is a surgical procedure that removes the primary tumor and its pseudocapsule, giving the gross appearance of having removed all of the viable tumor.

†LSS is a radical or wide en bloc resection for STS that requires a 1- to 3-cm normal tissue margin allowing the limb or extremity to remain intact. Amputation is avoided.

Disadvantages include the following:

1. Difficulties with postirradiation surgical wound healing may be more likely.
2. The precise extent and description of the tumor resulting from resection and direct observation are not available.[8,24,27]

Postoperative radiation therapy has also been effective for situations in which preoperative treatment is not feasible. Techniques include external beam therapy, brachytherapy, intraoperative electron beam treatment, or some combination of these. These modalities may also be used to boost preoperative doses.

With external beam therapy a shrinking-field technique is generally used. The initial field should include the entire compartment and/or wide margins up to 10 cm. The second volume treated is coned down to the tumor itself with narrower margins (+/− 5 cm). The final volume is the primary tumor volume plus a 2 to 3-cm margin. The scar should receive the full dose by inclusion tangentially or boosted with bolus or electrons. No regional lymph nodes except rhabdomyosarcomas, synovial sarcomas, and epithelioid sarcomas are included with radiation therapy techniques. Total circumferential radiation of extremities must be avoided by leaving at least a 1- to 3-cm strip of skin and soft tissue to avoid future excessive fibrosis and edema [8,18] (Fig. 2-3).

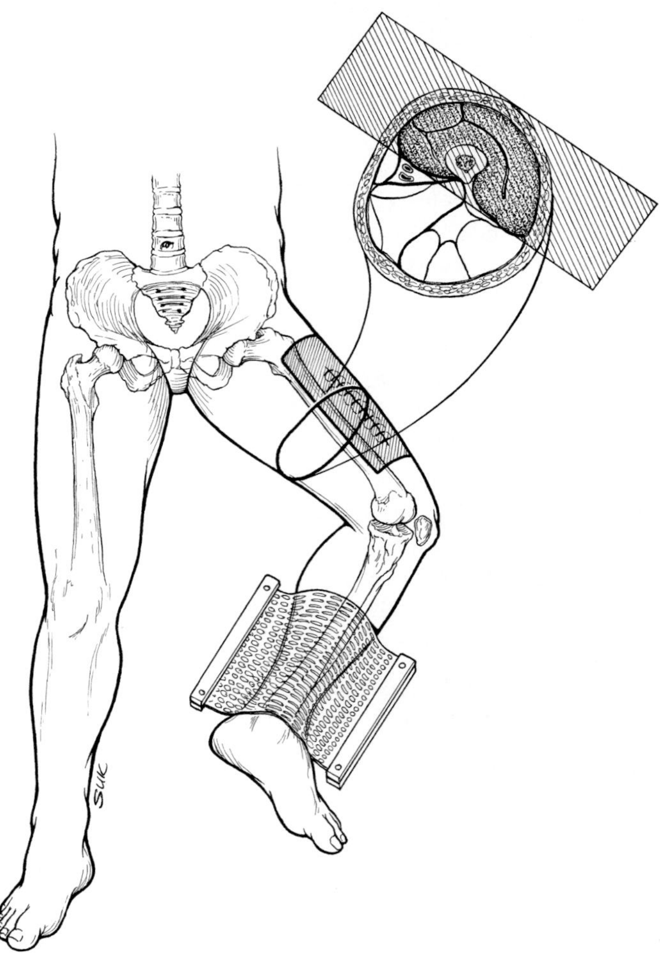

Fig. 2-3 Appropriate treatment position demonstrating access to the tumor compartment.

Brachytherapy is generally accomplished with catheters placed in the tumor bed at the time of the resection. Iridium 192 is loaded into the catheters after the fifth postoperative day to avoid wound healing problems.[5,26,34] Brachytherapy with iridium 192 is also a useful alternative for selected patients who have a recurrent extremity STS.[23] Iodine 125 is another radioactive source used in brachytherapy applications; it usually involves limited and selected patients with retroperitoneal and head and neck STS.[13,17] A trial of high-dose-rate remote brachytherapy for rhabdomyosarcoma involving selected organ sites in infants and young children has achieved some success in local control and organ preservation. Nag, Grecula, and Ruyman[21] recommend limiting this modality to controlled clinical trials until sufficient time has elapsed to observe long-term results. The brachytherapy dose depends on the way it fits in the comprehensive treatment plan and the site involved.

Intraoperative electron beam radiation is another adjunctive modality for selected patients. This technique affords the delivery of a high dose to areas at risk with the advantage of sparing normal adjacent tissues. Doses are usually between 1000 and 2000 cGy, with a range of electron beam energies from 9 to 15 MeV.[31,32]

Overall, STS requires high doses of radiation to achieve local control and long-term survival. A preoperative dose is usually limited to 5000 cGy with 180- to 200-cGy daily fractions. Postoperative shrinking fields generally deliver a total dose of 6500 cGy with field reductions at 4500 to 5000 cGy and 5500 to 6000 cGy. With the use of a boost the total dose may exceed 7500 cGy.

Chemotherapy. The use of chemotherapy has demonstrated some substantial advances, but optimal regimens do not appear to be established. A variety of drug programs have been investigated in which some patients have enjoyed relatively long periods of remission. The agents most often used in varying protocols include a combination of doxorubicin and dacarbazine: **CYVADIC** (cytoxan, vincristine, Adriamycin, and dacarbazine), **ADCZ** (doxorubicin, dacarbazine, cisplatin, and vincristine), **iM** (ifosfamide methotrexate), and **MAID** (methotrexate, doxorubicin, ifosfamide, and dacarbazine). Controlled studies will continue to investigate sophisticated advances in combined modalities to improve the overall survival and quality of life in patients with STS.[8,9,27]

Role of radiation therapist

The technical competence of the radiation therapist is assumed. Although an understanding of the academic, scientific, and intellectual aspects of STS should not be minimized, the obligation to apply that information with meaningful caregiving skills is the therapist's opportunity to provide comprehensive attention for the patient. The predilection for this primary to occur in younger populations in anatomical sites where disfigurement is often a threat may require educational and communication techniques unique to children, teenagers, young adults, and middle-aged patients. An assessment of the patient's physical, emotional, and coping status is essential in daily interactions with patients and their families.

Education. Wilkinson[34] reported that 25% to 35% of clients indicate dissatisfaction with the information received about their treatment and nursing care. Information about health care procedures reduces anxiety, pain, distressing side effects, and length of the hospital stay.

Taenzer and Fisher's study[31] indicated that providing patient education is one of the skills radiation therapists use most often. The educator role of the radiation therapist extends beyond dispensing information. It is an ongoing, integral part of the treatment process that includes the patient, family, and other health care team professionals. Just as traditional teachers use goals, objectives, and testing mechanisms in the educational process, therapists need to establish goals and objectives that are patient directed and then verify (test) patients for comprehension and understanding. Implementing these goals and objectives is a part of a formal or informal patient care plan custom designed to meet the needs of each patient.

Communication. Disfigurement, loss of limbs, decreased motor functions, or a threat of any of these leads to heightened emotional responses typically described by cancer patients as feelings of denial, frustration, anger, depression, fear, grief, bereavement, rejection, and loss of control. Although Taenzer and Fisher [31] also indicated that therapists reported offering emotional support and referrals to other professionals as nontechnical skills used quite frequently, they also indicated these skills were among the most difficult for them to acquire and use effectively.

Listening, attending, following, reflecting, touching, and questioning skills provide the basis for effective communication with the patient. Openness and assertiveness offers the patient a comfortable invitation to talk. Patients list talking to others as a therapeutic activity used in coping strategies for dealing with their cancers.[25] This is generally not different for patients with an STS diagnosis.

Assessment. Patient assessment and interventions obviously include the patient's pathophysiological and emotional status. The cancerocidal doses administered to achieve local control require a regular assessment of the skin's integrity. Monitoring of the anticipated erythema and dry and moist desquamation may require a decision to withhold treatment until the radiation oncologist verifies confirmation to proceed. Many STS patients are immunocompromised because of concomitant chemotherapy. Close observation for symptoms of infection and regular notation of blood counts with appropriate interventions described by institutional policy is the therapist's responsibility. An evaluation of the patient's nutritional status and performance rating may also indicate the need for an intervention referral.

As patients find emotional mechanisms to cope with the distress of an STS diagnosis, the radiation therapist should have the ability to recognize and support helpful responses. Identifying destructive responses is also important. Fawzy and Fawzy[13] describe reactions to behavioral, cognitive, and affective states that may be adaptive or maladaptive. These reactions are categorized as active-behavioral, active-cognitive, or avoidance methods. Radiation therapists need to be comfortable with supporting healthy coping mechanisms and develop strategies to help patients alter destructive behaviors with appropriate referrals to other professionals when needed.

The radiation therapist's broad-based patient care responsibilities include the knowledge and understanding of STS as a malignant process and treatment delivery competency. The radiation therapist is the patient's advocate in the coordination of referrals for all aspects of conditions relevant to the patient's disease status and treatment.

Review Questions

Multiple Choice

1. The epidemiology of STS includes which of the following parameters?
   a. The estimated incidence in the U.S. is ± 10,000 new cases per year.
   b. The incidence is more common in children than adults.
   c. A slight predilection exists for incidence in females compared with males.
   d. The incidence in the Pacific Northwest is significantly higher than other areas of the U.S.

2. Although the exact etiology of STS is unknown, which of the following factors have been implicated?
   a. Prior irradiation for benign diseases
   b. Appearance as a second primary 5 to 15 years after high-dose radiation therapy for other cancers
   c. The predisposition of von Recklinghausen's disease for certain STSs.
   d Prior exposure to defoliant chemicals
3. Favorable and unfavorable signs identified as prognostic indicators for STS include which of the following?
   I. Histology
   II. Size
   III. Site
      a. I only
      b. I and II only
      c. II and III only
      d. I, II and III
4. What is the correlation of Stage II STS with favorable-unfavorable signs?
   a. 3 favorable signs, 0 unfavorable signs
   b. 3 favorable signs, 1 unfavorable sign
   c. 3 favorable signs, 2 unfavorable signs
   d. 0 favorable signs, 2 unfavorable signs
5. Generally, a Stage IA STS may be assumed to have which of the following:
   a. Any tumor grade with a primary ≤5 cm.
   b. A tumor grade 1 with a primary ≤5 cm.
   c. A tumor grade 2 with a primary ≤5 cm.
   d. A tumor grade 3-4 with primary ≤5 cm.
6. Advantages of preoperative radiation therapy for STS include:
   a. Decreased difficulty with postirradiation surgical wound healing
   b. Availability of the precise extent and description of the tumor
   c. Possibility of a larger treatment volume
   d. Less aggressive surgery possible because of tumor regression
7. Intraoperative electron beam radiation usually involves energies ranging from 9 to 15 MeV with doses of which of the following?
   a. 1000 to 2000 cGy
   b. 1500 to 2500 cGy
   c. 2000 to 2500 cGy
   d. 2500 to 3000 cGy
8. Generally, a postoperative radiation shrinking-field technique plans the first field reduction at which of the following?
   a. 3000 to 3500 cGy
   b. 3500 to 4000 cGy
   c. 4000 to 4500 cGy
   d. 4500 to 5000 cGy
9. With the use of a shrinking-field technique and a boost, the total dose for STS may exceed which of the following?
   a. 6000 cGy
   b. 6500 cGy
   c. 7000 cGy
   d. 7500 cGy
10. STS metastasis occurs primarily by which of the following?
    I. Local invasion along adjacent, anatomically defined planes
    II. Hematological pathways to the lung and other sites
    III. Extension to regional lymph nodes
       a. I only
       b. II only
       c. I and II only
       d. I, II and III

Questions to Ponder

1. Consider the relationships between the surgical procedures used and radiation therapy planning for a patient who has an extremity STS. Describe, for example, the rationale for postoperative radiation therapy after a wide resection.
2. For extremity STS, incomplete total circumferential radiation with an external photon beam is recommended to avoid future excessive fibrosis and edema. What is the biological rationale for implementing this technique?
3. Despite the evidence that lymphatic involvement of STS is rare, the radiation therapy technique selected for rhabdomyosarcomas, synovial sarcomas, and epithelioid sarcomas frequently includes the regional lymph nodes. Discuss the rationale for this exception.
4. A shrinking-field external beam is generally used for the treatment of an STS with radiation therapy. Discuss the biological rationale for this technique. Why are the recommended dose ranges effective? Why is a boost with bolus or electrons to the scar frequently required?
5. The most common primary sites for STSs are the extremities (± 50%). The remaining sites may occur anywhere in the extraskeletal anatomy. Use the embryological and morphological ancestry of STS to explain the reason for this.

REFERENCES

1. American Cancer Society: *Cancer facts and figures,* Atlanta, 1996, The Society.
2. Barkley H et al: Treatment of soft tissue sarcoma by pre-operative irradiation and conservative surgical resection, *Int J Radiat Oncol Biol Phys* 14:693-699, 1988.
3. Basso-Ricci S et al: An extravisceral soft tissue sarcoma: effectiveness of radiation treatment and problems of radiotherapy and radiosurgical treatment, *Panminerva Med* 34(2):69-76, April-June 1992.
4. Beahrs OH et al, editors: *AJCC manual for staging of cancer,* ed 3, Philadelphia, 1988, JB Lippincott.
5. Brennan MF et al: The role of multi-modality therapy in soft tissue sarcoma, *Ann Surg* 214(3):328-336, September 1991.
6. Costa J et al: The grading of soft tissue sarcomas: results of a clinico-histiopathologic correlation in a series of 163 cases, *Cancer* 53:530-541, 1984.
7. Dannaher CL, Taniburro CH, Yam LT: Occupational carcinogenesis: the Louisville experience with vinyl chloride-associated hepatic angiosarcoma, *Am J Med* 70(2):279-287, February 1981.
8. Doosenbury KE, Thompson RC, Levitt SH: Extremity soft tissue sarcoma in adults. In Levitt SH, Khan FM, Potish RA, editors: *Levitt and Tapley's technological basis of radiation therapy: practical clinical applications,* ed 2, Malvern, Pennsylvania, 1992, Lea & Febiger.
9. Eilber FR, Eckhardt J, Morton DL: Advances in the treatment of sarcomas of the extremity: current status of limb salvage, *Cancer Suppl* 54(11):2695-2701, 1984.
10. Eilber FR et al: Progress in the recognition and treatment of soft tissue sarcoma, *Cancer* 65:660-666, 1990.
11. Enneking WF: A system for staging musculoskeletal neoplasms, *Clin Orthop* 204:9-24, 1986.
12. Enneking WF: Staging of musculoskeletal neoplasms: current concepts of disease and treatment of bone and soft tissue tumors, Heidelberg, Germany, 1984, Springer-Verlag.
13. Fawzy FI, Fawzy NW: Intervention for cancer patients, Gen Hosp Psych 16:151-191, 1994.
14. Gutin PH et al: Brachytherapy of recurrent tumors of the skull base and spine with I-125 sources, *Neurosurgery* 20(6):938-945, June 1987.
15. Jameel-Ahmed M et al: Soft tissue sarcomas in Kuwait: a review of 114 patients, *Clin Rad* 38(1):27-29, January 1987.
16. Kang H et al: Soft tissue sarcoma and military service in Vietnam: case-control study, *J Natl Cancer Inst* 79:693-699, 1987.
17. Karakousis CP et al: Feasibility of limb salvage and survival in soft tissue and survival in soft tissue sarcomas, *Cancer* 57(3):484-91, 1986.
18. Kumar PP, Good RR: Interstitial I-125 implantation in the treatment of retroperitoneal soft tissue sarcoma: report of a case, *Acta Radiol Oncol* 25(1):37-39, January-February 1986.
19. Lawrence TS, Lichter AS: Soft tissue sarcomas (excluding retroperitoneum). In Perez CA et al, editors: *Principles and practice of radiation oncology,* ed 2, Philadelphia, 1992, JB Lippincott.
20. Lawrence W et al: Adult soft tissue sarcomas' pattern of care: survey of the American College of Neoplasms, *Ann Surg* 205:349, 1987.
21. Nag S, Grecula J, Ruyman FB: Aggressive chemotherapy, organ preserving surgery and high dose rate remote brachytherapy in the treatment of rhabdomyosarcoma in infants and young children, *Cancer* 72(9):2769-2776, November 1993.
22. Nitti D et al: Management of primary sarcomas of the retroperitoneum, *Eur J Surg Oncol* 19(4):355-360, August 1993.
23. Nori D et al: Role of brachytherapy in recurrent extremity sarcoma in patients treated with prior surgery and irradiation, *Int J Radiat Oncol Biol Phys,* 20(6):1229-1233, June 1991.
24 Posner MC, Brennan MF: Soft tissue sarcomas. In Holleb AI, Fink DJ, Murphy GP, editors: *The American Cancer Society textbook of clinical oncology,* ed 1, Atlanta, 1991, The American Cancer Society.
25. Raleigh E: Sources of hope in chronic illness, *Oncol Nurs Forum* 19(3):443-446, 1992.
26. Rosenberg, SA, Suit HD, Baker LH: Sarcomas of soft tissues. In De Vita VT, Hellman S, Rosenberg SA, editors: *Cancer: principles and practices of oncology,* vol 2, ed 2, Philadelphia, 1982, JB Lippincott.
27. Rosier RN, Constine III LS: Soft tissue sarcoma. In Rubin P, McDonald S, Qazi R, editors: *Clinical oncology: a multi-disciplinary approach for physicians and students,* ed 7, Philadelphia, 1993, WB Saunders.
28. Shiu MH et al: Brachytherapy and function-saving resection of soft tissue sarcoma arising in the limb, *Intl J Radiat Oncol Biol Phys* 21(6):1488-1492, November 1991.
29. Silverberg E, Boring C, Squires T: Cancer statistics, *Cancer* 40:7-24, 1990.
30. Simon MA, Enneking WF: The management of soft tissue sarcomas of the extremities, *J Bone Joint Surg* 58-A:317-327, 1976.
31. Taenzer P, Fisher P: Psychosocial issues in radiation therapy, *Can J Med Radiat Technol* 20(2):81, 1989.
32. Tepper JE, Suit HD: The role of radiation therapy in the treatment of sarcoma of soft tissue, *Cancer Invest* 3(6):587-592, 1985.
33. Wijnmaalen A et al: Angiosarcoma of the breast following lumpectomy, axillary node dissection and radiotherapy for primary breast cancer: three case reports and a review of the literature, *Int J Radiat Oncol Biol Phys* 26(1):135-139, 1993.
34. Wilkinson S: Confusions and challenges; *Nurs Times* 88(35):25, 1992.
35. Willett CG et al: Intra-operative electron beam radiation for primary locally advanced rectal and rectosigmoid carcinoma, *J Clin Oncol* 9:843-849, 1991.
36. Willett CG et al: Intra-operative electron beam radiation therapy for retroperitoneal soft tissue sarcoma, *Cancer* 68(2):278-283, 1991.

BIBLIOGRAPHY

Wist E et al: Primary retroperitoneal sarcoma: a review of 36 cases, *Acta Radiol Oncol* 24(4):305-310, July-August 1985.

Zelefsky MJ et al: Limb salvage in soft tissue sarcoma involving neurovascular structures using combined surgical resection and brachytherapy, *Int J Radiat Oncol Biol Phys* 19(4):913-918, October 1990.

Zornig C et al: Retroperitoneal sarcoma in a series of 51 adults, *Eur J Surg Oncol* 18(5):475-480, October 1992.

Zornig C et al: Soft tissue sarcoma of the extremities and trunk in the adult: report of 124 cases, *Langenbecks Arch Chir* 377(1):28-33, 1992.

CHAPTER

3

Bone Tumors

Jean Roane

Outline

Bone tumors
- Epidemiology
- Etiology
- Prognostic indicators
- Anatomy and lymphatics

Clinical presentation
Detection and diagnosis
Staging
Treatment techniques
Role of radiation therapist

Key terms

Anaplastic
Articular cartilage
Diaphysis
Epiphyseal line
Epiphyses
Histiocytes
Hyperparathyroidism
Lytic
Necrosis
Osseous
Osteoblastic
Osteomyelitis
Paget's disease
Periosteum

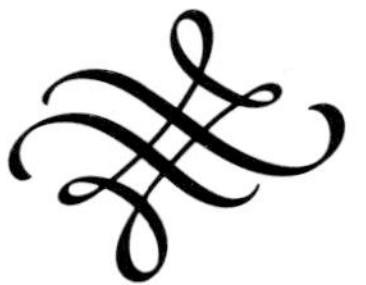

Bones or **osseous** tissue make up the skeletal system and give the body its shape, form, and ability to move. Bones possess the exceptional ability to support and protect softer tissues in the body. They also serve as a reservoir for fats, minerals, and other substances vital to blood cell production. *Bone tumors* refer to malignancies involving the bone, but they may also include collective tissues such as cartilage, joints, and blood vessels surrounding the bone. Bone marrow, responsible for blood cell production, is not spared from the attack of malignant cells.

The two types of bone tumors examined in this chapter are primary and metastatic. Malignant primary bone tumors do not constitute a major health hazard compared with other neoplastic disorders. In 1996 an estimated 2500 new cases of primary bone cancer were reported, with approximately 1380 deaths resulting from this disease. In contrast, the number of metastatic bone cancers arising in various skeletal areas from other primary disease sites was far greater than the number of primary bone tumors.[1]

Primary bone tumors create a diagnostic challenge for pathologists, radiation and medical oncologists, radiologists, and orthopedic surgeons. This challenge occurs because these tumors have a vast array of presentations and biological behaviors. Throughout this chapter the difficulty in diagnosing and treating these tumors will become apparent. Also, because this disease often strikes children, its devastating effect on the patient and family becomes quite clear.

The bone tumors covered in this chapter include osteogenic sarcoma (osteosarcoma), chondrosarcoma, fibrosarcoma, malignant histiocytoma, malignant giant cell tumors, multiple myeloma, metastatic bone disease, and Ewing's sarcoma.

BONE TUMORS
Epidemiology

The incidence of bone cancer (Table 3-1) is highest during adolescence (3 instances per 100,000 people). Bone tumors comprise 3.2% of malignancies in children under the age of 15. The incidence falls to 0.2 per 100,000 for people between the ages of 30 and 35, then slowly rises until its rate for those age 60 equals that for adolescents.[12]

Multiple myeloma, a nonosseous malignant tumor arising in the marrow, should be considered a primary bone tumor. Included in this classification, multiple myeloma becomes extremely significant, comprising approximately 35% to 43% of such tumors. Multiple myeloma is usually seen in middle-aged and older adults, peaking in the fifth and seventh decades. However, in this age bracket, multiple myeloma must be differentiated clinically and radiographically from metastatic carcinoma.[12]

Osteosarcoma, the most common osseous malignant bone tumor, is generally a tumor of adolescents and occasionally young adults, comprising about 20% of all bone tumors. Dahlin reported that it made up 28% of such tumors in his series.[9]

The next most common type of bone tumor comprises approximately 13% of the category and is known as *chondrosarcoma.* Although they may be primary tumors, chondrosarcomas can also occur as secondary malignancies developing in preexisting benign lesions.[12]

Fibrosarcoma (a rare form of bone malignancy) accounts for less than 4% of primary malignant bone tumors. In contrast, malignant fibrous histiocytoma has many of the same behaviors and is occasionally associated with bone infarctions or previous bone irradiation. Primary bone sarcomas are rare and more commonly show up as soft tissue sarcomas.[4,12]

Giant cell tumors of the bone generally arise in the metaphysis or epiphysis of long bones in young adults. These tumors most often arise around the knee and comprise approximately 0.5% of bone tumors. The majority of these tumors are extremely aggressive benign tumors, with a small percentage (about 7%) accounting for malignant lesions. Malignant giant cell tumors are most commonly seen in the context of previous radiation treatment portals for benign giant cell tumors. Approximately 10% of irradiated benign giant cell tumors ultimately transform into a malignancy.[12]

Metastatic bone disease accounts for approximately 60% to 65% of malignant bone lesions. Quite often, patients have a bone lesion resulting from the primary site located elsewhere in the body. Common primary sites are the prostate, breast, lung, kidney, and thyroid; a small percentage of bone lesions are from unknown origin. Metastatic carcinoma occurs most frequently in the spine and pelvis and becomes less frequent as the anatomical site becomes farther from the trunk. Metastatic bone lesions distal to the elbow or knee are extremely rare. They occur more often in the foot than in the hand. The primary tumor associated with these distal metastases is lung carcinoma.[12]

Ewing's sarcoma accounts for approximately 7% of bone tumors and affects a wide age range. This disease can strike anyone from the age of 5 months to 60 years, peaking in children from 11 to 17 years of age. Approximately 90% of patients are diagnosed before the age of 30, with the tumor rarely appearing in children under the age of 3. Ewing's sarcoma is rarely seen among African-American and Chinese people.[1,12]

After osteosarcoma, Ewing's sarcoma is the most common primary malignant bone tumor in children and adolescents. This disease accounts for about 3% of childhood cancers; approximately 200 instances occur per year in the United States. This disease appears to be more predominant in males than females and affects taller people more frequently than shorter individuals.[9,12]

Etiology

Areas of prolonged growth or overstimulated metabolism appear to have a direct link with the site of the neoplasm. This is seen in adult tissues affected by metabolic stimulation from long-standing **Paget's disease** (a condition character-

Table 3-1 Incidence of bone tumors

Bone Tumor	Incidence rate
Osteosarcoma (excluding myeloma)	20% of all primary malignant bone lesions
Chondrosarcoma	10%-20% of all primary malignant bone lesions
Fibrosarcoma	2%-6% of all primary malignant bone lesions
Malignant fibrous histiocytoma	0.78% of all primary malignant bone lesions
Giant cell tumors	0.5% of all primary malignant bone lesions
Multiple myeloma	35%-43% of all primary malignant bone lesions
Metastatic bone lesions*	60%-65% of all malignant bone lesions
Ewing's sarcoma	7% of all primary malignant bone lesions

Modified from Moss WT: *Radiation oncology,* ed 6, St. Louis, 1989, Mosby.
*Not a component of primary bone lesions. Represents a majority of all malignant bone lesions.

ized by excessive and abnormal bone reabsorption and formation), **hyperparathyroidism** (a condition caused by an abnormal parathyroid gland, resulting in a loss of calcium from the bones), chronic **osteomyelitis** (an infection of the bone or bone marrow), old bone infarcts, and fracture callous.[12] Cells that are proliferating or rapidly dividing (as occurs during the repair of bone tissue) tend to be more prone to a malignant transformation.

Another etiological factor linked to the formation of osteogenic sarcomas, chondrosarcomas, and fibrosarcomas is radiation. Also, bone-seeking radioisotopes from occupational (old radium dial painters) and medicinal uses need to be considered as a possible factor in diagnosing these tumors. Based on laboratory observations, another suggestion is that the role of infectious agents in bone cancers (particularly osteogenic sarcomas) has been indicated.[12]

The etiology of Ewing's sarcoma is unknown, but some studies have suggested some cytogenetic abnormality in the tumor. This concept could explain the higher-than-expected frequency of an osteosarcoma developing in an irradiated field in patients. Research is ongoing with the hope of a better understanding of this disease process and therefore more success in its treatment.[9]

Prognostic indicators

The prognosis for a patient with primary bone cancer depends on several factors. These include the location of the tumor, histological grade of the tumor, presence or absence of disseminated disease, and age and gender of the patient.

The prognosis of patients who have osteogenic sarcoma depends solely on the histological grade of the malignancy and the presence or absence of metastases at the time of presentation.[2] A study done by the Mayo Clinic cited five unfavorable prognostic factors and four favorable factors.[9] The unfavorable factors are (1) treatment before 1969, (2) a duration of symptoms less than 6 months, (3) male gender, (4) a lesion in proximal extremity, and (5) a patient under 10 years old. The favorable factors are (1) extremity lesions being better than axial primaries because of accessibility, (2) a longer duration of symptoms, possibly indicating a more indolent disease, (3) a smaller tumor size, and (4) a longer time interval between the presentation and appearance of the first metastatic lesion.

The prognostic indicators for patients with chondrosarcoma include the histological grade, size of the tumor, cell type, and location. In addition, the stage of the disease, patient's age, degree of local aggressiveness, and presence or absence of pain at the time of presentation all play a part in determining how well the patient functions with the disease.[9]

The prognostic indicators for fibrosarcomas include the histological grade, the location in the bone (medullary or periosteal), and whether the lesions arise de novo (anew) or are secondary to a preexisting bony condition.[9]

Malignant fibrous histiocytoma of the bone carries a poorer prognosis than that of soft tissue. The disease is extremely aggressive and overall entails a poor prognosis for any patient with the disease.[9]

Patients diagnosed with multiple myeloma and showing signs of advanced renal disease have a poorer prognosis than those diagnosed before the disease affects the kidneys. According to a study done by the Southwest Oncology Group (SWOG), the median survival time was 26 months for patients under the age of 55, and 20 months for patients over 65. Other indicators may shorten the survival or remission duration of these patients. These indicators include severe anemia, hypercalcemia, and high tumor cell volume. Based on the prognostic indicators, patients diagnosed early in the disease process are much more likely to have a longer survival or remission duration.[9]

Prognostic indicators in patients who have Ewing's sarcoma include the location of the tumor, the amount of extension by the time the patient is diagnosed, and whether the patient is male. Pelvic tumors carry a poorer prognosis because of the greater incidence of extraosseous extension.[9]

The most important prognostic factor with Ewing's sarcoma is the extent of the disease at the time of the diagnosis. Several variables are directly or indirectly related to this factor, making difficult the determination of the independent significance of any factor. Patients who have a grossly metastatic disease at the time of the diagnosis usually experience a poor outcome. Early studies have shown that patients with bone or bone marrow involvement did not do as well as patients with limited pulmonary involvement. However, progress is being made in the treatment of patients who have metastatic disease. Another prognostic factor is the extension of the soft tissue component of the primary tumor, producing a less favorable prognosis than that in patients with limited or no soft tissue involvement. In addition, because it involves the bone (greater or less than 8 cm), the size of the primary may influence the likelihood of a successful outcome. High serum levels of lactic dehydrogenase appear to be associated with a poor outcome, possibly because they reflect the tumor burden or activity of the tumor. A high leukocyte count may also be associated with an increased risk of tumor recurrence.[12]

Another important factor with Ewing's sarcoma is the site of the involvement, which is relevant to the success of therapy. The involvement of the pelvis or sacrum is associated with a worse prognosis than that of the proximal extremities (i.e., humerus and femur) or central sites such as the ribs and vertebrae. These sites are less favorable than the involvement of a distal extremity site, which makes treatment much easier. The local recurrence rate in the primary site is 15% for children with extremity lesions, 47% for children with rib primaries, and 69% for children with pelvic tumors.[12]

Anatomy and lymphatics

The high incidence rate of bone tumors in children supports the assumption that these neoplasms arise in areas of rapid growth. The most common site of a primary bone sarcoma is near the growth plate (Fig. 3-1). A typical long bone, as illustrated in Fig. 3-1, consists of the **diaphysis** (the main shaft of the bone), two **epiphyses** (the knoblike portions at either end

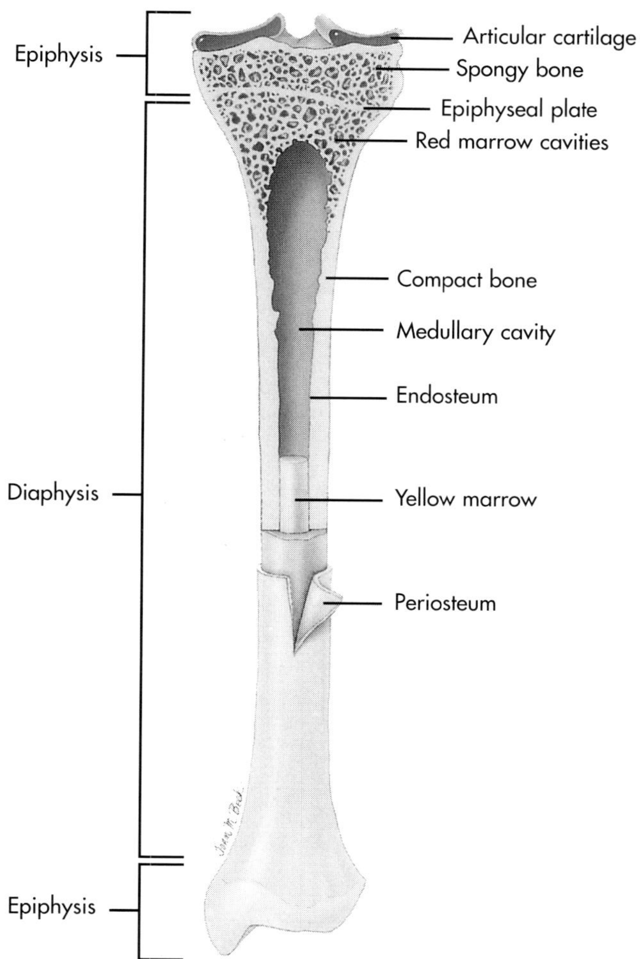

Fig. 3-1 A longitudinal section of long bone showing diaphysis, epiphyses, and articular cartilage. (From Thibodeau GA, Patton KT: *Anatomy and physiology,* ed 15, St Louis, 1996, Mosby.)

of the bone), **articular cartilage** (a thin layer of hyaline cartilage covering the joint surface of the epiphyses), and the **periosteum** (the hard dense covering of the bone). The growth plate is the area in long bones where rapid cell proliferation and remodeling activity takes place. This is known as the **epiphyseal line**. Because they possess large growth plates, the distal femur and proximal tibia are the two most common locations for bone tumors.[12]

Osteosarcomas are most commonly found in the distal femur or proximal tibia. The third most common site is the proximal humerus. Lesions appear in other areas, such as the proximal femur, distal tibia, and fibula, with rare occurrences in the vertebrae, ilium, facial bones, and mandible. In one study of patients 24 years or older, 41% of the lesions were found in flat bones associated with Paget's disease.[9]

Chondrosarcomas usually occur in areas such as the shoulder girdle, proximal femur, and proximal humerus. Just like osteosarcomas, chondrosarcomas are rarely found in the distal extremities. However, chondrosarcomas most commonly involve the femur, with some types involving the femoral shaft arising from preexisting benign conditions.[9]

Fibrosarcomas, malignant fibrous histiocytomas, and giant cell tumors of the bone often arise in long, tubular bones. These bones usually include the femur and tibia.[9]

Ewing's sarcoma can be present in virtually any bone but is most frequently seen in the lower half of the body. It can occur in any part of the bone but is most commonly seen in the diaphysis. Metaphyseal involvement occurs less often, and epiphyseal involvement is rare.[9] For treatment purposes the entire medullary cavity (the cavity of the bone that contains fats or yellow marrow) of the affected bones should be considered. Generally, extension occurs through the bony cortex into the soft tissue, giving rise to a large, soft tissue component. In axial lesions the soft tissue mass is quite often larger than the intraosseous component.[2]

Lung metastases are the most frequent result of hematogenous spread of Ewing's sarcoma. These metastases are frequently present at the time of the diagnosis, or the lung becomes the site of initial relapse. Lymph node involvement appears uncommon, although some studies suggest more frequent involvement may be evident with routine node sampling done during diagnosis and staging of processes. For the present, however, the true incidence of nodal involvement remains an unanswered question.[2]

Multiple myeloma can occur in any bone with **lytic** (areas of bone destruction) bone lesions showing up on diagnostic radiographs. However, the vertebral pedicles are rarely involved in patients who have multiple myeloma, compared with patients suffering from metastatic carcinoma.[9]

Metastatic bone disease most often involves the vertebral bodies, pelvic bones, and ribs. However, with widespread metastases, lesions are sometimes found in the humerus, femur, scapula, sternum, skull, clavicle, or ribs. Although the distal extremities are quite often spared from metastatic disease, lesions in the foot are more common than in the hand and usually result from a primary lung carcinoma.[2]

Lymphatic spread of most bone tumors is not of great concern unless the tumor arises in the trunk of the body. There the lymph vessels and nodes are more prominent and a greater chance exists of the tumor invading the lymph system. If this occurs, the microscopic tumor cells can be carried to other parts of the body through the lymphatic system.

Clinical presentation

The most common presenting factor with bone tumors is pain in the affected area. This may be accompanied by some swelling and locally engorged veins in instances of neglect. Patients with osteosarcoma usually complain of nonspecific pain and swelling in the involved area that begin insidiously and progress over a few months. Weight loss and symptoms related to anemia are also late complaints. Pathological fractures are not commonly seen in patients with osteosarcoma.[9]

Chondrosarcomas, fibrosarcomas, malignant fibrous histiocytomas, and giant cell tumors of the bone have symptoms similar to those of osteosarcomas, and the duration of the symptoms may be somewhat longer. Pain usually correlates with the degree of histological aggressiveness of the disease, and rapid worsening of symptoms may indicate the histological grade or cell type. Pathological fractures are common in malignant fibrous histiocytomas and fibrosarcomas. Also seen are neurological abnormalities in vertebral lesions, a decreased range of motion of the involved extremity, and muscular atrophy.[9]

Patients with Ewing's sarcoma also complain of pain and swelling in the affected area. The symptoms are frequently present for several months before a diagnosis is made. Patients with axial lesions especially have a prolonged duration of symptoms. In about 60% of patients a palpable mass is evident, demonstrating the propensity for this tumor to break through the cortex and involve surrounding tissue. Other symptoms include a fever, weight loss, and generalized fatigue. Occasionally, the presence of lung metastases may cause symptoms that encourage the patient to seek medical treatment early.[2,12]

Detection and diagnosis

Patients generally have pain that tends not to be activity related and may be worse at night. A complete history of the patient is important to determine the exact duration of the symptoms. Also, an indication of a previous carcinoma may suggest a metastatic etiology of a new bone lesion. Physicians also must keep in mind that a previously radiated area may result in a sarcoma. A long history (usually lasting years) of symptoms from a long bone lesion may indicate a benign condition, whereas symptoms that rapidly progress over weeks or a few months usually signify a higher likelihood of a malignant process.[6,12]

Because of the rarity of primary bone tumors, early detection is extremely difficult. The incidental finding of a bone lesion on a diagnostic radiograph is unusual. Usually, only persistent pain in a bone initiates a physician's investigation. Because pain is present early in the course of malignant lesions and they usually progress rapidly, incidental discoveries of these lesions are rare, making an early diagnosis difficult.[12]

The most important tool for a diagnosis and prognosis of a bone tumor is the radiograph. A variety of parameters are associated in accurately diagnosing a bone lesion. Some of these parameters are the permeative pattern, the sunburst periosteal reaction, the onion-skin periosteal reaction, and whether the lesion is osteolytic or **osteoblastic** (pertaining to bone-forming cells). All of the above indicate a bone lesion's level of advancement, its aggressiveness, and its rate of growth. (Fig. 3-2 illustrates several lytic lesions of the humerus caused by metastatic renal cell carcinoma. Fig. 3-3 shows the presence of a Ewing's sarcoma of the upper humerus.)

Computed tomography (CT) has been extremely helpful in establishing the extent of the tumor in the bone and determining the presence or absence of soft tissue masses. However, magnetic resonance imaging (MRI) has replaced CT in many instances (Fig. 3-4). MRI is used particularly in instances of highly malignant bone tumors because of the accurate detail it exhibits concerning the relationship of normal tissues and neurovascular structures with the tumor tissue. This is essential in planning a surgical biopsy and treatment. MRI is also a great means of showing with high sensitivity the reactive zone of the tumor in the bone and demonstrating marrow edema adjacent to tumor tissue.

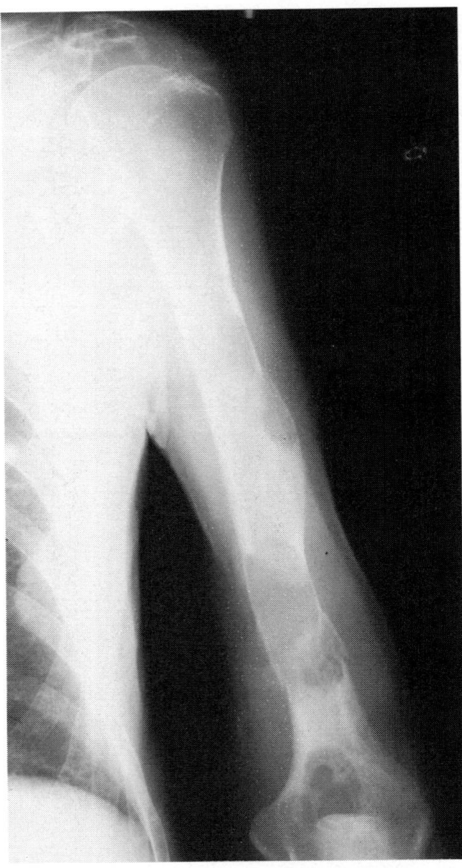

Fig. 3-2 Several lytic lesions are present throughout the humerus of this patient with metastatic renal cell carcinoma. Note the destruction of the periosteum along the mid- and lower portion of the shaft.

Bone scans using technetium 99 have played an important role in bone tumor evaluation. Fig. 3-5 demonstrates the diagnostic importance of a bone scan in a patient with metastatic prostate cancer. These scans are extremely sensitive and can detect tumor foci in bone not yet visualized on diagnostic radiographs. Therefore the extent of the tumor in the bone and the presence of skip metastases can be demonstrated accurately. Bone scans can also identify distant bony metastases even though they are extremely uncommon in primary bone tumors. For multiple myeloma, however, bone scan results are frequently negative and may underestimate the extent of the disease.[9]

The diagnosis of Ewing's sarcoma involves many diagnostic and some surgical procedures. The most important of these is the surgical biopsy. This procedure should be suffi-

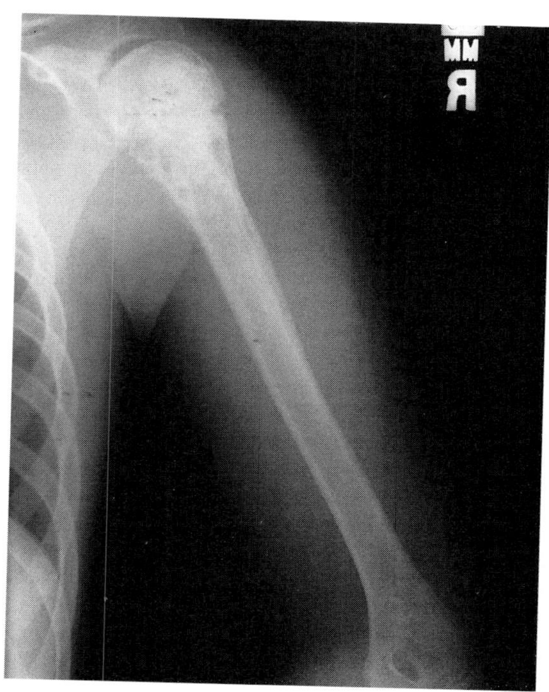

Fig. 3-3 Ewing's sarcoma of the upper right humerus. Note the diffuse permeative destruction of the bone, with pereosteal reaction involving the proximal portion of the humerus.

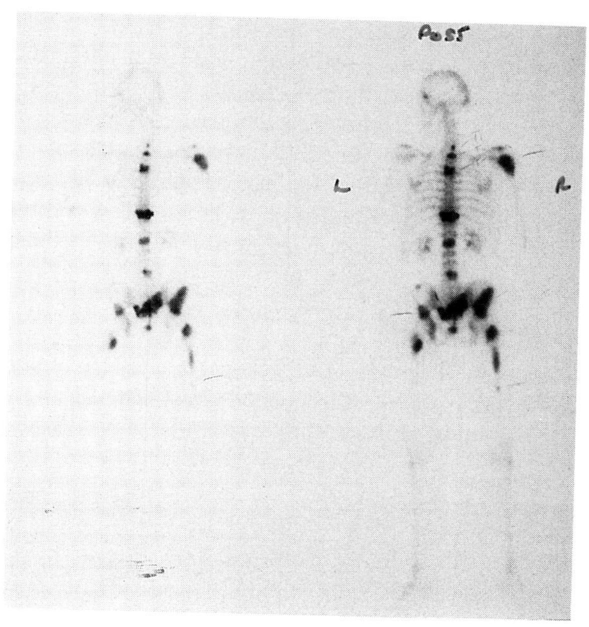

Fig. 3-5 This patient with metastatic prostate cancer has a diffuse disease in the right shoulder, vertebral column, and pelvic area. Bone scans with the use of technetium 99 play an important role in detecting the presence of metastatic disease. Both the anterior and posterior projections demonstrate several areas of increased uptake (dark areas) of the technetium 99.

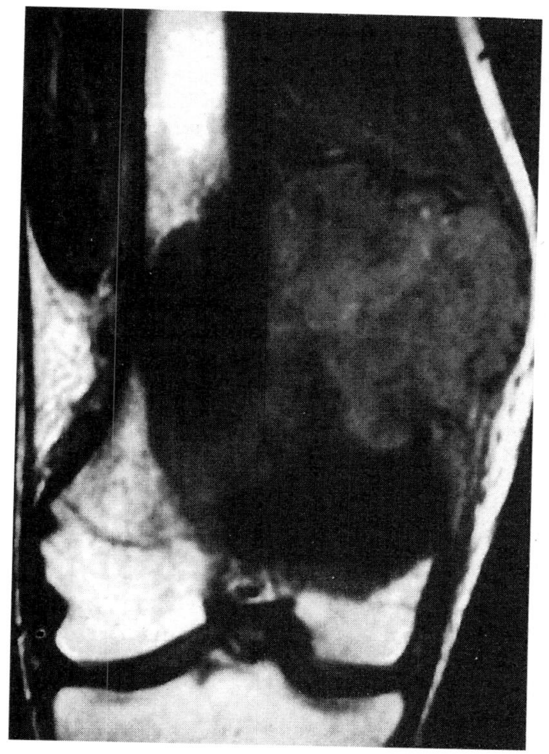

Fig. 3-4 An MRI scan of an osteogenic sarcoma of the distal femur showing the intermedularry and soft tissue extent of the tumor. (From Stark DD, Bradley WG Jr: *Magnetic resonance imaging,* ed 2, St Louis, 1991, Mosby.)

cient enough to confirm a pathological diagnosis. The biopsy site and approach must be discussed with the surgeon and radiation oncologist before the procedure is performed. If the biopsy incision is poorly placed, the delivery of optimal irradiation therapy may be technically impossible. Many patients have a considerable soft tissue mass, which can undergo a soft tissue biopsy rather than a biopsy of intraosseous tissue. A soft tissue biopsy is much easier and avoids further weakening of the bone, the integrity of which is already compromised by the tumor. This is especially true in patients who have lesions of weight-bearing bones due to the potential of a pathological fracture.

A radiographic assessment of the primary lesion is necessary to demonstrate an expanding destructive lesion in the diaphysis. The classical appearance of Ewing's sarcoma on radiographs shows a periosteal reaction in the form of periosteal elevation with extension through the cortex, giving an onion-skin appearance. CT and MRI have been extremely beneficial in assessing the disease extent.[12] Because of the propensity for Ewing's sarcoma to metastasize to the lungs, a CT scan of the lungs and a radiograph of the chest must be obtained.

Staging

No universally accepted staging system exists for primary bone sarcomas. The Enneking staging system classifies tumors according to the grade (G), local extent of the disease (T), and presence or absence of distant metastases (M). The box on p. 50 serves as a probable system to be used in the future.[6]

In the following sections, specific treatment techniques are discussed regarding osteogenic sarcoma, chondrosarcoma, fibrosarcoma, malignant fibrous histiocytoma, giant cell tumors, multiple myeloma, Ewing's sarcoma, and metastatic bone disease. In addition, more detailed information is provided for each of the histologies. Emphasis is on the role of radiation therapy as it relates to treatment, although for some primary bone lesions, radiation therapy plays a minor role (if any) in the treatment plan.

Treatment techniques

Osteogenic sarcoma. Osteogenic sarcoma is a relatively rare tumor but is the most frequently encountered malignant primary bone tumor. The hallmark of this disease is osteoid, or immature, bone produced by a malignant, proliferating spindle cell stroma. This disease is the most common bone tumor encountered in the first 3 decades of life, with the peak incidence rate occurring in girls 13½ years old and boys 14½ years old. The peak incidence rate corresponds respectively with growth spurts. Tall people and those affected with Paget's disease are at a higher risk.[12]

The most common metastasis from osteogenic sarcoma occurs in the lung. This seems to occur in about 80% of patients within 1 to 2 years after the initial diagnosis. However, with the introduction of more aggressive surgical techniques and newer chemotherapeutic agents, researchers hope to extend the disease-free status of patients. In addition, with the aggressive resection of pulmonary nodules, these patients are potentially curable.[2,12]

The most important prognostic indicator in patients diagnosed with osteogenic sarcoma is the presence or absence of metastases at the time of the diagnosis. Other factors requiring consideration are the duration of the symptoms, size of the tumor, gender of the patient, and site of the lesion. If the duration of the symptoms has been more than 6 months, this may indicate a more indolent disease, which may respond well to aggressive surgical and chemotherapeutic treatment. Reason dictates that the smaller the tumor, the more easily it can be surgically removed and the less chance it has to metastasize. The disease appears more often to attack males and those under the age of 10 at the time of the diagnosis. These patients do not seem to do as well as others. Also, lesions that occur in the extremities (usually the lower extremity) rather than in the axial primaries are more favorable. This has to do with the easy accessibility for surgical removal of the tumor to obtain localized control. Fig. 3-6 demonstrates the classic sunburst pattern seen radiographically, which is caused by the outward extension of bony spicules.

The treatment of osteogenic sarcoma requires a multidisciplinary approach. The mainstay of treatment for this disease is the attainment of local control. Because this tumor is relatively chemosensitive and radioresistant, the management of the primary tumor is the surgical removal of all gross and microscopic tumor. When possible, this is achieved most easily by amputation with a wide margin of normal tissue taken at the time of the surgery. The tumor's recurrence in the stump is usually attributed to skip lesions of the tumor in the affected bone separated from the primary tumor by several centimeters of normal bone. Historically, disarticulations were used to prevent this. Because of the introduction of adjuvant chemotherapy and improved CT and MRI scanning, the removal of entire bones is not necessary unless doing so is dictated by the location and extent of the tumor.[12]

Subamputative and limb-sparing surgery have been used in patients who have osteogenic sarcoma to reduce the functional and psychological morbidity of amputation. In this procedure the bone involved with the tumor is removed and replaced by an artificial prosthesis or bone graft. This procedure can only be performed if the vascular and neurolog-

Enneking Staging System for Bone Sarcomas

Grade

LOW GRADE (G1)
- Parosteal osteosarcoma
- Endosteal osteosarcoma
- Secondary chondrosarcoma
- Fibrosarcoma, low-grade
- Atypical malignant fibrous histiocytoma
- Giant cell tumor
- Adamantinoma

HIGH GRADE (G2)
- Classic osteosarcoma
- Radiation-induced sarcoma
- Paget's sarcoma
- Primary chondrosarcoma
- Fibrosarcoma, high grade
- Giant cell sarcoma

Local extent

INTRACOMPARTMENTAL (T1)
- Intraosseous
- Parosseous
- Intrafascial

EXTRACOMPARTMENTAL (T2)
- Soft tissue extension
- Extrafacial or deep fascial extension

Distant metastases

MO=No distant metastases
M1=Distant metastases present

Stage grouping

Stage	G	T	M
1A	G1	T1	M0
1B	G1	T2	M0
IIA	G2	T1	M0
IIB	G2	T2	M0
III	G1 or G2	T1 or T2	M1

Modified from Moss WT: *Radiation oncology*, ed 6, St. Louis, 1989, Mosby.

ical integrity of the limb is not compromised. In many instances, preoperative chemotherapy is used to reduce the size of the tumor to make limb-sparing surgery possible. However, the disease-free survival rate of patients with limb-sparing surgery is much the same as that with patients who have undergone an amputation. Subamputative and limb-sparing surgery is limited to patients with tumors of the lower extremity and those who have completed most of their growth. For patients with lesions of the humerus, any preservation of function in the hand can significantly improve long-term functional results.[12]

Before 1972, chemotherapy for osteogenic sarcoma was ineffective. In 1972, however, doxorubricin (adriamycin) or high doses of methotrexate followed by leucovorin were shown to produce objective tumor regression in 42% of patients. Since then, these two agents have been the basis for adjuvant chemotherapy. The early studies showed the importance of treatment with full-dose doxorubricin. Cisplatin has also proved to be an active agent in treating this type of tumor.[7,12]

Radiation therapy is not a treatment of choice for patients with osteogenic sarcomas. These tumors are radioresistant, and doses required for a clinical response often result in severe tissue damage and subsequent amputation. However, radiation has been used in patients for whom surgery is not feasible, but a cure with this approach is unusual. Radiation has been used to control or prevent pulmonary metastases but is of limited value in this setting. Palliative radiation therapy can be beneficial for pain control or the temporary control of metastases.[12]

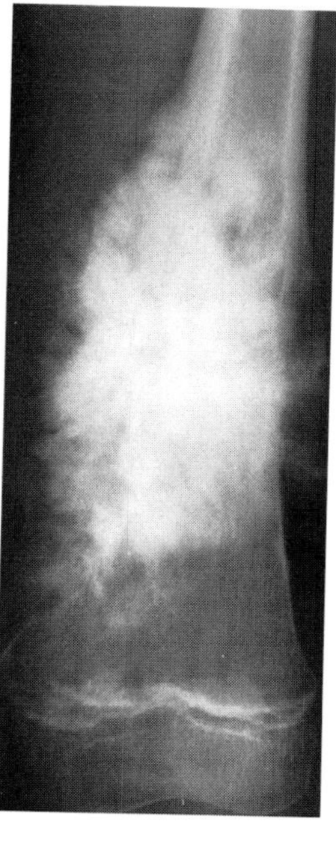

Fig. 3-6 Osteogenic sarcoma of the distal femur demonstrates a classic sunburst pattern caused by the outward growth of bony spicules. (From Eisenberg RL, Dennis CA: *Comprehensive radiographic pathology,* ed 2, St Louis, 1995, Mosby.)

Chondrosarcoma. Chondrosarcomas are malignant mesenchymal neoplasms that produce cartilage but no osteoid. The lesions are graded from 1 to 3, with 3 being the most **anaplastic** (exhibiting a loss of cell differentiation). Grading is an important prognostic indicator in this disease. The number of mitoses and the degree of cellularity are important in determining the grade of these tumors.[9]

A histological analysis of these tumors may indicate an invasion of the adjacent joint and infiltration beyond the x-ray margin of the tumor in the marrow cavity. Areas of **necrosis** (dead tissue), cyst formation, and hemorrhage may also be present. The average tumor size can range from 2 to 32 cm, with soft tissue extension possible.[9]

Low-grade chondrosarcomas do not tend to metastasize but do tend to recur locally. When this happens the tumor continues to grow and eventually evolves into a high-grade tumor. These tumors tend to metastasize to the lungs, giving the patient a poorer prognosis and thus making control more difficult.[2]

The prognosis of patients with chondrosarcomas depends on two factors. One factor is the histological grade of the tumor. Low-grade chondrosarcomas are locally invasive and do not metastasize, making this tumor easier to control. High-grade tumors, in contrast, have a high frequency of metastasis, particularly to the lungs. The other prognostic indicator is the tumor's location. If the tumor is located peripherally, it is easily accessible for surgical intervention; but if it appears in the pelvis or sacral area, surgery may not be possible. Fig. 3-7 shows a large chondrosarcoma of the distal femur.

The treatment of choice for this disease is the surgical removal of the entire tumor mass, with adequate bone and soft tissue margins. Radiation therapy does not usually play a role in treating these patients because of the radioresistant qualities of this type of tumor. However, in patients with an

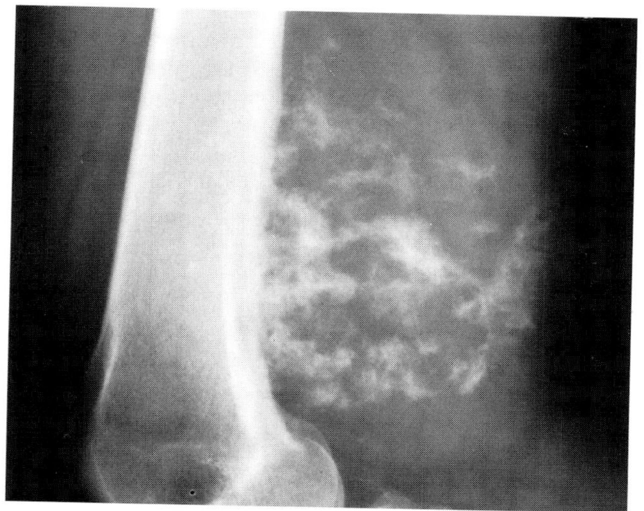

Fig. 3-7 A large chondrosarcoma located in the area of the distal femur. Note the prominent dense calcification of the lesion. (From Eisenberg RL, Dennis CA: *Comprehensive radiographic pathology,* ed 2, St Louis, 1995, Mosby.)

inoperable disease, radiation therapy has been used to a dose of 40 to 70 Gy with some response. To date, chemotherapeutic agents do not appear to have any substantial effect on this disease. Radioactive sulfur has been used in the past in patients who have an inoperable disease, but it has been abandoned because of its ineffectiveness and toxicity.[2,12]

Fibrosarcomas. Fibrosarcomas are locally aggressive lesions with a metastatic potential related to histological grade. High-grade lesions behave much like classic osteogenic sarcomas, whereas low-grade lesions appear less aggressive. These lesions are found mostly in the distal femur, followed in frequency by the proximal tibia and proximal humerus. The pelvis can be involved more often than in osteogenic sarcomas, and tumors of the jaw are not uncommon.[2,8]

Prognostic indicators for fibrosarcomas include the histological grade, the location in the bone, and whether the lesion arises de novo or secondary to a preexisting bony condition. The overall outlook for these patients is poor because of the tendency toward higher grade histology.[9]

Treatment for fibrosarcomas consists of an aggressive surgical procedure using wide or radical excision. Because these tumors have a high incidence rate of recurrence, even with aggressive surgery, postoperative radiation is now recommended. Fibrosarcomas are not highly radiosensitive, but irradiation is recommended for inoperable tumors, postoperative residual disease, and palliation. Doses of 66 to 70 Gy using a shrinking-field technique are recommended if radiation therapy is necessary to control a skeletal fibrosarcoma.[8]

Malignant fibrous histiocytoma. Malignant fibrous histiocytomas arise from **histiocytes** (a type of macrophage or phagocytic cell found in loose connective tissue) and may arise in bone or soft tissue of any part of the body. This is an extremely aggressive tumor, and like other soft tissue sarcomas, it metastasizes hematogenously (via the circulatory system) to the lungs. Metastases have also been found in the lymph nodes, liver, and bone. In addition, these tumors constitute a significant proportion of postradiation sarcomas.[12] The prognosis of patients with this disease is determined by the size and depth of the tumor and the presence or absence of metastases at the time of the diagnosis.

Treatment of soft tissue tumors includes wide surgical excision of the tumor, followed by radiation therapy or surgical resection without irradiation. These tumors tend to be radiosensitive, sometimes responding to doses as low as 10 Gy, but doses of 50 to 60 Gy are required for a cure. The suggestion has also been made that adjuvant chemotherapy may significantly improve the prognosis and decrease the metastatic rate.[12]

Malignant fibrous histiocytoma of the bone requires radical surgical resection, amputation, or disarticulation. Trials are underway that include radical or limited surgical procedures combined with preoperative or postoperative chemotherapy. Responses and occasional cures have been reported in patients receiving definitive radiation therapy with and without chemotherapy. Radiation therapy has also been reported as having a beneficial palliative response in some of the affected patients.[8]

Giant cell tumors. Giant cell tumors of the bone are malignant tumors made up of a stroma of spindly or ovoid cells, in addition to numerous multinucleated giant cells dispersed throughout the tumor tissue.[2] This tumor usually involves pain, swelling, and tenderness at the lesion site. The most common site for these tumors is in and around the knee. Approximately half the lesions occur at the distal femur, and half occur at the proximal tibia. Additional common sites for this tumor are the proximal humerus, proximal femur, sacrum, and other pelvic areas.

Giant cell tumors of the bone usually occur predominantly in the third and fourth decades of life, with some occurrences during the second decade of life. However, this condition is extremely rare for children below the age of 10. These tumors tend to recur locally. Metastases show up rarely, but when they do, the most affected area is the lung.

The histology of giant cell tumors is generally low grade, with areas of focally malignant cells present in the examined specimen. These lesions are treated locally because of their low propensity to metastasize. Occasionally, however, even these low-grade tumors have metastasized with a histological diagnosis of pulmonary nodules. These nodules sometimes occur as isolated, solitary nodules with a frequently encountered benign giant cell tumor. A fully malignant, Grade III, giant cell tumor is rarely encountered. Only about 10% of these tumors are fully malignant at the time of the initial diagnosis. However, about 20% of giant cell tumors become malignant after they have recurred locally. In addition, giant cell tumors have been reported to become fully malignant after the application of radiation therapy to obtain local control. It is unclear whether this transformation is a result of the natural history of this tumor or radiation therapy is truly an oncogenic agent. However, the occurrence of fully malignant giant cell tumors with metastatic capabilities may be an indication that radiation therapy causes malignant transformation or just is not adequate therapy to eradicate this tumor. The latter is probably closer to what can be expected because this tumor is a spindle cell sarcoma known to be radiosensitive.[2]

The prognosis of a patient who has a giant cell tumor of the bone depends primarily on the location and histology of the tumor. Tumors located in the extremity and those of low-grade histology are easily accessible for surgical intervention and have a low propensity to metastasize. Those located in the pelvic region are harder to excise; therefore local control is difficult.

The treatment of choice for giant cell tumors of the bone is surgical removal of the tumor. Benign giant cell tumors can be treated in several different ways, including curettage and bone grafting with or without cauterization, filling of the cavity with cement, application of liquid nitrogen after curettage, or surgical excision if functional results permit. Malignant giant cell tumors require a more radical surgical procedure, followed by the use of adjuvant chemotherapy. Radiation therapy is reserved for control of inoperable tumors or for palliation of symptomatic areas in patients with advanced malignant disease.[8]

Multiple myeloma. A multiple myeloma is a malignant plasma cell tumor that has several different forms. The forms constitute a spectrum from small, localized lesions to a diffuse, disseminated disease. The most frequent presentation of this disease is a disseminated disease with the involvement of multiple skeletal sites. Common complaints of patients with multiple myeloma include bone pain, bleeding, infections, and easy fatigability. These patients tend to experience anemia, with thrombocytopenia and/or granulocytopenia appearing in approximately one third of the patients. Multiple myeloma incidence increases with age and peaks during the sixth and seventh decades of life.

Multiple myeloma is characterized by an increased proliferation of plasma cells of varying degrees of differentiation. Plasma cells are found primarily in the tissues and organs of the lymphoreticular system, especially in the bone marrow, lymph nodes, liver, and upper respiratory and gastrointestinal tract mucosa. The suggestion has been made that plasma cells may be derived from B lymphocytes, which develop from primitive reticular stem cells found scattered throughout all tissues, thus making it possible to find these tumors in nearly any tissue or organ.[9]

Myeloma is a low-growth fraction tumor with only a small percentage of tumor cells in cycle at any time. This means that the time before patients need treatment can range from 1 to 3 years, with the actual time of treatment ranging from 1 to 10 years or more.[9]

Plasma cell tumors secrete a measurable amount of paraprotein, which constitutes a unique tumor marker. The serum level or paraprotein correlates with the tumor cell burden. This can be helpful in determining the prognosis of patients diagnosed with multiple myeloma.[9]

Because plasma cells circulate through the blood and lymph systems, multiple myeloma can appear in a localized area or may be disseminated anywhere in the body. Therefore, because of its nature, multiple myeloma does not metastasize to any specific organ. In addition, multiple myeloma can act in an indolent manner or be extremely aggressive. Fig. 3-8 illustrates the classic radiographic appearance of aggressive multiple myeloma.

Patients who have advanced renal disease in addition to multiple myeloma have a poorer prognosis. Those over 65 years of age have a median survival time of 20 months, whereas those under 55 years of age have a median survival time of 26 months, according to the SWOG. Other findings associated with shortened median survival times or remission durations include severe anemia, hypercalcemia, elevated blood-urea nitrogen, elevated M protein, hypoalbuminemia, and a high tumor cell burden. In addition, patients responding rapidly to treatment have a shorter median survival time and remission duration than patients responding more slowly. A correlation also exists between the survival median time and myeloma cell mass at the time of presentation.[9]

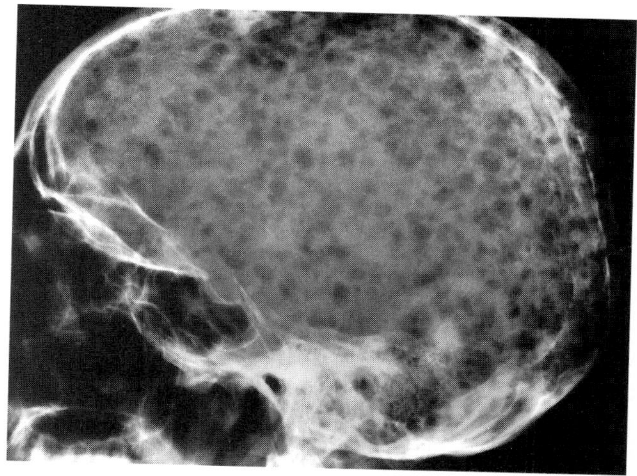

Fig. 3-8 An abundance of lytic lesions are scattered throughout the skull in this patient with multiple myeloma. Flat bones (like the skull, vertebrae, ribs, and pelvis) tend to be more affected. (From Eisenberg RL, Dennis CA: *Comprehensive radiographic pathology,* ed 2, St Louis, 1995, Mosby.)

The treatment that best palliates patients with multiple myeloma is chemotherapy and radiation therapy. A curative treatment for this disease has not yet been established. The use of alkylating agents (a type of chemotherapy) combined with prednisone has been effective for the palliation of these patients. However, some controversy exists on the length of time patients should stay on this drug regimen because continued therapy can lead to refracting anemia or the development of secondary acute leukemia. In contrast, the cessation of therapy can cause a relapse, and patients may not respond as well to retreatment.

Radiation therapy plays an important role in the management of patients with multiple myeloma. At one time, however, radiation therapy was the only effective mode of treatment for this disease. With the introduction of effective chemotherapy agents, radiation therapy is now an adjuvant therapy for multiple myeloma. Radiation therapy is indicated with the presence of the following criteria[9]:

1. For primary treatment in localized presentations (i.e., solitary plasmacytomas of bone and extramedullary plasmacytomas)
2. For the palliation of pain caused by bone lesions from disseminated disease not controlled by chemotherapy
3. For the prevention of pathological fractures in weight-bearing bones
4. For the relief of spinal cord compression or nerve root compression

With the use of irradiation to treat localized lesions, the field must be planned carefully so that the entire lesion is treated. Also, generous margins should be used in the treatment of osteolytic lesions of the long bones. For this reasons MRI has been supportive in guiding the radiation oncologist to locate, plan, and treat the ultimate portal for a lesion. The physician needs to treat the entire lesion but spare as much normal tissue as possible.[2] Fig. 3-9 represents a single posterior treatment field for disease in the sacrum and lumbar vertebrae.

Surgery does not play an important role in the treatment of multiple myeloma but is used in certain instances. If a patient has a pending pathological fracture, an orthopedic surgeon may want to stabilize the bone before initiating radiation therapy. Also, for paraspinal masses, which can be extremely large and cause paralysis and pain, a neurosurgeon may want to debulk the tumor before radiation therapy is initiated.

Total-body irradiation has been used in instances in which patients have been unresponsive to all alkylating chemotherapeutic agents. This mode of treatment is rarely practical and is a last resort to treat unresponsive patients. Also, patients with multiple myeloma already have blood systems and immune systems compromised by chemotherapy and probably would not tolerate total-body irradiation.

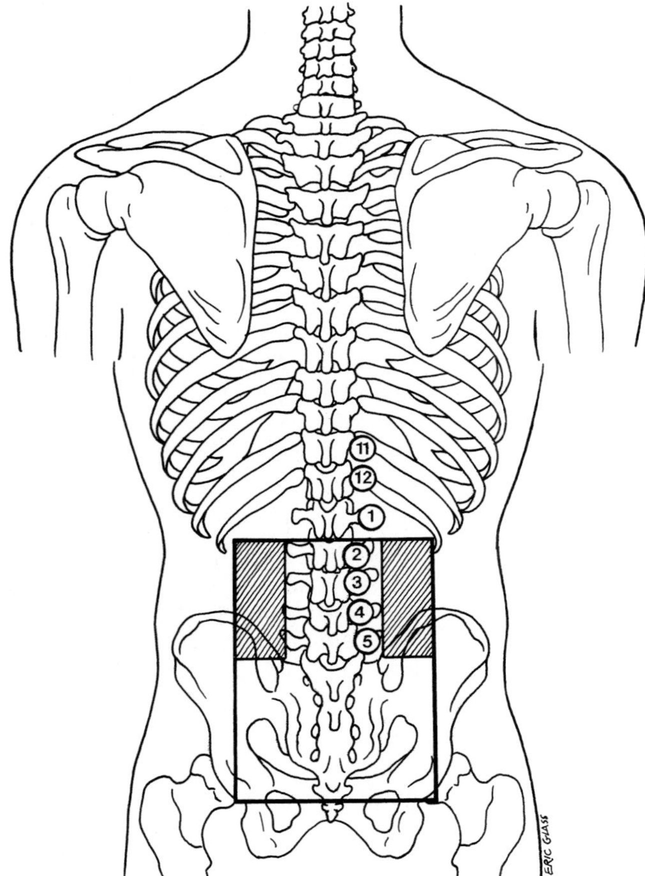

Fig. 3-9 A schematic representation of a single posterior treatment field for metastatic disease in the sacrum and lumbar vertebrae. The shaded areas represent shielding blocks used to spare normal tissue. The circled numbers correspond to thoracic and lumbar vertebrae.

Supportive care for these patients is extremely important and should not be forgotten. This type of care includes treatment for anemia, hypercalcemia, azotemia, and frequent infections. These patients cannot be cured, so in addition to palliative therapies for the relief of pain, support care is necessary for giving these patients some quality of life for whatever time they may have left.

Ewing's sarcoma. Ewing's sarcoma is a highly malignant, nonosseous tumor that usually arises in the bone but occasionally in soft tissue. It is the most common bone tumor in children under 10 years of age and second only to osteogenic sarcoma in the second decade of life. Because this tumor is more radiosensitive, radiation therapy plays a major role in the management of this disease.[12]

In 1921 James Ewing distinguished this tumor by virtue of its composition with small, round cells rather than with the spindle cells of osteosarcoma. Ewing's sarcoma has a propensity to metastasize, but with combined chemotherapy, surgery, and radiation therapy, the outlook for patients with this tumor is much more promising.[2,12] Fig. 3-10 illustrates the distribution of primary sites in Ewing's sarcoma.[2]

Most patients with Ewing's sarcoma appear to have a localized disease. However, the use of surgery or radiation therapy alone is unlikely to obtain curative results because of the presence of micrometastases. For this reason the use of chemotherapeutic agents has become increasingly effective in eliminating these cells and assisting in obtaining local control. Chemotherapy has been useful in reducing the need for radical surgery or high-dose, large-volume irradiation. The ultimate goal for patients with Ewing's sarcoma is the eradication of the entire tumor and the preservation of as much function as possible at the same time. The aggressiveness and optimal integration of all three modalities remains to be determined. Because 15% to 35% of patients have demonstrable metastatic disease at the time of the diagnosis, long-term survival is unobtainable even with aggressive treatment, including transplantation.[12]

A surgical biopsy with the use of optimal techniques is necessary to establish the diagnosis. As previously noted, care must be taken in this procedure so that the bone is not further compromised. Therefore biopsies should be taken from the soft tissue component if possible. The nature of surgery on the primary tumor is determined by its location, the extent of the disease, and the presence or absence of known metastases. Although surgeons vary in their approaches, data suggest that selective interventions are the most appropriate. Aggressive surgery (including amputation and, if possible, limb-sparing procedures) should be used if a severe pathological fracture is present or a potential for substantial growth impairment exists as a consequence of radiation therapy. The surgical resection of expendable bones can achieve local control without an undue functional deficit. For patients with bulky tumors (usually greater than 8 cm), radical surgery can be performed but not without great morbidity. In this instance, limited surgery with little normal tissue margin or microscopically positive margins followed by radiation therapy is at least efficacious in achieving local control. Another strategy is presurgical chemotherapy, with the definitive surgical procedure followed by radiation therapy if necessary. For a favorable distal extremity lesion, surgery or radiation therapy can be successful, keeping in mind that micrometastases may be present and curative results may not occur.[12]

Ewing's sarcoma is a radiosensitive tumor; therefore, radiation therapy plays a major role in treating patients with this condition. The potential to achieve local control depends on the location and extent of the tumor. Radiation therapy combined with chemotherapy has been successful in treating 90% of the patients with distal extremity lesions, 75% with proximal extremity lesions, but only 65% with central lesions. Radiation therapy is used in light of the surgical procedures deemed appropriate, keeping in mind the morbidities that can be encountered by one or both modes of treatment. For distal extremity lesions in nonexpendable bones or for the subtotal or marginal resection of a bulky tumor, radiation therapy is the most appropriate mode of treatment.[12] Patients with metastatic Ewing's sarcoma to the lungs and other sites benefit from radiation therapy. This treatment helps in overall disease control.

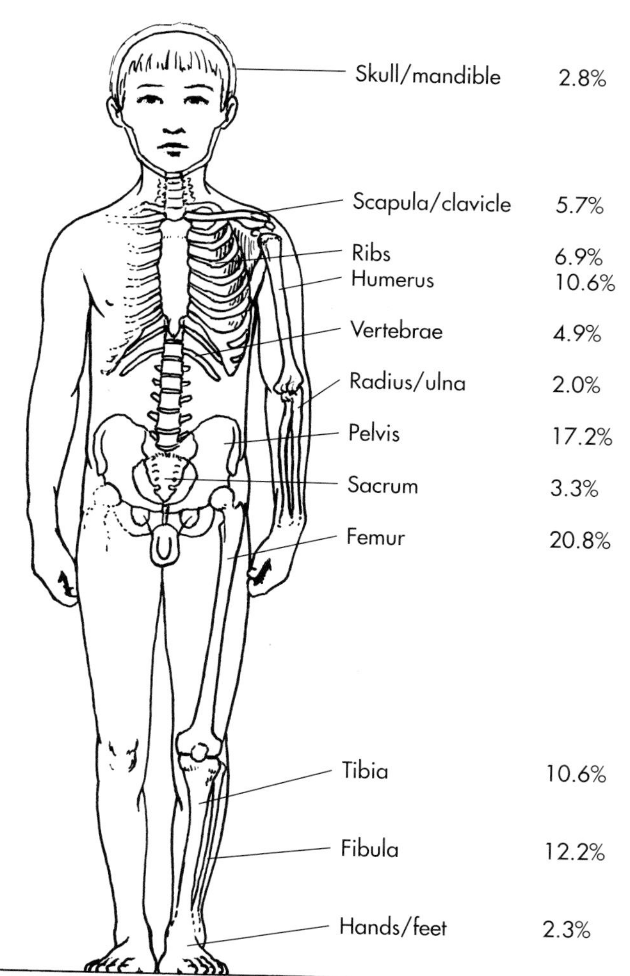

Fig. 3-10 The distribution of primary sites in Ewing's sarcoma. (Frequency data from DeVita VT Jr, Hellman S, Rosenberg SA: *Cancer: principles & practice of oncology,* Philadelphia, 1993, JB Lippincott.)

The administration of radiation therapy has been refined as a result of improvements in chemotherapy and imaging techniques, as well as information regarding local tumor recurrence. The traditional volume included a generous margin around the soft tissue component and the entire bone, with successive reductions to doses of 55 to 60 Gy. Recent data support the exclusion of one epiphyseal center at the opposite end of the bone from an eccentrically located lesion with peak doses of 50 to 60 Gy, depending on the tumor bulk and surgical procedure. Important considerations include the treatment of the surgical scar to kill any cancer cells present and the shaping of fields to maintain lymphatic drainage and avoid fluid buildup in the extremity.[12]

Ewing's sarcoma is also an extremely sensitive tumor to chemotherapy, with a significant response rate to numerous single agents. These agents include the following: high-dose melphalan, cyclophosphamide, doxorubicin, vincristine, 5-fluorouracil, ifosfamide, etoposide, and actinomycin D. Multiagent chemotherapy plays an important role in improved systemic and local control, resulting in better overall survival rates. Several regimens have been evaluated, with the four most successful including cyclophosphamide, doxorubicin, vincristine, and actinomycin D. High-dose use of the more active agents (cyclophosphamide and doxorubicin) has played a major role in improving disease-free survival rates. Although chemotherapy typically follows surgery and is administered in part before radiation therapy, selected situations may warrant chemotherapeutic administration before surgery to shrink a tumor for easier removal.[12]

Bone marrow transplantation may be a promising treatment for patients whose prognosis is poor. Studies are underway that use bone marrow transplantation in the hope of gaining positive results for patients with metastases at the time of the diagnosis.

Metastatic bone disease. The majority of malignant bone lesions are metastatic. The radiation therapist treats more patients with metastatic bone disease than patients with primary bone lesions. The development of bone metastases in cancer patients is a common and often catastrophic event. Bone metastases give rise to pain, pathological fractures, frequent neurological deficits, and forced immobility, causing a significant decrease in the quality of life for these patients. Patients with breast, prostate, kidney, thyroid, and lung carcinomas are likely to develop bone metastases sometime during the course of the disease.

Increasing pain that develops gradually over a few weeks or months is the most frequent symptom associated with bone metastases. The pain becomes localized and progressively severe during this time and may be worse at night. In patients who have multiple sites of bony metastases, pain may be associated with weight bearing. In this situation, radiographs are necessary to rule out a pathological fracture and determine whether surgical intervention is necessary. Pain may also be positional and relieved simply by shifting weight from the involved area. Bone involvement may also cause pain by nerve entrapment resulting from tumor expansion and pressure on the nerve by the direct destruction of bone. This type of pain occurs in patients with vertebral involvement or sacral metastases caused by the radicular nature of the pain. A careful and extensive neurological work-up is necessary because vertebral destruction is quite often associated with extradural spine disease, which can result in spinal cord compression. Early treatment of a partial or complete spinal cord block is crucial to prevent paralysis and sensory loss. This is one of the few emergency procedures encountered in radiation oncology.

Although metastatic bone cancer is rarely life threatening, maintaining a certain quality of life for these patients becomes quite important. Relieving the pain, decreasing the amount of narcotic medication, and maintaining ambulation are the first and most vital steps for improving the quality of the patient's life. Patients with metastatic bone cancer survive for many years with the disease; therefore, all aspects of their care should be considered in the initial management plans.

Bone metastases occur as the cells from the primary tumor spread through lymph and/or blood vessels to sites that permit new tumor growth. The appearance of a solitary bony metastasis on a radiograph is unusual but indicative of the eventual development of other metastases. The areas most frequently involved include the vertebral bodies, pelvic bones, and ribs. In patients with widespread disease, lesions in the humerus, femur, scapula, sternum, skull, or clavicle are not uncommon. For this reason, the physician must obtain a complete metastatic work-up on these patients to accurately assess the extent of the disease. This work-up may include bone, CT, and MRI scans; blood tests; and diagnostic radiographs.

The radiographic appearance of bony metastases takes on different aspects according to the type of lesion. Osteolytic lesions have ragged margins and may appear as a granular, mottled-looking area on an x-ray film. If the margins are smooth, a benign process must be considered. In comparing Figs. 3-11 and 3-12 a difference is evident between the ragged and smooth outlines of the tumor, generally indicating a benign or malignant process. Multiple myeloma and breast, kidney, and thyroid carcinomas commonly produce lytic lesions. The loss of outline of one or more pedicles may

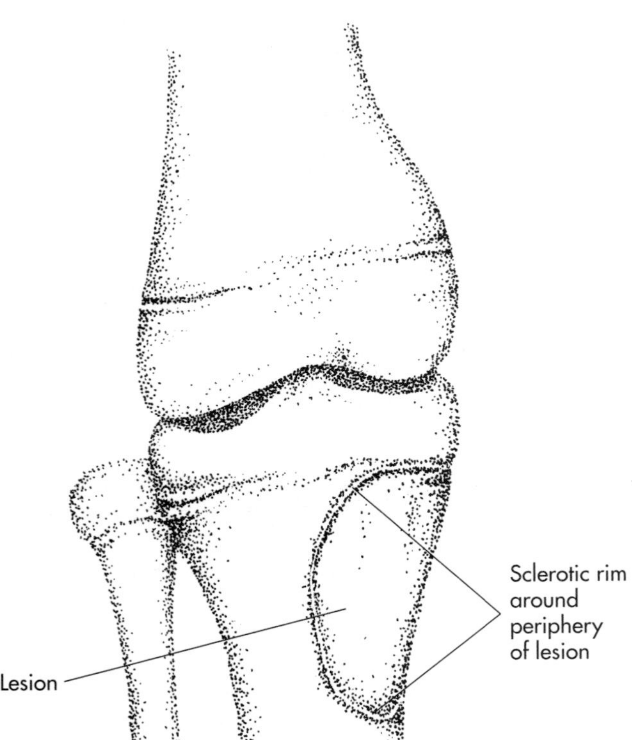

Fig. 3-11 A benign appearance of bone tumors demonstating a sclerotic rim around the periphery of the lesion.

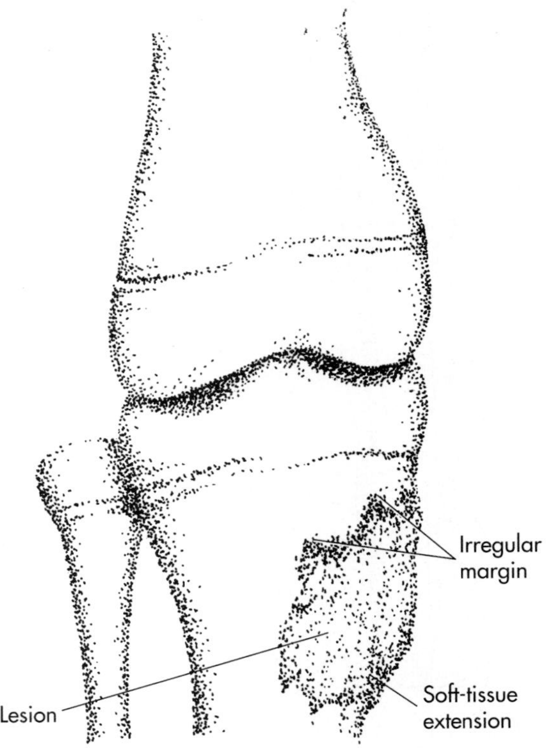

Fig. 3-12 A malignant appearance of bone tumors demonstrating an irregular margin with soft tissue extension.

be the earliest indication of vertebral body involvement in the spine. If a patient has multiple bone lesions without a known primary tumor site, multiple myeloma must be considered. However, in patients who have multiple myeloma the pedicles of the spine are not usually involved.[2]

Another appearance of metastatic bone disease is an osteoblastic lesion (Fig. 3-13, *A* and *B*). These lesions are usually sclerotic foci characterized by increased radiographic density. They may appear as isolated, rounded foci or diffuse sclerosis involving a large area in the bone. The involved area usually appears as an area of increased density radiographically. The majority of patients with osteoblastic lesions have metastatic breast or prostate cancer.[2]

Several factors play a role in determining the natural history of metastatic bone cancer. The presence of bone metastases generally predicts the eventual progression of disease, with the rate of progression varying tremendously, depending on the following factors: host resistance, tumor doubling time, and tumor responsiveness to systemic treatment. The extent of the disease at the time of the diagnosis varies greatly, depending on the primary site and whether metastases are evident. Patients who have a solitary asymptomatic

A

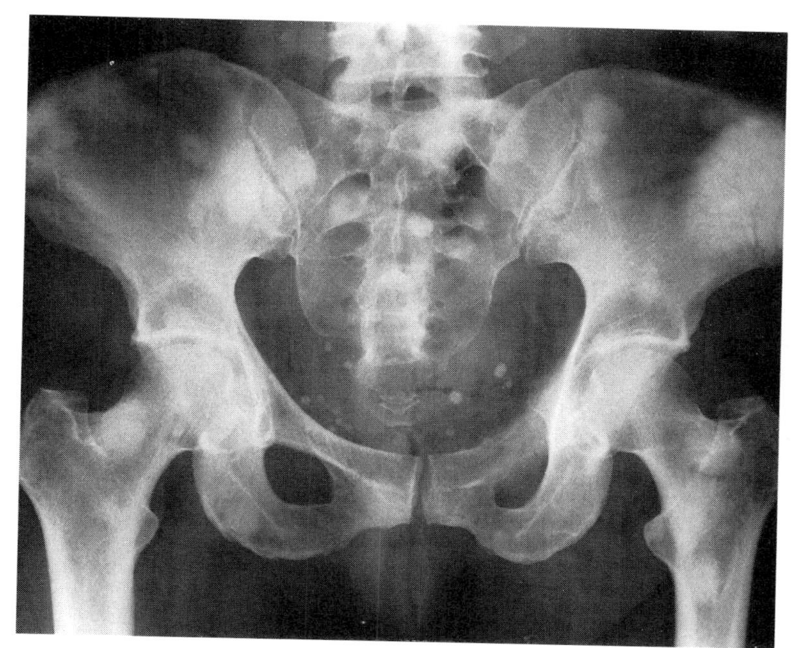

B

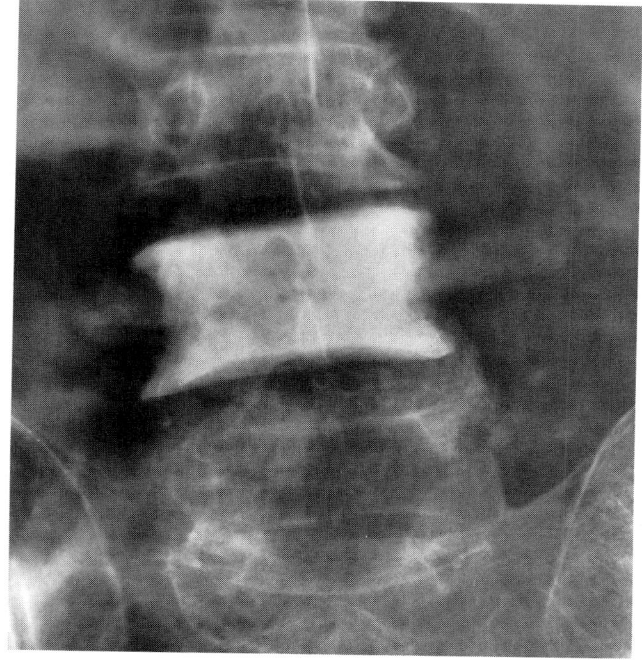

Fig. 3-13 **A,** Osteoblastic metastases from bladder cancer (areas of increased density) involving the pelvis and proximal femurs. **B,** Osteoblastic lesion of L4 metastatic from prostate cancer. (From Eisenberg RL, and Dennis CA: *Comprehensive radiographic pathology,* ed 2, St Louis, 1995, Mosby.)

lesion during the initial work-up may have a longer survival time than patients who have pain and widespread metastases. The median survival time for patients with malignant melanoma metastatic to bone is about 3½ months, whereas patients with cervix and colon cancer metastatic to bone have a median survival time of 13 and 18 months, respectively. Patients with breast and prostate cancer metastatic to bone may have a prolonged survival time because of combined chemotherapy and hormonal therapy. If patients do not respond to systemic therapy, local irradiation can provide pain control and local control of the lesion.[12]

The prognosis of patients who have metastatic bone disease depends on the primary site, histology, and degree of metastasis at the time of the diagnosis. For this reason a complete metastatic work-up is necessary before the initiation of any treatment. Some patients may benefit most from chemotherapy, whereas others may benefit more from radiation therapy, surgery, or a combined effort of systemic and local therapies. Many patients with metastatic bone cancer will undoubtedly die from their disease, so the focus must be on giving them the best quality of life for the time they have left. For these types of situations, teamwork on the part of physicians, oncologists, therapists, and nurses becomes extremely important.

The treatment of bone metastases is concentrated on the palliation of pain and the prevention of fractures to weight-bearing bones. Because patients with metastatic bone cancer usually experience a great deal of pain, narcotics to alleviate discomfort are used, possibly resulting in oversedation and constipation. Therefore the introduction of other modalities is necessary for the treatment of bone pain. To accomplish an effective method of treatment, a careful evaluation of the tumor type, extent of the disease, degree of symptomatology, and physical status of the patient must be completed.[2]

The use of radiation therapy is important in the local control of the lesion, relieving pain and preventing the loss of function of the bone or bones involved. However, radiation therapy does not address the systemic disease, which may require hormonal or chemotherapy, depending on the histology of the primary site. Surgery becomes an option for these patients when the stabilization of a weight-bearing bone is needed or when debulking of an extradural mass is necessary to relieve excruciating pain. Radiation therapy is usually introduced after the surgical procedure to obtain local control.[12]

Radiation portals need to encompass all involved areas but spare uninvolved tissue when possible. If stabilization has been performed surgically, radiation therapy should be initiated as soon as the wound has healed. The portal should include the fixation device and any micrometastases that may have been dislodged during the surgical procedure. However, a strip of soft tissue should be left unirradiated to preserve lymphatic drainage.[12]

The treatment of bone metastases involving the pelvis and vertebrae needs to be carefully planned. The portal should encompass the area involved with the tumor yet avoid uninvolved bone (to spare bone marrow) and other normal tissue. In the treatment of the spine, the portal should include the symptomatic vertebrae, with a one-vertebral-body margin above and below the involved vertebrae. If necessary, custom-made blocks can be used to shield uninvolved bone and reduce the amount of small bowel in the field.[12]

The introduction of strontium 89 has provided excellent results in bone-pain relief for patients with prostate and breast cancer metastatic to bone. Strontium 89 is a radiopharmaceutical agent used for the palliation of metastatic bone pain. It is a pure beta-emitter that causes minimal irradiation of the normal tissues. This agent localizes to osteoblastic areas or skeletal metastatic lesions from the primary cancer. The radioisotope has a therapeutic half-life of 50.5 days; therefore, its therapeutic effect may last up to 15 months. Approximately 1 to 3 weeks may pass before the patient notices any substantial effect. A physician administers strontium 89 to patients on an outpatient basis. The agent is introduced via a slow intravenous push into a peripheral vein. The usual dose is 4 mCI or 4 ml. Patients receiving strontium 89 may experience a mild flushing sensation during the administration process, but otherwise they feel nothing.

Because this agent can cause a slight reduction in platelet and white blood cell counts 5 to 6 weeks after treatment, patients must have a complete blood count taken before the administration of strontium 89. The patient's blood counts are monitored at certain intervals to ensure the physician the counts are stabilized.

Patients have been noted to experience a flarelike pain reaction for 2 to 4 days after the injection. They should, however, experience some pain relief in 1 to 3 weeks, with most patients responding for 3 months. After that time, strontium 89 may be readministered every 90 days.

Patients who have been injected with strontium 89 need to be reassured that they are in no way harmful to other people. This agent is confined within the body, and bodily contact is permitted. Strontium 89 is eliminated by the body, primarily in the urine, within the first 48 hours. This agent is being used more often because of the positive results that have been obtained.[4]

Metastatic bone cancer is the most widely seen type of bone cancer. The most important results in the treatment of these patients are pain control and improvement of their quality of life. Radiation therapy is an effective tool in the palliation of bone pain caused by metastatic disease. In many instances, the patient's pain and use of high doses of narcotics can be reduced.

Side effects. The two major categories of complications seen most frequently are acute and late effects. Patients treated with radiation therapy and chemotherapy at the same time may experience more acute side effects. The use of these two modalities together or in succession is not uncommon. The type and severity of the side effects depend on many factors, such as the type of disease, chemotherapeutic agents, and anatomical site of the radiation therapy portal. Aggressive systemic treatment (chemotherapy) may cause acute problems, including fever, neutropenia, mucositis, nausea, vomiting, and diarrhea. In addition to erythema in the irradiation field, these acute side effects are often enhanced by irradiation, depending on the location and size of the radiation fields. The use of radiation therapy in the treatment of primary bone cancer is limited. If metastatic bone disease is treated, patients may experience some nausea, vomiting, and diarrhea if the treatment portal includes any of the stomach or bowel. This is avoided when possible by limited fields or the blocking of these tissues.

Knowing when to withhold treatment (until a physician can be consulted) because of factors such as skin breakdown or a low blood count (white blood cell count $<2000/mm^3$ or platelets $<50,000/mm^3$) is critical to effective patient care. In the treatment of patients with metastatic cancer to the bone, care must also be taken to observe and evaluate the patient's condition for further metastatic spread of the disease. This can be done by questioning the patient and family members and observing the patient.

Subacute and late changes of edema, fibrosis, contractures, and growth arrest can often be avoided or minimized through the use of an optimal technique. If radiation is used in children, the treatment portal may include the growth plates for the treatment of long bones causing growth deficits. Patients treated with doses of 60 to 65 Gy have been known to develop oteosarcoma in bones previously treated for Ewing's sarcoma. Another complication is the development of leukemia in these patients who have been treated with megavoltage techniques and chemotherapy. Acute and late cardiac damage have been noted in patients who have received doxorubicin; this is a major consideration for planning a patient's course of treatment (limiting radiation doses to the heart). In addition, sterility, endocrine dysfunctions, and an increased risk of hemorrhagic cystitis are concerns of physicians planning a course of treatment for patients receiving pelvic irradiation combined with cyclophosphamide.[2]

Patients undergoing treatment for Ewing's sarcoma are clearly at great risk for developing second primaries, leukemias, cardiac damage, and many other problems. Therefore continued follow-up for an indefinite time is necessary to intervene before the complication becomes uncontrollable. Despite the efforts of all the physicians involved, many of these patients ultimately die a premature death as a result of the disease or a complication resulting from treatment. At the time of the diagnosis, all of the complications (acute and long term) need to be considered before a course of treatment is planned. Modifications may be necessary for obtaining the best technique while trying to prevent some of the complications. In general, the side effects experienced by patients with primary bone cancer are fairly well tolerated.

Because the amputation of a limb is sometimes necessary to control the disease, the use of prosthetic devices allows patients to lead a somewhat normal life. If, however, patients survive into adulthood, they are at a high risk for developing a second malignancy. This makes follow-up care and close monitoring of these patients extremely important.

Role of radiation therapist

The therapist's relationship with the patient is based on trust, professionalism, and knowledge of the disease. Patients usually establish trust in the staff members quite early in the course of treatment. This is especially obvious when patients confide in the therapist for information about the disease, side effects, and technical aspects of the treatment. The therapist's willingness to educate the family regarding the treatment process and its side effects reassures patients of their individuality in the radiation therapy setting. Everyone involved in the care of the patient needs to fully understand the importance of daily treatments and the nature and severity of expected side effects. In this section, several roles of the radiation therapist are discussed, including the following areas: education, communication, assessment, and management of accessory medical equipment.

Education. Information concerning the management of the patient's disease is partially the responsibility of the radiation therapist. Helping the patient understand the goals and objectives of treatment and the potential side effects is achieved through education (providing information and teaching). Printed information available through the National Cancer Institute or the American Cancer Society is one helpful method in providing general information about the disease process, potential side effects, and nature of the treatment. Radiation therapists should follow up regarding this information during the first few days of the patient's treatment. The therapist needs to know whether the patient has had time to look over the pamphlets and whether the patient has any questions regarding the information.

In a study by Rainey,[10] two groups of patients undergoing their first course of radiation therapy were tested regarding the information they received. One group participated in a 12-minute slide-tape presentation that explained the way the department personnel, equipment, and related technical procedures worked together to produce a treatment plan and deliver a prescribed dose of radiation therapy. The other group of 30 patients received a brochure to read. The data collected in the study showed that patients in the slide-tape group displayed increased understanding, lower anxiety levels, and better coping skills than the group receiving the brochure only. However, at the end of the treatment, both groups demonstrated equal levels of knowledge regarding their treatment. According to the data from the study, radiation therapy patients desire knowledge about their treatment, and continued intervention can have a positve effect on the patient.

Patients depend on the therapist to explain the technical aspects of the treatment. This explanation may include a brief description of the machine's components, movements, and noises. Weekly port films, scheduled blood tests, and the importance of the patient remaining still during the treatment should be communicated. Patients should be allowed time to reflect on the information before their understanding is checked.

Some patients desire more information than others about their treatment. In fact, some patients may do research at the library or on the internet regarding the role of radiation therapy, surgery, and chemotherapy in the management of their disease. Other patients want to know as little as possible and leave all the details to the cancer management team or another family member. Some patients are just too sick to take an active role in their own care. The therapist should provide as much or as little information as appropriate. If unable to answer a patient's question right away, the therapist should refer the patient to another member of the cancer management team or provide an answer later.

Communication. Radiation therapy, more than other areas of medicine, can cause fears, misunderstanding, and anxiety in many people. This is partly due to its early use to palliate the "dying" patient and a general lack of knowledge by most of its curative potential. Some people today confuse the older role of radiation therapy as they try to understand its application in their own lives. Proper communication and education can help overcome these fears and misunderstanding.

Some patients are quite good at keeping their real needs from the people who can help them the most. Because patients are afraid the disease is progressing, they minimize their symptoms, become more passive, and communicate less, fearing that more information may mean more bad news. Patients may be embarrassed to tell staff members about financial difficulties, transportation problems, or fears of treatment. Because they are in contact with patients daily, radiation therapists may be sensitive to the subtle comments from patients indicating a financial or emotional need. Several patient and family responses to radiation therapy are described by Weintraub.[13] These responses include a fear of treatment, implications of daily treatment, a loss of control over health and destiny, treatment-related side effects, and the financial implications of treatment. Consistent and effective communication on the part of the therapist can alleviate many of the fears and anxieties associated with the cancer diagnosis and treatment.

Assessment. Appraising and evaluating the patient's condition before, during, and after daily treatment is important for good cancer management of bone tumors and even more so for patients treated with metastatic bone cancer. Questioning and observing the patient before treatment can provide information on the condition of the patient's skin, bone or soft tissue pain, fatigue, or other acute side effects associated with the treatment. In the treatment of patients with metastatic cancer to the bone, care must also be taken to observe and evaluate the patient's condition for further metastatic spread of the disease.

Monitoring the patient during the administration of treatment is important to ensure the patient's safety and adequate dose distribution. This is especially true for pediatric patients who may need anesthesia, depending on the age of the patient and extent of the disease. Time spent with the patient and/or family after the treatment can provide an excellent opportunity to appraise and evaluate the patient's condition. The therapist needs to spend individual time with each patient, answering questions, assessing needs, and providing a listening ear. In addition, the radiation therapist must recognize medical emergencies such as allergic reactions, medical disorders, and cardiac arrest.

Monitoring medical equipment. Patients treated for bone tumors may range from the extremely old (those with metastatic disease) to the extremely young (those with Ewing's sarcoma). The needs of these patients and the accessory medical equipment used also varies. This equipment may include intravenous fluids, oxygen, a urinary catheter, a chest tube, or even a shunt to drain excess fluid. Care must be taken to position and monitor the various types of equipment. More than likely, children and hospitalized patients such as those treated for widespread bone metastases will require more intense monitoring of accessory medical equipment.

Case Study

CASE I

A 36-year-old woman with a 1-year history of symptoms initially experienced a cracking sensation along the anterior left horizontal ramus of the mandible after opening her mouth widely. When pain developed with the cracking, she sought medical attention. The physician advised her to wait 2 weeks to see if the pain resolved. After 1 month, she returned to the physician because of increased pain. Radiographs demonstrated a suspicious lytic lesion. The patient agreed to a biopsy, which revealed an osteogenic sarcoma of the mandible.

Through consultations with the medical oncologist, surgical oncologist, and radiation oncologist, a plan of action was established. The plan called for the patient to receive two cycles of chemotherapy initially, followed by a surgical resection, two more cycles of chemotherapy, radiation therapy to the mandibular bed, a bone graft implantation, and two more cycles of chemotherapy.

The patient received her first two cycles of chemotherapy, which included Adriamycin, platinum, high-dose methotrexate, and leucovorin. She tolerated the chemotherapy fairly well, except for some morbidity from the platinum. She was then scheduled for the surgical resection, with the placement of an appliance to retain the shape of her face. She tolerated this procedure and adapted to the prosthesis quite well. After an adequate recuperation period the patient received another cycle of chemotherapy, followed by radiation therapy. She received a dose of 5000 cGy over a 5-week period.

The physician advised the patient to return for routine follow-up visits because of the aggressive nature of her disease. She followed his advice diligently, keeping her appointments as scheduled. This patient continues to be disease free three years after treatment.

CASE II

A 52-year-old woman with a 2-year history of left calf pain and a 1-week history of dyspnea sought medical attention because the shortness of breath she experienced made work difficult. On examination the physician observed labored breathing by the patient and a mass in the left calf. The physician ordered a chest x-ray film and left lower leg radiographs. The chest x-ray film revealed multiple bilateral pulmonary metastases with consolidation in the right lower lung base. The left lower leg radiograph indicated a soft tissue mass that was suspicious for a malignant process. Biopsy results revealed a well-differentiated fibrosarcoma of the left calf, and pulmonary washings were positive for metastatic sarcoma.

An additional metastatic work-up included a CT scan of the chest, abdomen, and pelvis; an MRI scan of the lower leg; and a bone scan. The CT scan of the chest revealed extensive bilateral pulmonary metastases with a localized right pleural effusion. The bone scan showed a vague increased uptake in the left lower leg over the proximal fibular shaft, compatible with a periosteal reaction from a sarcoma. The MRI of the left lower leg revealed a 10×15 cm lesion deep in the posterior aspect of the left lower leg. The tumor abutted the proximal tibia and midtibia, with no evidence of cortical destruction. The patient's disease was staged as follows: T_2 N_O M_1 (lung).

Given all the options, the patient decided against surgery because of the morbidity involved; removal of the tumor would result in a large surgical deficit. She had an extensive vacation planned to visit family that she had not seen in several years, and it was important for her not to have difficulty walking.

The patient was immediately started on six cycles of chemotherapy using the following drugs: mesno, Adriamycin, isophosphamide, and DTIC (MAID). She tolerated the chemotherapy quite well, complaining of fatigue, alopecia, nausea, and vomiting (controlled with antiemetics). Her hematological status remained stable throughout the six cycles of drugs. After the completion of chemotherapy a repeat MRI scan of the lower leg and a chest x-ray film were obtained with positive results. The MRI scan demonstrated a significant reduction in the size of the tumor. The chest x-ray film revealed an excellent response with almost complete resolution of the bilateral pulmonary metastases and a complete resolution of the right localized pleural effusion.

Because the patient continued to complain of pain in the left lower leg, she was referred to the radiation oncology department for a consultation. The radiation oncologist considered all the options, including surgical intervention. Because surgery required the removal of the gastrocnemius muscle (lower calf muscle), causing a functionally impaired foot drop, the radiation oncologist decided to administer radiation therapy for the palliation of pain. High doses of radiation are needed to adequately control this disease. Therefore the radiation oncologist planned to deliver 5000 cGy in 20 fractions at 250 cGy per fraction, which is a slightly accelerated fractionation because the patient had a planned vacation. If after 5000 cGy was reached her chest x-ray film demonstrated the disease to be in remission, an additional 1250 cGy would be delivered to a reduced field. The patient tolerated her treatments quite well with minimal side effects. The patient had less pain and was encouraged to take her vacation and return for a follow-up.

After returning from her vacation (which was about 2 months after the completion of her treatments) the patient returned for a check-up. Her only complaint was swelling and limping of the left ankle after prolonged walking. The radiation oncologist ordered a chest x-ray, which demonstrated the growth of the pulmonary nodules and some right pleuritic pain. She was sent home and told to call if she had any further problems before her follow-up in 1 month.

Within 3 weeks time, the patient developed some expressive aphagia and was brought into the hospital for a metastatic work-up. A CT scan of the brain revealed a large, solitary lesion in the left frontoparietal region. The patient was started on a high-dose regimen of steroids and palliative radiation therapy to her whole brain. After 3 days of treatment the patient's physician discontinued the treatments. The patient subsequently succumbed to central nervous system disease 2 days later, just 5 months after her initial diagnosis.

CASE III

A 15-year-old female experienced an injury playing field hockey. She had a bruise and some soreness of the right pelvic area. After a few weeks the bruise and soreness persisted, so her parents started taking her to their family chiropractor. This went on for approximately 4 months with no relief. The girl's parents then made an appointment for her to see a physician. After a physical examination the physician noted a large right pelvic mass obscuring the right iliac crest. This prompted an immediate investigation. An ultrasound of the pelvis was obtained, revealing a right pelvic mass. Radiographs of the pelvis were then ordered and demonstrated an onion-skin appearance of the bone involving the right iliac crest with extensive soft tissue involvement, indicating a possible Ewing's sarcoma. Arrangements were then made to obtain a biopsy of the area for confirmation of the diagnosis. This was carried out a few days later, and the diagnosis of Ewing's sarcoma was confirmed.

Within the next few weeks, several consultations were scheduled with surgical oncologists, medical oncologists, and radiation oncologists. A metastatic work-up was performed during this time. The patient and her parents decided to initiate chemotherapy using vincristine, Adriamycin, and Cytoxan in hopes of reducing the size of the tumor, which measured 10 × 15 cm. If chemotherapy resulted in regression of the tumor, surgical intervention would be considered.

The patient was started on her first course of chemotherapy, and after 2 months a dramatic regression in the soft tissue disease was noted. The tumor measured 3 × 2 cm, making surgery feasible. She was asymptomatic, except for alopecia from the chemotherapy, and had no complaints of limping or difficulty walking. She was then referred back to the surgical oncologist.

Because of the location of the tumor, surgical intervention was possible but not without risks. If the patient chose surgery, she would have a large scar around her waist and probably significant functional deficit of the right leg. The use of surgery would, however, increase the chance of local control and decrease the chance of a second malignancy caused by radiation therapy. With that information in mind, the patient and family were sent for a radiation oncology consult so they could make a decision on her extended management.

The radiation oncologist explained the immediate and long-term effects of radiation therapy. These included a possible second malignancy, intestinal obstruction, fatigue, diarrhea, and cramping. Considering all the information provided by the surgical and radiation oncologists, the patient opted for radiation therapy.

The plan was to deliver 4500 cGy through opposed anteroposterior/posteroanterior (AP/PA) portals with a 4-cm margin. After 4500 cGy was reached the area would receive a boost to 5580 cGy through opposed oblique portals to spare the anterior bowel. The patient tolerated the treatments fairly well, except for some hematological depletions as a result of radiation therapy and chemotherapy being given at the same time. These depletions required unscheduled hospital admissions and transfusions.

Approximately 2 months after the completion of the treatment, she had a follow-up visit. No complaints were noted from the radiation therapy directly, but fatigue lingered partly because of the chemotherapy and radiation therapy. The decision was made for the patient to continue with her scheduled course of chemotherapy, with careful monitoring of her blood values.

Approximately 6 months after the initial diagnosis the patient was admitted for her final round of chemotherapy and was doing well. She tolerated her chemotherapy treatments without much morbidity and was discharged home. She was still disease free 1 year later.

Review Questions

Multiple Choice

1. The incidence rate of bone cancer is highest during which of the following?
   a. Infancy
   b. Adulthood
   c. Adolescence
   d. Equal for all ages
2. A nonosseous malignant tumor of the marrow is which of the following?
   a. Fibrosarcoma
   b. Chondrosarcoma
   c. Osteosarcoma
   d. Multiple myeloma
3. Bone lesions resulting from primary sites elsewhere in the body are which of the following?
   a. Osteosarcoma
   b. Multiple myeloma
   c. Metastatic disease
   d. Chondrosarcoma
4. The most common site of a primary bone sarcoma is which of the following?
   a. Epiphyseal
   b. Metaphyseal
   c. Diaphyseal
   d. None of the above
5. Neoplasms are seen in adult tissues affected by metabolic stimulation from which of the following?
   a. Long-standing Paget's disease
   b. Long-standing fracture
   c. Long-standing sarcoma
   d. Long-standing metastasis
6. Prognostic indicators for patients with primary bone cancer include all except which of the following?
   a. Age
   b. Gender
   c. Location
   d. Weight

7. The most common site of metastasis from primary bone cancer is which of the following?
   a. Brain
   b. Bowel
   c. Lung
   d. Distal extremities
8. Malignant plasma cell tumors are known as which of the following?
   a. Multiple myeloma
   b. Giant cell tumors
   c. Fibrosarcoma
   d. Melanoma
9. Which of the following is used in treating metastatic bone disease resulting from primary prostate or breast cancer?
   a. Technetium 99
   b. Iodine 131
   c. Strontium 89
   d. Iodine 125
10. The most common prognostic factor in Ewing's sarcoma is which of the following?
    a. Gender
    b. Age
    c. Extent of the disease at the time of the diagnosis
    d. Height

Questions to Ponder

1. Explain why patients with Ewing's sarcoma of the pelvis carry a poorer prognosis than patients with the same tumor of an extremity.
2. Define *skip metastases* and explain how radiation therapy can be used to treat these lesions.
3. Describe the shrinking-field technique and how it is used to control skeletal lesions.
4. Explain the difficulty in diagnosing primary bone tumors and the challenge that physicians face.
5. Define *limb-sparing surgery,* and describe its use in treating primary bone tumors.

REFERENCES

1. American Cancer Society: *Cancer response system, malignant bone tumors,* #406057, Atlanta, 1996, The Society.
2. DeVita VT Jr, Hellman S, Rosenberg SA: *Cancer: principles & practice of oncology,* Philadelphia, 1993, JB Lippincott.
3. Holleb AI, *Clinical oncology,* Atlanta, 1991, The American Cancer Society.
4. Maine Medical Center, Nursing Service: Strontium 89, 1994, The Center.
5. Marieb E: *Human anatomy & physiology,* Redwood City, California, 1989, Benjamin-Cummings.
6. Moss WT: *Radiation oncology,* ed 6, St Louis, 1989, Mosby.
7. Niederhuber J E: *Current therapy in oncology,* St Louis, 1993, Mosby.
8. Perez CA: *Principles & practice of radiation oncology,* Philadelphia, ed 1, 1987, JB Lippincott.
9. Perez CA: *Principles & practice of radiation oncology,* Philadelphia, ed 2, 1992, JB Lippincott.
10. Rainey L: *Effects of preparatory patient education for radiation oncology patients,* Cancer 56: 1056-1061, 1985.
11. Rubin P: *Clinical Oncology,* Atlanta, 1983, The American Cancer Society.
12. Rubin P: *Clinical Oncology,* Philadelphia, 1993, WB Saunders.
13. Weintraub FN: Coping with cancer treatment: family response to radiation therapy. In Dow KH, and Hilderly LJ, editors: *Nursing Care in Radiation Oncology,* Philadelphia, 1992, W. B. Saunders.

BIBLIOGRAPHY

Rubinstein Z Morag B: The role of radiology in the diagnosis and treatment of osteosarcoma. In Katznelson A, Nerubay J, editors: *Osteosarcoma: new trend in diagnosis and treatment,* New York, 1982, Alan R Liss.

Sapherson DA, et al: Atypical progression of multiple myeloma with extensive extramedullary disease, *J Clin Pathol* 47(3): 269-271, 1994.

Sim, FH, Ivans JC, Pritchard DJ: Surgical treatment of osteogenic sarcoma at the Mayo Clinic, *Cancer Treat Rep* 62:205, 1978.

Thomas PRM, et al: The management of Ewing's sarcoma: role of radiotherapy in local control, *Cancer Treat Rep* 68:703, 1984.

Trigg ME, Glaubiger D, Nesbit ME: The frequency of isolated CNS involvement in Ewing's sarcoma, *Cancer* 49:2404, 1982.

Urtasum RC, McConnachie PR: Disappearance of osteosarcoma after irradiation: immunological observations, *J Conad Assoc Radiol* 27:80, 1975.

Van-de-Graff, et al: Primary spinal epidural extraosseous Ewing's sarcoma, *Cancer* 68 (3), 1991.

Watts, HG: Introduction to resection of musculoskeletal sarcomas, *Clin Orthop* 153:31, 1980.

Weichselbaum, RR, Cassady JR: Radiation therapy in osteosarcoma. In Jaffe N, editor: *Solid tumors in childhood,* Boca Raton, Florida, 1983, CRC Press.

Zucker, JM, et al: Intensive systemic chemotherapy in localized Ewing's sarcoma in childhood, *Cancer* 52:415, 1983.

CHAPTER

4

Lymphoreticular System

Sally V. Green

Outline

Key terms

Akimbo
Ann Arbor staging system
Autologous bone marrow transplants
B symptoms
Contiguous
Mantle field
Oophoropexy
Paraaortic field
Peyer's patches
Pruritis
Reed-Sternberg cell
Staging laparotomy
Total nodal irradiation
Waldeyer's ring

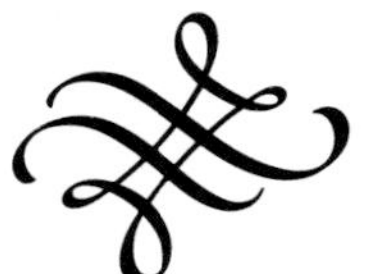

Lymphomas are the predominant cancers of the lymphoreticular system. The two main categories of lymphomas are Hodgkin's disease and non-Hodgkin's lymphoma. Thomas Hodgkin, an English pathologist, identified lymphoma in 1832 as a clinical entity distinct from inflammation. By the end of the nineteenth century, Hodgkin's disease was distinguished from leukemias and other lymphomas. In this century, researchers such as Brill, Symmers, Mallory, Rappaport, Lukes, Collins, Dorfman, and Bernard have continued to further classify and define this extremely diverse group of diseases of the lymphoreticular system.

HODGKIN'S DISEASE

Hodgkin's disease is a type of lymphoma. However, it is treated as a separate category because, unlike lymphomas, it spreads predictably in a systematic or **contiguous** pattern through the lymph system. The **Reed-Sternberg cell** must also be present in the lymph nodes of Hodgkin's patients. This cell is a giant connective tissue cell containing one or two large nuclei. The presence of this cell determines whether the diagnosis is Hodgkin's or non-Hodgkin's lymphoma.

Epidemiology

In the United States approximately 7500 new cases of Hodgkin's disease were reported in 1996, with 1510 deaths.[1] Hodgkin's disease accounts for only 6% of the newly diagnosed cancers per year. Approximately 500 more cases occurred in men than in women, indicating a slight male predominance. Worldwide, Hodgkin's disease is more frequent in developed countries than in undeveloped countries. To date, no explanation exists to account for this phenomenon.

Hodgkin's disease occurs in young people, most commonly those between the ages of 11 and 30, with the median age being 26 years at the time of the diagnosis. Another peak of incidence takes place between 75 and 80 years of age. Hodgkin's disease is rare in children under 10 years of age.

Etiology

The causes of Hodgkin's disease remain a mystery to researchers, who have not yet found conclusive evidence linking Hodgkin's disease to environmental or occupational exposure. Although clusters of patients with Hodgkin's disease are present in some communities, data have been insufficient to determine whether the origin of the disease is viral or contagious. However, components of the Epstein-Barr virus genome are in the cellular deoxyribonucleic acid (DNA) of the Reed-Sternberg cells involved in this disease. A link between a prior infection with the Epstein-Barr virus and Hodgkin's disease has been investigated. (The Epstein-Barr virus is found in the cell cultures of Burkitt's lymphoma and is associated with infectious mononucleosis). Defective T-cell functioning has also been identified as a risk factor.

Prognostic indicators

The histology of this disease has the least effect on the prognosis of a particular patient, whereas the stage of the disease has the greatest effect. In other words, the later the stage, the worse the prognosis. In the later stages, more bulky disease is present, and the risk of a relapse after treatment is greater with increased bulky disease.

More males than females are diagnosed with Hodgkin's disease, and the prognosis is also slightly worse for males. Gender may also influence the choice of treatment, based on a consideration of toxicities to the reproductive system. Fertility may be preserved in most men through the use of radiation therapy, but not with alkylating agents. In women the ovaries cannot be completely protected during radiation therapy, and some women experience menopause after radiation therapy. Youth is a favorable prognostic factor, with younger patients (those in their teens to twenties) doing better than older patients, who cannot tolerate the aggressive treatment. Hodgkin's disease is likewise difficult to manage in children because of the need to limit radiation therapy fields as a result of the effect on a child's growth processes. The extent of the disease, the presence of **B symptoms,** the number of sites of involvement, the presence of the disease in the lower abdomen, splenic involvement, and an elevation of serum markers (such as erythrocyte sedimentation rate) are all factors influencing the natural history of the disease.

Anatomy and lymphatics

A review of the lymphatic system is important for understanding the nature of Hodgkin's and non-Hodgkin's lymphomas. The lymph system originates in the lymphatic capillaries. The capillaries merge to form the lymphatic vessels, which in turn lead to the collecting ducts that unite with the veins in the thorax.

Interstitial fluid enters the lymphatic capillaries, where it is called *lymph*. The vessels formed by the merging capillaries are similar to veins in structure. These vessels lead to the lymph nodes, which contain large numbers of lymphocytes whose function is essential to the immune system.

The kidney-bean-shaped lymph nodes are less than 2 cm in length and enclosed by a capsule of white fibrous connective tissue. The lymph nodes occur in chains or clusters along the lymphatic vessels. The primary function of the lymph nodes is the production of lymphocytes and the filtration of foreign particles and cellular debris from the lymph before it is returned to the circulatory system. The major lymph nodes (Fig. 4-1) are as follows:

1. Waldeyer's ring and cervical, preauricular, and occipital lymph nodes
2. Supraclavicular and infraclavicular lymph nodes
3. Axillary lymph nodes
4. Thorax (includes hilar and mediastinal nodes)
5. Abdominal cavity (includes paraaortic nodes)
6. Pelvic cavity (includes iliac nodes)
7. Inguinal and femoral lymph nodes

After leaving the nodes, the lymph vessels merge to form the larger lymphatic trunks. The trunks drain lymph from large regions of the body and are named for the regions they serve, including the following: lumbar trunk, intestinal trunk, intercostal and bronchomediastinal trunks, subclavian trunk, and jugular trunk. The lymphatic trunks join one of two collecting ducts: the thoracic or right lymph duct. Then the lymph reenters the venous system just before the blood returns to the right atrium of the heart. The thymus and spleen are lymphatic organs whose functions are closely related to the lymph nodes. The thymus contains large numbers of lymphocytes (called *thymocytes*), most of which remain inactive. However, some develop into T lymphocytes, which play a part in the immune process.

The spleen is the largest lymphatic organ. It resembles a large lymph node in its structure, but its cavities are filled with blood instead of lymph. It functions as a blood reservoir. The chambers of the spleen are called *lobules.* Within these lobules are white and red pulp tissues. White pulp is distributed throughout the spleen in small islands. This tissue is composed of lymphatic nodules similar to those found in the lymph nodes filter. The red pulp contains many red blood cells and phagocytes. These phagocytes engulf and destroy foreign particles. Therefore the spleen filters the blood similar to the way lymph nodes filter lymphatic fluid, but through the action of the phagocytes, it destroys damaged red blood cells and the remains of ruptured cells carried in the blood. Of course, the lymphocytes help in the body's defense against infection.

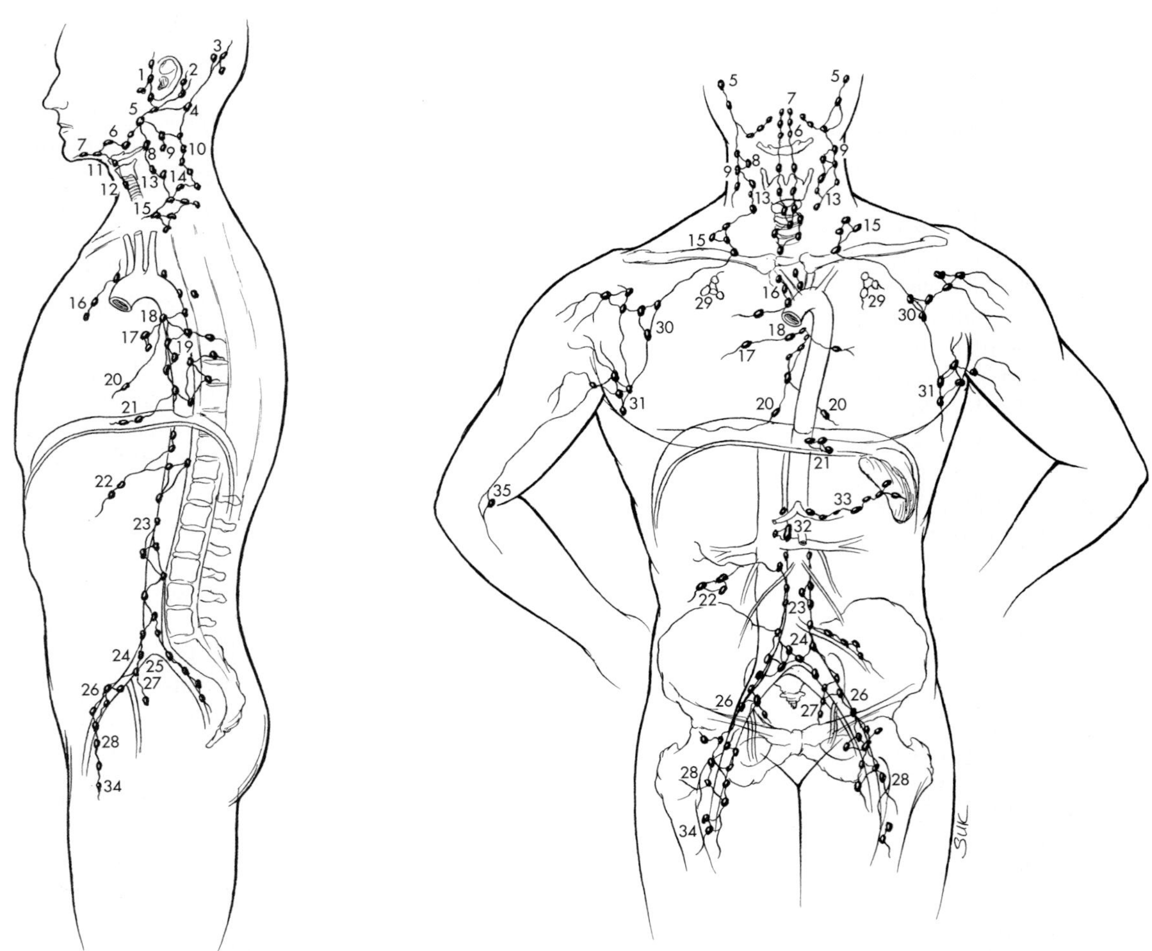

Fig. 4-1 Major lymph node regions of the body. Of particular importance in Hodgkin's disease patients are the spleen and the cervical, supraclavicular, infraclavicular, axillary, hilar, mediastinal, and paraaortic nodes.

Clinical presentation

Hodgkin's disease usually appears as a painless mass that the patient discovers. The most common sites of presentation are in the neck and supraclavicular regions. Mediastinal masses are usually detected on a radiograph of the chest The majority of patients have the disease above the diaphragm.

Approximately one third of the patients also experience the following systemic symptoms: unexplained fevers (over 38° C, or 100.4° F), drenching night sweats, and weight loss of 10% of their body weight in 6 months. These are referred to as *B symptoms*. Generalized **pruritus** (severe itching) and/or alcohol-induced pain in the disease-involved tissues may also be included as B symptoms but are present only in some instances.

Sometimes Hodgkin's disease is discovered during pregnancy, but pregnancy per se has no effect on the natural history. Pregnancy is merely coincidental because of the age group of the patients. Patients testing positive for the human immunodeficiency virus (HIV) are not at a greater risk than the general population for developing Hodgkin's disease. However, if an HIV-infected patient contracts Hodgkin's disease, the disease appears at a more advanced stage and the patient experiences the B symptoms. Treatment for these patients is a challenge because of their poor tolerance for chemotherapy and the occurrence of opportunistic infections.

Detection and diagnosis

Enlarged lymph nodes in the neck, clavicular, or axilla regions are usually the first indication of Hodgkin's disease. As mentioned before, a mediastinal mass is usually discovered on routine chest radiograph. Occasionally, these patients experience a cough, shortness of breath, or chest discomfort. The enlarged node may be the only symptom a patient experiences. However, about one third of the patients have the B symptoms.[4] An enlarged spleen or abdomen, bony tenderness, and pleural effusion indicate a later stage of Hodgkin's disease. Enlarged groin nodes can be an early symptom, although Hodgkin's disease rarely originates in the groin.

The diagnostic work-up includes a complete history and physical examination. Standard laboratory studies should include a complete blood and platelet count, liver and renal function tests, a blood chemistry, and thyroid function tests. Occasionally, patients display anemia, leukopenia, lymphopenia, or thrombocytosis, which may be indicative of bone marrow involvement. A serum alkaline phosphatase level is a nonspecific marker of tumor activity, hepatic bone marrow disease, or bone disease.

Radiographic studies should include a chest x-ray examination, computed tomography (CT) scan, or magnetic resonance imaging scan (MRI) of the thorax for disease detection and treatment planning. A bipedal lymphangiogram is the best assessment method for detecting retroperitoneal lymph node involvement because this test is more sensitive than the CT scan in localizing these nodes. A gallium scan or bone scan is optional but helpful in evaluating the mediastinum and residual disease after treatment.

A bone marrow biopsy should be restricted to patients with B symptoms or subdiaphragmatic disease. Only a 5% chance exists of bone marrow involvement with patients who have Hodgkin's disease.

Before the onset of the CT scan, a **staging laparotomy** was a standard procedure. The laparotomy included a detailed inspection of the abdomen, a splenectomy, selected lymph node biopsies, and liver and bone marrow biopsies. It is a major surgical procedure that requires skill, time, and effort on the part of the surgeon. The purpose for the laparotomy is to determine the extent of the disease, which indicates whether a patient is a candidate for radiation therapy alone. A laparotomy is not necessary if the disease already mandates the use of chemotherapy. Splenectomies are controversial because of the danger of sepsis and the increased risk of secondary leukemia in patients who have also received chemotherapy or radiation therapy. [6] Improved radiographic imaging techniques such as CT, MRI, and ultrasound can in many instances produce similar results to the laparotomy. Some researchers consider MRI superior to CT because it is able to detect bone marrow involvement and lymphadenopathy.[9] Because these imaging modalities are increasingly more available, the use of the staging laparotomy has declined since the late 1970s.

Patients who are candidates for a laparotomy are those who have a high probability of disease below the diaphragm. The spleen is quite involved when the high paraaortic nodes are involved. It is also at risk with lymphocyte depletion or mixed cellularity histologies. The liver biopsy should be done when splenic involvement occurs, but the liver is rarely involved if the spleen is not. A peritoneoscopy with multiple liver biopsies is a viable alternative to the laparotomy. However, a peritoneoscopy cannot view the retroperitoneal lymph nodes.[12] If a physician relies on clinical evidence alone in deciding on a laparotomy, this clinical evidence can be misleading. According to DeVita,[5] the clinical evaluation alone of the splenic involvement is highly inaccurate. Approximately half of the patients believed to have splenic disease, as indicated by the clinical evaluation, will have it at the time a biopsy is taken. In addition, about 25% of the patients thought to have normal spleens will have Hodgkin's disease in the spleen.

Pathology

As mentioned previously, Hodgkin's disease is identified pathologically by the presence of the Reed-Sternberg cell. The following four histological subtypes are designated by the Rye classsification of the Lukes and Butler system:

1. Lymphocyte predominance Hodgkin's disease (LPHD)—This subtype, the most favorable of the four, occurs frequently in young people (those less than 35 years old) and appears with early stage disease. In this subtype are excess normal-appearing lymphocytes and a scarcity of abnormal cells. Fewer than 10% of these patients experience any of the symptoms.
2. Nodular sclerosis Hodgkin's disease (NSHD)—This is the most common subtype in the United States. The mediastinum is often involved in NSHD, and about one third of the patients experience B symptoms. These patients tend to have a less favorable natural history.
3. Mixed cellularity Hodgkin's disease (MCHD)—With MCHD, patients suffer from advanced disease and tend to be slightly older than patients in the previous subtypes. The natural history is worse than NSHD.
4. Lymphocyte depletion Hodgkin's disease (LDHD)—This is the least common subtype in the United States. It occurs in older patients and occurs with advanced disease and B symptoms. LPHD carries the worst prognosis of the four subtypes.

Staging

The **Ann Arbor staging system** has been the accepted method of classification for Hodgkin's disease since 1971 (see the box on p. 68).

These stages can be subdivided into A or B groups. An *A* indicates the lack of general symptoms. For example, Stage IIA may indicate that two or more node regions are involved in the thorax and that the patient has not experienced any of the symptoms, such as fever, night sweats, and weight loss. The presence of these symptoms is indicated by a *B* next to the stage number (e.g., Stage IB). The A or B symptoms can occur in any stage. However, the presence of B symptoms usually indicates a worse prognosis.

Routes of spread

Hodgkin's disease has a predictable pattern of spread, and 90% of the patients have contiguous spread. In other words, the cancer has begun spreading to the adjacent node or region. The rapidity of the growth and spread of the disease, however, are not predictable.

Spread to the viscera occurs after spread to the adjacent lymph nodes. Obviously, visceral spread indicates a higher stage and worse prognosis.

The spleen becomes involved in late stages, and the likelihood of disseminated disease increases with splenic involvement. The liver and/or bone marrow are at increased risk with splenic involvement. Hodgkin's disease can also spread to the lungs and skeletal system in the late stages. It rarely involves the organ systems of the upper aerodigestive tract, central nervous system, skin, gastrointestinal tract, **Waldeyer's ring,** or **Peyer's patches.**

Treatment techniques

Radiation therapy is the primary method of treatment for Hodgkin's disease. Surgery is used *only* for a biopsy to grade and stage the disease or debulk large tumors. Chemotherapeutic agents are used in advanced cases, usually in combination with radiation therapy. Since 1902 patients with Hodgkin's disease have been treated with radiation, but it was not until the 1960s that the current methods were devised by Henry Kaplan et al. at Stanford University. The Stanford group used supervoltage radiation to treat the total lymphatic regions, or **total nodal irradiation.**

The objective of total nodal irradiation is to treat the contiguous lymphatic chains with a cancerocidal dose. The patients are treated with anterior and posterior fields to the supradiaphragmatic lymph nodes (**mantle field**) (Fig. 4-2) and to the subdiaphragmatic lymph nodes (**paraaortic field**). The subdiaphragmatic field always includes the paraaortic nodes, but the extent of the disease determines whether the pelvic, retroperitoneal, and inguinal nodes are also treated. The mantle and paraaortic fields are most commonly treated sequentially, with a break in treatment occurring between fields to enable the patient to recover from the side effects of treatment. These fields require meticulous treatment planning, simulation, and frequent verification films.

A dose of 3500 to 4400 cGy delivered by 6- to 10-MV photons is considered the optimum dose to the mantle and paraaortic fields. A minimum dose is 3000 to 3600 cGy. Fractionation typically is 750 to 1000 cGy per week, delivering 150 to 200 cGy per day, depending on the patient's tolerance to the radiation. The parallel opposed fields are evenly

AJCC Staging Classification for Hodgkin's Disease

Stage I	Involvement of single lymph node region (I) or localized involvement of a single extralymphatic organ or site (IE).
Stage II	Involvement of two or more lymph node regions on the same side of the diaphragm (II) or localized involvement of a single associated extralymphatic organ or site and its regional lymph node(s) with or without involvement of other lymph node regions on the same side of the diaphragn (IIE).
NOTE: The number of lymph node regions involved may be indicated by a subscript (e.g., II_3).	
Stage III	Involvement of lymph node regions on both sides of the diaphragm (III), which may also be accompanied by localized involvement of an associated extralymphatic organ or site (IIIE), by involvement of the spleen (IIIS), or both III(E + S).
Stage IV	Disseminated (multifocal) involvement of one or more extralymphatic organs, with or without associated lymph node involvement, or isolated extralymphatic organ involvement with distant (nonregional) nodal involvement.

From Beahrs OH et al, editors: *AJCC manual for staging of cancer,* ed 4, Philadelphia, 1992, JB Lippincott.

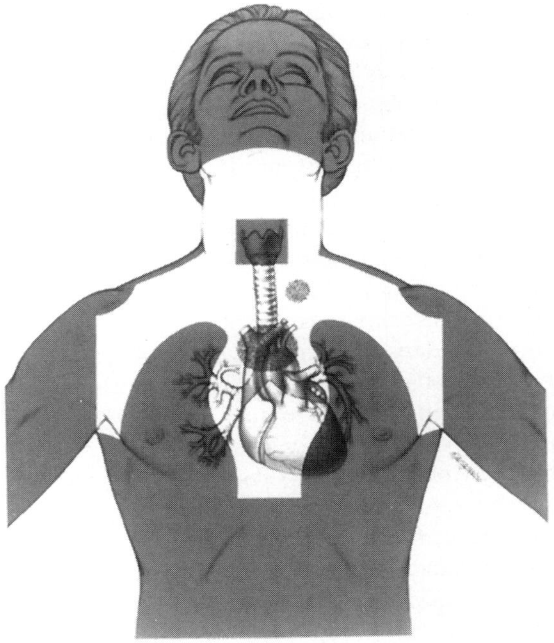

Fig. 4-2 A typical mantle field for the treatment of Hodgkin's disease. Note the blocking of healthy lung tissue and humeral heads. An anterior larynx block and posterior cervical spine block are optional, depending on the location of the affected nodes. The treatment is with parallel opposed anterior and posterior fields. (From Cox JD: *Moss' radiation oncology,* ed 7, St Louis, 1994, Mosby.)

weighted with a ratio of 1:1. The key to this technique is the prophylactic treatment to the clinically uninvolved nodes.[11]

Chemotherapy may be used for any stage but is most commonly used in unfavorable Stages I and II (A or B) and Stages III and IV. The use of chemotherapeutic drugs has led to an improved prognosis for these patients. Originally, the MOPP regimen was developed for patients with Hodgkin's disease.[5] Nitrogen mustard (or mechlorethamine), vincristine, procarbazine, and prednisone comprise the MOPP regimen, but acute toxicities from the chemotherapy were a problem. Side effects included nausea, vomiting, peripheral neuropathy, constipation, leukopenia, and thrombocytopenia. Several regimens that are less toxic have been developed more recently. The regimen of doxorubicin (or Adriamycin), bleomycin, vincristine, and decarbazine (ABVD) has been as effective, if not better, than the MOPP regimen. Other regimens currently in use include the following: VBM (Velban, bleomycin, and methotrexate) and NOVP (Novantrone, Oncovin, vinblastine, and prednisone). An investigational regimen called the *Stanford V* is composed of nitrogen mustard, Adriamycin, Oncovin, bleomycin, etoposide (VP-16), and prednisone.[7]

Chemotherapy is the initial treatment to reduce the bulky disease in these stages. Radiation therapy treatments to limited fields follow the chemotherapy. Sometimes a split course of chemotherapy and radiation is prescribed, with alternating of the treatments. Radiation doses for combined modality treatments vary between 2500 and 4000 cGy. MOPP and ABVD regimens can be delivered alternately to prevent cells from developing a resistance to a particular drug.

Treatment field design, and techniques

Mantle field. A mantle field is illustrated in Fig. 4-2. It includes all major lymph node regions above the diaphragm: submandibular, occipital, cervical, supraclavicular, infraclavicular, axillary, hilar, and mediastinal. Anteriorly, the superior border is at the inferior portion of the mandible, and the inferior border is at the level of the insertion of the diaphragm (usually around T-10). Posteriorly, the superior border includes the occipital nodes, and the inferior border is the same as it is anteriorly (approximately T-10). Laterally, the axillary nodes are included.

Precise blocking is extremely important in this field. As much healthy lung as possible should be spared by blocking the lungs anteriorly and posteriorly; however, adequate margins need to be designed around sites of involvement. Some lung will be radiated because the mediastinal and hilar nodes must be included in this field. Humeral head blocks are also important to prevent future bone destruction, and a larynx block should be included anteriorly unless bulky disease is adjacent to the larynx. Posteriorly, a cord block may be needed, depending on the total dose. A posterior cord block may be used from the outset of treatment or added at 4000 cGy, unless it is contraindicated by the location of the primary tumor.

The cardiac silhouette is irradiated to a dose of 1500 cGy, but then a block shielding the apex of the heart should be added. After 3000 to 3500 cGy a subcarinal block (5 cm inferior to the carina) should also be added to shield more of the pericardium and heart.

If the pulmonary hilar nodes are involved and the patient is treated with radiation alone, partial transmission blocks should be used to deliver a low dose of 1500 to 1650 cGy to the lungs. This is considered an adequate dose for the treatment of occult, microscopic disease.

A large mediastinal mass necessitates modifications of the typical mantle field. In such instances, as the tumor decreases in size, wider lung blocks are added to protect as much lung tissue as possible. With such a mass, treatment is given more slowly: 150 cGy per day to 1500 cGy, followed by a 7- to 14-day break to allow for tumor regression and a redesign of the blocks.

Structures included in the Waldeyer's ring are seldom involved in patients with Hodgkin's disease. However, with such involvement the preauricular nodes must be treated. A small Waldeyer's ring field is also treated when cervical nodes (which are superior to the thyroid notch) are involved. Parallel opposed photon fields, or unilateral 6-MeV or 9-MeV electrons, are used to treat the Waldeyer's ring. The advantage of the electron field is that it spares the contralateral parotid gland. A typical dose to the preauricular nodes is 3600 cGy. Care must be taken to abut the borders of this field with the superior border of the mantle field and to ensure that the teeth are outside of the Waldeyer's ring field.

The mantle treatment may be delivered as an isocenter setup if the size of the patient allows such an isocentric configuration. The treatment distance on some mantle fields needs to be extended to increase the field dimensions. Many of the older linear accelerators have limitations on the field dimensions that are set. For example, if the maximum field size that may be set at 100 cm is 40 × 40 cm and the actual treatment field needs to be 44 × 44 cm, the treatment distance must be extended to 110 cm source-skin distance (SSD). The method to determine the new treatment distance SSD is a simple direct proportion based on the geometrical principle of similar triangles: $44/40 \times 100 = 110$ (new extended SSD). Of course, the time or monitor units need to increase to compensate for the decreased intensity of the beam from extending the distance.

With treatment at extended distances (particularly with older couches), alternating the position of the patient between anterior and posterior fields is usually necessary. For example, the patient is supine for the anterior field and prone for the posterior field. The newer couches, however, accommodate the extended distances better, and the patients may be treated isocentrically without turning over during treatment. However, problems with posterior gapping of the borders between the mantle and paraaortic fields can arise when the patient remains supine. For the treatment of the mantle fields the patient lies supine (for anterior)

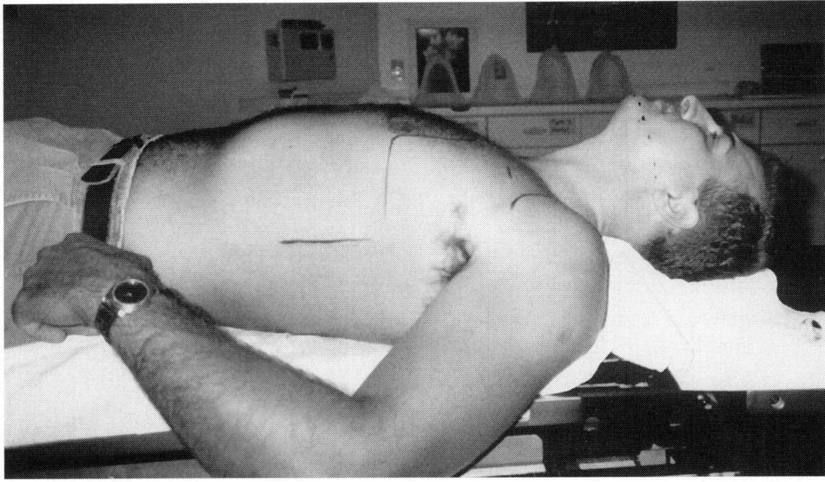

Fig. 4-3 Typical patient positioning for a mantle field. Note the position of the arms (akimbo), the chin position, and the leveling marks on the patient's side.

with the arms **akimbo** (elbows bent) and hands on the hips (Fig. 4-3) or above the head. The chin must be extended as much as possible to prevent exposure to the mouth, particularly from the posterior field. Treatment in the prone position for the posterior field forces the chin superiorly and eliminates the exit dose to the oral cavity. Body molds are helpful in reducing body movement and increasing the patient's comfort.

Inhomogeneous dose distribution. Because of the large field size, treatment at an extended distance, irregular-shaped blocks, and slanting body contours, an inhomogeneous dose distribution occurs in mantle treatments. Because the SSD and depth to the cervical, supraclavicular, axillary, and mediastinal lymph nodes vary so dramatically, so do the doses to these regions. Irregular field calculations need to be done to accommodate for the irregularities. Clarkson developed a method for determining the various doses to the lymphatic regions, and Johns and Cunningham provided further development. This method of calculation is named the *Clarkson integration* and provides estimated doses with an accuracy of about 1-3%.

To determine these various doses, the absorbed doses at various locations of interest in a treatment field are calculated by adding the dose contributions from the scattered radiation to those from the primary radiation. These contributions are derived through the use of zero area tissue-air ratios to predict the dose from the primary radiation and scatter-air ratios to estimate the dose from scattered radiation. [8] Further explanation can be found in Volume 2, Chapter 12 of this textbook series.

Today, this rather lengthy and complex calculation is rarely done by hand except as a didactic exercise. Most radiation therapy centers have computerized dosimetry software programs that calculate these point doses with the use of the Clarkson integration method.

After the doses to various points of interest have been calculated and summarized, a clinical decision must be made. The cervical and supraclavicular lymph node doses are typically higher than the daily and total prescribed doses, whereas the mediastinal doses are more likely to be lower. These dose discrepancies can be handled in numerous ways.

Compensators. One method for reducing the dose variance between the various anatomical points is the use of a compensator during the daily treatment. Compensators, or tissue-compensating filters, are designed and constructed so they compensate for differences in doses at various locations. They are made out of a variety of metals, usually brass blocks, lead, or Lipowitz metal. Compensators are constructed so more metal is placed in the areas of higher dose to absorb the radiation, and less or no metal is placed in the lower dose regions. Compensators are simple to use and easily mounted directly above or below the blocking trays during the daily treatment. The use of compensators to reduce dose variation is desirable because of the positive biological effect of reduction in variation of the daily and total doses between points.

Shrinking-field technique. Another way to reduce the total dose gradient between the various points of interest is the shrinking-field technique. This technique requires additional blocking as each anatomical site reaches the desired or total prescribed dose. The daily dose to each site remains the same, but the additional blocking alters the total doses. If a site needs to continue beyond the prescribed total dose, the additional treatments may be added to that site. This method has a slightly different biological effect on the tissues as a result of the varying daily doses.

Weighting. Most often the daily dose is divided equally, with half delivered to the anterior field and half to the posterior field. This typical division of the dose is referred to as *equal weighting*. The delivery of unequally weighted dose ratios, such as 2:1 or 3:1, is possible and sometimes desirable. For example, a 2:1 weighting for a daily dose of 180 cGy means that 120 cGy would be delivered to the anterior field and 60 cGy to the posterior field. If the patient's disease is more anterior, the weighting of the doses is desirable. A further benefit of this strategy is that it lowers the spinal cord dose.

Subdiaphragmatic fields. The most common treatment of the subdiaphragmatic fields is the treatment of the paraaortic nodes and the spleen or splenic pedicle when no evidence of subdiaphragmatic disease is present. The inferior border of the mantle field determines the superior border, with a gap between to avoid overdosing of the spinal cord. The inferior border is typically L4 or L5, or below the bifurcation of the aorta (Fig. 4-4).

The classic total nodal irradiation technique includes an inverted Y field. Included in the inverted Y field are the retroperitoneal, common iliac, and inguinal lymph nodes. The full inverted Y is seldom treated as a prophylactic measure, but it is treated for subdiaphragmatic disease. Sometimes it is also used for Stage IB or IIB disease. If the pelvis is not included in the treatment fields, the radiation method is referred to as *subtotal lymphoid irradiation*.

Blocking in the subdiaphragmatic fields is also extremely important because of the presence of the liver, kidneys, and bone-marrow-producing pelvic bones and reproductive organs. A low dose to the liver is delivered with partial transmission blocks of 50% to deliver 2000 to 2200 cGy if: (1) the spleen is involved, (2) radiation alone is used as a primary treatment, or (3) the liver is involved.

A lymphangiogram is a valuable tool in delineating the precise location of the lymph nodes to enable the most precise blocking. The ovaries overlie the iliac lymph nodes; therefore an **oophoropexy** can be performed during the staging laparotomy to avoid infertility. During this procedure the ovaries are clipped behind the uterus. A midline block of 10 HVL may then be placed to shield the gonads. In male patients, no special blocking is used to protect the testes unless the inguinal and femoral nodes are irradiated. In such instances, the dose to the testes may be as high as 10%. This dose can be reduced to 0.75% to 3% with the use of a 10-HVL midline block. The inguinal and femoral nodes are treated only if disease appears in these nodes or adjacent to them.

Gapping methods. When extremely large fields are treated above and below the diaphragm, an appropriate separation, or gap, must be left between the fields on the skin surface to account for the normal divergence of the edges of the beams. Typically, this can be accomplished by calculating the gap with the basic geometrical principle of similar triangles. The objective is to have the field edges match at midplane. If too much of a gap is left on the skin between the fields, the field edges will match much deeper than midline and a low dose region will occur just above the match line. If too little of a gap is measured on the skin surface, the opposite will occur. The field edges will match at a much shallower depth in the body, creating a high-dose region from the match line and below (Fig. 4-5).

Side effects. Acute side effects of treatment are numerous because of the size and extent of the fields. The most common side effects are as follows:

- Fatigue
- Occipital hair loss (may be permanent, depending on the dose)
- Mild skin erythemia
- Sore throat
- Altered taste (especially with preauricular nodes)
- Transient dysphagia from radiation-induced esophagitis
- Dry cough
- Nausea
- Occasional vomiting
- Diarrhea (rare)

Most of the side effects are managed by good nursing care, which may include an antiemetic, the application of nongreasy skin creams, protection from sunlight, additional rest, an altered diet (soft, bland foods and no alcohol), throat lozenges, and diarrhea medication. Because the course of treatment is relatively short for each phase of treatment, patients with Hodgkin's disease usually manage their side effects well.

Late-stage complications depend on the treatment technique, total dose, and irradiated volumes. Most of the complications result from the mantle field treatment. They include the following:

- Mild radiation pneumonitis (depending on the volume of the lung treated) 6 to 12 weeks after the end of treatment
- Hypothyroidism in one third of the patients
- Herpes zoster
- Xerostomia, which requires careful, permanent dental care
- Radiation carditis, which occurs in fewer than 5% of the patients
- Lhermittes syndrome, which is a transient complication consisting of numbness, tingling, or electric sensations (caused by the head flexion)

Each of these complications requires individual management. In addition, an increased chance of a second cancer (usually leukemia) exists after treatment with alkylating agents, but leukemia rarely occurs after radiation treatment alone. Secondary solid tumors have a latent period of 7 to 10 years and may be related to the radiation or chemotherapy treatments. Patients seem to be at increased risk for lung and breast cancer after mantle treatment.

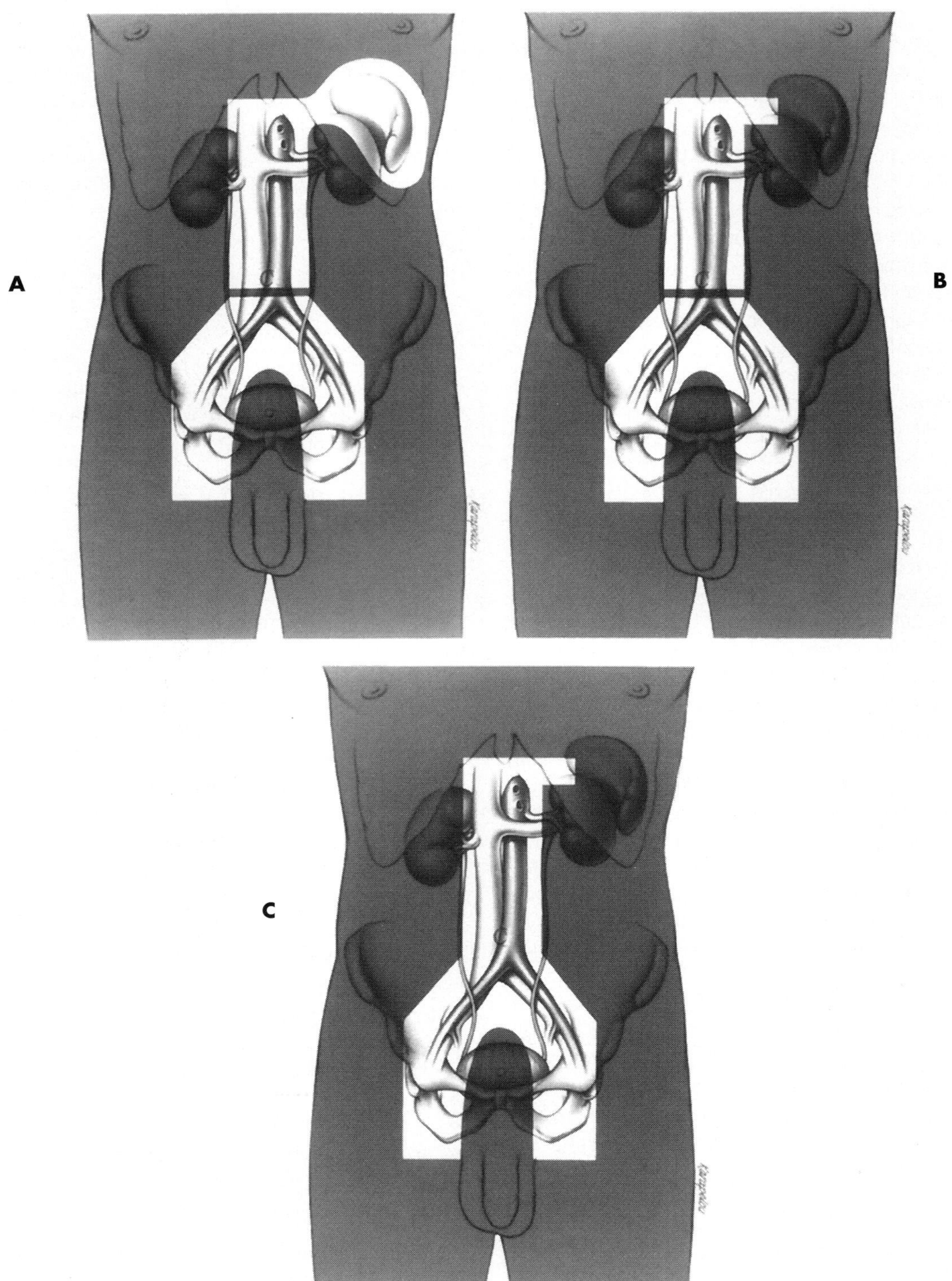

Fig. 4-4 Several treatment alternatives for subdiaphragmatic field arrangements. **A,** The paraaortic field must include the spleen if the spleen is still intact. The pelvic irradiation is done only if subdiaphragmatic disease is present and can be administered separately from the paraaortic fields to improve patient tolerance. **B,** Paraaortic treatment including the lymph nodes of the splenic pedicle after a splenectomy. **C,** Field arrangement when the paraaortic and pelvic fields are treated simultaneously. This is the classic inverted Y technique. (From Cox JD: *Moss' radiation oncology,* ed 7, St Louis, 1994, Mosby.)

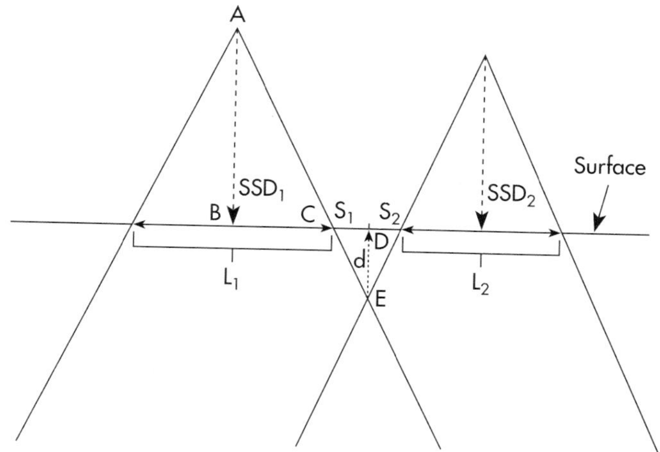

Fig. 4-5 A schematic illustration of the geometry of two adjacent beams that match or join at a given depth, *d*. L_1 and L_2 are the field lengths; SSD_1 and SSD_2 are the source-skin distances. Triangles *ABC* and *CDE* are similar triangles.
Therefore $\frac{CD}{DE} = \frac{BC}{AB}$ and $\frac{S_1}{d} = \frac{L_1}{2} \times \frac{1}{SSD_1}$ (From Khan KM: *The physics of radiation therapy,* ed 2, Baltimore, 1994, Williams & Wilkins.)

Xerospermia can result in men after pelvic irradiation if no precautions are taken. With precautions the sperm count diminishes during treatment but returns to normal levels afterward. The MOPP, but not the ABVD, regimen causes sterility in men.

In women over 30 years old, even with oophoropexy and well-planned pelvic irradiation precautions, the scattered dose may be sufficient to decrease ovarian functions and cause menopausal symptoms. Younger women do not experience these menopausal symptoms. Chemotherapy also affects women similarly. Combined chemotherapy and radiation therapy, however, may affect menstrual function and fertility in younger women.

Psychosocial problems that patients with Hodgkin's disease commonly experience include depression (associated with the low energy levels during treatment), marital difficulties, and a decrease in sexual interest. Patients who have recovered from Hodgkin's disease often have been denied coverage by insurance providers because of an increased risk of later disease.

Results of treatment

The results of treatments cited in this section are from studies conducted at Stanford University from 1974 to 1988 on 1231 patients.[11] This is one of the largest studies of patients who have Hodgkin's disease.

Stages I and IIA. The majority of studies indicate that patients have a 10-year survival rate of approximately 90% with radiation therapy as the only form of treatment. In the Stanford study of 385 patients, 90% of these patients had supradiaphragmatic disease and were treated with mantle radiation from 3600 cGy to 4400 cGy plus a prophylactic paraaortic-splenic pedicle field from 3000 cGy to 4000 cGy. The 10-year relapse-free rate was 75% to 80%. The most favorable presentation is Stage IA (lymphocyte predominant) limited to the high neck with a negative lymphangiogram or nodular sclerosing limited to the intrathoracic nodes. Patients who received combination chemotherapy and radiation had the same survival rate as those who received radiation therapy alone. These combined-modality patients had a lower relapse rate but experienced more severe chronic side effects.

Stages I and IIB. Patients receiving radiation therapy alone have a similar survival rates to patients in Stages I and II A. The 10-year relapse-free rate is 78% to 88%. However, the subgroup that experiences fevers and weight loss has a 10-year-survival relapse-free rate of 48% to 57%, regardless of the type of therapy.

Stages I and II, with bulky mediastinal involvement. Patients in this group have no difference in survival rates as Stages I and IIA, but their relapse rates are as high as 50%. These patients are at special risk for developing complications related to treatment. Usually, chemotherapy is used first to reduce the mediastinal disease and allow for more narrow lung radiation therapy fields.

Subdiaphragmatic Stages I and II. Approximately 10% of patients with Hodgkin's disease have this type of disease. In such instances the subdiaphragmatic fields are treated with the inverted Y and splenic fields. If the spleen is not involved, radiation alone may be used, but treatment above the diaphragm should also be included. If the spleen is involved, the disease should be treated as if it were Stage III.

Stage IIIA. A summary of 11 studies that used combined chemotherapy and radiation showed a 10-year survival rate of about 80 to 90% for patients. With radiation alone the 10-year survival rate declined to 68% to 80%.

Stage IIIB or IV. Systemic MOPP or ABVD is the treatment of choice. The 10-year survival rate is 43% to 51%. In centers that used radiation as an adjunct to chemotherapy, the survival rate for patients increased to 66% to 77%.

Pediatric cases are treated with combined chemotherapy and low-dose radiation therapy (1500 to 2500 cGy). The 5-year survival rate for children in all stages is 90%.

Treatment for relapse must be individualized. Generally, patients who received radiation alone are candidates for chemotherapy. Some researchers recommend the delivery of low-dose radiation (1500 to 2500 cGy) to the previously treated areas after chemotherapy and 3500 to 4400 cGy to the previously untreated areas.

Role of radiation therapist

For patients who have Hodgkin's disease the radiation therapist plays a vital role not only in delivering the radiation, but also in assisting with side-effect management education and offering psychological support during treatment.

Of course, the first priority of the therapist is the accurate delivery of the prescribed radiation dose. Positioning the patient consistently is vital for the accuracy of the treatments. Each day, the therapist must be sure the patient's chin is out of the treatment field and that the superior border lies just inferior to the mastoid tip. The therapist should also check the humeral head blocks for accuracy by palpating the head of the humerus. Leveling marks on the side of patients assist in ensuring that the patient is lying consistently flat. The use of horizontal marks on the shoulders (in alignment with the central axis) as a positioning guide for the arms is also quite helpful. For treatment of the paraaortic field the gap measurement must be done precisely and daily to prevent an overdose or underdose (Fig 4-5).

Accuracy in block placement can mean the difference in shielding disease or in delivering an unnecessary dose to healthy tissue. Custom blocks should always be fabricated because of the complex blocking. Fig. 4-6 demonstrates the use of shielding in a minimantle field. However, institutions differ as to whether they mount the blocks. Some clinics prefer to leave the blocks unmounted because of the frequency that the blocking is changed. Either way, verification films should be taken weekly to ensure accuracy.

Because of the addition of cord blocks, cardiac blocks, and shrinking fields, the maintenance of accurate records is critical. Clear and precise notes should be written in the charts, indicating all blocking changes. Verification films should be taken before changes in blocking, especially before the addition of the cord block.

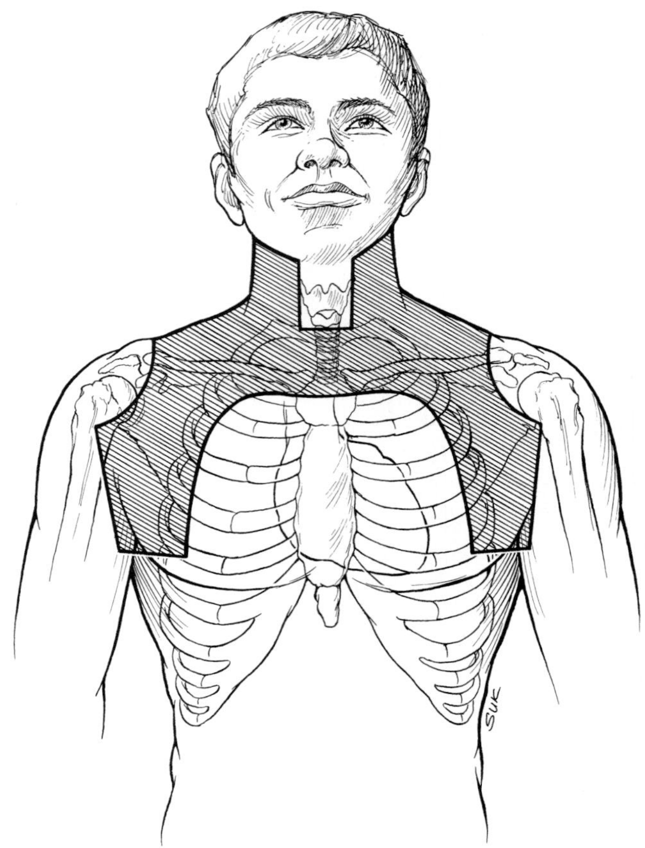

Fig. 4-6 A minimantle, or supramediastinal mantle field, for disease limited to the cervical, supraclavicular, or axilla regions. Note the use of blocks to shield the lungs. Treatment is delivered anteriorly and posteriorly with parallel opposed portals.

The blood counts require rigorous monitoring because the bone-marrow-producing bones are in the fields. Again, the therapist should pay close attention to the counts and ensure that they are taken as prescribed.

Communication is the second priority of a good therapist. The patient must be informed about daily procedures and any additional occurrences, such as port films or new blocking. As the treatment progresses, the therapist plays an important role in the management of side effects. Frequently, the therapist is told first of these side effects. According to institution policies, the therapist may advise the patient regarding the way to handle the side effects or refer the patient to a nurse, dietitian, or physician. Communication with the family (and other professionals involved with the patient's care) about the side effects is also important.

Because of the daily contact with the patient, the therapist is in the position of evaluating the patient's physical and emotional needs . Many times, referral to another agency or individual (such as a social worker, support group, or chaplain) is appropriate.

Case Study

A 28-year-old white female was treated for Hodgkin's disease in 1986. At the time of diagnosis the patient, J.K., had been in good health up to 6 weeks before her initial consultation. She had swelling in her lower neck. A biopsy was taken in August 1986 and revealed NSHD. Her weight had remained stable, she had no energy loss, and she did not exhibit any B symptoms. At the time of the biopsy a chest radiograph also revealed a mediastinal adenopathy, classifying J.K.'s disease as Stage IIA.

The patient had a tonsillectomy at age 4. In 1979 she had a benign lymph node removed from the high cervical area. She smoked lightly in high school and has an occasional glass of wine. She had no family history of cancer, although her maternal grandmother had a bilateral mastectomy for reasons unknown to the patient.

In addition to the biopsy and chest radiograph, a liver function test and CT scan were performed. The outcomes were negative for any abdominal involvement. Therefore the conclusion was made that a bone marrow biopsy was unnecessary. During physical examination the physician did not find any organomegaly, masses, inguinal adenopathy, nor epitrochlear lymphadenopathy. J.K. was also presented to a tumor board. The tumor board recommended a lymphangiogram to serve as an additional diagnostic procedure and assist in the treatment planning. The consensus of the tumor board was that radiation alone would be the optimal treatment for this patient.

J.K. was treated with parallel-opposed mantle fields to 4140 cGy in 25 fractions (180 cGy per day) over 35 elapsed days with 6-MV photons. The mantle field measured 33 × 29.5 cm anteriorly and 31 × 29.5 cm posteriorly, both at 105 cm source-skin distance (SSD). She was treated in the supine position for the anterior field and the prone position for the posterior field.

After a month break from the completion of the mantle fields, she received radiation therapy to the paraaortics and spleen anteroposterior/posteroanterior (AP/PA) to 3960 cGy in 22 fractions over 29 elapsed days. This field measured 25 × 17 cm and was treated at 105 SSD in a spade field configuration. The superior border was T-10, and the inferior border was between S-1 and S-2.

During the mantle field treatment, J.K. experienced severe nausea and vomiting, beginning after the third fraction. Compazine was given without much relief, followed by Reglan at 1620 cGy (9 fractions). The Reglan brought some minor relief, but on the fifteenth treatment, intramuscular injections of HexaBetaline were given and resulted in dramatic improvement. During this time, J.K. lost 10 pounds and experienced headaches, a sore throat, and a dry mouth. She also had difficulty swallowing. She was instructed to drink tepid liquids, and she was given throat lozenges and Tylenol #3. By the end of the mantle treatment course, she had regained two of the pounds she had lost.

J.K. tolerated her paraaortic treatments better. When she returned 1 month after the completion of the mantle field, she was feeling better, was eating well, and had good energy levels. She experienced some nausea and vomiting, which were relieved by Reglan at 3060 cGy. Her total weight loss during the last half of treatment was only 3 3/4 pounds.

About 1 month after the completion of her treatments, J.K. experienced a herpes outbreak on her right chest wall, which cleared in about a week. She experienced no other late or chronic side effects.

In 1988 J.K. gave birth to a second child. In 1991 a suspicious nodule appeared in her neck and was removed. The biopsy revealed it to be benign. She remains free of any evidence of disease 8 years after the diagnosis.

NON-HODGKIN'S LYMPHOMA

Non-Hodgkin's lymphoma (NHL) is the second type of cancer of the lymph system and may arise anywhere that the lymph travels. Malignant lymphomas occur in the lymph nodes, a group of lymph nodes, an organ such as the stomach or lung, or any combination of these. NHLs differ from Hodgkin's disease in several ways, including the following:

1. They occur primarily in older persons. The median age is 50.
2. They can originate in the lymph nodes or in extranodal tissue.
3. They are more likely to spread randomly, rather than orderly as Hodgkin's disease does.
4. They encompass a wide variety of diseases, which the experts continue to attempt to classify into appropriate categories.

Epidemiology

The incidence of lymphomas has increased 65% since the 1970s. The most recent projections from the American Cancer Society estimate 52,700 new cases in the U.S. in 1996 and 23,300 deaths from NHL in 1996.[1] The male-to-female ratio is similar to that of Hodgkin's disease in that there is a slight male predominance ratio of 1.7:1. Worldwide, the incidence of NHL varies greatly from country to country. For example, Burkitt's lymphoma is common in Africa and New Guinea but rare in other countries, although patients with acquired immunodeficiency syndrome (AIDS) tend to get this form of lymphoma. NHLs are rare in rural Poland but common in non-Jewish Israel.

Etiology

There seems to be increasing evidence of a viral association with lymphomas. Burkitt's lymphoma, Mediterranean lymphoma, and T-cell leukemia/lymphoma have viral features. Serological (blood) studies have shown an association between human T-cell leukemia/lymphoma virus (HTLV-1) and T-cell leukemia/lymphoma. The HTLV-1 virus has been isolated in patients with T-cell lymphoma/leukemia in Japan. NHL is also seen with increasing frequency in patients who have AIDS and in other immunosuppressed patients, such as those having heart and kidney transplants.

People exposed to ionizing radiation are at a greater risk of developing lymphomas. There is an increased incidence of lymphocytic and histiocytic lymphoma in atomic bomb survivors who were exposed to 100 cGy or more. Patients who received radiation therapy for ankylosing spondylitis (a chronic inflammatory disease affecting the spine, which was formerly treated with radiation) are at risk for contracting lymphomas. There is also an increased incidence in patients who take phenytoin to control seizures, in agricultural workers exposed to herbicides, and in industrial workers exposed to solvents and vinyl chloride. Patients who have received chemotherapy are also at an increased risk of developing NHL.

Aside from the histology of the disease, age is an important prognostic factor. The younger the patient, the better the prognosis because older patients have less tolerance to the treatment.

Clinical presentation

The signs and symptoms of NHL are similar to those of Hodgkin's disease. Unlike Hodgkin's disease, however, NHL may arise in a wide variety of sites, most commonly in the lymph nodes, gastrointestinal tract, and the Waldeyer's ring. Lymphomas of the central nervous system commonly occur in AIDS patients.

Clinically, lymphomas can appear as enlarged nodes or are discovered when the patient has symptoms related to the site and extent of tumor involvement. For example, shortness of breath or a cough is symptomatic of lung involvement. Abdominal pain or a change in bowel habits may indicate pelvic disease. Symptoms of brain involvement are headaches, vision problems, and seizures. Disease outside the lymph system is more common in intermediate- and high-grade lymphomas. Generally, when the lymphoma occurs outside the nodes, such as in the gastroinestinal tract or central nervous system, the course of disease is worse. The Waldeyer's ring is the least worrisome of all of the extranodal sites.

Systemic symptoms (as seen in Hodgkin's disease patients) are rare, occurring in only 10% to 15% of the patients at the time of presentation, and no conclusive evidence exists as to whether the presence of symptoms plays a part in the overall prognosis. Distinguishing the importance of the histology from that of the stage of disease is difficult.

Detection and diagnosis

The diagnostic work-up defines the extent of the disease and assists in the decision on the treatment course. The history and physical examination are, of course, the standard first steps, as are the bone marrow biopsy and cytological evaluations. Included in the blood tests are a complete blood count, an HIV test, a blood chemistry, a urinalysis, serum lactate dehydrogenase (LDH), liver function tests, and serum alkaline phosphatase. A chest radiograph; a CT of the abdomen, pelvis, neck and chest; and a bone scan are also part of the first line of diagnostic tests.

Sometimes a staging laparotomy or peritoneoscopy with a liver biopsy are done, especially if a late stage of disease is suspected. The staging laparotomy procedure is as controversial for lymphoma patients as for Hodgkin's disease patients. Many times it does not influence the decisions regarding therapy; therefore the laparotomy is difficult to justify.

Further diagnostic tests may include a gallium whole-body scan, upper gastrointestinal or small bowel series. A CT scan of the brain may be recommended if previous tests or symptoms indicate possible disease at these sites. A lymphangiogram of the pelvis and abdomen are done if the CT scan shows abnormal results.

Most of the lymphoma patients are older and have advanced disease. Their age is another reason for the choice of the CT scan in lieu of the laparotomy. If the CT scan shows normal results, a lymphangiogram is still valuable because it gives specific information about the status of the retroperitoneal nodes. If radiation therapy becomes a mode of treatment, the lymphangiogram is extremely valuable in localizing the treatment fields. The gallium scan is useful after treatment for the evaluation of residual masses.

Pathology

The two types of cells in the lymph system are B cells (which make antibodies) and T cells (which are responsible for the regulation of the immune system). The majority of lymphomas in the United States are of B-cell origin.

Features that best predict the prognosis of lymphomas are size, shape, and pattern of the cells. Small and round or angulated cells are called *cleaved cells.* Others may be large or combinations of small and large. Intermediate-sized lymphocytes with rapidly dividing cells are characteristic of aggressive, high-grade lymphomas.

In the normal lymph nodes are microscopic clusters or follicles of specialized lymphocytes. In lymphomas, some lymphocytes arrange themselves in a similar pattern called a *follicular,* or *nodular, pattern.* These lymphomas and small cell lymphomas tend to be low grade and follow a chronic course with an average survival time for patients of 6 to 12 years.

The more aggressive lymphomas (intermediate and high grade) lose their normal appearance by the diffuse involvement of tumor cells that are usually moderate or large sized.

Lymphomas can be histopathologically classified as nodular (or follicular) and diffuse, with 40% appearing as nodular and 60% as diffuse. The nodular lymphomas are of B-cell origin and tend to run an indolent course with prolonged survival. Although many patients have advanced disease, the median survival for patients with nodular or follicular types is 5 to 7 years. Nodular lymphomas usually appear below the diaphragm, and the involvement of the mesenteric lymph nodes is common. Children seldom get nodular lymphomas, nor do these lymphomas commonly involve the Waldeyer's ring.

Diffuse lymphomas can be of B- or T-cell origin and run a more aggressive course. Ironically, they usually appear with more localized disease, but they spread quickly to other nodes and extranodal sites. There is also an increase in bone marrow and Waldeyer's ring involvement. The lymphatics are the most common site of recurrence with either type.

Grading. The establishment of a grading system for NHL has continually evolved since the 1950s because research continually reveals new characteristics of this complex disease process. The Rappaport classification (Table 4-1), which was established in the 1950s, distinguished patients by survival differences. Not only did this system require the expert interpretation of biopsy results, but it was developed when relatively little was known about the functions of the immune system and contained scientific inaccuracies, such as the term *histiocytic* for tumors of transformed lymphocytes. In addition, lymphomas commonly progress from low to high grade during the course of the disease. This factor also makes the Rappaport system less significant.

In the 1970s the Lukes-Collins classification replaced the Rappaport system. The Lukes-Collins system distinguished the B-cell and T-cell lymphomas as separate entities.

The International Working Formulation classification system was adopted for use in 1982. It is a clinicopathological system that represents a compromise categorization based on clinical behavior. The Working Formulation (Table 4-1) system defines 10 subtypes according to morphology, clinical features, and prognosis. It uses the broad divisions of low, intermediate, and high grade to categorize the diseases. For example, the follicular (nodular) histologies are in low and intermediate grades and therefore have a better prognosis than the diffuse histologies. The Working Formulation system emphasizes morphological differences as proposed by Lukes and Collins and takes into account the incidence of multiple histological types that are frequent in lymphomas.

No classification system of NHL is likely to be permanent. Already, new subtypes have been identified that do not fit well into the Working Formulation system. Peripheral T-cell lymphoma is one such subtype.

Staging

Categorizing lymphomas into staging systems is as complex as grading them. As research continues, particularly with HIV patients, additional light is shed onto this disease process. Although the Ann Arbor system is most commonly used for the staging of NHLs, it is not completely satisfactory. In contrast to Hodgkin's disease, many patients with NHL have advanced disease. The Ann Arbor system also fails to account for bulky disease, which plays a significant role in lymphomas because many patients have advanced disease but experience relatively long-term survival rates.

Table 4-1 Histopathological classifications of malignant lymphomas (ML)

Rappaport Classification	Working Formulation
Nodular	**Low grade**
Lymphocytic, well differentiated*	ML, small symphocytic*
Lymphocytic, poorly differentiated	ML, follicular, small-cleaved cell
Mixed, lymphocytic and histiocytic	ML, follicular, mixed small-cleaved and large cell
Histiocytic	
Diffuse	**Intermediate grade**
Lymphocytic, poorly differentiated	ML, diffuse, small-cleaved cell
Mixed, lymphocytic and histiocytic	ML, diffuse, small and large cell
Histiocytic	ML, diffuse, large cell
	High grade
Histiocytic	ML, large cell immunoblastic
Lymphoblastic†	ML, lymphoblastic†
Undifferentiated (Burkitt's lymphoma)‡	ML, small noncleaved cell (Burkitt's lymphoma)‡

Modified from U.S. Armed Forces Institute of Pathology, Washington, DC, 1966; and National Cancer Institute: The non-Hodgkin's lymphoma pathologic classification project: summary and description of a working formulation for clinical use, *Cancer* 49:2112-2135, 1982.
ML, Malignant lymphoma.
*Indistinguishable from chronic lymphocytic leukemia (CLL).
†Indistinguishable from acute T-cell leukemia (ALL).
‡ Indistinguishable from acute β-cell leukemia (ALL).

Although the diaphragm plays an important role in the staging of Hodgkin's disease, it is insignificant in the progression of lymphomas. Therefore a major factor in the Ann Arbor system is inconsequential in NHLs.

Treatment techniques

In determining treatment, the physician must take into account the patient's age and general health, the extent of the disease, and the disease subtype. The most common practice is to administer chemotherapy with or without radiation for most patients. Although it *may* be curative in patients who have localized extranodal NHL, surgery is never recommended as the sole means of treatment. The stage and grade, more than the particular treatment regimen, determines the ultimate outcome of treatment.[11]

Localized disease involving only one site or two immediately adjacent sites, with the tumors less than 10 cm in diameter and no systemic symptoms, has a high likelihood of cure. This may be true for all subtypes, but the majority of studies have been conducted on diffuse, histologically aggressive lymphomas.

More than 50% of patients with diffuse, large cell NHL in Ann Arbor Stage I can be cured with radiation therapy alone.

However, they must undergo extensive staging procedures, including a laparotomy, to establish this stage, and frequently this procedure is not advisable because of the patient's age. Therefore, chemotherapy is also given for most of these patients.

Single-agent chemotherapy can be administered. Vincristine is commonly used as a single agent. However, multiagent chemotherapy has been much more effective. [5] Formerly, the most common treatment for Stage I and non-bulky Stage II diffuse, aggressive NHL was the CHOP regimen (cyclophosphamide, doxorubicin, vincristine, and prednisone), given in three or four cycles and followed by radiation therapy to the involved site and adjacent lymph nodes. The dose of chemotherapy can be reduced by half when radiation therapy immediately follows chemotherapy.

Since CHOP was introduced in the 1970s, there has been no apparent change in mortality from lymphomas in the United States.[2] Therefore new regimens have been developed, including the following[5,7]:

1. C-MOPP (cyclophosphamide, vincristine, procarbazine, and prednisone)
2. BACOP (bleomycin, doxorubicin, cyclophosphamide, and vincristine)
3. COMLA (vyvlophosphamide, vincristine, methotrexate with leucovorin rescue, and cytarabine)
4. mBACOD (high-dose methotrexate, bleomycin, Adriamycin, Cytoxan, and Oncovin and dexamethasone)
5. ProMace-CYTABOM (prednisone, high-dose methotrexate, Adriamycin, Cytoxan, etoposide [VP-16], cytosine arabinoside, and bleomycin and Oncovin)
6. MACOP-B (methotrexate with leucovorin rescue, Adriamycin, Cytoxan, Oncovin, prednisone, and bleomycin)

Procarbazine has proved effective for the treatment of diffuse histiocytic and lymphoblastic lymphomas, but it has not been effective for nodular lymphomas.

Cure is rare for patients with disseminated, low-grade NHL. However, patients who are asymptomatic at the time of the diagnosis can be monitored closely without therapy until symptoms occur, and a substantial portion of these patients have spontaneous remissions. If the symptoms can be improved or the patient is unwilling to proceed without therapy, treatment usually includes radiotherapy, single-agent chemotherapy, or a combination chemotherapy regimen with or without radiation therapy. Complete remissions can be achieved in most patients, and the remissions tend to last for extended periods. Interferon-α has been used successfully in combination with CHOP. Patients receiving this treatment have a longer remission time and a higher rate of survival than those treated with CHOP alone.

Autologous bone marrow transplants are also being conducted on patients with low-grade NHL and those having relapses. In this type of transplant, patients receive their own bone marrow, which has been treated and stored. Early results of trials are quite encouraging. [4]

Current data indicate that 60% to 80% of adults with diffuse, aggressive NHL in Stage II to Stage IV can achieve complete remissions. Long-term, disease-free survival can be achieved in 30% to 50% of these patients. Larger doses of chemotherapy are given to patients who have histologically aggressive disease.[11]

Patients infected with HIV are particularly prone to NHLs. These lymphomas usually have a B-cell origin, are often associated with the Epstein-Barr viral genome in the tumor, and frequently occur in unusual extranodal sites such as the brain. Although it is also common in this population, Burkitt's lymphoma is not usually associated with immunosuppression. Unfortunately, because of their already suppressed immune system, these patients do not tolerate treatment well. If no opportunistic infection occurs, the patients can tolerate some therapy and often respond well to treatment. The choice of chemotherapeutic agents for this population remains controversial.

Radiation therapy. The role of radiation therapy in the treatment of lymphomas varies substantially from that in the treatment of Hodgkin's disease. Although NHLs are sensitive to radiation, only a small portion of patients obtain a cure if treated with local or regional radiation alone. NHLs include a wide variety of clinical diseases. For example, lymphoma in children and lymphoma of the bone, lung, and Waldeyer's ring are all quite different and require different therapeutic approaches. The regimens vary from local field irradiation to whole-body irradiation and from single-agent chemotherapy to aggressive multidrug therapy. Combination chemotherapy, radiation, and bone marrow transplantation is a regimen used to treat relapse.

Because lymphomas are radiosensitive, they regress quickly; however, radiation does not always alter the natural history of these diseases. In the study of treatment regimens, true survival and disease-free relapse must be distinguished.

Typically, radiation is given to the site of involvement, with coverage to the draining nodal groups on the same side of the diaphragm. Although total nodal radiation can be used for Stages I and II, it is not a common practice in the United States. The reason for this is that, although longer disease-free survival accompanies total nodal radiation, there is no change in overall survival rates.

Radiation therapy is a standard management for Stage I and II low-grade lymphomas, especially for patients under 40 years of age. At least 4000 cGy is recommended.[7] For extranodal disease or a large Stage I lymphoma, 5000 cGy should be given.[11] The field should include the draining lymph nodes. Results are still inconclusive as to whether adjuvant chemotherapy is beneficial or radiation therapy to the opposite side of the diaphragm is necessary for early-stage lymphomas.

For Stage III and IV low-grade lymphomas, several options for treatment are available, including the following: [11]

1. No initial treatment for patients without symptoms—These patients must be carefully monitored. (This option is not frequently used in the United States.)
2. Single drug therapy, usually oral chlorambucil or Cytoxan
3. Combination chemotherapy with CVP (Cytoxan, Oncovin, and prednisone), C-MOPP, or CHOP

New treatments being investigated include the use of interferon-α (an antitumor agent) alone, in combination with chemotherapy, or as an adjuvant to chemotherapy; monoclonal antibodies; and high-dose chemotherapy with fractionated total-body radiation followed by bone marrow transplantation.

If a patient relapses, the same chemotherapy is often used. However, two additional agents have proved effective in the treatment of relapses: fludarabine and 2-chlorodeoxyadenosine (2-Cd-A). High-dose rate chemotherapy, radiation, and bone marrow transplantation are also used for the treatment of relapse in Stages I and II. Radiation alone may also be used to reduce bulky disease and/or to relieve pain.

The 5-year survival rate is 90% for patients in Stages I and II and 80% for those in Stages III and IV. The average survival time for patients with low-grade lymphomas is 6 to 12 years.

Intermediate-grade lymphomas can be divided into favorable and unfavorable tumors. Favorable tumors are those less than 4 to 10 cm in diameter in which the lactate dehydrogenase level is normal and no B symptoms are present. For patients with favorable Stage I & II disease, treatment options include the following:[7]

1. Chemotherapy alone (CHOP)
2. Chemotherapy and radiation therapy
3. Primary radiation alone to the site, particularly if the patient is unable to tolerate the chemotherapy

The 5-year survival rate for patients with Stage I intermediate-grade lymphomas is 80% to 90% and 70% to 80% for patients in Stage II. [7]

Unfavorable lymphomas in Stages I, II, III, and IV are treated with combination chemotherapy. Regimens include CHOP, mBACOD, ProMace-CYTABOM, and MACOP-B. The survival rate is significantly lower for these patients than it is in the earlier stages. A 5-year survival rate of 40% to 50% is the norm for these patients.[7]

High-grade and lymphoblastic lymphomas usually receive multiagent chemotherapy with prophylactic central nervous system radiation. Stage IV patients have extensive disease, usually bone marrow involvement and/or central nervous system involvement and a high lactate dehydrogenase level. Generally, these patients have done poorly with conventional therapy and may benefit from intensive chemotherapy and radiation, followed by bone marrow transplantation.

The 5-year survival rate is 80% for patients with limited disease and 20% for patients with extensive disease involving the bone marrow or central nervous system.

AIDS-associated lymphomas are usually intermediate- and high-grade lymphomas and are highly aggressive. Of course, the condition of the patient dictates the treatment.

If given total nodal irradiation at high doses, patients with Stage III nodular lymphomas achieve a 33% remission rate after 10 years. However, with diffuse lymphomas, only 10% of the patients survive 10 years after total nodal radiation. Chemotherapy (either a single alkylating agent or a combination of agents) is usually used for this stage.

Radiation doses must be over 3500 cGy to achieve the least probability of recurrence. Typically, the doses are 4000 cGy to 5000 cGy, especially for diffuse lymphomas. For palliation, 2500 cGy can be used. For localized radiation the entire lymphatic region with appropriate margins should be treated.

Unless the disease originates in the mediastinum, mediastinal spread is rare. The mantle technique is commonly used in instances of mediastinal involvement. A minimantle or supramediastinal mantle is appropriate if no mediastinal disease or upper abdominal disease is present. Anteriorly, the inferior border for a minimantle field should be at the level of the inferior portion of the head of the clavicles; posteriorly, it should be at the inferior surface of the shaft of the clavicles (Fig. 4-6).

Preauricular nodes are frequently involved in the diffuse lymphomas and are at high risk in patients with cervical adenopathy. In such instances, these nodes should be treated with a prophylactic dose of 3600 cGy, administered in right and left lateral ports over 4 weeks.

Subdiaphragmatic treatment. Mesenteric lymph node involvement is common with lymphomas occurring inferior to the diaphragm. In such instances, the whole abdomen is treated with the following four field techniques[11](Fig. 4-7).

1. An AP/PA field extending from the dome of the diaphragm to the iliac crest (unless the tumor is at the level of the iliac crest, and then the the field continues to the floor of the pelvis) is treated initially. The lateral portions of the ileum should be blocked to protect the iliac bone marrow, and the right lobe of the liver and the kidneys should also be protected. Over 2 to 3 weeks, 1500 cGy should be delivered at a rate of 150 cGy per day.
2. After the AP/PA course of treatment, the upper abdomen is treated from lateral fields, based on the initial isocentric setup. If abdominal disease is massive, the pelvic portion may continue with an AP/PA configuration. The posterior margin of these fields should be anterior to the kidneys but should include

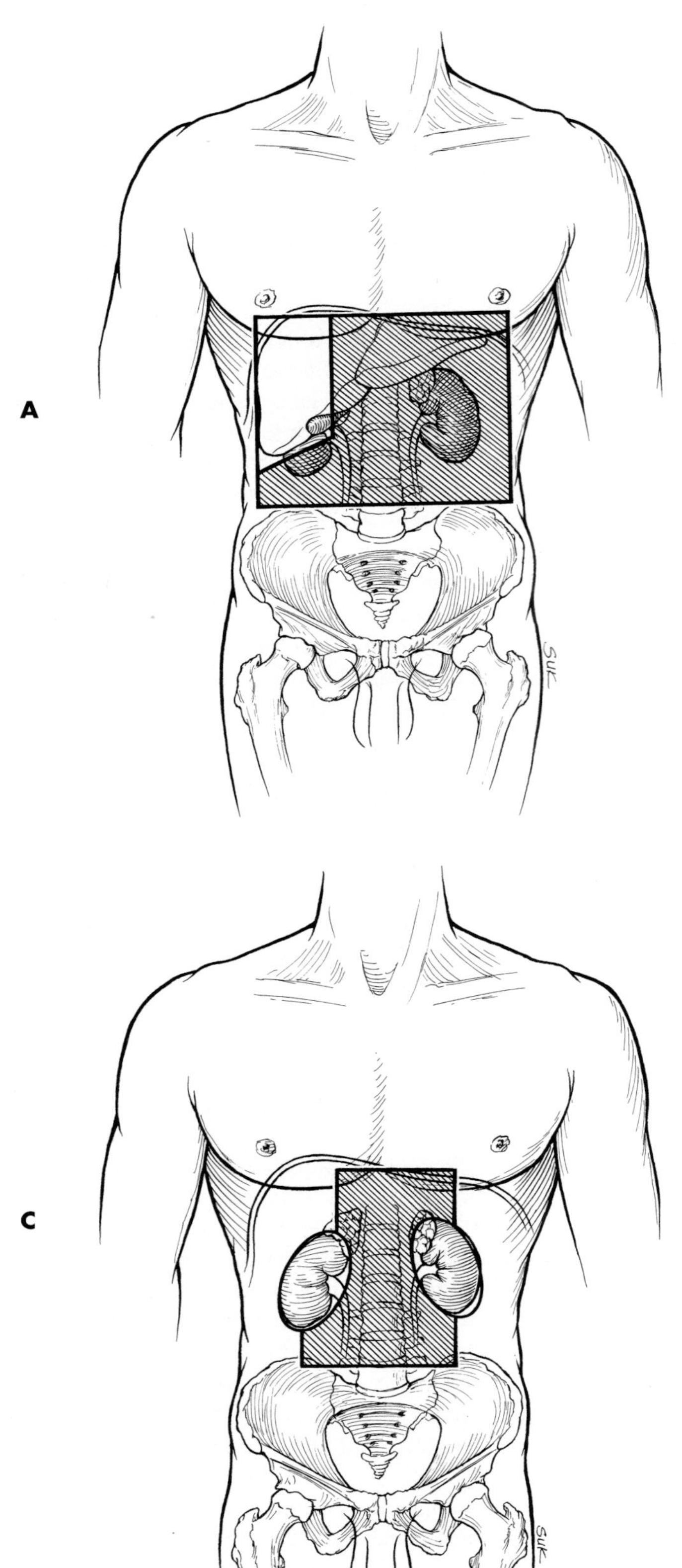

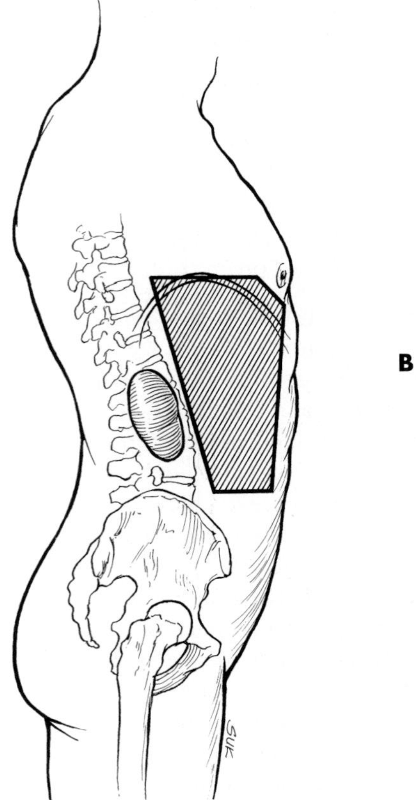

Fig. 4-7 The abdominal field configurations for treatment of the paraaortic and mesenteric lymph nodes. **A,** AP/PA abdominal field. This portion is treated only to 1500 cGy because of exposure to the kidneys. **B,** Lateral fields then follow to spare the kidneys. The total dose to the lateral fields should be 1500 cGy. **C,** AP/PA paraaortic fields with 5-HVL kidney blocks. The total dose to all three fields is 4500 cGy.

the paraaortic nodes. Anteriorly, the field should include the anterior abdominal wall. Another 1500 cGy over a 2-week period should be given, bringing the total dose to 3000 cGy over 4 to 5 weeks.

If the disease is on the posterior abdominal wall, the kidneys cannot be shielded. If the kidneys lie in the same plane as the paraaortic nodes, the lateral fields should be omitted.

3. Finally, a wide AP/PA paraaortic field (10 to 12 cm) is treated with kidney blocks, delivering 1500 cGy in another 2-week period. The lateral margins of such a field should extend from the lateral margins of one kidney to the lateral margins of the other, with 5 half-valve layer (HVL) kidney blocks.

The total dose delivered to the whole abdomen is 4500 cGy in 6 to 7 weeks. Pelvic irradiation may continue on an AP/PA basis throughout this period of abdominal irradiation if blood counts permit. Midline blocks should be no higher than the symphysis pubis.

When total-body irradiation is used for palliation in advanced cases of nodular lymphocytic lymphoma or nodular mixed lymphoma, 150 cGy to the midplane should be delivered over 5 weeks. Two or three fractions should be delivered weekly for a total of 30 cGy per week. The major complications of such treatment are thrombocytopenia or leukopenia. The platelet counts must be closely watched, with counts taken before each treatment.

Central nervous system and gastric lymphomas. NHL is about 60 times more common in AIDS patients than in the general population.[3] These patients typically have high-grade and large cell immunoblastic-type lymphomas and Burkitt's lymphoma. These lymphomas commonly occur in the central nervous system, with two thirds appearing with cerebral disease. Extranodal sites are also common in these lymphoma-AIDS patients.

Surgery is necessary for a diagnosis, but an excision is not necessarily therapeutic. Radiation therapy improves the median survival time, but only to 15 months. A typical radiation field is a whole-brain field with extension to the upper cervical spinal cord and occasionally the orbit if it is at risk. Doses above 5000 cGy may lead to longer survival rates. Chemotherapy can be effective if the patient's immune system is not already severely depressed.[11]

Lymphomas of the gastrointestinal tract are the most common of the extranodal lymphomas. They are most commonly diffuse, large cell lymphomas. They appear with gastric symptoms, and a diagnosis is obtained via an endoscopic biopsy. The regimens recommended for such cancers are surgery and chemotherapy, a biopsy, chemotherapy and radiation therapy, or a biopsy and radiation therapy. One third of the patients have unresectable disease at the time of surgery. Surgery delays chemotherapy administration and causes morbidity from the functional loss of the stomach. A 10% mortality rate accompanies this surgery.[11]

Bone marrow transplants have been conducted increasingly with lymphoma patients. Allogenic or autologous transplants can be done. Frequently, these transplants are performed if the therapy for relapse or primary disease has failed. Typically, bone marrow transplants are done for aggressive cell types.

Side effects. The side effects of radiation therapy treatment for lymphomas depend on the areas treated. For example, if a patient receives radiation in a mantle or the Waldeyer's ring field, the side effects will be a dry mouth, difficulty swallowing, a loss of appetite, mucositis, mouth sores, a Monilia infection, altered taste, redness of the skin, a sore throat, possible hair loss, transient dysphagia from esophagitis, and a dry cough.

Management of these side effects therefore includes eating small, frequent meals and avoiding extremely hot or cold fluids or alcohol. Good skin care includes the use of aloe vera or an approved topical application if the skin begins to redden. The patient must be cautioned, however, not to have the skin care product on at the time of treatment because of increased skin irritation. For this reason, many centers do not recommend any skin creams until after the radiation therapy. Corn starch, however, is allowed and works effectively at relieving skin irritations.

Abdominal treatment is sure to cause nausea and vomiting. Antiemetics such as Compazine and Tigan should be taken 30 minutes before the treatment to control the vomiting or nausea. The use of tetrahydrocannabinol (THC) or Marinol (marijuana) is sometimes prescribed to control the nausea and improve the appetite for these patients. Fatigue is also common in this group of individuals, and plenty of rest should be encouraged. Patients who work full time should be strongly encouraged to limit their work hours during treatments. Also, help at home in dealing with family stress (e.g., child care and meal preparation) should be investigated.

If the pelvis is treated, diarrhea may occur, depending on the dose. In such instances a low-fiber diet should be recommended, and diarrhea medications may be indicated.

Vomiting and low blood counts are the primary side effects of total-body irradiation.

Chronic effects of NHL treatments are caused more by the chemotherapeutic drugs than by the radiation therapy. Alkylating agents used in the treatment of NHL and Hodgkin's disease cause sterility and the risk of a second cancer (usually leukemia). One study group indicates a 2% risk of a second cancer 7 years after treatment and a 9.9% risk after 9 years. No risk is involved if the patient is treated by radiation alone to limited fields.

Results of treatment

Patients with Stage I and II nodular lymphomas have excellent survival rates with radiation therapy alone. In these instances, treatment on the opposite side of the diaphragm is unnecessary. The patients have an 80% to 100 % 5-year survival rate, assuming that no abdominal disease is present. However, if a surgical staging has not been done, both sides of the diaphragm should be treated.

Patients with localized Stage I and II large cell lymphomas typically receive adjuvant chemotherapy after the site of involvement is treated. Some groups use chemotherapy without adjuvant radiation as the primary treatment with good results, but these groups generally experience increased morbidity.

Patients with high-stage, indolent, nonaggressive lymphomas have several options. These options include no treatment, combination chemotherapy, combination chemotherapy and radiation therapy, low-dose total body irradiation (TBI) total lymph node irradiation, and chemotherapy with TBI and bone marrow transplantation.

In Stage III nodular lymphoma patients, a 5- to 10-year survival rate exists, with conservative management of patients who do not have symptoms and are feeling well. The treatment for these patients tends to be a small-field, low-dose radiation therapy for symptom relief. Patients who receive intensive chemotherapy have good responses but high rates of relapse.

Patients with nodular mixed lymphomas receive good results (possibly cures) with the C-MOPP regimen.

Total lymphoid radiation for Stage III has resulted in a 30% freedom-from-relapse rate at 10 years; results are the same for whole-body radiation. Similar results occur for Stage IV, but total nodal radiation is not considered appropriate for these patients.

For Stage III and IV diffuse histology, chemotherapy is the mainstay, with the C-MOPP or BACOP regimens being used. Of the patients in this group, 40% achieve long-term freedom from relapse.

Results of other histological types are less optimistic.

Role of radiation therapist

The radiation therapist's role in treating the lymphoma patient is quite similar to that for the Hodgkin's disease patient. Accuracy is the primary concern. If abutting fields are present, the therapist should be careful to match fields or measure gaps with extreme accuracy.

The therapist must be aware of the importance of blocking the critical structures in the fields (i.e., spine, liver, and kidney). Keeping precise records is vital, and clear notes should be written to indicate blocking changes. Port films should be taken before the onset of blocking changes, particularly in regard to the liver and kidney blocks because these structures have extremely low tolerances to radiation. (The liver 's maximum tolerance is 3000 cGy, and the kidney's maximum tolerance is only about 2300 cGy.) Therefore precision in block placement is paramount.

Blood counts should be taken regularly for these patients. Monitoring these counts and ensuring that the blood is drawn often become the duty of the therapist.

Because they tend to be older than the Hodgkin's disease patients, lymphoma patients may have worse overall health and may rely on the therapist for additional assistance in moving around the room. As with all patients, communications and instructions must be clear. Communication is critical, not only with the patients, but also with their families, especially as side effects require management.

SUMMARY

New forms of NHL are being identified as a result of advances in immunological molecular diagnosis and the use of special techniques. Enteropathy-associated (small intestine disorder) T-cell lymphomas and mantle-cell-derived lymphomas are two such diseases.

Further investigation has shown nodular lymphocyte predominant Hodgkin's disease to be a B-cell proliferation that may progress to a high-grade B-cell NHL. Also, many cases of lymphocyte depletion Hodgkin's disease have been reclassified as *T-cell NHL.* The relationship between Hodgkin's disease and non-Hodgkin's large cell anaplastic lymphoma has likewise become increasingly blurred. Therefore current research continues to shed new light on these disease processes, which increasingly are appearing more interrelated than ever before.

Treatment advances are also being continually developed. The hope is that the prognosis will improve for patients in all the categories of lymphomas.

Case Study

M.T. is a 30-year-old woman with intermediate-grade, large cell NHL. In September she developed chest pain, which worsened until December, when she had a chest x-ray examination. A 10.5-cm mediastinal mass was discovered on the radiograph. A biopsy then revealed the intermediate-grade, large cell lymphoma. At the time of the work-up, M.T. experienced superior vena cava syndrome. Chemotherapy began shortly. ProMace-CYTABOM was delivered in six cycles, the last of which ended in April of the following year. The patient tolerated the chemotherapy well.

Chest radiographs and CT scans showed the near total resolution of the mediastinal mass, and no evidence of tumor involvement existed outside the chest.

M.T. has no family history of carcinoma. She works as an accountant and does not use cigarettes nor alcohol. She has not experienced any of the following: headaches, dizzy spells, nausea, vomiting, shortness of breath, coughing, diarrhea, constipation, and abdominal pain. Her appetite and energy level are good. In addition, she does not exhibit cervical, supraclavicular, axillary, or inguinal adenopathy.

Because of the size of the initial mass, limited radiation therapy was given to the involved field only. Over 31 days, 3960 cGy of 6-MV photons were delivered in 22 fractions to the involved field. M.T. experienced fatigue at 1080 cGy, which was unusual for such a limited field of treatment and after only six fractions. However, the fatigue resolved within the week, and the patient felt much better by the twelfth fraction. She experienced an unrelated bladder infection, which was cleared up with Bactrim D.S.

After the completion of the radiation, she was seen in follow-up in August of the same year. To date, she has not experienced any further side effects nor any chronic effects. M.T. has been disease free since this time.

Review Questions

Essay

1. Name the lymph nodes included in a mantle treatment.
2. What are B symptoms? Approximately what percentage of Hodgkin's disease and non-Hodgkin's lymphoma patients experience these symptoms?
3. List the four histological subtypes of Hodgkin's disease. Which is the most favorable, and which is the least favorable?
4. What are the typical borders of a mantle field? What is the typical daily and total dose given for a mantle field and for the paraaortic field?
5. What are the common side effects from a mantle treatment? How are these side effects managed?
6. Name two common grading systems for NHLs, and explain their differences.
7. What type of lymphomas have the longest survival rates for patients?
8. Name three chemotherapeutic regimens commonly given to treat NHLs.
9. List two newer modalities of treating late-stage NHLs.
10. What radiation dose should be given for the management of Stage I low-grade lymphomas (without chemotherapy).

Questions to Ponder

1. Compare and contrast the differences between Hodgkin's disease and NHL, including the causes, clinical presentation, routes of spread, prognosis, and treatment modalities.
2. Why is the Ann Arbor staging system appropriate for Hodgkin's disease but difficult to apply to NHLs?
3. Which is the greater prognostic factor, the stage or the histological subtype in Hodgkin's disease? How does this differ in NHLs?
4. For the treatment of a subdiaphragmatic lymphoma with a four-field abdomen technique, which structures need to be blocked or protected?
5. What is total nodal irradiation? Describe the fields involved. Why is this technique more commonly used with Hodgkin's disease patients than with NHL patients?
6. What considerations must the therapist keep in mind daily when setting up a Hodgkin's disease patient for a mantle field and for a paraaortic field?

REFERENCES

1. American Cancer Society: *Cancer facts and figures,* Atlanta, 1996, The Society.
2. Armitage JO: Treatment of non-Hodgkin's lymphomas, *N Eng J Med,* 328:1023-1029, April 8, 1993.
3. Beral V et.al: AIDS-associated non-Hodgkin's lymphoma, *Lancet* 337:805-809, April 6, 1991.
4. Bolwell B: Autologous bone marrow transplantation for Hodgkin's disease and non-Hodgkin's lymphoma, *Semin Oncol* 21(suppl 7):86-95, 1994.
5. DeVita VT et al: *Cancer: principles and practice of oncology,* ed 2, Philadelphia, 1982, JB Lippincott.
6. Dietrich PY et al: Second primary cancers in patients continuously disease-free from Hodgkin's disease: a protective role for the spleen? *Blood* 84:1209-1215, August 15, 1994.
7. Dollinger M et al: Everyone's guide to cancer therapy, ed 1, Kansas City, 1991, Sommerville House Books.
8. Hendee WR: *Radiation physics,* St Louis, 1970, Mosby.
9. Hoane BR et al: Comparison of initial lymphoma staging using computed tomography (CT) and magnetic resonance (MR) imaging, *Am J Hematolo,* 47:100-105, October 94.
10. Longo DL et al: The calculation of actual or received dose intensity: a comparison of published methods, *J Clin Oncol* 9:2042-2051, 1991.
11. Perez CA, Brady LW: *Principles and practice of radiation oncology,* ed 2, New York, 1992, JB Lippincott.
12. Sweet DL et al: Hodgkin's disease: problems of staging, *Cancer,* 42(suppl):957-968, August 1978.

BIBLIOGRAPHY

Armitage JO et al: Salvage therapy for patients with lymphoma, *Semin Oncol* 21 (suppl 7):82-85, August 1994.

Bonadonna G: Modern treatment of malignant lymphomas: a multidisciplinary approach, *Ann Oncol* 5(suppl 2):5-16, September 5-16, 1994.

Cox J.D: *Moss' radiation oncology,* ed 7, St Louis, 1994, Mosby.

Dasher B, Wiggers N, Vann AM: *Portal design in radiation therapy,* ed 1, Atlanta, 1994, RL Bryan.

Gladstein E, Kaplan HS: *Determination of tumor extent and tumor localization of Hodgkin's disease and non-Hodgkin's lymphomas: technical basis of radiation therapy practical clinical consideration,* Philadelphia, 1984, Lea & Ferbiger.

Gonzalez C, Mederios J: Non-Hodgkin's lymphomas and the Working Formulation, part 2, *Contemp Oncol,* pp.43-55, February 1993.

Hole JW: *Human anatomy and physiology,* ed 2, Dubuque, Iowa, 1981, Wm C Brown.

Holleb AI, Fink D, Murphy GP: *American Cancer Society textbook of clinical oncology,* ed 1, Atlanta, 1991, American Cancer Society.

Horning SJ et al: The Stanford experience with combined procarbazine, Alkeran and vinblastine (PAVe) and radiotherapy for locally extensive and advanced stage Hodgkin's disease, *Ann Oncol* 3:747-754, 1992.

Kaminski MS et al: Radioimmunotherapy of B-cell lymphoma with (131 I) AntiB (Anti CD-20) antibody, *N Engl J Med,* 329:459, August 12, 1993.

Khan KM: *The physics of radiation therapy,* ed 1, Baltimore, 1984, Williams & Wilkins.

Lymphoma classification—where now? *Lancet,* 339:1084-1085, May 2, 1992.

Sonneveld P et al: Full-dose chemotherapy for non-Hodgkin's lymphoma in the elderly, *Semin Hematol* 31 (suppl 3):9-12, April 1994.

CHAPTER

5

Leukemia

Susan Belinsky
Cathy Turley
Theresa Grady

Outline

Historical perspective
Pertinent anatomy
Acute lymphocytic leukemia
- Epidemiology
- Etiology
- Prognostic indicators
- Clinical presentation
- Detection and diagnosis
- Pathology
- Staging and classification
- Treatment techniques

Acute myelogenous leukemia
- Epidemiology
- Etiology
- Prognostic indicators
- Clinical presentation
- Detection and diagnosis
- Pathology
- Staging and classification
- Treatment techniques

Chronic lymphocytic leukemia
- Epidemiology
- Etiology
- Prognostic indicators
- Clinical presentation
- Detection and diagnosis
- Pathology
- Staging and classification
- Treatment techniques

Chronic myelogenous leukemia
- Epidemiology
- Etiology
- Prognostic indicators
- Clinical presentation
- Detection and diagnosis
- Pathology
- Staging and classification
- Treatment techniques

Role of radiation therapist

Key terms

Auer rods
Dysplopia
Ecchymoses
Epistaxis
Leukoencephalopathy
Menorrhagia
Nadir
Papilledema
Petechiae
Pluripotent
Progenitors
Pruritus
Purpura
Stomatitis
Striae

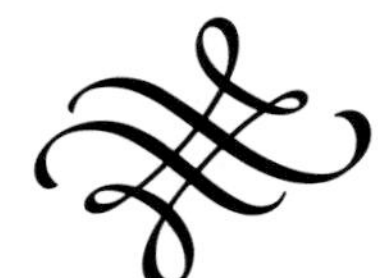

Leukemia is a heterogeneous group of neoplastic diseases of the hemopoietic system affecting approximately 8.6 persons per 100,000.[8] It is broadly divided into acute and chronic types, based on the disease's natural history. Acute leukemia progresses quickly and is characterized by the autonomous proliferation of undifferentiated cells in the bone marrow, whereas chronic leukemia is distinguished by a slower progression of disease and the uncontrolled expansion of mature cells. Acute and chronic leukemias are further subdivided into myelogenous leukemias (those arising directly or indirectly from hemopoietic stem cells) and lymphocytic leukemias (those arising from other cells populating the bone marrow). Therefore consideration of three factors (natural history of the disease, degree of cellular maturation, and dominant cell line) results in the four main subtypes of leukemia (Table 5-1): acute lymphocytic leukemia (ALL), chronic lymphocytic leukemia (CLL), acute myelogenous leukemia (AML, which is sometimes referred to as *acute nonlymphocytic leukemia,* or *ANLL*), and chronic myelogenous leukemia (CML).

Table 5-1 The four main subtypes of leukemia

Natural history of the disease	Lymphocytic	Myelogenous
Acute	ALL	AML
Chronic	CLL	CML

HISTORICAL PERSPECTIVE

The first documented description of a case of leukemia appears to be that of Alfred Velpeau, a French surgeon, who in 1827 recorded his observations. Dameshek and Gunz[3] described the case:

> His patient, a 63-year-old florist and seller of lemonade, who had abandoned himself to the abuse of spirituous liquor and of women without, however, becoming syphilitic, fell ill in 1825 with a swelling of the abdomen, fever, and weakness. He died soon after admission to the hospital and was at autopsy found to have an enormous liver and spleen, the latter weighing ten pounds. The blood was thick, like gruel...resembling in consistency and color the yeast of red wine.

In 1844 Alfred Donné reported his microscopic observations of leukemia cells in his treatise *Cours de Microscopie.* His studies included the examination of a postmortem sample of blood from a woman who had suffered from a large abdominal tumor and diarrhea as well as samples collected in vivo from other patients. Donné is credited with the first known observation of leukemic cells and the establishment of the disease as a hematological condition.[5]

In 1845 Rudolf Virchow, a German physician, referred to the blood taken from a patient with splenic enlargement and massive accumulations of white blood cells as *weisses blut* (white blood). In 1847 Virchow first used the term *leukemia.* A decade later, Virchow described two types of leukemia: splenic and lymphatic. The advent of staining techniques in microscopy in the late nineteenth century permitted the morphological subdivision of the myelogenous and lymphocytic leukemias.[11]

Because of the unique nature of each of the four subtypes of leukemia, they are discussed separately in this chapter.

PERTINENT ANATOMY

Leukemia develops during the formation of the constituent elements of the blood and lymphocytes. The hemopoietic process through which mature erythrocytes, neutrophils, eosinophils, basophils, monocytes, and platelets are formed and the lymphopoietic process through which lymphocytes are formed begin at the most primitive level with the **pluripotent** stem cells. These cells have a self-renewing capability and generate differentiating cells of multiple lineage. The cells of the pluripotent stem cell pool differentiate into either myeloid or lymphoid stem cells (Fig. 5-1). The myeloid stem cell pool provides the **progenitors** for the six types of blood cells, whereas the lymphoid pool provides the progenitors for the classes of lymphocytes. In the normal course of differentiation and maturation, these cells eventually become fully mature, functional blood cells and lymphocytes. During leukemic development the production of the hemopoietic or lymphopoietic progenitors is uncontrolled and greatly accelerated, resulting in incomplete or defective cellular maturation. Acute leukemia involves the rapid proliferation of primitive, undifferentiated stem cells, whereas cellular differentiation is largely preserved in chronic leukemia.

The symptoms of leukemia result from the leukemic cells' interference with normal processes. The leukemic cells accumulate in the bone marrow, impairing the body's normal production of adequate supplies of red blood cells, white blood cells, and platelets. The decrease in the number of these necessary blood components in the circulating blood results in anemia, thrombocytopenia, neutropenia, and the related symptoms of fatigue, pallor, bleeding, and infection.

With the acute leukemia subtypes the accumulating leukemic cells are immature or have undergone a defect in maturation. ALL is characterized by the invasion of the bone marrow by leukemic lymphoblasts. AML results from the proliferation of defective or incompletely matured cells derived from the pluripotent hemopoietic stem cell pool.

In chronic leukemia the maturation of the cells is preserved, but unregulated proliferation results in the accumula-

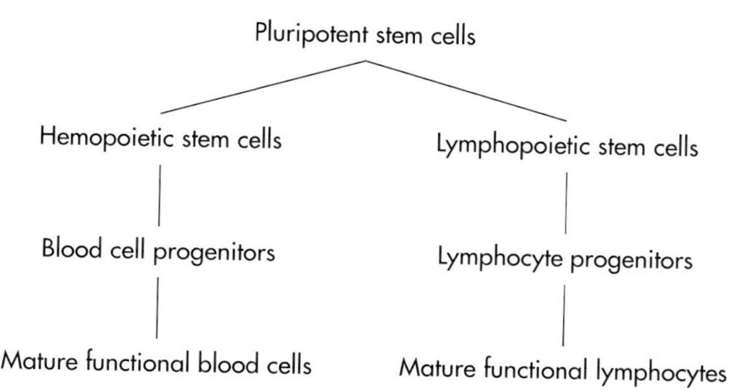

Fig. 5-1 Hemopoiesis and lymphopoiesis.

tion of leukemic cells in the bone marrow. CLL is a disorder of morphologically mature, but immunologically less mature, lymphocytes. An increased proliferation of these short- and long-life lymphocytes and the prolonged survival of the long-life lymphocytes results in an enormous accumulation of these cells in the marrow, blood, lymph nodes, liver, and spleen. This causes an enlargement of the involved organs and a decrease in bone marrow function. CML involves the replacement of marrow cells with mature myeloid cells that are insensitive to the normal proliferation control mechanisms.

ACUTE LYMPHOCYTIC LEUKEMIA

Epidemiology

The acute subtypes account for approximately 50% of all instances of leukemia in the United States, affecting about five persons per 100,000.[7] ALL is the most common of the pediatric malignancies, and nearly 80% of children with acute leukemia have the ALL subtype.

ALL is primarily a disease of children, with its incidence peaking between the ages of 2 and 6 years. It is relatively uncommon in persons over the age of 15. The incidence of ALL is higher among males than females. The disease is more common among whites than blacks and has a higher incidence among Jews than non-Jews.

Etiology

The causes of acute leukemia are unknown. Physical and chemical agents have been associated with increased instances of leukemia. The markedly higher incidence of acute leukemia among survivors of the atomic bomb explosions in Japan has suggested that ionizing radiation may play a role in leukemogenesis. Japanese atomic bomb survivors had a ten- to fifteen-fold increase in the incidence of acute leukemia, with a greater increase in the incidence of ALL than AML. Benzene derivatives and other hydrocarbons and alkylating agents such as cyclophosphamide have been associated with an increased risk of acute leukemia.

Heredity appears to play a role in the development of acute leukemia. If one identical twin is diagnosed with acute leukemia, the risk of the other twin developing the disease within 6 months is approximately 20%. Down syndrome is associated with a fifteen- to twenty-fold increased risk of acute leukemia.

Naturally occurring retroviruses and the human T-cell lymphotropic virus have been implicated as causative agents in instances of adult ALL but not childhood ALL.

Prognostic indicators

More than 95% of patients with ALL can be expected to experience a complete remission, although the duration of the remission and subsequent potential for cure appear to be related to a number of factors, including clinical variables such as age and white blood count (WBC) at the time of the diagnosis. ALL in children younger than 2 and older than 10 years carries a poor prognosis. The prognosis is the worst for an infant under age 1. In adult ALL, advancing age is an adverse prognostic sign, with patients older than 50 years faring worse than younger patients. An initial leukocyte count of less than 10,000/mm^3 is more favorable than a count of 20,000 to 49,000/mm^3. A WBC greater than 50,000/mm^3 is the least favorable.

Other features with prognostic value include central nervous system leukemia at the time of the diagnosis, a mediastinal mass, massive organomegaly and/or adenopathy, and biological qualities of the leukemic cells such as the immunophenotype, cytogenetics, and deoxyribonucleic acid (DNA) content. Poor performance status, impaired organ function, and low serum albumin levels are unfavorable prognostic indicators.

Clinical presentation

The symptoms of ALL at the time of presentation stem from the suppression of the normal blood components that causes anemia, thrombocytopenia, neutropenia, and associated symptoms. A nonspecific flulike malaise is common, with fatigue and pallor resulting from the anemia. Thrombocytopenia is manifested by oozing gums, **epistaxis** (nose bleeds), **petechiae** (tiny red spots on the skin caused by the escape of small amounts of blood), **ecchymoses** (discoloration of the skin caused by the escape of blood into tissues), **menorrhagia** (excessive menstrual bleeding), and excessive bleeding after dental procedures. Neutropenia causes an increased susceptibility to respiratory, dental, sinus, perirectal, and urinary tract infections. Other common symptoms at the time of presentation are liver, splenic, and testicular enlargement. The disease at times may mimic rheumatoid arthritis with joint swelling, bone pain, and tenderness, often causing a child to limp or refuse to walk. Unlike AML, the symptoms of ALL rarely occur more than 6 weeks before the diagnosis. Vomiting, headaches, **papilledema** (swelling of the optic disc), neck stiffness, and cranial nerve palsy are indicative of central nervous system involvement.

Detection and diagnosis

A blood cell count is one indicator for detecting ALL. Thrombocytopenia and anemia occur in the majority of the patients (two thirds) at the time of the diagnosis. Leukocyte counts vary from low to high. An abnormal increase in white cells indicates a poor prognosis.

Immunophenotyping includes a morphological evaluation, special stains, an electron microscopy, and surface marker studies. It can establish a diagnosis in 90% of the patients.

A bone marrow aspiration biopsy is necessary to make a definitive diagnosis. The amount of leukemic blast cells is the determinant for a definitive diagnosis. A biopsy revealing greater than 5% leukoblasts is positive for leukemia.

Other abnormalities may be present at the time of the diagnosis. These include hyperuricemia and several metabolic abnormalities, hyperkalemia, hypomagnesemia, hypocalcemia, and hypercalcemia. Of the patients identified with having ALL at the time of the initial diagnosis, 30% have low serum levels of immunoglobulins.

Leukemic infiltrates of the liver, periosteum, and bone may be present. A mediastinal mass may be present in some high-risk patients. This can be demonstrated on a chest radiograph.

Extramedullary leukemia is important in regard to relapse. The two most common sites for extramedullary leukemia are the central nervous system and testes. A diagnosis of these two sites is obtained through a cytologic examination and a wedge biopsy, respectively.

Pathology

ALL is characterized by an unregulated proliferation of lymphoblasts. The disease cells limit the production of other healthy cells by overcrowding and inhibiting cell growth and differentiation.

Staging and classification

The two major means to classify ALL are based on the morphological appearance and immunological surface markings. The morphological classification used is the FAB (French-American-British) system. This classification divides lymphoblastic leukemias into three levels (L1, L2, and L3). These divisions of ALL are based on the cell size, nuclear shape, number, prominence of nuclei, and amount and appearance of cytoplasm. These levels are as follows:

L1—A small cell with a high nucleus, a regular cytoplasm ratio, or a clefted cell and small, inconspicuous nucleoli

L2—Larger blast cells with irregular nuclear membranes, one or more prominent nucleoli, and a relative abundance of cytoplasm

L3—Large lymphoblasts with round to oval prominent nucleoli and basophilic cytoplasm

The majority of pediatric ALLs are L1. L3 carries a poor prognosis and is associated with B-cell ALL.

Immunological classification identifies the surface-marking characteristic of blast cells. Approximately 25% of patients with ALL are categorized by T-cell, B-cell, or preB-cell markers. About 70% of the patients are classified with null-cell type ALL. The null-cell type has subcategories, the majority of which fall into the common type. This null-cell type reacts to an antibody made from a surface antigen generally found in ALL cells. This antigen is referred to as *CALLA*, or *common leukemia-associated antigen.*[2]

Treatment techniques

Treatment techniques used for ALL are radiation therapy, chemotherapy, and bone marrow transplantation. These three modalities are used alone or in combination with each other.

If radiation therapy is administered, four different techniques may be used for treating ALL. The patient may receive total body radiation with the dose totaling 1200 cGy. For 3 consecutive days, 200 cGy is given two times a day (b.i.d.). This dose is used to immunosuppress the patient in combination with a bone marrow transplant.

The dose rate set on the treatment unit is 10 cGy per minute, prescribed at midplane at the central region, the umbilicus. This low dose rate is necessary to spare late-responding tissues. These tissues include all visceral organs. The most common example is the lung.

A helmet field may be used to encompass the meninges. This is a prophylactic treatment for ALL. The helmet dose is 1800 cGy, delivered 200 cGy each day for 9 consecutive days.

The central nervous system technique is a combination of a helmet and spine fields. This technique is used to treat positive cells in the cerebral spinal fluid. The helmet field is treated to a total dose of 2400 cGy. The dose is delivered 150 cGy each day for 16 days. This is combined with a field to encompass the entire spine. The spine receives a total of 1500 cGy, with 150 cGy each day for 10 days.

The final treatment technique for ALL is a testes field. This field receives 400 cGy for a single fraction and is commonly used with total body irradiation treatment.

The chemotherapy treatment techniques used in treating ALL are divided into three groups: induction, consolidation, and maintenance therapy. Induction therapy involves the use of intrathecal methotrexate, cytarabine, and hydrocortisone. These chemotherapeutic agents are given immediately after the diagnosis to eradicate all detectable leukemia. Consolidation therapy uses intrathecal methotrexate and begins after remission has been achieved. Maintenance therapy involves the use of intravenous mercaptopurine, methotrexate, vincristine, and prednisone.

The use of these drugs and regimens may vary among institutions. Protocols are also frequently updated and changed as new information is discovered. All the treatment techniques and devices discussed in this chapter are those used at Tufts-New England Medical Center's Radiation Oncology Department. Most radiation oncology facilities use similar types of treatment techniques.

Another treatment technique for ALL is bone marrow transplantation. Bone marrow transplantation, which was considered an experimental procedure until about 15 years ago, is the treatment of choice for several diseases, including ALL, AML, and CML. The procedure involves the harvesting of healthy marrow from a suitable donor. The marrow is then infused into a patient whose diseased marrow has been destroyed or ablated by chemotherapy or total body irradiation. The transplanted marrow finds its way into bone marrow cavities and begins supplying the patient with normal, healthy hemopoietic cells.

The most desirable donors are identical twins because they are generally identical to the patients for all transplantation antigens. Allogeneic transplants, available to 20% to 30% of patients, use human leukocyte antigen (HLA) histocompatible siblings as donors. In recent years, bone marrow registries have been developed to locate and use nonrelated histocompatible donors. Some success has been achieved with the use of marrow from donors in whom only a partial match of transplantation antigens is present.

For potential bone marrow donors, risks are small and primarily related to anesthesia. The aspiration of bone marrow is a technically simple transplant procedure done in the operating room under sterile conditions and anesthesia. Multiple aspirations are drawn from the donor's anterior and posterior iliac crests. A small amount of heparin is used to prevent clotting.

The marrow recipient is treated before the transplant with a large dose of cyclophosphamide and total body irradiation or with chemotherapy alone (busulfan and cyclophosphamide). These measures reduce the leukemic cell load and impair the host's ability to reject the donor marrow. After an intravenous injection the donor marrow cells migrate to the recipient's marrow cavities and begin to produce normal cells in the blood in 2 to 4 weeks.

Autologous bone marrow transplants involve the reinfusion of a patient's own marrow that has been harvested and cryopreserved while the patient was in remission. Leukemic cells are removed from the collected marrow through the use of monoclonal antibodies directed against cell-surface antigens that are expressed on leukemic blasts but not on normal stem cells.

Factors that lead to failure in bone marrow transplants are recurrent leukemia (primarily in autologous donors) and graft versus host disease, which occurs in about 50% of patients. This condition may exist only as a slight skin rash, or it may progress to a life-threatening syndrome involving the skin, liver, and/or gastrointestinal tract.[10]

Field design and critical structures. With total body irradiation the field size used is 40 × 40 cm. This is the largest jaw size that can be set on the treatment unit. The gantry is then placed in the lateral position. The patient sits in the diamond-shaped box with the knees toward the chest, the arms by the side, and the forearms on the side of the knees (Fig. 5-2). The arms are placed in this position to act as compensators for the lungs. This position is necessary to place the entire person in the beam. The diamond-shaped box is about 5 feet from the gantry, so the light field covers the exact outer rim of the box, ensuring total coverage of the patient. The patient's eyes and face should be looking straight ahead.

Half of the treatment is given in this manner. Then the box, which is on wheels, is rotated 180 degrees. The second half of the treatment is given to the patient's other side. The patient is treated from the right and left lateral positions. After the completion of one lateral treatment field, the box is rotated manually 180 degrees and the other lateral is treated.

Thermoluminescent dosimeters (TLDs) are placed between the patients ankles, knees, and thighs once during a treatment to check midline doses. To even the dose over the uneven surfaces of the body, lead compensators are placed on a Lucite tray in the beam. The compensators are positioned over the thinnest body parts, such as the head and neck area, as well as the foot and ankle areas.

The field design for a helmet field is derived from specific anatomical landmarks; the field size should cover the meninges and C2, with falloff around the head (Fig. 5-3). The patient lies supine on a plastic head cup for stability and comfort. The lenses of the eyes should be blocked with an adjustable block.

The spinal cord is a critical structure for the treatment of the head to the level of C2. (The helmet should be used as

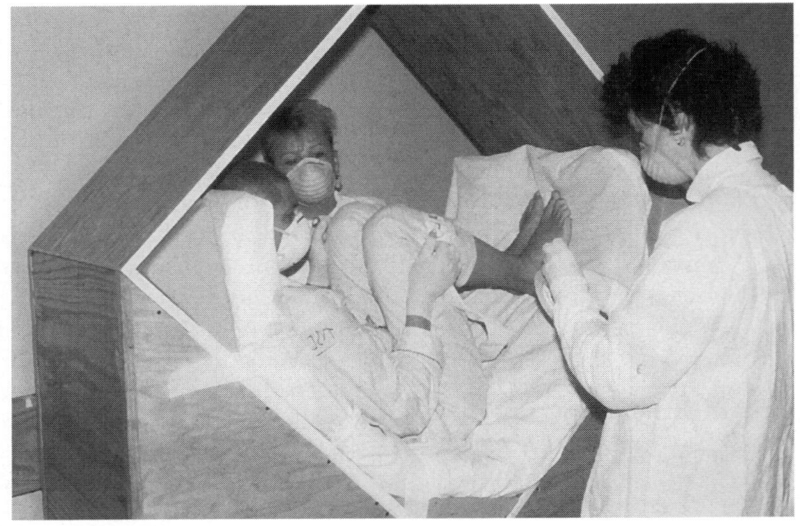

Fig. 5-2 New England Medical Center's custom-made immobilization device for total body irradiation.

was just described.) With spinal cord involvement, there should be a recorded dose for this particular site.

For the treatment of the central nervous system, the patient is placed in the prone position. Numerous head holders, such as the Smithers or Osborne holders (Fig. 5-4), comfortably stabilize the head. The patient's chin should be tucked slightly to avoid a crease in the neck (Fig. 5-5). This is a critical match area and should be flat with no skin folds.

The field arrangement is in two volumes. The first field arrangement is the cranial volume, which includes two lateral parallel opposed ports with the helmet field design arrangement. The second volume is the spinal field, which contains the entire spine. To encompass the entire spine, the field may have to be treated in two parts. A gap calculation must be done for the two fields. The match is at the level of the spine. In addition to the gap calculation just mentioned, another is done for the match of the spine and helmet field. The gap calculations are done to ensure coverage of the entire central nervous system with no cold spots. (See Volume I, Chapter 16, Treatment Procedures.)

The field size of these beam arrangements depends on the contour of the patient. The field must include the entire spine and the whole brain, including C2.

Another technique used to ensure that all the meninges are being treated is the feathering technique. With this technique the junctions are shifted by changing the lengths of all fields. This is done daily with three different match lines. The marks are differentiated by three colored marks drawn on the patient's skin. These marks correspond to the same colored pens used to record information in the treatment chart.

The only border that must remain stable is the posterior border of the spine. A block is positioned at the posterior border of the spine for stability. As the length of the fields shifts, the border with the blocked area remains stable.

The critical structures included in a central nervous system field are the lenses of the eyes, which are blocked with a moveable clinical block. The spinal cord is another critical structure, which receives a 1500 cGy dose.

Testes radiation for the treatment of ALL is usually in combination with total body irradiation. The field design is a simple setup. The patient lies supine in a lithotomy position, and a field is set up to encompass the entire organ. The testes field is treated with electrons.

The treatment techniques just presented are from one institution. Variations exist to each technique and the devices described. The leukemic sites treated are the same from one institution to another.

Side effects. Patients receiving total body irradiation experience numerous side effects. The gastrointestinal side effects include nausea, vomiting, diarrhea, anorexia, and malaise. Mucosa of the mouth, pharynx, bladder, and rectum may be affected. Normal secretions are inhibited and their functions impaired. The integumentary side effects include

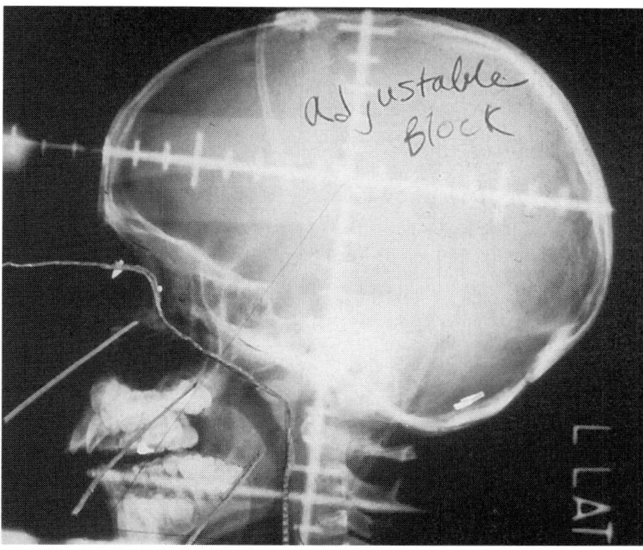

Fig. 5-3 Simulation film for a helmet field that covers the meninges encompassing C2.

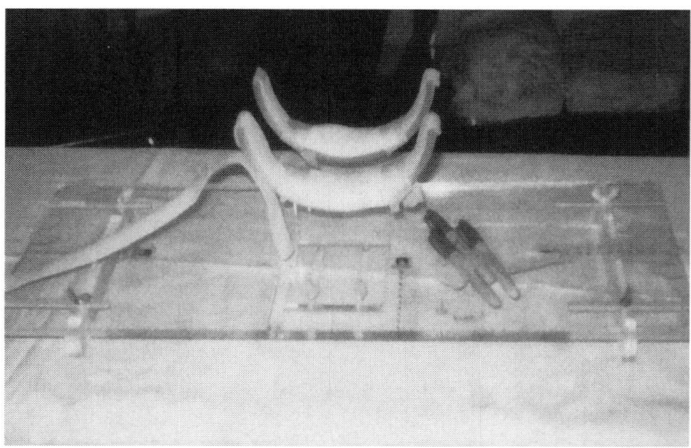

Fig. 5-4 A Smither's headholder for total central nervous system treatments.

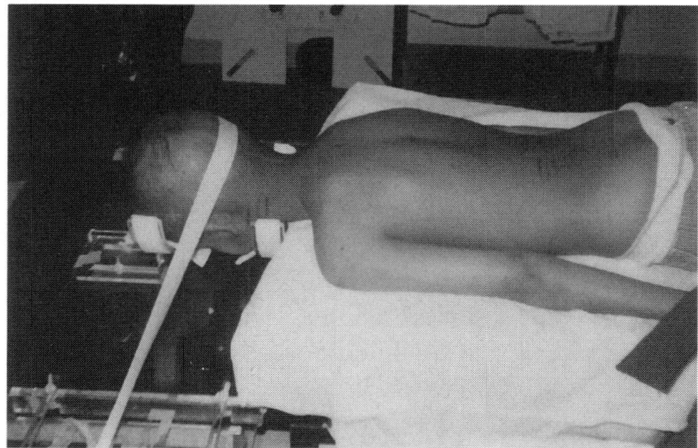

Fig. 5-5 A patient immobilized through the use of the Smither's headholder.

skin reactions, itching, tingling, bruising, and dry and inelastic skin that cracks easily. Alopecia can occur, as well as blanching or erythema of the skin and mucous membrane. A respiratory-related side effect is interstitial pneumonitis. These effects are all acute and subside in time.

Chronic side effects include permanent sterility and cataracts of the eyes (easily reversed with surgery). Hepatic fibrosis and radionecrosis of the genital tissue, muscle, and kidney are also chronic side effects.

The side effects for helmet and central nervous system radiation are skin reactions and hair loss for the integumentary system. The hemopoietic reactions are a decrease in blood counts and **leukoencephalopathy**, demyelinating brain lesions. Nausea and vomiting are the gastrointestinal side effects. The effect on the central nervous system is somnolence syndrome, characterized by drowsiness and malaise that is self-limiting. Serious injury to the tissue or blood vessels in the brain can lead to lethargy, seizures, spasticity, paresis, difficulty with movements, and Lhermittes sign.

Lhermittes sign may develop if the spine receives radiation treatment. This syndrome is characterized by a sensation of an electric shock in the arms, legs, or neck when the patient flexes the neck. These are the acute symptoms of helmet and central nervous system radiation.

The chronic side effects include neuropsychological deficits, intellectual deficits, and cataract formation. Growth retardation and hypothalamic-pituitary dysfunction are a result of irradiation to the brain and central nervous system. Hypothalamic-pituitary dysfunction is an abnormality in the hormonal secretions that include growth hormones, thyroid hormones, adrenal hormones, and sex-related hormones.

Myelopathy is another side effect causing irreversible injury to the spinal cord. Secondary tumors are also seen as a late effect. These tumors can be benign or malignant.

Chemotherapy has many side effects. The results from the cytotoxicity for each drug are different. The effects of vincristine are anorexia, constipation, and a metallic taste in the mouth. Neurological effects include jaw pain, **dysplopia** (double vision), vocal cord paresis, impotence, general motor weakness, and loss of deep tendon reflexes. The effects on the skin are alopecia and dermatitis.

Prednisone is a hormone, the effects of which are an exaggeration of normal physiological action, hypertension, muscle weakness, diabetes, and fluid retention. Gastric irritation, osteoporosis, and a modification of tissue reactions leading to infection or slow tissue healing are other side effects of prednisone.

L-asparaginase causes gastrointestinal reactions such as anorexia, nausea, and vomiting. Neurological reactions such as lethargy, progressive malaise, headaches, and confusion often result from this drug. Immunological reactions can be seen secondary to a decreased number of lymphoblasts. The blood chemistry as a result of this agent has the following abnormalities: hypoalbuminemia, hyperglycemia, or altered blood-clotting factors. Elevated blood urea levels or pancreatic enzymes are also seen. Fever and chills are common side effects of this drug.

Daunorubicin causes bone marrow depression and gastrointesintal problems such as abdominal pain and **stomatitis,** inflammation of the mouth. Cardiovascular effects are dose limiting, causing serious myocardial toxicity. The integumentary side effects are alopecia, hyperpigmentation, a skin rash, and loosening of the nails. Reproductive effects are mutagenic and teratogenic. Renal toxicity and hepatotoxicity are common.

With methotrexate, patients develop a rapid onset of bone marrow depression, with **nadir** (the lowest point) occurring in 10 to 14 days. Side effects include nausea, vomiting, stomatitis, pharyngitis, diarrhea, and renal dysfunction. Alopecia and a rash with associated erythema and **pruritus** (itching) are integumentary effects. Brown pigmentation of the skin and photosensitivity are other effects. Infertility and congenital malformation may result from this drug.

Case Study*

A 12-year-old male with recurrent ALL is being considered for total body irradiation before a bone marrow transplant. At age 3, he exhibited easy bruisability, fatigue, and coughing. Blood work performed at this time revealed a high white blood cell count, anemia, and thrombocytopenia. A bone marrow aspiration that extracted marrow from the patient's anterior iliac crest was done. A diagnosis of ALL was made at that time. After the diagnosis a chest x-ray examination was done to check for mediastinal involvement, thymic enlargement, and pleural effusion. The results were negative.

His first course of treatment was chemotherapy. He received systemic chemotherapy and intrathecal methotrexate and was placed in remission.

Approximately 14 months later, the patient exhibited testicular swelling. He received modified chemotherapy and radiation to his testes and remained in remission.

About 10 months later, the patient developed a nonproductive cough and a low-grade fever. These symptoms were treated with antibiotics, and they resolved. Approximately 3 months later, he showed increased fatigue and a nonproductive cough. A complete blood count (CBC) at this time was significant for a white count of 400,000 with 19% blasts. He had an immature T-cell, FAB classification of L2. A chest radiograph taken at that time revealed a mediastinal mass. He also exhibited hepatosplenomegaly.

The patient was scheduled to receive a regimen of vincristine, Adriamycin, prednisone, cytarabine (ara-C), and L-asparaginase. His family was tested, and his brother had a human leukocyte antigen (HLA) match. The patient has been

*Courtesy Tufts-New England Medical Center's Radiation Oncology Department.

enrolled in an in-house protocol for bone marrow transplantation, high-dose Cytoxan, and total body irradiation, followed by a bone marrow transplant.

ACUTE MYELOGENOUS LEUKEMIA

Epidemiology

The incidence rate of AML is five times greater than that of ALL.[9] AML occurs with equal frequency in all decades of life but is slightly more common in patients over 50 years of age. In contrast to ALL (the predominant pediatric leukemia), approximately 80% of adults with leukemia have the AML subtype. AML's incidence is slightly higher among males, with the gender difference being more obvious in older patients.[4]

Etiology

Risk factors for AML are similar to those for ALL. Exposure to ionizing radiation appears to increase a person's risk for developing the disease. An increased incidence of AML has occurred in military personnel at Nevada bomb test sites, patients treated with radiation for ankylosing spondylitis, menorrhagia, and thymic enlargement. Patients receiving Thorotrast (thorium dioxide) for radiologic examinations showed an increased risk of AML.

Fanconi's anemia and Bloom syndrome (genetic disorders with a chromosome breakage tendency), as well as exposure to benzene and alkylating agents, have been associated with AML risk.

Prognostic indicators

Unfavorable prognostic variables of AML are similar to those of ALL. Unfavorable signs include an age greater than 50 years, myelodysplastic syndrome, a poor performance status, impaired organ function, and low serum albumin. Children with AML have a poorer prognosis than those with ALL. As with ALL, a white blood cell count (WBC) of less than 20,000/mm^3 is more favorable than a WBC of 20,000 to 49,000/mm^3. A WBC of greater than 50,000/mm^3 is the least favorable. For AML the age, tumor burden at the time of diagnosis, and drug sensitivity of the leukemic cells are more important than cell morphology in predicting survival.

Clinical presentation

The onset of AML may be abrupt, although most patients experience a 1- to 6-month prodromal period, during which symptoms are present. As with ALL, symptoms at the time of presentation include nonspecific flulike symptoms. Fatigue, pallor, and dyspnea on exertion are secondary to anemia. Petechiae, **purpura** (hemorrhage under the skin), epistaxis, gingival bleeding, and gastrointestinal or urinary tract bleeding may result from reduced platelet production. Neutropenia may result in a susceptibility to local infections, such as skin abcesses, or systemic infections with accompanying fever, chills, and site-specific symptoms. The sensation of an enlarged spleen may be present.

Detection and diagnosis

Specific tests for detecting AML include complete blood cell counts; differential leukocyte, platelet counts; and blood smears. Abnormal blood counts lead to the detection of AML. Thrombocytopenia, anemia, and an increased leukocyte count should be suspect in patients with these conditions. Another form of detection is that of chromosomal abnormalities, which occur in 30% to 50% of patients with AML.

The circulation of **Auer rods** (structures present in cytoplasm myeloblasts, myelocytes, and monoblasts) in the leukemic cells is central to the diagnostic finding of AML. A definitive diagnosis is made via a bone marrow aspiration and biopsy. In AML the bone marrow is hypercellular. The diagnosis is made based on the percentage of blast cells. If more than 30% blast cells are present, acute leukemia is the diagnosis. A staining procedure is the final step to determine a differential diagnosis of AML. In summary, a diagnosis of AML is based on the circulation of Auer rods in leukemic cells, an increase in leukemic blast cells, and a decrease in normal precursors.

Immunophenotyping that includes a morphological evaluation, special stains, an electron microscopy, and surface marker studies can establish a diagnosis in 90% of AML patients. Morphological evaluations are based on monoclonal anitbodies reacting with a surface antigen that is expressed on the membrane of the leukemic cell.

Pathology

The pathogenesis of AML is derived from the unregulated proliferation of early precursor cells that have lost the ability to differentiate in response to hormonal signals and cellular interactions. This proliferation or clonal disease involves the hemopoietic stem cells or pluripotent cells. The result is a gradual accumulation of undifferentiated cells in marrow or other organs.

These undifferentiated cells have a decreased proportion of blast cells in the S or M phase of the cell cycle compared with normal bone marrow blast cells. Because of this decrease of blast cells in these specific phases, the cells do not reach maturity or are defective at maturity.

Staging and classification

For a morphological evaluation the FAB system is used. AML is categorized in different maturation states, from M0 (undifferentiated) to M7 (megakaryocytic). They are as follows[4]:

M0—Minimal evidence of maturation exists.

M1—The cells tend to have fine azurophil granules and may have few Auer rods. Minimal evidence exists of differentiation along the rest of the granulocytic or monocytic lineages.

M2—The number of blast cells is greater than 30%, and the proportion of monocytic precursors with less than 20% cells have abundant cytoplasm and moderate to marked granularity.

M3—The APL predominant cell is heavily granulated with azurophil granulation. Many cells have bundle of Auer rods whose nucleus is often bilobed or kidney shaped.

M4—The myeloid precursors or other granulocytic precursors are between 20% and 80% of the nonerythroid nucleated cells. The monocytic cells comprise 20% or more of the nonerythroid nucleated cells.

M5—The proportion of granulocyte precursors is less than 20%.

M6—Fewer than 30% of the cells are of myeloid or monocytic lineage, and more than 50% are megaloblastic erythroid precursors.

M7—This state is often associated with extensive marrow fibrosis that has an increase in reticulin or collagen.

Other classifying techniques include cytochemical, immunological and chromosomal studies.

Treatment techniques

The treatment techniques for AML are radiation therapy, chemotherapy, and bone marrow transplantation. These three techniques are used in a combined fashion.

Radiation therapy is administered to the whole body (total body irradiation). It is given b.i.d. for 3 days, with a total dose of 1200 cGy. (See the ALL treatment technique section on pp. 87-88 for further details.)

The chemotherapy treatment techniques for treating AML are divided into three groups: induction, consolidation, and maintenance. The drugs used in induction chemotherapy are cytosine arabinoside, daunorubicin, and doxorubicin. Cytarabine is used for consolidation therapy. Maintenance therapy includes 6-thioguanine, vincristine, and prednisone.

Bone marrow transplantation is the final treatment technique used in treating AML. (See pp. 87-88 for a description of the bone marrow transplantation procedure.)

Field design and critical structures. The field design and critical structures are described in the section on ALL on pp. 88-89.

Side effects. Bone marrow depression in 4 to 7 days and immunological suppression are the hemopoietic side effects of cytosine arabinoside and cytarabine. Nausea, vomiting, esophagitis, stomatitis, diarrhea, and ulceration are common gastrointestinal problems. Renal effects include urinary retention and thrombophlebitis. Rashes and alopecia are skin reactions. In reproduction, mutagenic and teratogenic problems arise.

Bone marrow depression also occurs after the use of daunorubicin. With this drug, common gastrointestinal problems are abdominal pain and stomatitis. Myocardial toxicity is the dose-limiting factor for daunorubicin. The integumentary effects are alopecia, hyperpigmentation of the nail beds, and sun sensitivity. Reproductive side effects are teratogenic or mutagenic. The urine turns red after one or two administrations.

The drug 6-thioguanine also produces bone marrow depression. Diarrhea, stomatitis, and anorexia are common gastrointestinal side effects. The skin may develop dermatitis. Reproductive side effects are mutagenic and teratogenic. Photosensitivity also occurs.

Case Study*

A 41-year-old mother of two is being considered for total body irradiation followed by bone marrow transplantation. She initially complained of heavy menstrual periods and progressive fatigue. She noted dyspnea on exertion, petechiae, and some gingival bleeding.

About 2 months later, a blood test was performed and she was found to have panocytopenia with a WBC of 900, the hematocrit at 17%, and 80,000 platelets. A bone marrow aspiration and biopsy showed myeloblasts, and the diagnosis of AML was made.

The patient received induction chemotherapy with cytosine arabinoside, daunorubicin, and doxyrubicin. This treatment was complicated by neutropenia, a fever, and a rash that she developed over her body.

She had her first consolidation 1 month later, with cytarabine combined with hydrocortisone. She tolerated this treatment well. Her maintenance therapy consisted of 6-thioguanine, vincristine, and prednisone. This treatment caused her diarrhea, anorexia, and dermatitis.

The patient now awaits her total body irradiation and bone marrow transplant. Her brother is a 5.6 human leukocyte antigen (HLA) match. She is being prepared for a bone marrow transplant and is having a second cycle of consolidation therapy.

CHRONIC LYMPHOCYTIC LEUKEMIA

Epidemiology

CLL is the most common leukemia. It affects between 1.8 and 3 persons per 100,000 and accounts for approximately 30% of the leukemia cases in the United States.[9] CLL is nearly twice as common as the chronic myelogenous subtype. The incidence of CLL increases with age, with 65 as the average age of onset. The disease is rare in persons under 35 years old. CLL affects approximately 5.2 persons per 100,000 between 35 and 59 years of age and 30.4 persons per 100,000 between 80 and 84 years of age. The disease affects twice as many males as females and is less common among Japanese and other Asian populations.[4] CLL occurs with equal frequency among black and white people.

Etiology

Heredity appears to play a role in the development of CLL. First-degree relatives of persons with CLL have a threefold increase in risk, and the familial clustering of CLL is the most notable of all the leukemias. Immunological factors such as

*Courtesy Tufts-New England Medical Center's Radiation Oncology Department.

immunodeficiency syndromes and viruses have been associated with CLL. Several small studies have attempted to determine a suspected link between CLL and chemicals (primarily carbon tetrachloride and carbon disulfide) used in the rubber industry. CLL is the only leukemia for which an association with radiation exposure has not been established. In addition, retroviruses have not been linked with this disease.[4]

Prognostic indicators

Prognostic factors for CLL include the stage at the time of diagnosis, age, doubling time of the peripheral blood lymphocyte count, and pattern of bone marrow involvement. The T-cell variety of CLL tends to run a more aggressive clinical course and results in shorter survival times.[10]

Clinical presentation

CLL most often occurs as incidental findings on blood tests taken during routine medical visits, with lymphocyte counts often equal to or higher than 10,000/mm^3. Patients are frequently asymptomatic, with abnormalities found only on peripheral blood smears and a bone marrow biopsy. Complaints include fatigue, fever, night sweats, and weight loss. Lymphadenopathy may be present in CLL, and the spleen is almost always enlarged. Complaints of uncomfortable neck masses are common at later stages.

Detection and diagnosis

Blood tests are used to detect CLL. Patients always exhibit lymphocytosis. Other manifestations of the disease are anemia and thrombocytopenia. Laboratory tests that determine monoclonal surface immunoglobulin and B-cell markers are important to the diagnosis. Phenotyping of leukemic lymphocytes reveals a B-cell origin in 95% of CLL cases.[2]

Other factors leading to the detection and diagnosis of CLL include the enlargement of lymph nodes and the spleen. Of patients with CLL, 50% have chromosomal abnormalities.

Pathology

The origin of CLL may be in the bone marrow lymphoid tissue.[2] A pathological examination of CLL reveals an increased proliferation of leukemic cells in the bone marrow, blood, lymph nodes, and spleen, with resulting organ enlargement and decreased bone marrow function.[4]

Staging and classification

One classification system for CLL is the Rai's staging system. With this system the three major prognostic groups used to categorize patients are as follows:

Stage 0—Low risk
Stages I and II—Intermediate risk
Stages III and IV—High risk

These stages are based on the presence of adenopathy, splenomegaly, anemia, and thrombocytopenia.[2] The majority of patients are in the intermediate-risk category, followed by an equal percentage for the other prognostic groups.

The Binet staging system categorizes patients into three stages based on the involvement of five specific anatomical sites: the cervical nodes, axillary nodes, inguinal nodes, spleen, and liver. These stages are as follows:

Stage A—No cytopenia and involvement of up to two sites
Stage B—Involvement of three or more sites
Stage C—Anemia, thrombocytopenia ,or both

Cytochemistry is used to classify CLL according to two subtypes: B-cell CLL and T-cell CLL.[4]

Treatment techniques

The optimal treatment for CLL is unknown. It is believed that some patients with an early stage of the disease will not benefit from treatment. Chemotherapy is administered for progressive anemia and thrombocytopenia. The drugs used are primarily alkylating agents, chlorambucil, or cyclophosphamide. They prevent the separation of the strands of DNA, which is necessary for cell replication.[1]

Other treatment techniques are radiation therapy and surgery. Palliative radiation therapy is used for localized masses of lymphoid tissue and/or the spleen. The treatment is given in an AP/PA fashion to a dose of 500 cGy, with 100 cGy per day for 5 days.

The surgery used for treating CLL is the splenectomy. An enlarged spleen causes cytopenia, which is the result of accelerated removal or excessive pooling of platelets or red blood cells. A splenectomy is used in a situation in which markedly enlarged spleen produces cytopenia.

Field design and critical structures. The field design for treating a spleen is clinical. The field must encompass the entire spleen with a 1-cm margin around the organ. Field setups are done through palpation or a fluoroscopy. Simulation is necessary to localize the spleen field and make sure the kidney is safely out of the field (Fig. 5-6). Iodinated contrast is used for this intravenous pyelogram procedure.

Side effects. Cloramabucil causes bone marrow depression. Gastrointestinal side effects include anorexia, nausea, and vomiting. Dermatitis and urticaria are other side effects. Reproductive side effects include mutagenesis, teratogenesis, and sterility.

Cyclophosphamide can cause leukopenia with nadir in 7 to 10 days. This drug is a potent immunosuppressant. Gastrointestinal side effects include nausea, vomiting, and diarrhea. The renal side effects are cystitis, hematuria, urinary frequency, and dysuria. The integumentary system is affected by alopecia and hyperpigmentation of the skin and nails. Reproductive side effects of this drug are fetal damage, sterility, and mutagenic effects.

Prednisone causes gastrointestinal peptic ulcers and pancreatitis. Metabolic responses include centripetal obesity, hyperlipidemia, hyperosmolar nonketotic coma, and immunosuppression. The neurological side effect is pseudotumor cerebri. Glaucoma and cataracts may also appear. Hypertension, skin **striae,** amenorrhea, and impaired wound healing are also side effects.

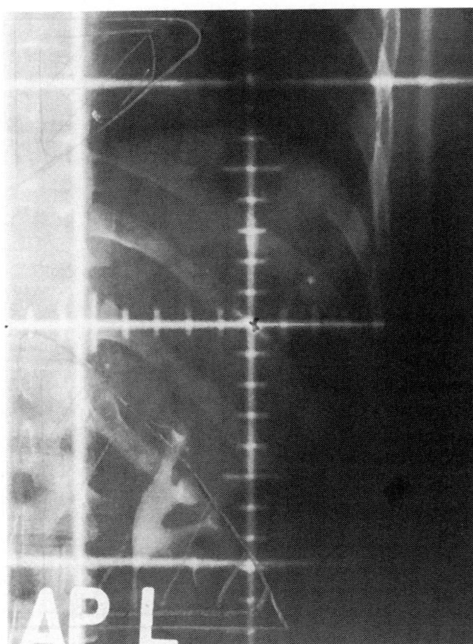

Fig. 5-6 Simulation film of a spleen field, excluding the kidney.

Case Study*

Mrs. W. is a 68-year-old woman who was diagnosed 2 years ago at age 66. She was being treated at a neighborhood health center for a thyroid condition. During a routine blood test, her differential count showed a lymphocytosis of 67% (10,800/mm^3 white blood). Her hematocrit had dropped from an average of 36 to 32.2. Therefore she was referred for further evaluation.

The patient's initial history revealed night sweats and a fever. She had chronic sinus congestion and hearing loss. She denied having a cough, shortness of breath, or chest pain, but she did note slight fatigue. Her spleen was enlarged.

Her physical examination showed clear lungs, no hepatosplenomegaly, and no arthritis. Her blood work showed a hemoglobin of 11.6 gm/100 ml, a hematocrit of 35.1%, a mean corpuscular volume (MCV) of 90.1, and unremarkable red blood count (RBC) morphology. Her WBC was 11.7 thousand per milliliter. These numbers showed the hemogloblin and hematocrit at the lower margins of normal. The lymphocytosis was consistent with CLL stage O. Peripheral blood lymphocyte markers were obtained, revealing 63% B cells. This is also consistent with CLL Stage O.

About 10 months after diagnosis, Mrs. W. developed neuropathy with pain and numbness of her feet. A neurologist examined her and found nothing. A few months later, she developed leg ulcers. At this point, she was started on a treatment of prednisone. Her pain improved, and her ankle ulcers all healed.

Mrs. W. is presently asymptomatic, and her prognosis is excellent.

*Courtesy Tufts-New England Medical Center's Radiation Oncology Department.

CHRONIC MYELOGENOUS LEUKEMIA

Epidemiology

CML accounts for approximately 20% to 30% of all leukemias. The incidence of this disease, which is rare in childhood and uncommon before the age of 20, peaks among persons in their midforties. A slight predominance of cases exists among males.

Etiology

The etiology of CML is unknown. Radiation and benzene exposure have been linked with the development of the disease, but no other environmental or genetic factors have been clearly implicated as causes. The identification of the Philadelphia chromosome by Nowell and Hungerford in 1960 and its presence in 95% of CML patients has led to much interest regarding its possible etiological role in this disorder.

Prognostic indicators

The prognosis for patients with CML is affected by numerous factors, including the spleen size, platelet count, hematocrit, gender, and percentage of blood myeloblasts. The disease typically transforms into an acute leukemia after a chronic phase of about 3 years, when the patient enters a blast crisis. A patient in the active phase of the disease has a median survival time of approximately 2 years.

Clinical presentation

The natural history of CML is divided into three stages: chronic, accelerated, and acute phase, or blast crisis. The early phase of the disease is usually insidious; clinical symptoms are generally mild and nonspecific. Malaise, fatigue, heat intolerance, sweating, and easy bruising are common complaints. Symptoms related to splenic enlargement include vague discomfort in the left upper quadrant (LUQ), early satiety, weight loss, and peripheral leg edema. Within 3 to 4 years, most patients undergo a transformation to a blast crisis. At this stage, all the organs of the body are invaded by leukemic blast cells, and the circulating blood count can reach several hundreds of thousands per cubic millimeter. During the blast crisis, symptoms include fever, bone pain, and more pronounced weight loss.

The active-disease phase of CML, as defined by the Chronic Leukemia Myeloma Task Force, is characterized by weight loss greater than 10% of the body weight in less than 6 months, fever, extreme fatigue, anemia, thrombocytopenia, organ involvement (other than lymph nodes, spleen, bone marrow, and liver), and progressive or painful enlargement of the spleen.

Detection and diagnosis

The detection and diagnosis of CML is difficult. This disease is insidious and generally not found, except incidentally. Specific indicators lead to a diagnosis. These abnormal indicators include mild to moderate anemia and leukocytosis. Myeloblasts, promyelocytes, and nucleated red cells, which indicate CML, are present in the blood. Bone marrow specimens reveal increased granulocytic and often megakaryocytic hyperplasia. Another indicator of CML is a low or absent leukocyte alkaline phosphotase (LAP) score. The most important diagnostic factor for detecting CML is the presence of the Philadelphia chromosome.

Pathology

CML pathogenesis is a result of abnormal hemopoietic stem cells that give rise to progeny that have the Philadelphia chromosome.[6] Because of the abnormal stem cell pool, an increased proliferation of granulocytic and megakaryocytic cells exists. Erythropoiesis is impaired.[2]

Staging and classification

The three distinct stages of CML are the chronic (or stable) phase, accelerated phase, and acute phase (or blast crisis). (For a further description of stages, see the clinical presentation section.)

Treatment techniques

The three treatment techniques for treating CML are radiation therapy, chemotherapy, and bone marrow transplantation. Radiation therapy is delivered to the spleen and total body. The treatment technique for the spleen is the same as that for CLL. (See the treatment techniques section for CLL on p. 93.) The treatment technique for total body irradiation is the same as that for ALL.

In chemotherapy the drugs used are busulfan and hydroxyurea. Busulfan is an alkylating agent given orally. It causes a gradual reduction of the leukocyte count toward normal, an increase in the RBC, and a decrease in the spleen size. Hydroxyurea blocks DNA synthesis by inhibiting a ribonucleotide reductase.

The final treatment technique for CML is bone marrow transplantation. (See the treatment technique section for ALL on p. 87-88.) Allogeneic bone marrow transplantation is the only curative treatment for CML. The success rate for patients is lower when they are in the accelerated phase, especially if they have developed a blast transformation.

Field design and critical structures. The spleen field design is explained in the CLL section on p. 93. The total body irradiation field design is explained in the ALL section on p. 88-89.

Side effects. The side effects of busulfan include pancytopenia and delayed bone marrow depression. Gastrointestinal side effects are diarrhea, nausea, and vomiting. Interstitial pulmonary fibrosis is a side effect to the lungs. In the integumentary system, alopecia, hyperpigmentation, and muscle wasting occur. In the reproductive system testicular atrophy and gynecomastia occur in males. Amenorrhea and sterility are other reproductive side effects. Cataract formation also occurs.

Hydroxurea affects the hemopoietic system, with bone marrow depression, rapid leukopenia, and erythrocytic abnormalities. The gastrointestinal side effects are anorexia and diarrhea. Facial erythema and maculopapular rash are integumentary reactions. The reproductive side effect is teratogenic.

Case Study*

A 17-year-old female with CML complained of a 1-month history of fatigue, easy bruising, and the passing of large blood clots during a menstrual period. Blood work was performed and revealed a WBC of 78,000/mm^3. A blood smear showed numerous myeloid forms consistent with CML. Her hematocrit was 35%, and her platelet count was 204,000/mm^3.

A bone marrow biopsy and aspiration were performed and found to be consistent with CML. Her LAP score was 36. Cytogenetics showed a translocation of the number 9 and number 22 chromosomes. This is consistent with a Philadelphia chromosome.

The patient was first given hydroxurea. She tolerated this well, aside from some mild anorexia and diarrhea. About 3 months later, the patient received 500 cGy to her spleen. This was followed by total body irradiation and a bone marrow transplant 1 week later.

ROLE OF RADIATION THERAPIST

Because of the systemic nature of the disease, chemotherapy is the frontline treatment for leukemia. Radiation therapy plays a relatively small, although significant, role in the management of this group of diseases. Therapists who work in health care facilities in which bone marrow transplants are not performed or specialized pediatric oncology services are not provided may see few leukemia patients. Issues relating to scheduling treatments and communicating with and providing support and reassurance for children and their parents must be taken into consideration in departments that routinely treat leukemia patients.

In treating children who have leukemia, therapists must be prepared to communicate with and provide support for the patients and their parents. The radiation oncology experience may evoke fear; the equipment is large and imposing, and the child has most likely undergone numerous painful medical procedures. Sufficient time should be allowed for an explanation of the procedures and the provision of necessary support. Creative methods of eliciting the

*Courtesy Tufts-New England Medical Center's Radiation Oncology Department.

cooperation of a young child (e.g., stuffed animals and rewards for holding still) and extreme patience may be necessary if anesthesia for daily treatment needs to be avoided. Exposure of the anatomical areas to be treated may cause emotional concern for a young patient and must be considered and respected by the treatment team. Therapists must be aware of the concerns of the patient's parents, who often have had to subject their child to painful medical procedures and are themselves coping with issues of denial, acceptance, and possible loss.

Last-minute changes and delays in scheduling often accompany the treatment of leukemia patients. Radiation therapists should be aware of these modifications and realize that the flexibility of daily treatment schedules is frequently necessary. Children who require anesthesia for their daily treatments not only need extra time and equipment for treatment, but also careful coordination of radiation oncology, anesthesia, and nursing schedules. The radiation oncologist may need to set up treatment fields daily for leukemia patients being treated for an enlarged liver or spleen. The radiation oncologist palpates the organ and modifies the field as needed. Patients being treated for the control of blood counts may need to have blood drawn and blood count results reported before each treatment. Extra time may be required for positioning and precise matching of multiple fields for central nervous system treatment.

Total body irradiation in preparation for bone marrow transplantation requires special attention and consideration by the radiation therapist. As much as 1½ hours need to be set aside in the treatment schedule for each of these procedures. If b.i.d. treatment is prescribed, major interruptions in the daily treatment schedule can occur, requiring the rescheduling of other patients' appointments. Because the bone marrow transplant patient's immune system is compromised, the treatment room and machine must be scrubbed with disinfectant before the patient's arrival. The treatment team must use reverse isolation techniques (i.e., gown, gloves, and mask). Extra time and patience is required to make sure the patient is in a position that can be maintained for the actual treatment. Because an extended source-skin distance (SSD) is required to achieve the necessary field size, the actual treatment ("beam on") time required to deliver the prescribed dose is often as long as 45 minutes. The patient may experience nausea during treatment. The treatment must then be interrupted, and the patient must be allowed to move and walk around until the nausea subsides. At that time the patient can be repositioned, and the treatment can be resumed.

Review Questions

Multiple Choice

1. Which of the following concerning CLL is not true?
   a. It is a disease of children.
   b. It resembles CML but with a malignant lymphoid cell line.
   c. It can be confused with lymphoma.
   d. Therapy is usually reserved until the patient is symptomatic.
2. Which of the following is a *specific characteristic* of CML?
   a. A disease of children
   b. Philadelphia chromosome
   c. Requirement of prophylactic central nervous system radiation
   d. Presentation with an enlarged spleen
3. Which of the following is not a common symptom associated with acute leukemia at the time of presentation?
   a. Fatigue
   b. Easy bleeding and bruisability
   c. Nausea and vomiting
   d. Fever
4. Which of the following leukemias has not been associated with previous radiation exposure?
   a. CML
   b. CLL
   c. AML
   d. ALL

Fill in the Blank

5. Two anatomical sites that are potential sanctuaries for leukemic cells are the __________ and the __________ __________.
6. The four main subtypes of leukemia are __________, __________, __________, and __________.
7. The primary treatment modality for leukemia is __________.
8. The most documented etiological factor for leukemia in humans is __________.

Essay

9. Name one way in which radiation therapy is used in the management of leukemia patients.

Questions to Ponder

1. Discuss the main factors that differentiate the four subtypes of leukemia.
2. Describe the various treatment techniques used for the four main subtypes of leukemia.
3. Describe the systems used to classify the leukemias.
4. Discuss the sanctuary areas in the treatment of leukemia.
5. Differentiate between detection and diagnosis in reference to the specific subtypes of leukemia.
6. Describe the different types of bone marrow transplantation techniques.

REFERENCES

1. American Cancer Society, *Cancer manual,* ed 8, Boston, 1990, The Society.
2. American Cancer Society: *Clinical oncology: a multidisciplinary approach,* ed 6, 1983, The Society.
3. Dameshek W, Gunz F: *Leukemia,* ed 2, New York, 1964, Grune & Stratton.
4. DeVita V, Hellman S, Rosenberg S: *Cancer principles and practice of oncology,* Philadelphia, 1993, JB Lippincott.
5. Freireich EJ, Lemak NA: *Milestones in leukemia research and therapy,* Baltimore, 1991, John Hopkins University Press.
6. Henderson ES, Han T: Current therapy of acute and chronic leukemia in adults, CA *J Clin* 36(6):322-350, 1986.
7. National Cancer Institute: *Annual cancer statisitics review,* NIH publication #88-2789, Washington, DC, 1988, US Department of Health and Human Services.
8. National Cancer Institute: *SEER cancer statistics review, 1973-1992: tables and graphs,* NIH publication #96-2789, Bethesda, Maryland, 1995, The Institute.
9. National Cancer Institute: *Surveillance epidemiology end results, incidence and mortality data,* NIH Monograph 57, Bethesda, Maryland, 1995, The Institute.
10. Thomas ED: Bone marrow transplantation, *CA J Clinici* 37(5): 291-296, 1987.
11. Wiernik PH et al: *Neoplastic diseases of the blood,* New York, 1991, Churchill Livingstone.

BIBLIOGRAPHY

American Cancer Society: *Clinical oncology,* Atlanta, 1991, The Society.

Brager BL, Yasko J: *Care of the client receiving chemotherapy,* Reston, Virginia, 1984, Reston Publishing.

Manual of oncologic therapeutics, Philadelphia, 1989/1990, JB Lippincott.

Rubin P: *Clinical oncology,* ed 7, Philadelphia, 1993, WB Saunders.

Taber's cyclopedic medical dictionary, ed 17, Philadelphia, 1993, FA Davis.

Tarbel N, Mauch P, Chin L: Total body irradiation. In *JCRT handbook,* Boston, 1994, Joint Center for Radiation Therapy.

C H A P T E R

6

Endocrine System

Tammy Newell
James D. Becht

Outline

- Thyroid cancer
  - Epidemiology
  - Etiology
  - Prognostic indicators
  - Anatomy
  - Physiology
  - Clinical presentation
  - Detection and diagnosis
  - Pathology
  - Staging
  - Routes of spread
  - Treatment techniques
- Pituitary tumors
  - Epidemiology and etiology
  - Prognostic indicators
  - Anatomy
  - Physiology
  - Clinical presentation
  - Detection and diagnosis
  - Pathology
  - Staging
  - Treatment techniques
  - Results of treatment
- Adrenal cortex tumors
  - Epidemiology and etiology
  - Prognostic indicators
  - Anatomy
  - Physiology
  - Clinical presentation
  - Detection and diagnosis
  - Pathology
  - Staging
  - Routes of spread
  - Treatment techniques
- Adrenal medulla tumors
  - Epidemiology and etiology
  - Anatomy
  - Clinical presentation
  - Detection and diagnosis
  - Pathology and staging
  - Routes of spread
  - Treatment techniques
  - Results of treatment
- Role of radiation therapist

Key terms

Adenohypophysis
Alopecia
Bitemporal hemianopsia
Chromophobe adenomas
Cold thyroid nodule
Cortex
Diffuse adenomas
Dysphagia
Hot thyroid nodule
Hyperthyroidism
Hypothyroidism
Infundibulum
Intrahypophyseal tumors
Intrasellar lesions
Invasive neoplasms
Isthmus
Latent period
Macroadenomas
Medulla
Microadenomas
Neurohypophysis
Sterotactic radiosurgery
Warm thyroid nodule

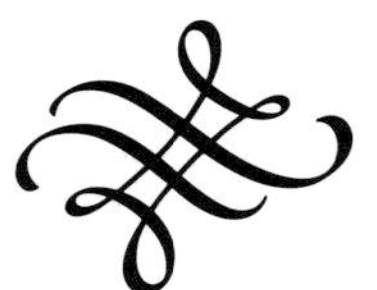

The endocrine system is composed of multiple glandular organs responsible for complex metabolic regulatory functions. The principal organs of this system include the following glands: pituitary (which resides in the sella turcica at the base of the brain), thyroid, and adrenal. Also included are the parathyroid glands and specialized cells in the pancreas called the *islets of Langerhans,* which are referred to as the *endocrine portions of the pancreas.* Each of these organs (or specialized portions of them) produces hormones under complex feedback-control mechanisms that affect various functions to meet ongoing metabolic needs and stresses of the organism. The master regulatory gland of this system is the pituitary. This gland produces many hormones under the influence of the hypothalamus, which directly affects the function of other endocrine organs. This sophisticated mechanism of stimulation and inhibition of endocrine organ function is critical for maintaining metabolic homeostasis (stability) and providing the organism with the ability to respond to various stresses.

Many disorders of the endocrine organs can result in disruption of this complex surveillance and response system. These disorders may be related to benign, congenital, degenerative, traumatic, autoimmune, or infectious processes that may affect the function of one or many organs in the endocrine system. The result can range from minor to potentially life-threatening dysfunction. Probably the most widely recognized endocrine dysfunction is insufficient insulin production by the islet cells of the pancreas, or diabetes mellitus. Although this is a complex multisystem disease, the abnormality in glucose metabolism caused by insulin deficiency can be disastrous. This situation is remedied through the supply of insulin via an injection to reestablish homeostasis of glucose metabolism.

The function of the endocrine system may also be affected by neoplastic change in the various glands. Although true primary malignancies of these organs are rare, they are important to consider because of the wide-ranging effects they can have on the organism as a whole. Metabolic function altered by neoplastic change in various endocrine organs can produce clinical syndromes that are often well recognized. These syndromes can lead the clinician to perform various diagnostic studies to confirm the suspicions related to an endocrine gland tumor. This chapter discusses neoplastic lesions of the thyroid, pituitary, and adrenal gland. Pancreatic tumors, which can display endocrine and exocrine function, are discussed in Chapter 10.

THYROID CANCER

Epidemiology

Although thyroid cancers are the most common of the endocrine malignancies (accounting for approximately 90% of all new cases and 63% of deaths), they represent only 1.3% of all cancers. Women have a higher incidence rate than men, with approximately a 2.3:1.0 ratio. Young adult females have a five-fold risk compared with males.[15]

Etiology

Unlike other endocrine glands for which the incidence of malignancy is rare, thyroid cancer has several recognized etiological factors.

External radiation to the thyroid gland, particularly before puberty, is the only well-documented etiological factor. Approximately 25% of the patients who receive between 2 cGy and several hundred cGy of external radiation to the thyroid gland develop thyroid carcinoma. These carcinomas are usually a low-grade papillary subtype. [31]

Many studies have been conducted on the inhabitants of Nagasaki and Hiroshima after the explosion of the atomic bomb in 1945. Out of 20,000 heavily and lightly exposed individuals examined every year since 1959, approximately 0.2% have developed thyroid cancer. Again, most of these have been papillary. [31]

After the radioactive fallout from a nuclear test in the Marshall Islands, the inhabitants have annually been studied systematically and compared with a nonexposed population. According to the results in 1974, 34 of 229 exposed persons developed thyroid lesions. Three of the total number of patients developed cancers. Those irradiated before the age of 20 showed the highest incidence rate of thyroid nodularity. [15]

The Chernobyl incident of 1986 has produced conflicting studies on the increase of thyroid cancer, probably because of the extremely short interval between radiation exposure and tumor occurrence. One study conducted $4^1/_2$ years after the Chernobyl reactor accident showed no significant difference in thyroid nodularity among persons residing in highly contaminated and control villages.[27]

However, another study's data confirm that the neoplasms increasingly diagnosed between 1986 and 1991 among children of the Republic of Belarus were thyroid carcinomas.[13] In the Cancer Registry of Belarus, 101 instances of thyroid cancer in children less than 15 years of age had been noted between 1986 and 1991, in contrast to only 9 cases between 1976 and 1985.[13]

External radiation for benign disease, especially in young patients, was a widespread practice in the United States in the 1930s, 1940s, and 1950s. X-rays or radium was used to treat benign conditions such as acne, tonsillitis, hemangiomas, and thymic enlargement. Young patients who received radiation for malignant conditions, such as mantle irradiation for Hodgkin's disease, demonstrated an increased risk of developing thyroid cancer.[15,26]

The **latent** (time) **period** between exposure and incidence of abnormalities varies with age. The average latent period in infants is 11 years, and in adolescents it is 15 to 30 years. Whether adults develop cancer at a higher rate after exposure is questionable.[16]

Prolonged stimulation of the thyroid gland with a thyroid-stimulating hormone (TSH) in laboratory animals has produced thyroid cancer. However, no human population studies have been done that support this hypothesis.[33]

Some other, less well-defined, factors include the following[3]:

- Long-standing, nontoxic colloid goiter in relation to papillary and anaplastic carcinoma
- The relationship of follicular adenomas as premalignant lesions to follicular carcinomas
- The role of genetics for medullary carcinoma*

Prognostic indicators

The extent of the disease at the time of the diagnosis is a major prognostic factor. Lesions confined to the gland have an overall better prognosis than those demonstrating capsular invasion.

*A large proportion of cases are familial, occurring as part of two complex endocrine syndromes: multiple endocrine neoplasia (MEN) IIa and IIb.

As far as the histological subtype is concerned, patients with well-differentiated thyroid carcinoma (papillary and follicular) have a better prognosis than those with undifferentiated carcinoma (anaplastic).

A study by Cady et al.[7] showed that age and gender plays a significant role in survival. Young patients with differentiated thyroid cancers do better than older patients displaying the same histological features. Basic risk groups were defined by age and gender alone. The low-risk group consisted of men 40 years of age and younger and women 50 years of age and younger. The high-risk group was composed of older patients.

Cady et al.[7] also found that the overall risk of recurrence for women under 50 years of age was 10%, and the risk of death was 3%. Among patients with recurrent or metastatic disease, only 30% died of their malignancy. For women over the age of 50 the respective figures were 32%, 30%, and 89%. These changes with age showed a high degree of statistical significance for women, but for men the significance was only borderline in terms of recurrence. A change in the death rate according to age was not significant in men.

Anatomy

The thyroid gland, consisting of a right and left lobe, lies over the deep structures of the neck; is close to the larynx, trachea, parathyroid glands, and esophagus; and is anterior and medial to the carotid artery, jugular vein, and vagus nerve.[6] (See Fig. 6-1 for the anatomy of the thyroid gland and its anatomical relationships to surrounding structures.)

The lateral lobes are approximately 5 cm in length and extend to the level of the midthyroid cartilage superiorly and the sixth tracheal ring inferiorly. These lobes are connected in the midline by the **isthmus** at the level of the second to fourth tracheal rings.The thyroid gland weighs approximately 25 g.[32]

Lymphatic capillaries are arranged throughout the gland and drain to many nodal sites. These sites include the internal jugular chain, Delphian node (anterior cervical node), pretracheal nodes, and the paratracheal nodes in the lower neck.[6,32]

Superior mediastinal lymphatics can be considered the lowest part of the cervical lymphatic system. If it is involved, this represents significant regional spread of disease.[6,32]

Physiology

The thyroid gland produces several hormones, including thyroxine (T-4) and triiodothyronine (T-3), which are responsible for metabolic regulation. Thyroidal function is regulated by pituitary and hypothalamic hormones, which respond to complex systemic feedback mechanisms based on metabolic needs. The TSH produced in the pituitary gland causes direct stimulation of thyroid cells to produce and release hormones that are critical for carbohydrate and protein metabolism.

The production of these hormones relies on the thyroid gland's ability to remove iodine from the blood. Without sufficient amounts of iodine, several clinical disorders can be observed from the resultant deficiency in thyroid-hormone production. Functional disorders of the thyroid gland are characterized by hyperactivity **(hyperthyroidism)** or underactivity **(hypothyroidism).**

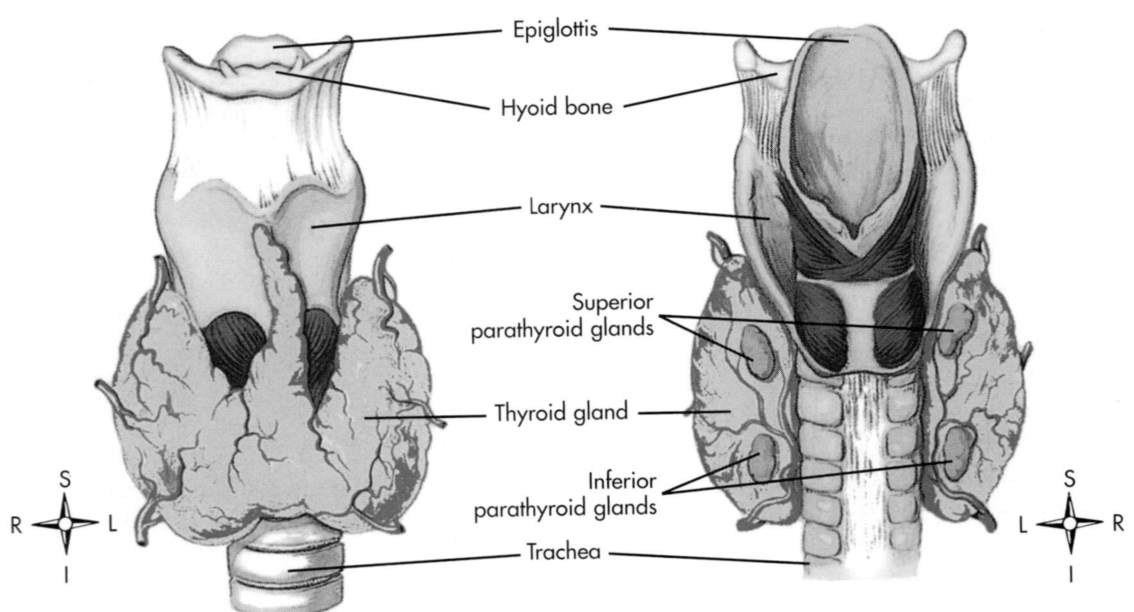

Fig. 6-1 Anatomy of the thyroid gland. (From Thibodeau GA, Patton KT, editors: *Anatomy & physiology,* St Louis, 1987, Mosby.)

Disorders from hypothyroidism can include the following[20]:

- Cretinism—This disorder appears in infants shortly after birth. Symptoms include stunted growth, abnormal bone formation, retarded mental development, a low body temperature, and sluggishness.
- Myxedema:—This disorder occurs if hypothyroidism develops after growth. Symptoms include a low metabolic rate, mental slowness, weight gain, and swollen tissues caused by excess body fluid.

Disorders from hyperthyroidism can include the following[20]:

- Graves' disease—This disorder is characterized by an elevated metabolic rate, abnormal weight loss, excessive perspiration, muscular weakness, emotional instability, and exophthalmos.
- Goiter—This disorder is a physical sign of an enlarged thyroid gland. Overstimulation by TSH causes an enlargement of thyroid cells. If this is associated with increased hormone production, it is referred to as *toxic goiter.*

In addition, a specialized subgroup of cells exists in the thyroid known as *C-cells.*These produce calcitonin, which is a hormone involved in calcium metabolism.

Clinical presentation

Most patients with thyroid cancer have a palpable neck mass, which is often detected during a routine physical examination. Almost 25% of young people with differentiated thyroid carcinoma present because of a palpable cervical lymph node metastasis as a result of occult primary thyroid cancer.[5] These occult-differentiated thyroid cancers can go undetected for years because of their indolent nature. A biopsy should be performed on persistent, enlarged lymph nodes found in children, teenagers, and young adults, with a clinical differential of Hodgkin's disease, benign inflammatory disease, or papillary carcinoma of the thyroid gland.[6]

Lesions in the thyroid gland should arouse suspicion if they exhibit extreme hardness, appear with fixation to deep structures or skin, and have recurrent laryngeal nerve paralysis (hoarseness).

Anaplastic carcinomas are usually large, hard, and fixed; grow rapidly; and occur in older patients. Patients can appear with symptoms related to compression and/or invasion of the esophagus, airway, or recurrent laryngeal nerves. Symptoms include pain, dysphagia, dyspnea, stridor, and hoarseness.[32]

A majority of patients with medullary carcinoma initially have an asymptomatic painless mass.[8,19,32] They may appear with systemic symptoms of diarrhea related to vasoactive substances produced by the tumor. This usually represents an advanced stage of the disease. (See Table 6-1 for clinical symptoms and signs of patients with thyroid carcinoma.)

Table 6-1 Clinical symptoms and signs in 106 patients with thyroid carcinoma

Symptoms and signs	Patients (66) with papillary carcinoma (%)	Patients (33) with follicular carcinoma (%)	Patients (7) with anaplastic carcinoma (%)
Hoarseness	9	15	55
Dysphagia	11	12	28
Pain and pressure	8	6	28
Dyspnea	3	6	43
Increasing size	56	75	85
Solitary nodule	60	65	14
Multinodular	33	20	70
Found in routine examination	27	30	0

Modified from Ureles AL et al: Cancer of the endocrine glands. In Rubin P: *Clinical oncology: a multidisciplinary approach for physicians and students*, Philadelphia, 1993, WB Saunders.

Detection and diagnosis

Clinical presentation cannot determine a diagnosis of carcinoma. For confirmation of the diagnostic suspicion of cancer, a biopsy (most important), specialized imaging studies, and laboratory testing are necessary.

Laboratory testing includes an analysis of the thyroglobulin and calcitonin levels.

Thyroglobulin levels cannot distinguish between a benign tumor and differentiated thyroid cancer.[15,35] Postoperatively, however, elevated levels indicate residual, recurrent, or metastatic differentiated thyroid cancer and can be correlated with I 131 imaging for the detection of thyroid cancer. As such, thyroglobulin levels may be useful for monitoring patients who have an established diagnosis of thyroid cancer.

Calcitonin levels that are elevated preoperatively indicate C-cell hyperplasia and/or medullary thyroid cancer.[14,15] Postoperative levels indicate residual, recurrent, or metastatic medullary thyroid carcinoma.

Imaging studies include radionuclide imaging, ultrasonography, computed tomography (CT), and magnetic resonance imaging (MRI). Each examination can provide useful information for the diagnosis of thyroid cancer.

Radionuclide thyroid imaging is commonly used to evaluate the function and anatomical location of a palpable thyroid nodule through the localization of hot or cold spots in the gland. By this means the detection of occult cancers in high-risk patients can be accomplished. This imaging technique can detect a primary lesion in patients with suspected regional and distant thyroid cancer metastases. In addition, radionuclide imaging can detect local-regional or distant metastases in patients with known thyroid cancer. Patients previously treated for thyroid cancer are typically monitored with repeat scans.

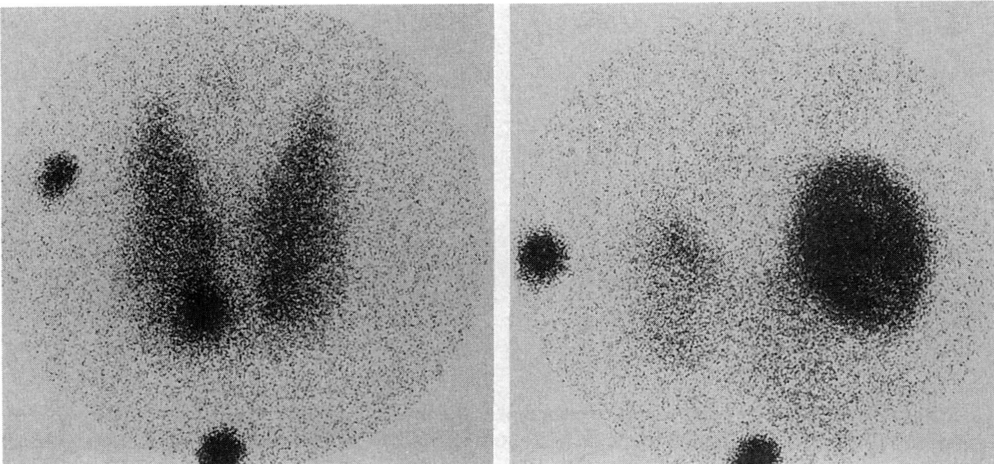

Fig. 6-2 Normal thyroid imaging. (From Bernier DR et al: *Nuclear medicine technology and techniques,* St Louis, 1994, Mosby.)

The four radiopharmaceuticals most commonly used for radionuclide imaging of the thyroid are I 131, I 125, I 123, and Tc 99m. A thyroid nodule can image in three ways: (1) **cold thyroid nodule** (no radionuclide uptake), (2) **warm thyroid nodule** (slightly higher concentration than the rest of the thyroid gland), and (3) **hot thyroid nodule** (radionuclide uptake much higher than the rest of the thyroid gland).[15] (See Fig. 6-2 for normal thyroid imaging and Fig. 6-3 for abnormal thyroid uptake.)

Most cold nodules are thyroid adenomas or colloid cysts, with only 15% to 25% representing thyroid cancers. If multiple cold nodules appear, the incidence of the malignancy drops to 5%.[15]

The incidence rate of cancer with warm or hot nodules is low and usually represents a functioning adenoma or areas of normal tissue in an otherwise diseased gland. Some metastatic, well-differentiated follicular carcinomas accumulate radioiodine. Most metastatic, differentiated thyroid tumors do not accumulate radioiodine until all normal thyroid tissue has been ablated. This happens because normal-functioning thyroid tissue preferentially accumulates iodinated radiopharmaceuticals relative to the tumor.

Ultrasonography can determine whether a nodule is solid or cystic. This technique is used as a complementary test to radionuclide imaging. A nodule found to be solid through ultrasonography has a 30% probability of being a cancer.[15,34]

A CT scan cannot differentiate between a benign or malignant lesion. However, it can show the local and regional extent of advanced or recurrent cancer.[32] CT can also help a radiation oncologist in treatment planning if the use of external beam radiation is anticipated.

MRI can be useful in depicting lesion margins, lesion extent, tissue heterogenicity, cystic or hemorrhagic regions, cervical lymphadenopathy, invasion of adjacent structures, and additional nonpalpable thyroid nodules.[15,23,28]

A needle biopsy in some circumstances can obviate surgery by differentiating malignant from nonmalignant lesions. Two types of needle biopsies are the needle aspiration cytology (performed with a small-gauge needle) and core needle biopsy (performed with a large-cutting biopsy needle of the Silverman type).

Both biopsies have a false-negative rate of up to 10%. A needle biopsy is invalid for follicular carcinoma because it cannot be diagnosed by cytological or histological criteria. However, a needle biopsy may play a role in the management of anaplastic thyroid malignancies and lymphomas because the diagnosis is more obvious.[6]

Pathology

Malignant thyroid neoplasms are divided into four categories: (1) papillary and mixed papillary-follicular, (2) follicular, (3) medullary, and (4) anaplastic. Rare tumors that account for less than 5% of thyroid malignancies include the following[15]:

- Lymphoma and plasmacytoma
- Squamous cell and mucin-producing carcinoma
- Teratoma and mixed tumors
- Sarcoma, carcinosarcoma, and hemangioendothelioma
- Metastatic carcinoma to the thyroid
- Thyroid cancer at unusual sites, including the median aberrant thyroid gland, lateral aberrant thyroid gland, and struma ovarii

Differentiated thyroid cancers include papillary, mixed papillary-follicular, and follicular carcinomas. These tumors arise from the thyroid follicle cell and can usually be treated with I 131 and thyroid hormone suppression.[15]

Papillary and mixed papillary-follicular cancers are the most common types of thyroid cancer, representing 33% to 73% of all malignant thyroid lesions. As previously men-

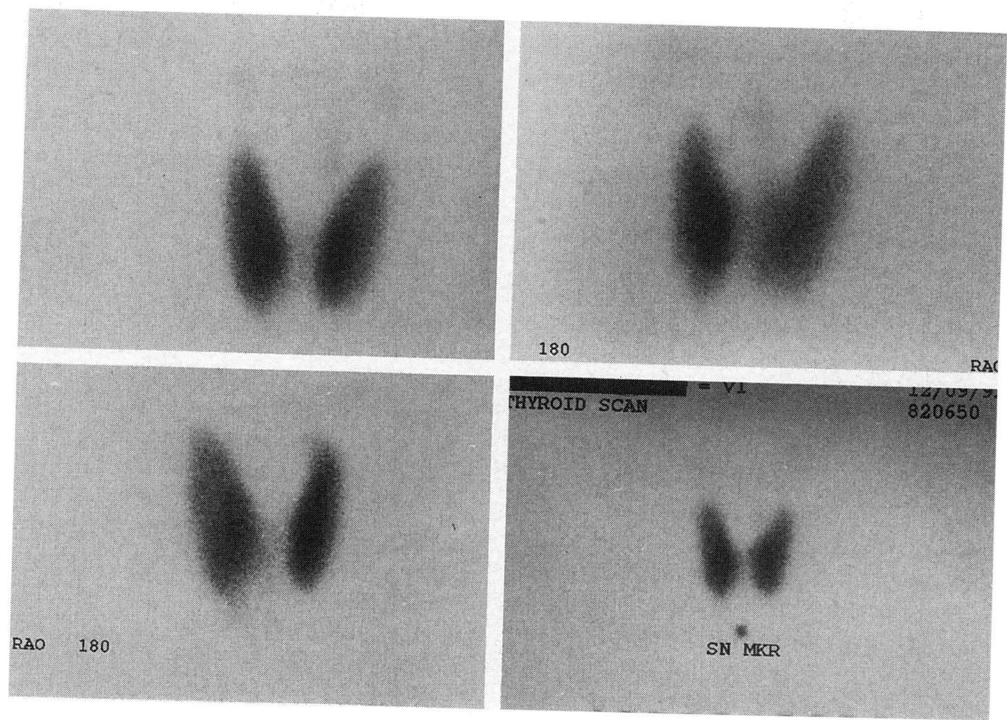

Fig. 6-3 Abnormal thyroid imaging. (From Bernier DR et al: *Nuclear medicine technology and techniques,* St Louis, 1994, Mosby.)

tioned, papillary carcinoma is the type most frequently seen in irradiated individuals. These tumors are slow growing, are nonaggressive, and have an excellent prognosis. This type of cancer is two to four times more common in females than males. The peak for occurrence is in the third to fifth decade of life, although the cancer can occur at any age. In children under 15 years of age, papillary carcinoma accounts for 80% of thyroid cancers.[15]

Follicular carcinoma accounts for 14% to 33% of all thyroid cancers. These tumors have the greatest propensity to concentrate I 131. They are two to three times more common in women than men, with the average age for a diagnosis from 50 to 58 years. They rarely occur in children. Follicular carcinoma has a worse overall prognosis than papillary carcinoma.[15,43]

Medullary thyroid cancer represents 5% to 10% of all thyroid cancers. About 80% of medullary thyroid cancers appear spontaneously, with 20% occurring as part of familial MEN syndromes (IIa, IIb, or III). No gender differentiation is seen between spontaneous and familial forms. With regard to age, however, spontaneous forms occur from the fifth decade on, whereas familial forms have been seen in patients less than 10 and as old as 80 years. Medullary carcinoma has a worse prognosis than papillary, mixed papillary-follicular, and possibly follicular cancers, although it has a better prognosis than anaplastic carcinoma.[15]

Anaplastic carcinoma carries the worst overall prognosis. It is more aggressive than the previously mentioned types, and a patient's life expectancy is usually short after the diagnosis is established. Anaplastic carcinoma represents 10% of all malignant thyroid lesions. The age of occurrence is from 40 to 90 years, with the incidence in women outnumbering that in men by four to one.[15]

Staging

The American Joint Committee on Cancer has staged thyroid cancers according to the histological type and age of the patient. (See Table 6-2 for the staging system.)

Routes of spread

Each pathological classification has its own route of spread, which ranges from slow growing to extremely aggressive.

Papillary and mixed papillary-follicular carcinomas metastasize to regional lymph nodes through lymphatic channels. At the time of operation, 50% to 70% of these carcinomas have cervical lymph node metastases, although the presence of positive regional lymph nodes does not significantly worsen the prognosis. Blood-borne metastases can occur.

Follicular cancers have a tendency to invade vascular channels and metastasize hematogenously to distant sites, including the bone, lung, liver, and brain. Lymph node metastases are uncommon.

Medullary thyroid cancer can vary from indolent to rapidly fatal growth patterns. Medullary carcinoma spreads regionally before displaying distant metastases, with up to 50% of patients having regional metastases at the time of the diagnosis. Metastases occur hematogenously and through

Table 6-2 Stage grouping*

Stage	Patients under 45 years old	Patients 45 years and older
Papillary or follicular		
I	Any T, any N, M_0	T_1, N_0, M_0
II	Any T, any N, M_1	T_2, N_0, M_0
		T_3, N_0, M_0
III		T_4, N_0, M_0
		Any T, N_1, M_0
IV		Any T, Any N, M_1
Medullary		
I	T_1 N_0 M_0	
II	T_2 N_0 M_0	
	T_3 N_0 M_0	
	T_4 N_0 M_0	
III	Any T N_1 M_0	
IV	Any T any N M_1	
Undifferentiated		
IV†	Any T Any N Any M	

Modified from Beahrs OH: *AJCC Manual for staging of cancer,* ed 4, Philadelphia, 1992, JB Lippincott.
*Separate stage groupings are recommended for papillary and follicular, medullary, and undifferentiated cancers.
†All cases are Stage IV.

lymphatic routes involving mainly the cervical nodes, lung, liver, and bone.

Anaplastic carcinoma displays local invasion of structures such as the trachea. Skin invasion is also seen, giving rise to dermal lymphatic metastases on the chest and abdominal walls. Regional neck nodes are often involved, although sometimes the primary tumor is so extensive that the regional node status is difficult to assess.[32]

Treatment techniques

Surgery. Papillary carcinoma and mixed papillary-follicular carcinomas are rarely invasive and seldom require the resection of the muscles of the neck, internal jugular vein, esophagus, or trachea. Radical neck dissections are warranted only if nodes are grossly involved with metastatic disease. Because papillary and mixed papillary-follicular carcinomas are usually indolent diseases, prophylactic or elective neck dissections are no longer performed. During radical neck dissections, special care is taken to spare the recurrent laryngeal, vagus, spinal accessory, and phrenic nerves. Care is also taken to preserve the parathyroid glands.[41]

For small, lateralized lesions that do not show extrathyroid involvement nor lymph node metastasis, lobectomy including the isthmus is required. Surgery for mixed papillary-follicular carcinoma is the same as that for papillary carcinoma, unless vascular invasion or blood-borne metastases are present, in which case the lesion is treated as follicular cancer.

For encapsulated follicular carcinoma confined in the thyroid, a lobectomy including the isthmus can often successfully control the disease. In early stages in which the spread to cervical lymph nodes is rare, prophylactic neck dissection is not needed. If a second lesion is present in the contralateral lobe, a total or near-total thyroidectomy is performed, usually with good results.[41] If follicular carcinoma is extrathyroidal or metastatic disease is present, a bilateral total thyroidectomy is mandatory.

For medullary carcinoma that is sporadic and intrathyroidal, a lobectomy plus isthmus removal is required. If the lesion has extended beyond the thyroid to involve lymphatics and/or soft tissue, a radical en bloc resection is required. Because regional lymph nodes occur in 50% of the patients, an elective neck dissection may be advisable.[41] In the familial form, in which the cancer is generally bilateral, a total thyroidectomy is warranted.

For undifferentiated (anaplastic) carcinoma, surgery is effective on only a few occasions. Surgery is often necessary to alleviate a central airway obstruction resulting from extrinsic compression of the larynx and upper trachea caused by this aggressive malignancy. A tracheotomy is usually required to preserve a patient's airway. Radical surgical attempts are not always justified or technically possible because growth into soft tissue and deeper structures of the neck is often present.[6]

For malignancies that metastasize to the thyroid (an extremely rare situation), the treatment varies with primary sites, including the larynx, esophagus, lung, kidney, rectum, and skin. A biopsy is usually needed to differentiate a metastasis from a primary thyroid cancer.

Side effects of surgery can include tumor hemorrhage, damage to parathyroid gland resulting in temporary or permanent hypoparathyroidism, and temporary or permanent vocal cord paralysis.

Radioactive iodine. Radioactive iodine is used to treat papillary, mixed papillary-follicular, and follicular cancers. Indications for radioactive iodine include the following:

- Inoperable primary tumor
- Thyroid capsular invasion
- Thyroid ablation after a partial or subtotal thyroidectomy
- Postoperative residual disease in the neck and recurrent disease
- Cervical or mediastinal nodal metastasis
- Distant metastasis

The routine use of I 131 after surgery in small, lateralized, well-differentiated cancers is debatable; thyroid suppression therapy alone may be adequate. Because normal thyroid tissue has a greater propensity than differentiated thyroid cancer to absorb iodine, the consensus seems to be that all normal tissue should be ablated to allow residual or metastatic disease to accumulate I 131. An ablation dose administered after a thyroidectomy may vary from 50 to 100 mCi. If a tracer dose of radioiodine reveals persistent

Guidelines for Patients Receiving Iodine 131 (I 131)

Planning

Order I 131 at least 48 hours in advance. Schedule the patient for hospital admission.

Room preparation

Charcoal filters in the room air system and an exhaust vent in the hallway
Plastic bag coverings for the telephone, food table, basin faucet handles, and nurse-call set
Disposable mats next to the bed, commode, and shower
Seat liners for the commode
Two radiation-waste containers in the room (laundry and foods or paper)

Patient preparation

Instruct the patient on the way to replace and dispose of covers and mats.
Instruct the patient to keep the outside door closed and the bathroom door open at all times.
Obtain vital signs and blood and urine samples before I 131 administration.

Administration

The patient must wear a hospital gown with a "chuck" around the neck and in the lap.
Personnel administering I 131 should wear gowns, gloves, and masks.
A vial containing I 131 should be vented in the nuclear medicine hood to allow any volatile I 131 to escape just before administration.
The patient should sit on the side of the bed in front of the I 131 in the lead vial on the covered table.
The patient should be instructed to open the vial with a T-bar, insert a drinking straw, and put a small amount of water in the vial (running water down the straw so it does not splash).
The patient should swish and then swallow several cups of water to rinse the I 131 from the oral cavity.
The patient should not remove the straw from the vial; the patient should bend the straw over and carefully replace the lead cap.

Initial survey

Within 15 minutes the radiation exposure rate should be measured at 1 m from the midline of the patient's abdomen in anteroposterior and lateral directions. The average should be calculated. The patient may be released when the same readings show less than 30 mCi of I 131—usually about 48 to 72 hours after the 100 mCi was given, but highly variable.
Posted on the room door must be a room diagram showing the safety shield's position, an inventory-survey form with the initial activity and exposure rate, nursing instructions, and a decontaminating form.
Urine should not be collected unless a lead container is available and there is specific reason.

Safety

Nursing recommendations: No pregnant nurses should care for patients receiving I 131. Nurses should not be assigned to care for more than one radioactive patient per month. At 30 mCi I 131 discharge, the exposure rate is 100 cGy/hr at 25 cm.
Visiting is discouraged. A limitation of ½ hr/day/visitor should be enforced. Children under 18 years and pregnant women should not be allowed to visit. Visitors should wear a gown, gloves, and a mask and should sit in a designated chair across the room. If visitors come close to the patient, they should sit behind a lead shield.
Patients should wear a hospital gown (not personal clothing [I 131 is found in breath and sweat]), and should leave bed only to go to the bathroom or a designated chair.
Patients should drink copious amounts of water to speed the release of unused radioactive agent, shower frequently, and flush the toilet several times after each use. Men should urinate seated.
No personal items should be used except those to be disposed of at discharge.
After discharge, the patient should sleep alone for 3 days and should not hold children closely for 3 days.

Modified from Greenfield LD: Thyroid tumors. In CA Perez, LW Brady, editors: *Principles and practice of radiation oncology,* Philadelphia, JB Lippincott.

thyroid activity after this procedure, a second ablation dose is needed. (See the box above for guidelines for patients receiving I 131.)

After all normal thyroid tissue is ablated, I 131 (for differentiated thyroid cancers) can be used to treat local and regional disease, as well as distant metastasis. Some of the side effects are listed in the box to the right.

Thyroid hormonal therapy. Thyroid hormone suppression therapy is routinely given for differentiated thyroid cancers, although its effectiveness remains unproved.

Side Effects of I 131

Inflammation of salivary glands
Nausea
Vomiting
Fatigue
Bone marrow suppression (only after repeated administrations)

Differentiated thyroid carcinoma grows under the stimulation of TSH. Thus, through the lowering of TSH levels, tumor activity should be decreased.[15]

A study by Cady et al.[7] showed no improvement of the survival time for TSH suppression as an adjunct to surgery for differentiated thyroid cancer. This failure to affect the survival time applied to all patients, regardless of age, gender, pathological type, or stage of the disease.[7]

External beam radiation. Responsiveness to external beam radiation varies according to histological type. Among differentiated thyroid cancers, papillary and mixed papillary-follicular carcinomas are more radiosensitive than follicular carcinomas. Medullary thyroid cancer is less radiosensitive than papillary carcinoma. In general, anaplastic carcinomas are completely unresponsive.

External beam radiation can be used alone or in conjunction with I 131 and surgery. Following are several indications for its use:

- Inoperable lesion
- Patient physically unfit for surgery
- Incomplete surgical removal of thyroid carcinoma
- Superior vena cava syndrome
- Skeletal metastases in which minimal accumulation of I 131 occurred
- Residual disease involving the trachea, larynx, or esophagus

In differentiated thyroid cancer for the curative treatment of inoperable localized disease or in patients with gross residual disease, tumor doses should be 6500 cGy in 7 weeks (180 to 200 cGy daily). The radiation field should include the entire thyroid gland, neck, and superior mediastinum. The dose to the spinal cord and other radiosensitive areas should be considered, with a cord block added around 4500 cGy. For metastatic bone involvement, doses of 3500 to 4500 cGy in 3 to 5 weeks are recommended.[15]

Several field arrangements can be used to deliver an adequate dose to the neck and mediastinum. Through anteroposterior/posteroanterior (AP/PA) portals, 4500 cGy can be given at the midplane to the neck and mediastinum. An additional dose (for a total tumor dose of 6500 cGy) can be delivered through anterior obliques or opposed oblique portals.

For the stimulation of a thyroid cancer patient, the head should be extended to avoid exposure to the mouth, with the use of an immobilization device for reproducibility. So that adequate tumor coverage is ensured, the tumor volume should be wired out, and a CT scan of the treated area should be obtained for treatment planning. Dose distribution must be considered through this area, especially for the cord dose.

For medullary carcinoma that has not extended below the clavicles, radiation therapy can be considered. The recommended dose is 5500 to 6500 cGy in 6 to 7 weeks. The treatment fields should encompass the primary lesion, bilateral cervical node chains, and superior mediastinum. For residual disease after a surgical resection, a dose of 5000 to 6000 cGy in 5 to 5$^{1}/_{2}$ weeks is recommended.

For bone metastasis, radiation therapy is warranted and often effective.

Anaplastic carcinoma is the least radiosensitive of all the thyroid cancers. Tumor control is seldom accomplished, even after a dose of 6000 cGy to the primary lesion, neck, and superior mediastinum.[15]

Case Study

A 34-year-old woman underwent a right hemithyroidectomy about 10 to 12 years ago for benign disease. Almost 2 years ago, the patient exhibited a cold nodule in the remaining left lobe of the thyroid gland. A needle aspiration biopsy showed only benign disease. Other than this asymptomatic nodule, the patient had no other symptoms. Because of its persistence, this left-sided nodule was excised. It showed follicular carcinoma with capsular invasion. No obvious vascular invasion was present. The patient was advised to have a complete lobectomy of the left thyroid gland or a I 131 ablation of the remaining thyroid gland. The patient elected surgical ablation.

Histopathologically, the resected lobe showed focal areas of residual follicular carcinoma with areas of infiltration into the stroma. A careful examination with the patient under anesthesia revealed no evidence of lymph node involvement. The patient received suppression therapy and afterward underwent an I 131 scan that showed residual uptake in the left neck, probably corresponding to the previous bed of the left thyroid lobe. No uptake was present on the right side, and there was no cervical lymph node involvement. No other activity was seen on the body scan. The patient was referred for I 131 thyroid ablation to the residual tumor in the left neck.

The acute risks of nausea and potential long-term risks of solid and hematological cancer induction was discussed with the patient. The precautions to be taken by the patient and her family, with specific regard to exposure to the children, were carefully outlined. The advised procedures were based on the National Council on Radiation Protection (NCRP) recommendations for people ingesting radioactive material for therapeutic purposes.

With her consent, the patient was given 30 mCi of I 131 via a capsule. The dose was relatively low because the patient effectively had a total thyroidectomy and was young. After observation for 1 hour without any nausea or vomiting and with the exposure rate being measured and recorded, the patient was discharged. A 6-month repeat thyroid scan showed no residual uptake in the left neck.

PITUITARY TUMORS

Pituitary tumors are less aggressive than many central nervous system tumors, although pituitary neoplasms still pose problems as a result of local growth causing compressive and destructive effects, as well as endocrine abnormalities caused by pituitary hormone dysfunction. The pituitary is composed of an anterior, posterior, and intermediate lobe. Tumors of the posterior and intermediate portion are virtually unknown. This section addresses tumors arising from the anterior pituitary gland, or adenohypophysis.

Epidemiology and etiology

Pituitary tumors are most always benign, with malignancies accounting for fewer than 1% of all pituitary tumors.[2] Neoplasms represent 10% of all intracranial tumors, although small, asymptomatic adenomas appear in approximately 25% of all pituitary glands examined at autopsy. With the increasing quality of diagnostic studies, these pituitary neoplasms are now estimated to account for 30% of all intracranial tumors.[36]

Pituitary adenomas can be classified as functioning or nonfunctioning, as related to the hormones they produce. Hormone production often serves as a diagnostic and treatment-response marker. Pituitary adenomas categorized as functioning are as follows:

- *Prolactin* (PRL)*-secreting tumors* are the most common, representing 65% of all functioning pituitary adenomas. These neoplasms grow large and show little tendency toward local invasion.[25,36]
- *Growth hormone* (GH)*-secreting tumors* represent 15% of all pituitary adenomas and are more likely to be locally invasive.[25]
- *TSH-secreting tumors* represent fewer than 1% of all pituitary adenomas.
- *Adrenocorticotrophic hormone (ACTH)-secreting tumors* are more likely to be invasive compared with the other functioning adenomas.[36]

Chromophobe adenomas, which are nonfunctioning, are usually larger than functioning tumors and tend to exhibit invasive characteristics.[29] Patients usually have visual symptoms caused by the compression of the optic chiasm or a headache, rather than syndromes associated with the hypersecretion of pituitary hormones. These syndromes are referred to in Table 6-3.

Pituitary tumors can occur at any age, from infancy to old age, although they are rarely found before puberty and are most commonly diagnosed in middle-aged and older patients.[22] No significant difference exists in the prevalence of adenomas among men and women.

Because of the rarity of malignant pituitary tumors, little knowledge exists of the etiology. Hardy, Beauregard, and Robert[18] have found an association between PRL-secreting tumors in women and the use of oral contraceptives. However, no clear etiological link has been determined.

Prognostic indicators

The prognosis depends on the type of adenoma and a combination of other factors, including the following: (1) the extent of the abnormalities (through mass effect or hormonal alterations), (2) the success of the treatment in normalizing endocrine activity and/or relieving pressure effects, (3) the morbidity caused by the treatment, and (4) the effectiveness of the treatments in preventing a recurrence.

Anatomy

The pituitary gland is 1.3 cm in diameter and located at the base of the brain. Attached to the hypothalamus by a stalklike structure (the **infundibulum**), the pituitary gland lies in the sella turcica of the sphenoid bone. The gland is divided structurally and functionally into an anterior lobe (**adenohypophysis**), a posterior lobe (**neurohypophysis**), and an intermediate lobe. The blood supply to the adenohypophysis is from several superior hypophyseal arteries, and the blood supply to the neurohypophysis is from the inferior hypophyseal arteries.[39]

The pituitary gland is close to critical structures of the central nervous system, such as the optic chiasm (superiorly) and the cavernous sinuses and their contents (laterally). (See Fig. 6-4 for the anatomical relationships.)

Related to topographical anatomy, the pituitary gland is positioned behind the temporal mandibular joint (TMJ) and midplane behind the nasal bone (i.e., between the eyes).

Physiology

Derived from the endoderm, the adenohypophysis forms the glandular part of the pituitary. The glandular cells (acidophils and basophils) are responsible for the secretion of seven hormones.

Acidophils secrete the following:

- GH—Controls body growth
- PRL—Initiates milk production

Basophils secrete the following:

- TSH—Controls the thyroid gland
- Follicle-stimulating hormone (FSH)—Stimulates egg and sperm production
- Luteinizing hormone (LH)—Stimulates other sexual and reproductive activity
- Melanocyte-stimulating hormone (MSH)—Relates to skin pigmentation
- ACTH—Influences the action of the adrenal cortex

The release of these hormones is stimulated or inhibited by the chemical secretions from the hypothalamus, which are called *regulatory,* or *releasing, factors.* The posterior lobe or neurohypophysis secretes oxytocin (which causes smooth muscle contractions) and antidiuretic hormone (ADH) or vasopressin, which regulates free water resorption in the kidneys.[39]

Clinical presentation

Hormonal effects. Functioning pituitary tumors retain hormone-producing capabilities, although they are unresponsive to regulatory mechanisms and produce hormones

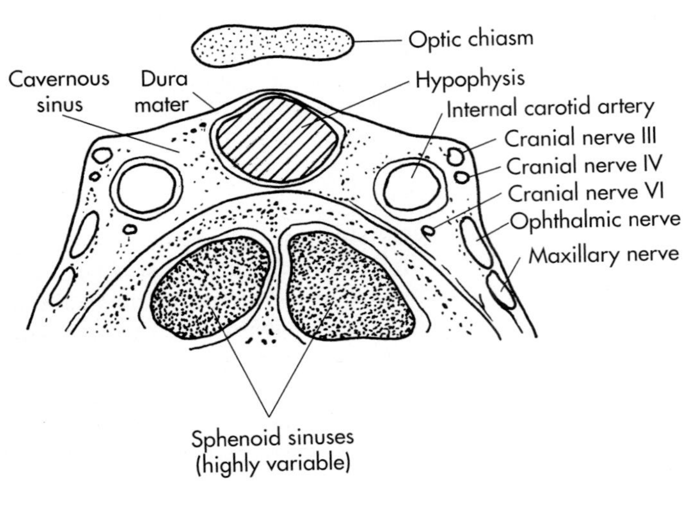

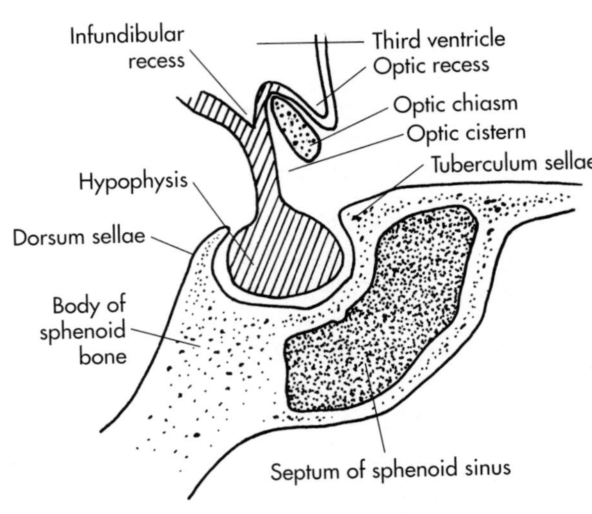

Fig. 6-4 Frontal and median planes of the pituitary fossa region. (Redrawn with permission from Perez CA, Brady LW, editors: *Principle and practice of radiation oncology,* Philadelphia, 1992, JB Lippincott.)

Table 6-3 Clinical effects of excess secretion of pituitary hormones

Hormones	Clinical effects
ACTH	Cushing's disease
GH	Giantism, acromegaly
Prolactin	Females: infertility Males: impotence, decreased libido
TSH	Hyperthyroidism

ACTH, Adrenocorticotrophic hormone; *GH,* growth hormone; *TSH,* thyroid stimulating hormone.

regardless of metabolic needs.[36] Hypersecretion of pituitary hormones results in varied clinical presentations, depending on the type of secreting tumor. PRL-secreting tumors produce clinical symptoms such as amenorrhea and galactorrhea, which is detected easier in premenopausal versus postmenopausal women. The hypersecretion of GH produces clinical symptoms such as weight gain; thickening of the bones; soft tissues of the hands, feet and cheeks; and overgrowth of the jaw and tongue. Patients are hypertensive and commonly complain of headaches and lassitude. This clinical syndrome is referred to as *acromegaly* if hypersecretion occurs after puberty and *giantism* if it happens before puberty.[38] (See Table 6-3 for more hypersecreting syndromes.)

In some instances, local compressive effects of the tumor in the pituitary itself may cause deficient production of hormones normally synthesized in the gland. Hormones that have target organs (such as ACTH [adrenals], TSH [thyroid] and FSH [ovaries and testes]) can cause an array of abnormalities that result from a loss of pituitary hormonal action.[12] These clinical manifestations are listed in Table 6-4.

Table 6-4 Clinical effects of hypopituitarism

Hormone	Target tissue	Clinical effects
ACTH	Adrenal cortex	Postural hypotension; impaired tolerance of stress (trauma, surgery); can lead to shock
Prolactin FSH LH	Gonads	Gonadal atrophy; loss of reproductive function; decreased gonadal hormones
TSH	Thyroid	Hypothyroidism (fatigue, slow or slurred speech, bradycardia, decreased reflexes, cold intolerance)
GH	Bones, muscles, organs	Decreased bone growth; lethargy; hypoglycemia

Modified from Donehower MG: Endocrine cancers. In Baird SB, McCorkle R, Grant M, editors: *Cancer nursing: a comprehensive textbook,* Philadelphia, WB Saunders.
ACTH, Adrenocorticotrophic hormone; *FSH,* follicle stimulating hormone; *LH,* luteinizing hormone; *TSH,* thyroid stimulating hormone; *GH,* growth hormone.

Pressure effects. The most common manifestation of an expanding pituitary lesion is headache, which occurs in 20% of all patients.[12,36] Local pressure on the lining of the sphenoid sinus and traction on the diaphragma sellae produce these headaches.

Visual acuity and field defects are other clinical manifestations and signify extension beyond the sella. Suprasellar extension of these tumors causes pressure effects on the inferior aspect of the optic chiasm, resulting in visual symptomatology, which is usually progressive. The presentation may be altered visual acuity, but more commonly, visual field defects are observed. The most common field defect is **bitemporal hemianopsia** (loss of peripheral vision). If pressure effects on the optic chiasm persist for significant periods, the result can be permanent visual field defects or blindness. In rare instances, these tumors can extend laterally into the cavernous sinuses (Fig. 6-4) and cause characteristic cranial nerve deficits.

Detection and diagnosis

Patients with functional tumors have characteristic endocrine abnormalities that are associated with the hypersecretion of hormones. The clinical syndromes from Table 6-3 prompt medical attention. Laboratory testing, which can directly measure hormone levels, can confirm pituitary hormone dysfunction and strongly suggest the diagnosis. The expanding growth of nonfunctioning tumors into the suprasellar area causes pressure symptoms such as headache, visual disturbances, and impairment of various cranial nerves.[22] These symptoms often bring the patient to medical attention and prompt diagnostic studies.

The principal imaging study for the pituitary gland is CT or MRI. MRI is superior to CT in delineating the extent of the tumor process relative to normal critical structures such as the optic chiasm, vascular structures, cranial nerves, and cavernous sinuses just lateral to the pituitary gland. (Fig. 6-4). MRI provides detailed anatomical information in transverse, sagittal, and coronal projections. This information is invaluable to the neurosurgeon and radiation oncologist in determining a therapeutic approach.

Pathology

Pituitary tumors are sinusoidal, papillary, or diffuse.[29] Although pituitary tumors appear encapsulated, no true capsule exists. Neoplasms are formed of tightly packed cells that remain separate from normal tissue without a membrane.

Neoplasms are classified according to size. **Microadenomas** are less than 1.0 cm, and **macroadenomas** are greater than 1.0 cm.[22,29] This classification is important because predictions of the prognosis can be made from the tumor size. Larger adenomas are surgically more difficult to remove with complete resections, and recurrence is more common in this group.

Pituitary tumors can also be classified according to their growth patterns (by expansion or invasion) and are separated into intrahypophyseal, intrasellar, diffuse, and invasive adenomas. **Intrahypophyseal tumors** stay in the pituitary gland, whereas **intrasellar lesions** grow within the confines of the sella. **Diffuse adenomas** usually fill the entire sella and can erode its wall. **Invasive neoplasms** have a more rapid growth rate and tend to erode outside the sella to invade neighboring tissues such as the posterior pituitary gland, sphenoid bone, and cavernous sinus. These neoplasms may even penetrate into the brain and third ventricle. Invasive adenomas are classified as malignant adenomas when metastases are present. Malignant adenomas metastasize via cerebrospinal fluid (CSF) or vascular pathways. This is extremely rare.

Hardy and Vezina's Tumor Classification

Grade I—Sella of normal size, but with asymmetry
Grade II—Enlarged sella, but with an intact floor
Grade III—Localized erosion or destruction of the sella floor
Grade IV—Diffusely eroded floor
Type A—Tumor bulges into the chiasmatic cistern
Type B—Tumor reaches the floor of the third ventricle
Type C—More voluminous tumor, with extension into the third ventricle up to the foramen of Monro
Type D—Extension into temporal or frontal fossa

Modified from Hardy J, Vezina JL: Transsphenoidal neurosurgery of intracranial neoplasm. In Thompson RA, Green JR, editors: *Advances in neurology,* vol 15, New York, 1976, Raven Press.

Staging

Because the majority of tumors are benign, no true staging exists. However, pituitary tumors have been classified into four grades according to the extent of expansion or erosion of the sella. This system also types tumors into four categories based on suprasellar extension (see the box above).

Treatment techniques

The primary goal of treatment is to normalize pituitary hormonal function or relieve local compressive and/or destructive effects of the tumor. In some instances, both factors must be ameliorated. This can be accomplished surgically, radiotherapeutically, medically, or with a combination of these modalities. An obvious secondary goal is to prevent recurrence.

Surgery. Surgery plays a significant role in the management of pituitary tumors. Before 1970, craniotomies were performed with an associated operative mortality rate of 2% to 25%. Currently, the less invasive transsphenoidal approach is widely used, decreasing the mortality rate to 0.9%. Complications of this surgery are CSF leakage, infection (meningitis), and visual pathway defects, with a combined morbidity rate of about 14%.[25] (See Fig. 6-5 for a depiction of the transsphenoidal approach.) In summary, the two main surgical approaches are the transfrontal approach (transfrontal craniotomy) and the transsphenoidal approach, which allows direct access to the pituitary gland without disturbance of the central nervous system structures.

Transsphenoidal surgery is reported to permanently control 70% to 90% of small adenomas. Results with larger adenomas are less satisfactory, although the debulking of large tumors decompresses vital structures.[36] Trans-

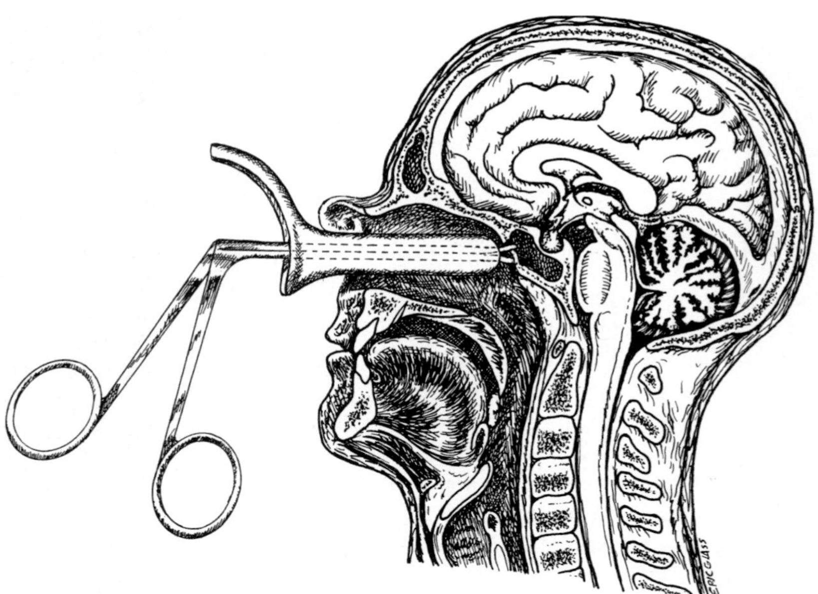

Fig. 6-5 Anatomical root for a transsphenoidal hypophysectomy.

sphenoidal surgery results in the improvement of visual field defects in 80% of patients. Only 4% of patients experience worsening of visual field defects with transphenoidal surgery. Results are the same with a craniotomy, with a higher percentage of visual impairment related to the surgical procedure.[24,40]

Characteristic hormonal abnormalities show favorable responses after surgery. If surgical intervention of functioning adenomas is successful, the response in terms of the normalization of hormone levels is almost immediate. Symptomatic relief is seen in 94% of patients with acromegaly, although the recurrence rate after 10 years is 8% to 10%. Results are generally satisfactory for patients with Cushing's syndrome (ACTH-producing adenomas). Although results vary, remission occurs in 80% to 86% of patients, with a recurrence rate over 10 years of 8% to 10%.[24] Similar, excellent results are achieved with PRL-secreting adenomas.

Radiation therapy. Surgery is often only one part of the overall management for a pituitary adenoma. Although the role of postoperative radiation therapy is controversial, it has been shown in various series to reduce recurrence rates compared with surgery alone. Radiation therapy alone has also been used to control pituitary tumors in patients who refused surgery or those who were medically unfit.

Postoperative radiation therapy is used as an adjunctive modality in the following circumstances:

- An incompletely resected invasive tumor
- Tumors demonstrating suprasellar extension with an associated visual field defect
- Large tumors in which the risk of attempted removal is relatively high
- Persistent hormonal elevation after surgery

Radiation therapy techniques. With any treatment technique a precise target volume must be defined through the use of MRI, CT, surgical, and clinical findings. The treatment volume should be slightly larger than the target volume, allowing for day-to-day variations in the treatment setup. The head must be immobilized to ensure reproducibility and accuracy. The patient's chin is usually tucked to avoid radiation exposure to the eyes. Lead markers on the outer canthus of each eye during simulation documents the eye position with respect to the radiation beam. The use of three tattoos (two lateral and one midline) aids in repositioning. Verification portals should be taken routinely to document the field location. (See Figs. 6-6 and 6-7 for examples of simulation and portal film.)

With the advent of high-energy megavoltage linear accelerators (i.e., 10 to 18 MeV) and multiple field treatment approaches, the dose-volume distribution to the pituitary gland has been greatly enhanced. This results in a more precise dose delivered to the tumor volume, a reduction in the dose to normal central nervous system structures, increased tumor-control probability, and decreased treatment-related morbidity.

The optimization of dose-volume distribution is illustrated in various treatment plans shown in Figs. 6-8, 6-9, and 6-10. These treatment plans show an obvious advantage of high-energy photons and multifield or rotational arrangements to accomplish the goal of optimizing the dose to the target tissue while minimizing the dose to nontarget, normal tissue. This is of paramount importance in the pituitary gland because of the critical normal tissue surrounding it. (See Fig. 6-11 for a treatment portal of a superimposed lateral and vertex.)

Other strategies not widely available are used to treat pituitary adenomas. These strategies include proton beam ther-

A

B

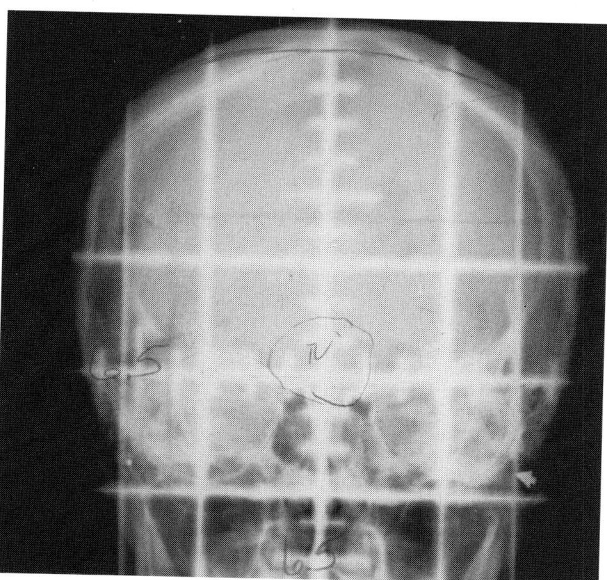

Fig. 6-6 **A,** Lateral simulation film illustrating the portal used for external irradiation of pituitary adenoma. **B,** AP simulation film.

apy and stereotactic radiosurgery. (See Volume I, Chapter 15.)

Proton beam therapy. Because of the proton beam's physical characteristics (i.e., a particulate beam versus a photon beam), the dose can be precisely delivered within millimeters of a defined target directly related to the beam's energy. This is a particularly attractive feature for treatment near critical structures such as the optic chiasm and the temporal lobe, areas in which an excessive radiation dose can produce devastating clinical consequences.

Stereotactic radiosurgery. **Stereotactic radiosurgery** uses a high-energy photon beam with multiple ports of entry convergent on the target tissue. This is typically done as a

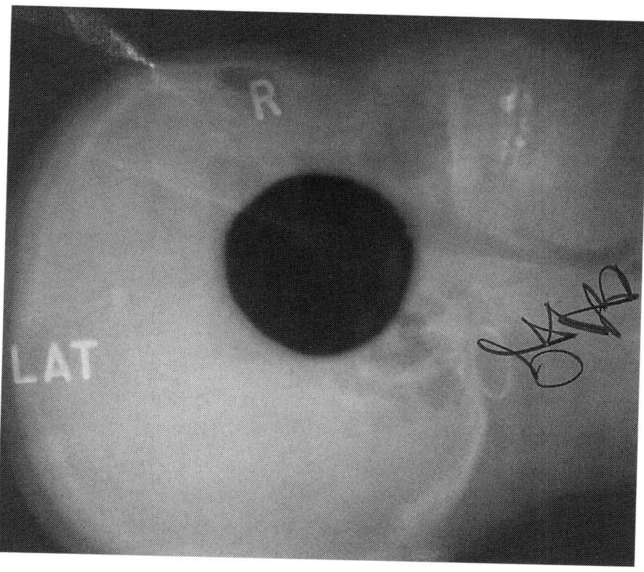

Fig. 6-7 Lateral verification film (portal image) on a therapy machine.

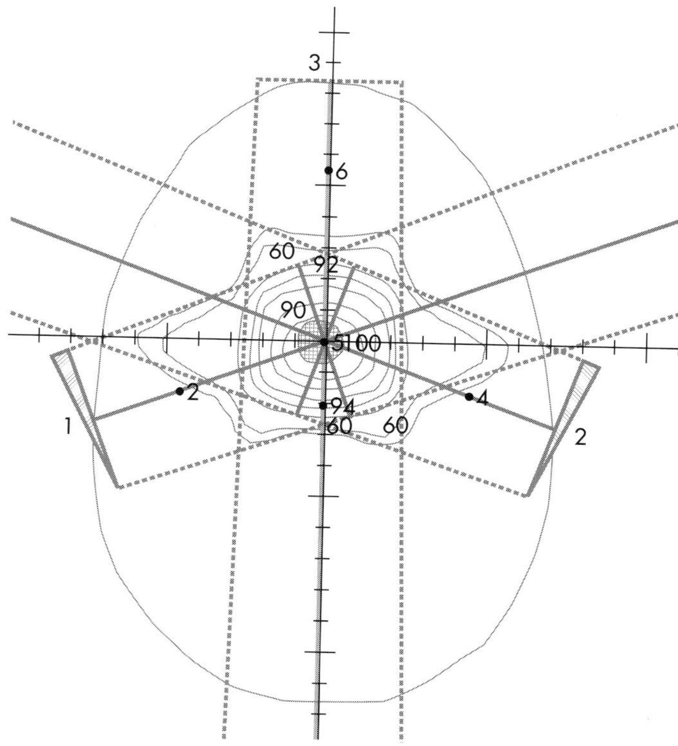

Fig. 6-8 Isodose curves for a 2-cm-diameter tumor volume, with the use of a 15-MV linear accelerator and three portal arrangement: an open vertex and two 110-degree posterior oblique, 30-degree wedge fields.

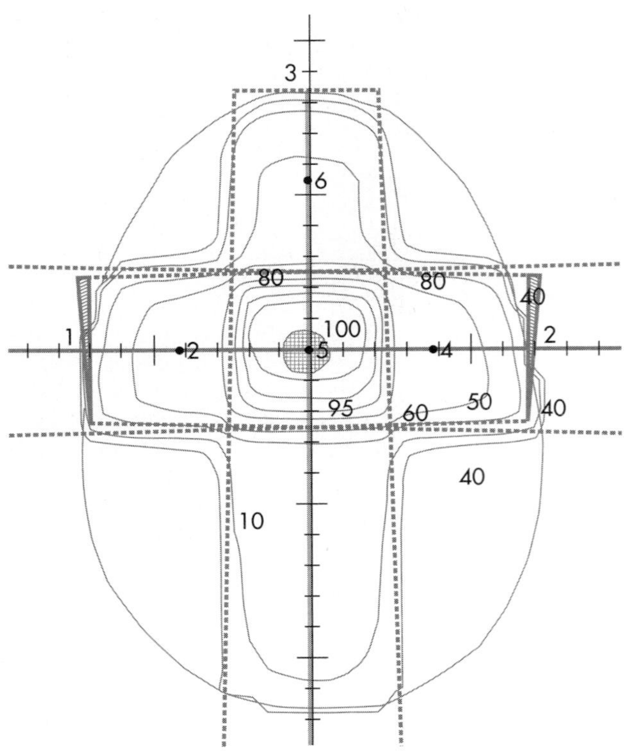

Fig. 6-9 Isodose curves for a 2-cm-diameter tumor volume, with the use of a 15-MV linear accelerator and three portal arrangement: open vertex and two lateral 15-degree wedge fields.

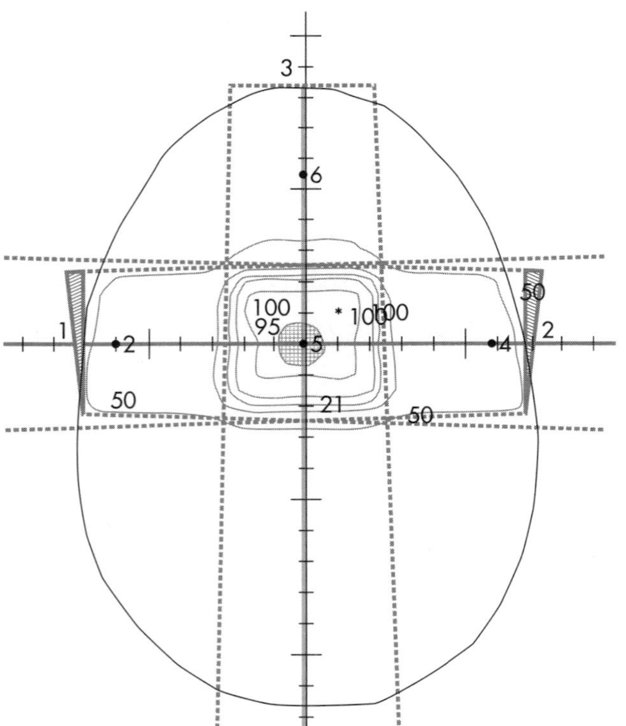

Fig. 6-10 Isodose curves for a 2-cm-diameter tumor volume, with the use of a 4-MV linear accelerator and three portal arrangement: open vertex and two lateral 30-degree wedge fields.

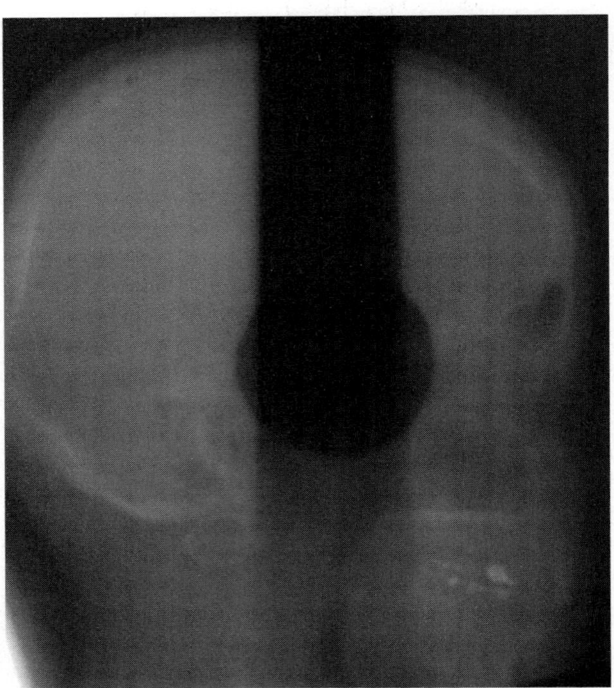

Fig. 6-11 A vertex therapy machine portal that is used to deliver a portion of dose without irradiation of the temporal lobes.

single, large fraction of treatment with the patient immobilized in a stereotactic head frame. After being rigidly positioned, the patient undergoes a planning CT scan to define the tumor volume and determine the multiports of entry. With the patient immobilized the entire time, this procedure takes several hours and requires several films on the treatment unit to ensure accuracy.

This technique may not be an optimal approach to this particular disease because pituitary neoplasms are benign and high single-fraction treatment can produce significant normal-tissue morbidity if an uncertainty exists regarding the target volume treated. With improved technology, stereotactic radiation may eventually be delivered as fractionated treatment, making it more desirable in this circumstance.

Results of treatment

The treatment of pituitary adenomas shows results that are quite favorable. Surgery for microadenomas is generally curative. Series with radiation therapy alone have demonstrated excellent disease-free survival rates of up to 85% at 5 and 10 years. A direct comparison between the results of different treatment approaches is difficult to make because of the various criteria used to select the optimal treatment, as previously described. However, surgery and radiation therapy alone or in combination clearly produce excellent results.

Case Study

A 32-year-old woman entered the emergency room with a history of headaches. During examination the patient demonstrated features of acromegaly. She had a 2-year history of progressively enlarging hands and feet and pain in the joints of the upper extremities. She noted that her shoe size increased from an 8 to a 10 over this period. She complained of amenorrhea for approximately the past year but denied any visual symptomatology.

As part of the initial work-up, a brain MRI scan showed findings consistent with a pituitary macroadenoma measuring about 1.5 cm in diameter and extending into the suprasellar cistern anterior to the optic chiasm. A slight elevation of the optic chiasm was present. The cavernous sinuses appeared free of tumor extension. The floor of the sella was eroded, and the tumor appeared to extend partially into the sphenoid sinus. The GH measurement preoperatively was in the 150 ng/ml range (normal range, 1 to 10 ng/ml), and a transsphenoidal hypophysectomy was advised.

After surgery the patient had a remarkable reduction in the GH level and a reversal of some of the clinical findings of acromegaly. However, with the persistent elevation of GH and radiographic (erosion of sella) and surgical findings (involving the sphenoid sinus), the patient was at an extremely high risk for recurrence of her adenoma. A course of radiation therapy directed at the pituitary fossa, sphenoid sinus, and cavernous sinus region was recommended to improve the probability of local control and normalization of the GH level.

In a supine, immobilized position the patient was treated via a three-field technique through the use of 6-cm-diameter circular fields with 10-MV photons. Right and left lateral opposed fields in combination with a superior vertex field angled 15 degrees off the horizontal were used. CT and MRI scans were performed through the treatment volume to aid in the treatment planning. This three-field arrangement was treated at 180 cGy per fraction. Equal weighting was provided from each field for 25 treatment fractions to accomplish 4500 cGy to the pituitary fossa, which included the sphenoid sinus.

The patient tolerated the therapy well but still complained of headaches and fatigue at the completion of the therapy. About 3 months after the external beam radiation therapy, the patient continued to show regression of her acral changes. This regression was characterized by thinning facial characteristics, smaller hands, and smaller feet. An MRI scan at that time showed no evidence of a tumor. During subsequent follow-up visits the patient continued to do well, with decreasing GH levels. Approximately 2 years after the therapy the patient's GH level was 3.0.

ADRENAL CORTEX TUMORS

Neoplasms of the adrenal glands are rare, with malignant tumors accounting for only 0.04% of all cancers.[11] Tumors arising in the adrenal glands are classified according to the portion of the gland from which they arise. This includes tumors arising from the cortex (outer portion of the gland) and those from the medulla (inner portion of the gland). The **cortex** and the **medulla,** which make up the adrenal gland (Fig. 6-12), have distinct histological features and physiological functions. In general, the cortex manufactures steroid hormones that are critical in metabolic regulation, and the medulla produces epinephrine (adrenalin) under the regulation of the autonomic nervous system.

Epidemiology and etiology

Adrenocortical tumors are extremely rare, with only 150 to 300 instances in the United states per year (of which, approximately 10% are malignant).[42] Men and women are affected equally, although hyperfunctioning malignancies are more common in women. Tumors arise more commonly in the left gland than the right. Although the median age is 50 years, the ages in two series ranged from 1 to 80 years.[10,11]

Adrenal adenomas are benign neoplasms that can be found in 2% of all adults, according to an autopsy series.[39] These adenomas are rarely associated with serious medical illness. However, in some circumstances these can cause hypersecretion of normally produced steroid hormones, giving rise to various clinical syndromes.

Prognostic indicators

The stage of the disease at the time of diagnosis closely parallels survival rates. The majority of patients have advanced disease at the time of presentation. Only 30% of patients have a tumor confined to the adrenal gland.[11]

The ability of the surgeon to achieve curative resection is another prognostic factor because surgery is the only modality that has demonstrated a significant effect on survival rates. All patients should have close postoperative surveillance for the detection of abdominal and distant metastases while they are still resectable.

A young age at the time of diagnosis is a favorable prognostic factor.

Anatomy

The adrenal glands are paired organs located on the superior pole of the kidneys. These glands have a yellow cortex and dark brown medulla. They derive their blood supply from the adrenal branches of the inferior phrenic artery, aorta, and renal artery.[4] The lymphatic drainage is to the paraaortic nodes. The normal adrenal gland weighs approximately 20 g.

Physiology

The adrenal cortex produces steroid hormones, including glucocorticoids, mineralocorticoids, and sex hormones, which are responsible for metabolic regulation. These hormones include cortisol, aldosterone, estrogen, and androgen. The cells of the adrenal cortex that manufacture these hormones are regulated by the ongoing stresses and needs of an individual's metabolism. The normal functioning adrenal cortex can respond instantaneously to meet metabolic demands and maintain homeostasis.

Clinical presentation

Because of the location of adrenal cortex tumors in the abdomen and the inaccessibility for physical examination, many patients develop symptoms of pain from advanced cancer. Alternatively, clinical manifestations of symptoms related to excess hormone production may prompt medical attention. Well-described syndromes are associated with the excessive production of hormones from the adrenal cortex. These are listed in Table 6-5.

In a series of 47 patients with adrenocortical carcinoma reported by Cohn, Gottesman, and Brennan,[9] symptoms relating to a nonfunctioning tumor included an abdominal mass in 77% of the patients, weight loss in 46%, fever in 15%, and distant metastases in 15%. Many patients have more than one symptom at the time of diagnosis. In the same series, symptoms relating to functional tumors included Cushing's syndrome in 26% of the patients, mixed Cushing's syndrome and virilization in 24%, virilization in 15%, and feminization in 9%.

Detection and diagnosis

Patients may exhibit functioning or nonfunctioning tumors. With functioning tumors the clinical syndromes from Table 6-5 often lead to the diagnosis and can be easily confirmed with laboratory testing. In nonfunctioning tumors, pain is the presenting symptom and is often associated with locally advanced disease.

The principal imaging study for the adrenal gland is CT or MRI. These scans often suggest the diagnosis of an adrenal neoplasm and demonstrate the local and regional extent of the disease. (See Fig. 6-13 for an abdominal CT scan of a suspected adrenal neoplasm). A definite tissue diagnosis requires a needle biopsy under CT guidance.

Pathology

Adrenocortical tumors are usually large, single, rounded masses of yellow-orange adrenocortical tissue. Because they are usually large at the time of diagnosis, they have considerable hemorrhage, necrosis, and calcification.[4]

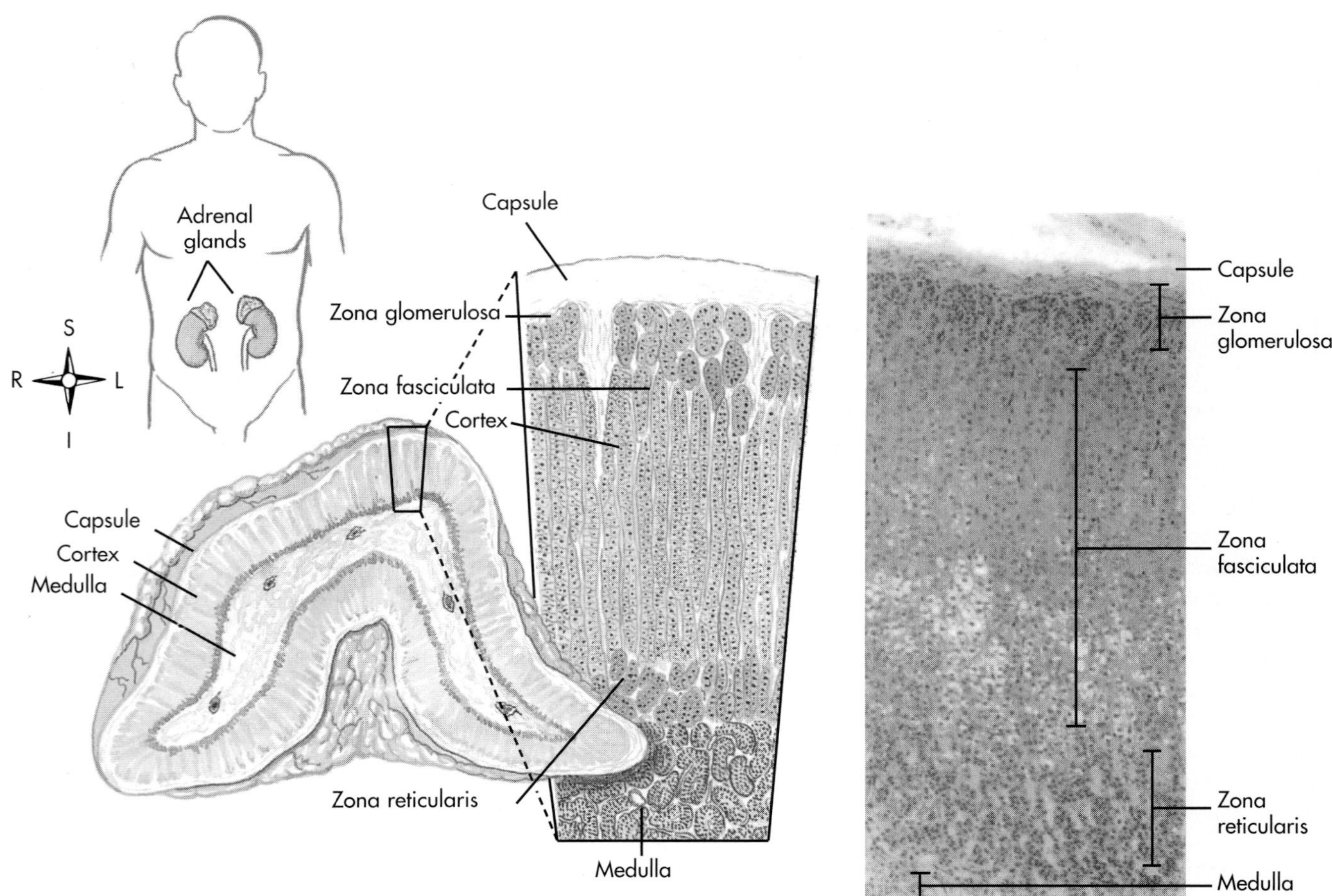

Fig. 6-12 Anatomy of the adrenal gland. (From Thibodeau GA, Patton TK, editors: *Anatomy and physiology,* St Louis, 1987, Mosby.)

Table 6-5 Clinical manifestations of adrenocortical hormone excess

Hormone	Syndrome	Clinical manifestations
Aldosterone	Conn's syndrome (aldosteronism)	Hypernatremia, hypokalemia, hypertension, neuromuscular weakness and paresthesias, electrocardiographic and renal function abnormalities
Cortisol (ACTH)	Cushing's syndrome	Acid-base imbalance, hypertension, obesity, osteoporosis, hyperglycemia, psychoses, excessive bruising, renal calculi
Sex hormones (testosterone, estrogen, and progesterone)	Virilization (in women)	Male pattern baldness, hirsutism, deepening voice, breast atrophy, decreased libido, oligomenorrhea
	Feminization (in men)	Gynecomastia, breast tenderness, testicular atrophy, decreased libido

From Donehower MG: Endocrine cancers. In Baird SB, McCorkle R, Grant M, editors: *Cancer nursing: a comprehensive textbook,* Philadelphia, 1991, WB Saunders.
ACTH, Adrenocorticotrophic hormone.

In a series of 38 patients conducted by Karakousis, Rao, and Moore,[21] tumors were graded according to the cells' resemblance to normal adrenal cortical cells. Well-differentiated (Grade I) tumors were distinguished from adenomas by the presence of capsular and vascular invasion and abnormal mitoses. The survival rate for Grade I and II tumors is significantly greater than that for Grade III tumors.

Staging

No true staging system exists because so few cases are reported. However, an example of a conventional staging system for adrenocortical carcinoma is presented in the box on p. 116. This system stages according to the size of the tumor and the extent to which it has advanced locally or distantly.

Routes of spread

Adrenocortical carcinomas can grow locally into surrounding tissues. However, these carcinomas may also spread to regional paraaortic nodes, lung, liver, and brain.[1,11]

Local invasion or distant metastases are often present at the time of diagnosis. In a series of 42 patients conducted by Didolkar et al.[11] metastatic disease was present at the time of diagnosis in 52% of the patients. Locally advanced disease was found in 40% of the patients. Tumors on the right side involved the kidney, liver, and vena cava (often by direct extension of the tumor). Tumors on the left side often involved the kidney, pancreas, and diaphragm.

Treatment techniques

Surgery is the treatment of choice. A complete resection is not always feasible because of invasion to adjacent vital

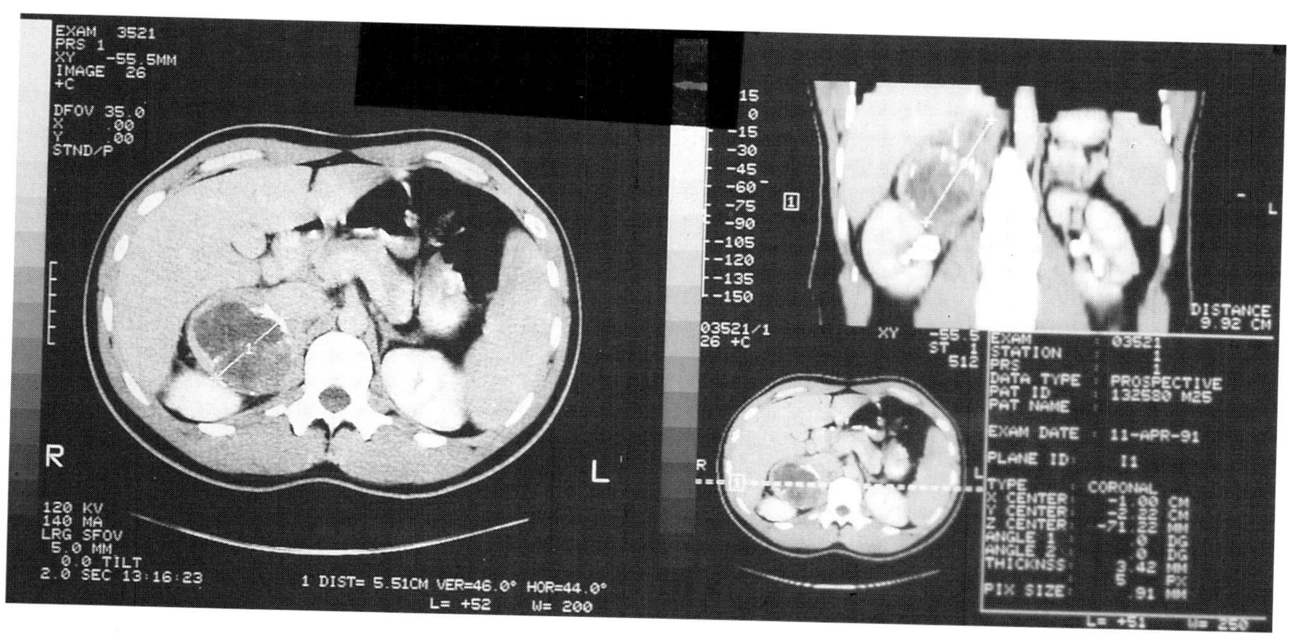

Fig. 6-13 An abdominal CT scan of a suspected adrenal neoplasm.

Proposed Clinical Staging System for Carcinoma of the Adrenal Cortex

T = extent of the primary tumor
- 1 = < 5 cm and confined to the adrenal gland
- 2 = > 5 cm but < 10 cm or adherence to the kidney
- 3 = > 10 cm or invasion of surrounding structures including the renal vein

M = Presence and type of metastases
- 0 = no demonstrable metastases
- 1 = regional lymphatics
- 2 = distant metastases, (e.g., liver, lung, bone)

R = Tissue remaining after resection
- 0 = tumor completely excised
- 1 = tumor entered at operation
- 2 = tumor tissue remaining after resection

D = Degree of histological differentiation
- 1 = differentiated, no capsular or vascular invasion
- 2 = moderately undifferentiated, capsular or vascular invasion
- 3 = anaplastic, capsular and and vascular invasion

Stage 1 = 3 or fewer; (e.g., T_1 M_0 R_0 D_1)
Stage 2 = 4 and 5; (e.g., T_2 M_0 R_1 D_2)
Stage 3 = 6 and 7; (e.g., T_3 M1 R_1 D_2)
Stage 4 = 8 or more; (e.g., T_3 M_2 R_2 D_3)

Modified from Bradley EL: Primary and adjunctive therapy in carcinoma of the adrenal cortex, *Surg Gynecol Obstet* 141:507, 1995.

structures such as the spleen, kidney, and parts of the pancreas. Although the resection of adrenal carcinomas is not always for cure, debulking results in decreased pain. Radiation therapy has a limited role, but it may be used as an adjunct to surgery to improve local control and for the palliative treatment of metastatic disease.

The use of systemic treatment in the management of adrenocortical cancer has been disappointing. Most reported series have evaluated patients with locally advanced or metastatic disease. Mitotane is an adrenolytic drug that has demonstrated limited but favorable responses. About a 40% response rate is observed in patients with advanced disease. Some studies have suggested that patients who receive mitotane as adjuvant treatment after surgical resection (i.e., without obvious evidence of metastatic disease) may realize significantly improved disease-free survival.[37] Whether this confers a true overall survival benefit or a delay in the development of metastatic disease is not clear.

Because of the rarity of this malignancy, cytotoxic chemotherapy has not been widely studied. However, some evidence suggests that agents having activity alone or in combination against adrenocortical carcinoma include Adriamycin, cisplatin, etoposide (VP-16), Cytoxan, and 5-fluorouracil (5-FU). The role of these agents in an adjuvant setting is far from clear.[17]

ADRENAL MEDULLA TUMORS

Epidemiology and etiology

Approximately 400 medullary tumors are diagnosed in the United States per year. These are called *pheochromocytomas,* and only 10% of these have cytologic features that are malignant.[42] The peak incidence of this tumor is in the fifth decade of life, but it can be seen at any age. These tumors may be bilateral in various familial syndromes and can be associated with MEN syndromes. In addition, this type of tumor has been observed in patients with von Recklinghausen's disease (Type I neurofibromatosis).

Anatomy

The anatomy of adrenal medulla tumors is discussed in the section on adrenal cortex tumors on p. 113.

Clinical presentation

A well-recognized clinical syndrome is associated with pheochromocytomas. The symptoms include hypertension, severe headache, nervousness, palpitations, excessive perspiration, angina, blurred vision, and abdominal and chest pain. These are mediated by the excessive production of epinephrine associated with these tumors. Symptoms vary little among benign and malignant tumors and are often sporadic.[4]

Detection and diagnosis

These tumors are suspected based on the clinical presentation. CT or MRI scans are used to assess the extent of disease. Laboratory testing, which measures urinary or plasma catecholamines (Vanillylmandelic acid [VMA] and precursors of epinephrine), can help confirm the diagnosis. A needle biopsy can establish a tissue diagnosis but may not be necessary if the clinical, radiographic, and laboratory findings support the diagnosis.

Pathology and staging

Adrenal medulla tumors are well-delineated, circumscribed tumors ranging from dark red, through gelatinous pink, to gray-brown or gray. The tumor size varies from 1 cm to 30 cm, with areas of hemorrhage and necrosis.[30]

Routes of spread

The metastatic pattern of malignant pheochromocytomas is similar to that of adrenocortical carcinoma.

Treatment techniques

Surgery is the treatment of choice for these tumors. Malignant tumors may grow extensively into surrounding structures, making a complete resection impossible. Persistent elevation of blood pressure indicates residual tumor or metastatic disease.[30]

The surgical resection of benign pheochromocytomas results in a normal life expectancy, and patients with malignant pheochromocytomas can be maintained for many years. Patients with extraadrenal malignancy have a poorer prognosis.

Results of treatment

Adrenocortical carcinoma. The outcome for patients treated with this disease is poor. The 5-year survival rates for all stages range between 25% and 40%. The stage at diagnosis and ability to resect the disease has a significant effect on its outcome. Because most patients (65% to 75%) have advanced-stage disease, the ability to accomplish a curative resection is minimized and survival rates decrease.[9]

Adrenal medulla-pheochromocytoma. Because the majority of these tumors are benign and the surgical resection is often complete, results of treatment are excellent. Most patients live a normal life span.

Case Study

A 26-year-old male was in a normal state of health until approximately 2 months before presentation, at which time he experienced right flank pain and sought medical attention. His past medical history was unremarkable, except that 7 years before, he had sustained a blunt, right-sided chest wall and flank injury. A physical examination demonstrated no evidence of cushingoid changes, hyperaldosteronism, or virilism (signs of a functioning tumor). His blood pressure was normal, and he denied having flushing, sweats, palpitations, and diarrhea.

As part of the initial work-up, an intravenous pyelogram (IVP) showed an apparent partially calcified mass above the right kidney that was pushing the kidney inferiorly and posteriorly. A CT scan was performed and showed a 10-cm mass that appeared to be involving the right adrenal gland region with obvious extrinsic compression of the right kidney. No direct invasion of the inferior vena cava was evident. Obvious hypodense regions and calcified areas were present in this apparent tumor mass. Neither adenopathy nor liver abnormalities were obvious. For a determination of the vascular supply of the tumor before surgery, an arteriogram was performed. It showed a single vessel with a trifurcate artery coming off the aorta serving this tumor mass. The venous phase of the arteriogram showed no gross invasion of the vena cava. Preoperative urinary VMAs and metanephrines (laboratory testing done to rule out pheochromocytoma) were normal. A preoperative chest x-ray examination was unremarkable.

According to the operative note, a rock-hard mass was encountered in the upper quadrant above the kidney overlying the entire right renal vein and inferior vena cava. This mass appeared to be involved with peritumoral inflammation and fibrosis. This was an extremely arduous resection secondary to the fibrous adherence to the local structures. A clear cleavage plane was established between the kidney and mass. However, dense adherence was encountered over the inferior vena cava, requiring a resection of a portion of the cava to remove the mass. A lymph node overlying the right renal vein was encountered and surgically resected. At the completion of the procedure, induration that spread in a sheetlike manner was behind the cava. The consensus was that additional resection was not possible.

The patient had an uneventful surgical recovery. Histologically, this proved to be a high-grade adrenocortical carcinoma. Because of concern for a residual tumor overlying the vena cava and in the retroperitoneal space behind the cava, the patient was sent for a radiation oncology consultation. The radiation oncologist felt that, because of the high nuclear grade of portions of this tumor, the patient was indeed at risk for local regional recurrence and that postoperative external beam treatment was indicated to secure the optimal probability of local control.

The patient was treated in the supine position with combined proton beam and megavoltage (10-MV photon) radiation therapy. The patient received a total dose of 6000 cGy. The photon portion of the treatment included the delivery of 3280 cGy via a parallel-opposed AP/PA pair of Cerrobend-shaped fields, weighted with a ratio of 1:1. Consecutively, 720 cGy in four fractions were given via a parallel-opposed lateral wedge pair of Cerrobend-shaped fields, weighted with a ratio of 2R:1L. The patient then received 2000 cGy from proton beam therapy. The characteristic properties of the proton beam allow a maximum target dose while limiting radiation exposure to surrounding structures. The patient was immobilized in a lateral decubitus position to spare the dose to critical structures such as the small bowel and stomach.

A high-resolution, contrast-enhanced CT scan with the patient in the treatment position was performed to delineate the primary target volume and neighboring critical dose-limiting structures. The dose to the spinal cord was 4600 cGy; the cauda equina received 4500 cGy, 30% of the right kidney received <4000 cGy, and the left kidney received less than 5 Gy.

Other than mild fatigue and mild intermittent nausea, the patient tolerated the treatment quite well. The patient was sent to a medical oncologist to discuss an adjuvant chemotherapy program. The patient received four cycles of adjuvant chemotherapy with cisplatin and Adriamycin over a 4-month period. Other than minimal weight loss and fatigue, the patient tolerated this treatment well.

Approximately 30 months have passed since the completion of the postoperative external beam radiation therapy. Since that time the patient has undergone a complete radiographic staging with a CT scan of the thorax, abdomen, and pelvis. There is no evidence of recurrence.

ROLE OF RADIATION THERAPIST

Education of the patient and family members during radiation therapy is aimed at helping the patient understand the goals and importance of treatment, as well as the potential side effects. Symptoms experienced during treatment are often difficult to endure and affect the patient's ability to consent to the completion of treatments. However, with the support of family and health care professionals and with information for controlling side effects, the patient can successfully complete a course of therapy. Open communication between the patient and supporting staff members (nursing, dietary, and social services) is of utmost importance in abating and controlling symptoms during and after a course of treatment.

The following are some potential side effects patients can experience while receiving radiation to glands of the endocrine system:

1. *Fatigue* is a common side effect of the majority of patients receiving radiation therapy. Daily treatments and biological effects of the disease and radiation can cause fatigue. Poor nutrition, depression, and family and financial worries are all contributing factors. Scheduling appointments around rest or meal times can aid in combating fatigue. The therapist should discuss the daily activity level with the patient to assess potential problems, and family members should be encouraged to assist in daily activities (e.g., meal preparation) to allow for rest time.

   Appointments with the social services department can subside financial worries and aid in emotional support. The therapist should encourage patients and family members to discuss their concerns and fears with each other.
2. *Skin* reactions can be painful and irritating to the patient. The therapist should advise the patient to avoid harsh creams, soaps, and lotions in the irradiated area. Hot water and sun exposure to the treated area should also be avoided. After a reaction starts the therapist should communicate with the physician, and depending on the degree of desquamation (dry or moist), a treatment break may be warranted.

   For patients who may have a tracheostomy a plastic cannula should replace a metal one, allowing it to stay in place during treatments. This will aid in preventing the enhancement of a skin reaction at the tracheostomy site.

   Loose-fitting clothes, especially cotton, should be worn to prevent rubbing and further irritation.
3. *Hair loss* **(alopecia)** can occur in the irradiated field as a result of the radiosensitivity of hair follicles. High-dose radiation may cause alopecia or delayed hair regrowth. The therapist should try to give the patient and family an appraisal for the potential and degree of hair loss and a time frame for its approximate occurrence. The therapist should inform patients to use mild shampoo and avoid excessive hair washing, which only dries and irritates the skin. In addition, the therapist should inform the patient and family that the new hair may have a different quality, texture, and color.

   If hair loss becomes significant, the use of a wig or turban may be indicated. Therapists should inform patients of national programs (e.g., "Look . . . Feel Better") that promote positive feelings and attitudes.
4. **Dysphagia** (difficulty swallowing) is often present in thyroid patients before the start of treatments as a result of the disease process. Early in the treatment, the patient may describe the feeling of "a lump in the throat." The therapist should encourage the patient to eat frequent meals consisting of high-protein and caloric foods. Eggnog, frappes, Ensure, Sustecal, and shakes supply high-protein and caloric intake and are soothing and easy to swallow.

The patient should be advised to avoid commercial mouthwash, hot food and drinks, smoking, spicy food, and alcoholic beverages. If available, a dietary consultation should be scheduled within 1 week of the start of treatments.

Visual changes due to the disease can also cause a patient to be depressed. Simple pleasures such as reading or watching television can no longer be enjoyed. Unfortunately, little can be done to alter these effects caused by damage to the optic nerve; even treatment may not reverse the damage already inflicted on the nerve. However, audio tapes of best-selling books are available and may offer some enjoyment to the patient. The therapist can also encourage a family member to take time out to read the daily paper or a novel to the patient. The therapist should try to encourage family participation so the patient does not feel left out.

Endocrine neoplasms can cause an array of previously discussed hormonal upsets, which can result in changes in emotions, appearance, and abilities. An altered body image can lower a patient's self-esteem. Patients with hair loss, hormonal syndromes, or acromegalic features may have misconceived notions of the way others perceive them. The therapist should be alert to these changes, allowing patients to express their feelings, promoting support from family members, and offering support to the family. Illness not only affects the patient, but also the family because aggression and anger is often directed toward the family members.

The therapist should offer outside counseling (e.g., "I Can Cope") that is aimed at supporting families and patients through difficult times. Seeing other patients in similar circumstances lets patients know that they are not alone, their feelings are normal, and help is available.

Before the initiation of radiation therapy, the therapist should discuss the treatment process with the patient and family. The therapist should inform them that holding still is of the utmost importance for the delivery of proper treatment. In addition, the therapist should assure them that, although alone in the room, the patient is being carefully monitored. The therapist should take them into the room, explain positioning procedures, show them the monitors and intercom, and clearly explain that the machine will stop and someone will come in if help is needed. The therapist needs to give them a sense of control. The more they understand, the less anxiety they will feel, making the overall treatment process more tolerable.

Before educating patients and their families, therapists should educate themselves. Therapists should read the consultation, know the basics, and be prepared to address any specific questions or concerns a patient may wish to discuss. The patient must feel comfortable and confident in the therapist, allowing for open communication and trust throughout the duration of the treatment. A lack of trust can inhibit communication and cause undue stress for the patient and family.

Therapists must present themselves in a professional manner. After all, patients are entrusting themselves to the therapist, with little understanding and with much apprehension for what is before them.

Review Questions

True or False

1. Pituitary cancers are the most common of the endocrine malignancies.
   True ___________ False ___________
2. A diagnosis of carcinoma of the thyroid gland can be made by clinical presentation alone.
   True ___________ False ___________
3. Prolactin-secreting tumors are the least common of all functioning pituitary adenomas.
   True ___________ False ___________

Multiple Choice

4. X-rays or radium was used in the past to treat which of the following benign conditions?
   a. Acne
   b. Rashes
   c. Tonsillitis
   d. All of the above
5. Which of the following is an indication for the use of radioactive iodine?
   a. Inoperable primary tumor
   b. Thyroid capsular invasion
   c. Distant metastasis
   d. All the above
6. What are the pituitary tumors that stay within the pituitary?
   a. Intrasellar
   b. Diffuse
   c. Intrahypophyseal
   d. Invasive

Fill in the Blank

7. The use of a high-energy photon beam with multiple ports of entry convergent on the target volume is ______________.
8. Pituitary tumors less than 1.0 cm are called ___________.
9. Adrenal cortex tumors arise more commonly in the ___________ adrenal gland.
10. For adrenal cortex tumors, ___________ of disease at the time of diagnosis correlates highly with survival rates.

Questions to Ponder

1. Discuss the diagnostic tests for a patient suspected of having a low-grade, early-stage malignancy.
2. Discuss the role of I 131 in the management of a patient with papillary or follicular cancer. Why is this iodine-based pharmaceutical useful in thyroid cancer?
3. Discuss the clinical syndromes that can be associated with adrenocortical carcinoma and the factors mediating these symptoms.
4. Explain which imaging studies should be suggested for a patient suspected of having an adrenal neoplasm.
5. Describe the critical structures in proximity to the pituitary gland and the effect of the tumor mass and pressure on these structures. Discuss the presenting symptoms related to the tumor mass and pressure on these structures.
6. Explain for a pituitary adenoma the criteria for postoperative radiation therapy management and the various radiation treatment techniques.
7. As a radiation therapist, discuss the way you would help a patient deal with the physical and emotional changes brought about by an endocrine malignancy. List some of the resources available to patients and their families.

REFERENCES

1. Alkire KT: Cancer of the pancreas, hepatobiliary and endocrine system. In Baird SB et al: *A cancer source book for nurses,* Atlanta, 1991, American Society Professional Education Publication.
2. Arafah B, Brodkey J, Pearson O: Acromegaly. In Santen R, Manni A, editors: *Diagnosis and management of endocrine related tumors,* Boston, 1984, Martinus Nijhoff.
3. Block MA et al: Clinical characteristics distinguishing heredity from sporadic medullary thyroid carcinoma, *Arch Sug* 115:142, 1980.
4. Brennan MF: Cancer of the endocrine system. In DeVita VT Jr, Hellman S, Rosenberg SA, editors: *Cancer principles and practice of oncology,* Philadelphia, 1987, JB Lippincott.
5. Buckwalter JA , Gurll NJ, Thomas CG Jr: Cancer of the thyroid in youth, *World J Surg* 5:15, 1981.
6. Cady B: Cancer of the thyroid. In Nealon TF Jr. editor: *Management of the patient with cancer,* Philadelphia, 1986, WB Saunders.
7. Cady B et al: Risk factors analysis in differentiated thyroid cancer, *Cancer* 43:810-820, 1979.
8. Chong GC et al: Medullary carcinoma of the thyroid gland, *Cancer* 35:695-704, 1975.
9. Cohn K, Gottesman L, Brennan M: Adrenocortical carcinoma. Presented at the Seventh Annual Meeting of the American Association of Endocrine Surgeons, Rochester, Minnesota, April 14-15, 1986.
10. DeAtkine AB, Dunnick NR: The adrenal glands, *Semin Oncol,* 118(2):131-139, 1991.
11. Didolkar MS et al: Natural history of adrenocortical carcinoma: a clinicopathologic study of 42 patients, *Cancer,* 1981
12. Donehower MG: Endocrine cancers. In Baird SB, McCorkle R, Grant M, editors: *Cancer nursing: a comprehensive textbook,* Philadelphia, 1991, WB Saunders.
13. Furmanchuk AW et al: Pathomorphological findings in thyroid cancers of children from the Republic of Belarus: a study of 86 cases occurring between 1986 ('post-Chernobyl') and 1991, *Histopathology* 21:401-408, 1992.
14. Graze K et al: Natural history of familial medullary carcinoma: effects of program for early diagnosis, *N Engl J Med* 299:980, 1985.
15. Greenfield LD: Thyroid tumors. In Perez CA, Brady LW, editors: *Principles and practice of radiation oncology,* Philadelphia, 1987, JB Lippincott.
16. Greenspan FS: Radiation exposure and thyroid cancer, *JAMA* 237:2089, 1977.
17. Hajjar RA, Hickey RC, Samaan NA: Adrenal cortical carcinoma: a study of 32 patients, *Cancer* 35:549, 1975.
18. Hardy J, Beauregard H, Robert F: Prolactin secreting pituitary adenoma: transsphenoidal microsurgical treatment. In Robyn C, Garter M, editors: *Progress in prolactin physiology and pathology,* Amsterdam, 1978, Elsevier/North Holland Biomedical Press.
19. Hill CS, Jr et al: Medullary carcinoma of the thyroid gland: an analysis of the M.D Anderson hospital experience with patients with the tumor, its special features, and its histogenesis, *Medicine* 52:141-171, 1973.
20. Hole JW Jr: *The endocrine system in human anatomy and physiology,* Dubuque, Iowa, 1981, Wm C Brown.
21. Karakousis CP, Rao U, Moore R: Adenocarcinomas: histologic grading and survival, J Surg Oncol 29:105-111, 1985.
22. Kovacs K, Horvath E: Pathology of pituitary tumors, *Endocrinology and Metabolism Clinics,* 16(3):529-551, September 1987.
23. Kroop SA et al: Evaluation of thyroid masses by MR imaging. Presented at the Radiological Society of North America 71st Scientific Assembly Annual Meeting, Chicago, November 17-22, 1985.
24. Laws ER Jr: Pituitary surgery, *Endocrinology and Metabolism Clinics,* September 1987.
25. Lingood RM: Tumors of the central nervous system. In Wang CC, editor: *Clinical oncology indicators, techniques and results,* Littleton, Massachusetts, 1988, PSG Publishing.
26. Mazzaferri EL et al: Papillary thyroid carcinoma: the impact of therapy in 576 patients, *Medicine* 56:171, 1977.
27. Mettler FA et al: Thyroid nodules in the population living around Chernobyl, *JAMA* 268(5):616-619, August 5, 1992.
28. Mountz JM, Glazer GM, Sissom JC: Evaluation of thyroid disease using MR imaging and scintigraphy. Presented at the Radiological Society of North American 71st Scientific Assembly Annual Meeting, Chicago, November, 1985.
29. Murali Rai: Tumors of the nervous system. In Nealon TF Jr, editor: *Management of the patient with cancer,* Philadelphia, 1986, WB Saunders.
30. Newsome HH Jr, Kay S, Lawrence W Jr: The adrenal gland. In Nealon TF, editor: *Management of the patient with cancer*, ed 3, Philadelphia, 1986, WB Saunders.
31. Parker LN et al: Thyroid carcinoma after exposure to atomic radiation: a continuing survey of a fixed population, Hiroshima and Nagasaki, 1958-1971, *Ann Intern Med* 80:600, 1974
32. Parsons JT, Pfaff WW: Carcinoma of the thyroid. In Million RR, Cassisi NJ, editors: *Management of head and neck cancer: a multidisciplinary approach,* Philadelphia, 1984, JB Lippincott.
33. Sambade MC et al: High relative frequency of thyroid papillary carcinoma in Northern Portugal, *Cancer* 51:1754, 1983.
34. Scheilbe W, Leopold GR, Woo VL: High resolution real-time ultrasonography of thyroid nodules, *Radiology* 13:413, 1979.
35. Schneider AB et al: Plasma thyroglobulin in detecting thyroid carcinoma after childhood head and neck irradiation *Ann Intern Med* 86:29, 1977.
36. Schreiber NW: Endocrine malignancies. In Groenwald SL, editor: *Cancer nursing principle and practice,* Boston, 1987, Jones and Barttlett.
37. Schteingart DE et al: Treatment of adrenal carcinoma, *Arch Surg* 117:1142-1146, 1982.
38. Shelin GE, Tyrrell BJ: Pituitary tumors. In Perez CA, Brady LW, editors: *Principle and practice of radiation oncology,* Philadelphia, 1987, JB Lippincott.
39. Tortora GJ, Anagnostakos NP: *Principles of anatomy and physiology,* ed 3, New York, 1980, Harper & Row.
40. Trautmann JC, Law ER Jr: Visual status after transsphenoidal surgery at the Mayo Clinic, 1971-1982, *Am J Ophthalmol* 96:200-208, 1983.
41. Wang Chi-an: Thyroid cancer. In Wang CC, editor: *Clinical radiation oncology: indications, techniques and results,* 1988, PBG Publishing.
42. Wittes RE: *Manual of oncologic therapeutic 1989/1990,* Philadelphia, 1977, JB Lippincott.
43. Wool MS: Management of papillary and follicular cancer. In Greenfield LD, editor: *Thyroid cancer,* Boca Raton, Florida, 1978, CRC Press.

BIBLIOGRAPHY

Cady B et al: The effect of thyroid hormone administration upon survival in patients with differentiated thyroid carcinoma, *Surgery,* 6(94):978-983, December, 1983.

Denny JD, Marty R, Van Herle AJ: Seumthyroglublin: a sensitive indicator of metastatic well differentiated thyroid carcinoma. Society of Nuclear Medicine Western Regional Meeting II, Las Vegas, 1977.

Hardy J, Vezina JL: Transsphenoidal neurosurgery of intracranial neoplasm. In Thompson RA, Green JR, editors: *Advances in neurology,* vol15, New York 1976, Raven Press.

Van Herle AJ: Pathophysiology of thyroid cancer. In Greenfield LD, editor: *Thyroid cancer* Boca Raton, Florida 1976, CRC Press.

CHAPTER

7

Respiratory System

Donna Stinson
Paul Wallner

Outline

Cancer of the respiratory system
- Epidemiology and etiology
- Anatomy
- Physiology
- Clinical presentation
- Detection and diagnosis
- Pathology
- Staging
- Routes of spread
- Treatment techniques
- Role of radiation therapist

Key terms

Accelerated fractionation
Accelerated hyperfractionation
Boost fields
Bronchogenic carcinoma
Carina
Conventional fractionation
Field-within-a-field
Hilum
Horner's syndrome
Hyperfractionation
Hypertrophic pulmonary osteoarthropathy
Karnofsky Performance Scale
Mediastinum
Mesothelioma
Orthogonal radiographs
Orthopnea
Pancoast tumors
Paraneoplastic syndromes
Shrinking fields

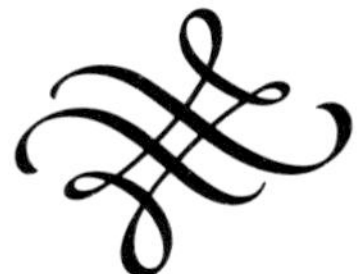

This chapter discusses lung cancer as it relates to the practice of radiation therapists. The focus is on **bronchogenic carcinoma,** although **mesothelioma** is explained in a limited fashion. Technically, bronchogenic carcinomas are lung cancers that arise in the bronchi. Frequently, however, the term is used to refer to lung cancers collectively. Etiology and epidemiology related to age, gender, causes, occupational exposure, and prognosis are highlighted. The section on the anatomy of the respiratory system describes the organs of the system, physiology, blood supply, and lymphatics. The signs and symptoms of lung cancer are discussed through clinical presentations of local, regional, and metastatic disease. Also discussed is the way lung cancer is detected and diagnosed. Various types of radiographic imaging techniques, laboratory studies, and relevant findings are identified. The details of pathology and staging (including histological cell types, location, and prognosis) are discussed. Direct, lymphatic, and hematogenic routes of spread are also described. Surgical and chemotherapeutic treatment techniques are discussed, with radiation therapy covered in detail. The section on field design and critical structures elaborates on the methods used for the definitive treatment of lung cancer and includes examples of the following: parallel-opposed fields, boost fields, multiple field combinations, frequently treated critical structures, off-axis points, customized beams, and doses. Side effects; clinical presentations; the therapist's role in patient education, communication, and assessment; and the use of accessory medical equipment are described.

CANCER OF THE RESPIRATORY SYSTEM

Epidemiology and etiology

Cancers of the bronchial tree, lung, and pleural surfaces represent the most common invasive malignancies in the United States. In 1994 an estimated 172,000 new cases were diagnosed and approximately 153,000 deaths were caused by the disease. Considered as a group, these malignancies represent almost one sixth of all new cancers in the United States and one fourth of all cancer deaths.[7]

Age and gender. Over the past 4 decades, an absolute increase has occurred in new cancers, with the peak presentation between the ages 55 and 65. In 1950 the male-to-female ratio was approximately 6:1, but an increase in female incidence has now produced a ratio of approximately 3:1. In 1987 lung cancer surpassed breast cancer as the leading cause of cancer-related deaths in women.

Causes. The most common cause of lung cancer is significant tobacco exposure, which is generally defined as more than one pack of cigarettes per day. Although tobacco product manufacturers have consistently denied absolute proof of the link, epidemiological data strongly suggest an unequivocal causal relationship. Also, an apparent dose-response consistency is related to a higher incidence of lung cancers with (1) an increased duration of smoking, (2) an increased use of unfiltered cigarettes, and (3) an increased number of cigarettes consumed.[39] The use of chewing tobacco, cigars, and pipes is generally associated with a higher incidence of malignancies in the upper aerodigestive tract rather than the lung.

Occupational exposure. Additional causative factors include fumes from coal tar, nickel, chromium, and arsenic, as well as exposure to various radioactive materials. Especially dangerous are agents with alpha emissions in their various daughter products, such as uranium and radon. The Environmental Protection Agency estimates that radon is the second leading cause of lung cancer in the United States and has recommended guidelines for various levels of radon exposure.

Radon may be present in various levels in soil. Also, depending on the type of home construction, ventilation, insulation, and size, radon may be found in high quantities inside parts of a home.

Pollution and genetic factors may be synergistic in their causative effect, adding to the risk above and beyond the various exposures indicated. However, these relationships are somewhat more difficult to prove.

Prognosis. Although numerous factors affect prognosis, the most significant variables include the following: (1) stage—extent of the disease (see the box on p. 123), (2) clinical performance status—measured by scales such as the **Karnofsky Performance Scale**[20] (see the first box on p. 124), and (3) weight loss[1]—especially greater than 5% of the total body weight over 3 months. Multiple studies have clearly demonstrated the independent nature of each of these variables in determining the prognosis. This effect is so marked that prospective clinical trials for definitive disease management frequently exclude patients who are in an advanced clinical stage (although the disease is apparently limited to the chest), patients with a Karnofsky Performance score of less than 70, or patients with weight loss greater than 5%. Individuals with advanced intrathoracic disease, extrathoracic extension, a Karnofsky score below 70, or weight loss greater than 5% rarely survive more than 2 years.

Malignant mesothelioma of the pleural surfaces has been increasing at a greater rate than other types of lung cancers presumably related to the long latent period existing between carcinogenic exposure and development of the disease. Approximately 8,000,000 individuals have been exposed to significant levels of asbestos (the primary etiological agent), and estimates suggest that by the year 2030, perhaps 300,000 new cases per year may be evident. Because asbestos exposure had previously occurred in primarily male-dominated industries, the incidence of mesothelioma is seen overwhelmingly in men. Nonoccupational asbestosis and asbestos-related mesothelioma may occur in women.[27]

Asbestos fibers inhaled primarily in industries such as mining, asbestos-material manufacturing and insulation, railroads, shipyards, pipe insulation, and gas mask producers are primarily associated with the production of mesotheliomas. Many types of asbestos particles exist, all of which have potential risks, but the longer and thinner strands produce more chemical reactivity and greater carcinogenesis.

Because metastatic disease to the lung represents a common occurrence for other primary tumor sites, the definitive establishment of the lung disease as primary or secondary is appropriate in most instances. This determination usually has significant implications for subsequent decisions regarding additional evaluation, management, and prognosis.

Anatomy

Organs of the system. The respiratory system consists of the nose, pharynx, larynx, trachea, and both lungs. Air is conducted from the nose, through the pharynx, larynx, and trachea, and into the lungs. Because cancers of the upper respiratory system (nose, pharynx, and larynx) are discussed in Chapter 8, only the anatomy of the trachea and lungs are included in this section.

The lower respiratory system consists of the trachea and lungs. The trachea is the major airway in the thoracic cavity. The wall is composed of rings of cartilage, smooth muscle, and connective tissue. Epithelial cells line the trachea. The trachea begins at the inferior border of the larynx and ends at the level of the fifth thoracic vertebrae (T5), where it bifurcates.[37] This place of bifurcation is called the **carina,** the area in which the trachea divides into two branches. Anatomically and radiographically, the carina corresponds to the level of the fifth and sixth thoracic vertebra (T5 and T6). At the bifurcation the trachea divides into the right and left primary bronchi. These bronchi begin a branching process that is similar to the structure of a tree (the bronchial tree).

AJCC Staging System for Lung Cancer

Primary Tumor (T)

- TX Primary tumor cannot be assessed, or tumor proven by presence of malignant cells in sputum or bronchial washings but not visualized by imaging or bronchoscopy
- T_0 No evidence of primary tumor
- Tis Carcinoma in situ
- T_1 Tumor 3 cm or less in greatest dimension, surrounded by lung or visceral pleura, without bronchoscopic evidence of invasion more proximal than the lobar bronchus
- T_2 Tumor with *any* of the following features of size or extent:
  - More than 3 cm in greatest dimension
  - Involves main bronchus, 2 cm or more distal to the carina
  - Invades the visceral pleura
  - Associated with atelectasis or obstructive pneumonitis that extends to the hilar region but does not involve the entire lung
- T_3 Tumor of any size that directly invades any of the following: chest wall (including superior sulcus tumors), diaphragm, mediastinal pleura, parietal pericardium; or tumor in the main bronchus less than 2 cm distal to the carina but without involvement of the carina; or associated atelectasis or obstructive pneumonitis of the entire lung
- T_4 Tumor of any size that invades any of the following: mediastinum, heart, great vessels, trachea, esophagus, vertebral body, carina; or tumor with a malignant pleural effusion

Lymph node (N)

- NX Regional lymph nodes cannot be assessed
- N_0 No regional lymph node metastasis
- N_1 Metastasis in ipsilateral peribronchial or ipsilateral hilar lymph nodes, including direct extension
- N_2 Metastasis in ipsilateral mediastinal or subcarinal lymph node(s)
- N_3 Metastasis in contralateral mediastinal, contralateral hilar, ipsilateral or contralateral scalene, or supraclavidular lymph node(s)

Distant metastasis (M)

- MX Presence of distant metastasis cannot be assessed
- M_0 No distant metastasis
- M_1 Distant metastasis

Stage grouping

Occult carcinoma	TX	N_0	M_0
0	Tis	N_0	M_0
I	T_1	N_0	M_0
	T_2	N_0	M_0
II	T_1	N_1	M_0
	T_2	N_1	M_0
IIIA	T_1	N_2	M_0
	T_2	N_2	M_0
	T_3	N_0	M_0
	T_3	N_1	M_0
	T_3	N_2	M_0
IIIB	Any T	N_3	M_0
	T_4	Any N	M_0
IV	Any T	Any N	M_1

Modified from Beahrs OH et al: *AJCC manual for staging of cancer*, ed 4, Philadelphia, 1992, JB Lippincott.

The **hilum** of the lung is the area in which the blood, lymphatic vessels, and nerves enter and exit each lung. The **mediastinum** refers to the anatomy between the lungs.

The primary bronchi are also called the *right and left main-stem bronchi.* The primary bronchi form branches of decreasing size until finally reaching the microscopic level where gases are exchanged. First, the main-stem bronchi form branches called the *secondary bronchi.* These lobar bronchi continue to divide into smaller, tertiary bronchi. Also called the *segmental bronchi,* these tertiary bronchi divide into smaller branches known as *bronchioles.* Bronchioles are microscopic structures that further divide into alveolar ducts. Many capillaries supply the alveolar ducts. Gases diffuse across the alveolar-capillary membranes. Oxygen and carbon dioxide exchanges take place at this microscopic level.[37]

Physiology

Ventilation is the term for oxygen and carbon dioxide exchange to the external environment (i.e., breathing). The physiology of the respiratory system begins as air is inhaled into the body. Air moves inferiorly along the trachea and enters the lungs at the main-stem bronchi. The bronchi divide into many branches. As the branching increases, the cartilage decreases and the amount of smooth muscle in the structures increases.

A respiratory unit is composed of the bronchioli, alveolar ducts, atria, and alveoli. Gas exchange takes place from these units to the lung capillaries and is called *external respiration.* Oxygenated blood moves from these capillaries and major vessels in the lungs to the heart, where it is pumped throughout the body. Oxygenated blood is carried in the arteries and then exchanged in cells throughout the body for deoxygenated blood. From the capillaries, further exchanges take place through the interstitial fluid to the cells. This is known as *internal respiration,* a process in which oxygen and carbon dioxide exchanges take place at the cellular level as a result of changes in pressure. Thus, carbon dioxide is removed from the cells, returned through the venous system

Karnofsky Performance Scale

100	Normal; no complaints; no evidence of disease
90	Ability to carry on normal activity; minor signs or symptoms of disease
80	Normal activity with effort; some signs or symptoms of disease
70	Self-care; inability to carry on normal activity or do active work
60	Requirement of occasional assistance, but ability to care for most personal needs
50	Requirement of considerable assistance and frequent medical care
40	Disability; requirement of special care and assistance
30	Severe disability; hospitalization indicated, although death not imminent
20	Extreme sickness; hospitalization necessary; active support treatment necessary
10	Moribund; rapid progression of fatal processes
0	Dead

Modified from Macleod CM, editor: *Evaluation of chemotherapeutic agents,* New York, 1949, Columbia University Press.

to the capillaries in the lungs, and finally exhaled through the respiratory units (alveoli → atria → alveolar ducts → bronchioli) to the external environment.[37]

Blood supply and lymphatics. The lymphatic system is important in lung cancer because it is one of the principal routes of regional spread. Lymph nodes and channels permeate the respiratory system. At many points the lymphatics anastomose (connect) with pulmonary arteries and veins. Lymphatics of the lungs are classified in several ways. They are grouped anatomically according to the TNM (tumor, node, metastases) staging system into mediastinal and intrapulmonic nodes[3] (see the box above on the right).

Mediastinal nodes are subdivided into five sets of nodes: (1) superior mediastinal, (2) tracheal, (3) aortic, (4) carinal and subcarinal, and (5) pulmonary ligament.[3] The superior mediastinal nodes are adjacent to the upper one third of the trachea. They are anterior and posterior to the innominate veins. The tracheal nodes are adjacent to the lower two thirds of the trachea. Tracheal nodes include the pretracheal (tracheobronchial), retrotracheal, and precarinal nodes. The aortic nodes include the subaortic, aorticopulmonary, and periaortic nodes. These nodes are near the ascending aorta and phrenic arteries. The carinal and subcarinal nodes are inferior to the carina. The pulmonary ligament nodes are in those ligaments and near the right and left pulmonary veins. Flow between the mediastinal nodes is complicated and difficult to predict. As an example, mediastinal nodes connect directly with the subcarinal, pretracheal, and diaphragmatic channels.[12] Lymphatic flow is influenced by lung pressures, the diaphragm, movements of the chest wall, and motions of other local organs and vessels.[17]

Respiratory System Lymphatics

Mediastinal nodes

1. Superior mediastinal
2. Tracheal
3. Aortic
4. Carinal and subcarinal
5. Pulmonary ligaments

Intrapulmonic (hilar, bronchopulmonic) nodes

1. Main-stem bronchus
2. Interlobar
3. Lobar

The other major group of lymph nodes of the respiratory system, intrapulmonic nodes, are composed of three subdivisions: (1) main-stem bronchus, (2) interlobar, and (3) lobar.[3] These nodes are also known as *hilar nodes* or *bronchopulmonic nodes.* The main-stem bronchus nodes are superior and inferior to the main-stem bronchus. The interlobar nodes are found between the lobes of each lung. The lobar nodes are located at the lobar bronchi.

The blood supply of the respiratory system is similar to that of the lymphatics. Many of the vessels have similar names. For example, the vessels that supply the trachea are called the *tracheal veins* and *arteries.*

The location of the lungs in relation to the circulatory system is important. In fact, the two systems are linked. The lymph channels that drain the heart flow into the mediastinal nodes at the level of the carina.[17] At the carina the lymphatic drainage of the lungs meets with the cardiac flow of the lymph. From this region of the bifurcation of the trachea, access to the circulatory system occurs as the flow enters the thoracic duct and aorta.

In addition, the lymph nodes have arterial and venous blood supplies. Cancer cells trapped in the lymph nodes form emboli that can leave the node through its own blood vessels.[17]

When bronchogenic carcinoma of the lung is treated with radiation, the fields generally include the tumor, draining blood, and lymph vessels. A simple field design, such as a mediastinum, includes all the lymphatics and blood vessels that flow in the area of the carina. Structures such as the hilum of each lung, aorta, thoracic duct, esophagus, vertebral bodies, and others are included in fields of this nature. The lungs, mechanics of respiration, blood, and lymphatic supplies are considered in planning a course of radiation therapy for patients with lung cancer.

Clinical presentation

The signs and symptoms of lung cancer are often insidious and especially difficult to differentiate from the symptoms of chronic obstructive pulmonary disease that often occur.

Presenting features are associated with (1) local disease in the bronchopulmonary tissues; (2) regional extension to the lymph nodes, chest wall, and/or neurological structures; and (3) distant dissemination.[6]

Local disease. Symptoms related to local disease extent are generally among the earliest complaints, with evidence of a cough in approximately 75% of patients. This cough may be severe and unremittent in 40% of the patients. Hemoptysis (blood associated with the cough) may be present in up to 60% of patients and may be the first sign of disease in up to 5% of patients. Approximately 15% of patients complain of a recent onset of dyspnea (shortness of breath), and a similar percentage exhibits chest pain.

Regional disease. Regional extension of disease (usually to the central mediastinal, paratracheal, parahilar, and subcarinal lymph nodes) may produce pain, coughing, dyspnea, and occasionally an abscess formation secondary to an obstructive pneumonia. Disease extension into the mediastinum may be manifested as dysphagia (difficulty swallowing) because of esophageal compression. Compression of the superior vena cava, especially in lesions of the right lobe extending into the mediastinum, may produce a **superior vena cava syndrome** associated with increasing dyspnea; facial, neck, and arm edema; **orthopnea** (an inability to lie flat); and cyanosis (a blue tinge to the lips). Hoarseness may occur as a result of compression or invasion of the recurrent laryngeal nerve, especially on the left side, where the nerve takes a somewhat longer course. Dyspnea may occur secondary to phrenic nerve involvement, producing diaphragmatic paralysis.

Less common are apex tumors of the lung. Apical tumors may be **Pancoast tumors,** but certain criteria other than anatomical location must be met. A patient with a true Pancoast tumor has a tumor in the superior sulcus and a clinical presentation that includes the following: (1) pain around the shoulder and down the arm, (2) atrophy of the hand muscles, (3) **Horner's syndrome,** and (4) bone erosion of the ribs and sometimes the vertebrae.[28] Pancoast tumors involve the cervical sympathetic nerves that cause Horner's syndrome. Classically, Horner's syndrome includes an ipsilateral (same-side) miosis (contracted pupil), ptosis (drooping eyelid), enophthalmos (recession of the eyeball into the orbit), and an ipsilateral loss of facial sweating. Arm and shoulder pain is caused by brachial plexus involvement, and these tumors may extend upward into the neck. Erosion of the first and second ribs may cause arm pain. Not all apical tumors are Pancoast tumors.

Metastatic disease. Distant metastasis is generally associated with anorexia (loss of appetite), weight loss, and fatigue. Approximately 2% of patients with lung cancer may demonstrate **paraneoplastic syndromes** that are thought to represent distant manifestations of the effect of chemicals or hormones produced by these tumors.[18] Typically, symptoms of paraneoplastic syndromes may affect nerves, muscles, and endocrine glands. These symptoms may be improved but rarely controlled for significant periods in the absence of primary tumor control. A frequently seen phenomenon associated with lung cancer is **hypertrophic pulmonary osteoarthropathy,** which is manifested by clubbing of the fingers' distal phalanges (Fig. 7-1). Although this finding is most frequently associated with benign, long-standing chronic obstructive pulmonary disease, it may be seen as a presenting sign of lung cancer.

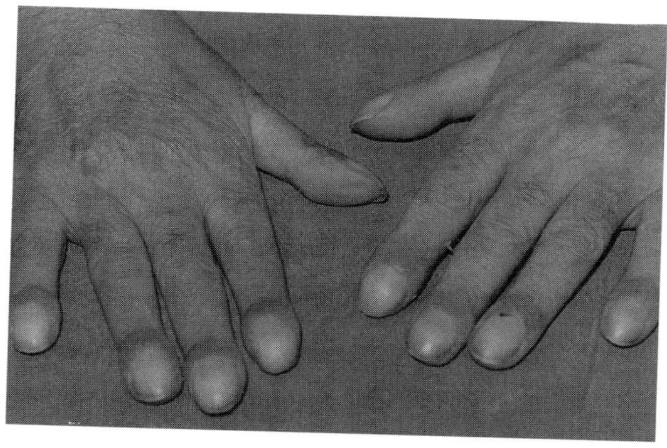

Fig. 7-1 Hypertrophic pulmonary osteoarthropathy (clubbing).

Individuals at high risk for the development of lung cancer because of habits such as tobacco consumption, occupational exposures, and/or significant exposure to passive smoke are often encouraged to consider routine chest x-ray screenings. A number of trials have been attempted through the use of annual chest x-ray screenings alone or with the addition of annual sputum cytologies. Most of these attempts to diagnose disease at an earlier stage have not been associated with significant improvement in long-term survival rates and have been largely abandoned, except in some industrial settings.

Detection and diagnosis

Radiographic imaging. Conventional chest x-ray examinations using posteroanterior and lateral projections remain the principal method of lung cancer detection, although estimates show that approximately 75% of the natural history of the disease has occurred at the time of first radiographic appearance.[32] Fig. 7-2 shows a radiograph of an abnormal anterior chest, whereas the computed tomography (CT) scan demonstrates that the tumor has already invaded the chest wall.

At the initial presentation the most frequent findings include a solitary soft tissue lesion, mediastinal widening secondary to lymphatic extension, parabronchial or parahilar lymphadenopathy, and pleural effusion (Fig. 7-3). Obstructive pneumonias may occur with endobronchial extension sufficient to produce bronchial obstruction. Solitary lesions are frequently irregular in contour and marginal distinctness. These lesions, if connected to a bronchus,

A

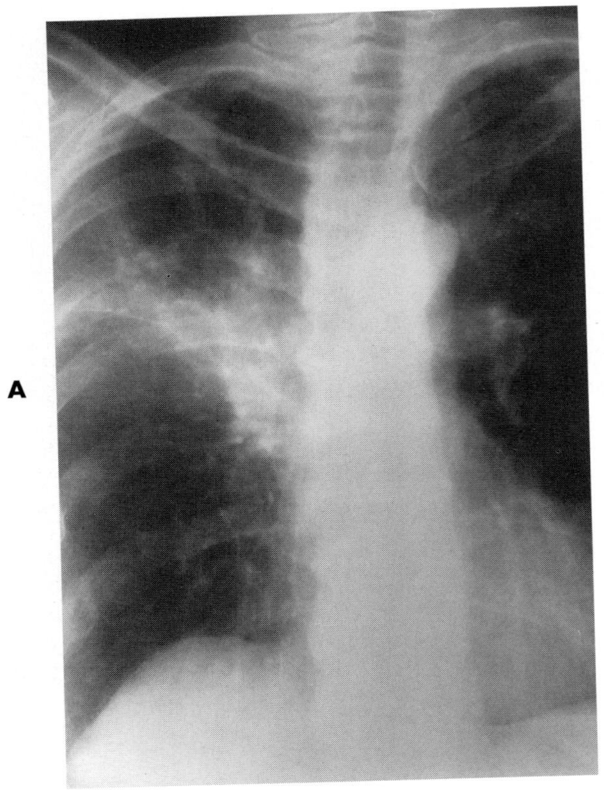

B

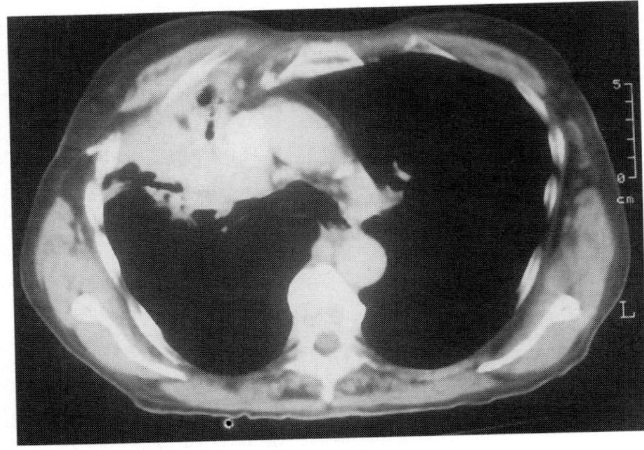

Fig. 7-2 **A,** A PA chest radiograph showing a right upper lobe tumor. **B,** A CT scan demonstrates the involvement of the chest wall.

A

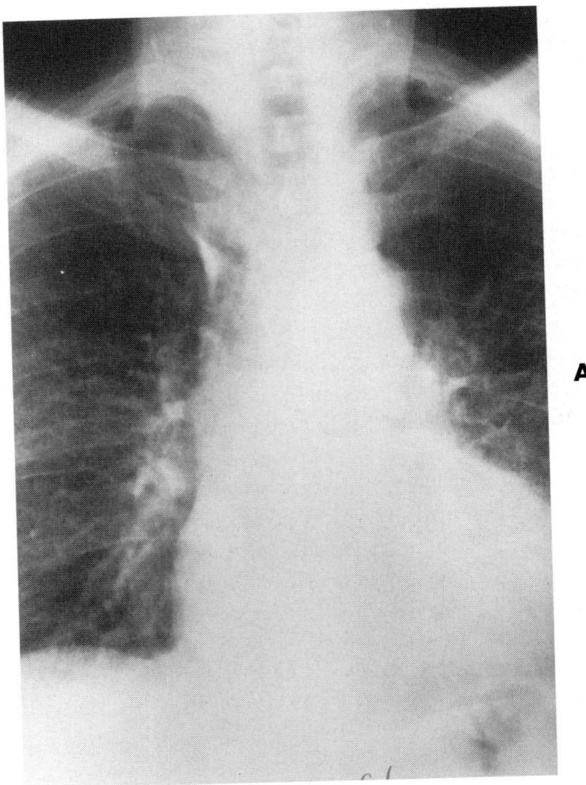

B

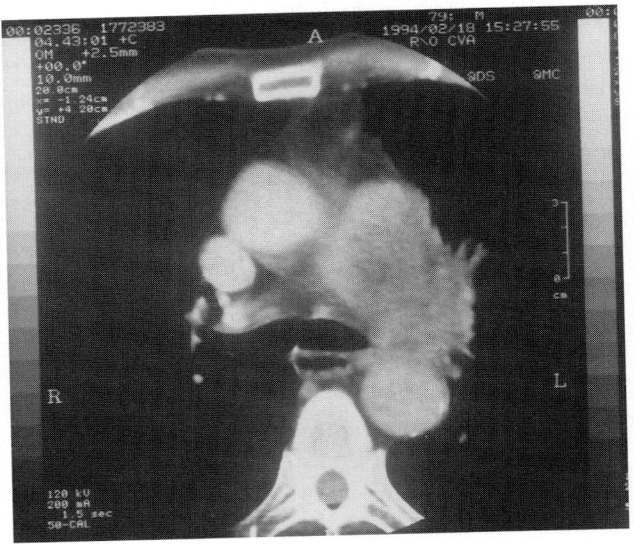

Fig. 7-3 **A,** A PA chest radiograph showing midline disease. **B,** A CT scan demonstrates the involvement of the mediastinum.

may eventually break down to produce a thick-walled abscess with an air-fluid level. Long-standing obstructive pneumonias may also lead to abscess formation.

Chest radiographs that are suspicious for lung cancer must lead to other diagnostic interventions. Because a histological (or cytological) diagnosis is essential for appropriate management decisions, the next steps in evaluation frequently include CT of the chest to evaluate the following: (1) the primary finding itself, (2) the possibility of other pulmonary lesions, (3) the involvement of mediastinal and paramediastinal structures, and (4) pleural or extrapleural thoracic involvement. Fig. 7-4 demonstrates a right upper lobe tumor that has invaded the midline structures, whereas the CT scan shows mediastinal extension.

CT examinations are often crucial in selecting sites for a biopsy. CT examinations should involve the upper abdomen

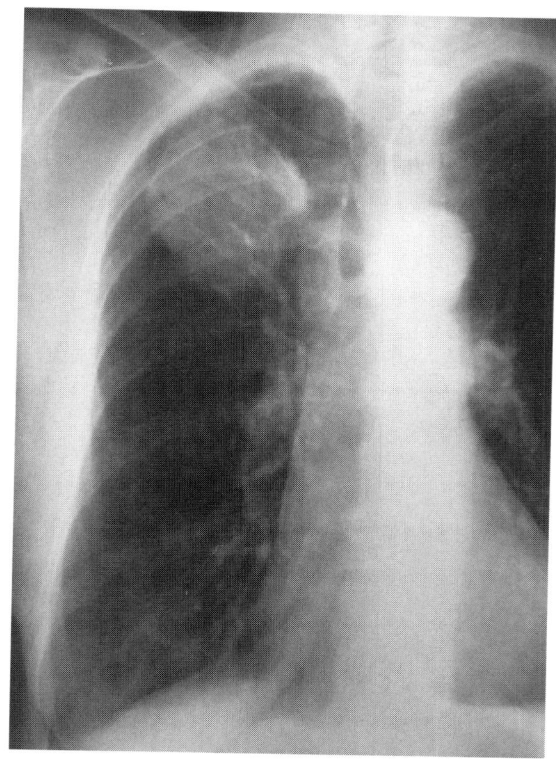

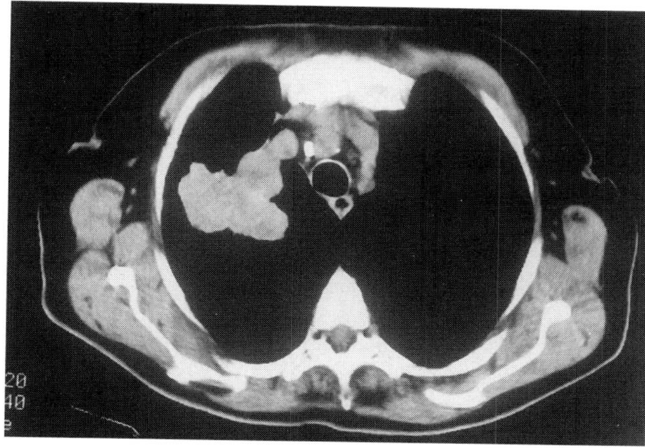

Fig. 7-4 **A,** A PA chest radiograph showing a right upper lobe tumor. **B,** A CT scan demonstrates the involvement of midline structures.

for an evaluation of the liver and adrenal glands, which are frequent sites of metastatic spread. CT scans have become an invaluable aid in the preoperative determination of resectability.

Patients in whom lesions are too peripheral for bronchoscopy or for whom bronchoscopy has failed to demonstrate endobronchial disease may be candidates for a CT-directed percutaneous fine needle aspiration (PFNA). This procedure is highly effective and associated with a small risk of pneumothorax. PFNA is frequently carried out on an outpatient basis with postprocedure time for monitoring of the respiratory status and blood pressure.

Magnetic resonance imaging (MRI) studies and positron emission tomography (PET) scans are being investigated, but at this time they seem to have an insignificant role in the pretreatment evaluation of the disease extent, except as it is related to spinal cord or epidural involvement. Evidence suggests that PET scanning may be valuable in posttreatment evaluation and differentiation of persistent-recurrent tumors versus treatment-related scar tissues.

Except for bone scans, radioisotope studies have been supplanted primarily by CT scans of various organs, with much greater sensitivity and selectivity resulting.

Laboratory studies. Pulmonary function studies are beneficial primarily for determining a patient's ability to withstand various types of treatment, especially because many of these patients have preexisting compromised pulmonary function from their chronic pulmonary disease.

Sputum cytology may be positive in up to 75% of patients with lung cancer. These cytologies are of limited use, however, because of the difficulty in determining the precise sites of disease based on expectorated sputum and because specific tissue subtyping may be difficult.[11]

Bone marrow biopsies are of limited value except in individuals who have small-cell, undifferentiated carcinoma of the lung in which up to a 40% incidence of bone marrow involvement exists.

A histological evaluation is generally sought and usually obtained through interventional routes that include surgery.

Surgery. Tumor histology is most frequently obtained through a fiber-optic bronchoscopy because up to 75% of lesions may be visible in this fashion. Endobronchial brushing, an endobronchial biopsy, or a transbronchial biopsy provides a true-positive diagnosis in over 90% of patients with visible lesions. The patency of bronchi and sites of bleeding can also be established.[31]

A pleural biopsy is used most frequently for pleural-based diseases such as mesothelioma. Thoracentesis (removal of fluid from the chest) or a pleural biopsy may be invaluable in the presence of pleural effusion because malignant effusion adversely affects the prognosis.

Numerous institutions are investigating the role of video-assisted thoracoscopy in the diagnosis and treatment of lung cancer. The procedure involves the insertion of a tube into the chest and visualization of intrathoracic contents on a television monitor. Video-assisted thoracoscopy may be especially beneficial with pleural-based disease or if no dominant masses are demonstrated. The procedure may also assist in staging.

A mediastinoscopy is frequently used for the evaluation of the superior mediastinal extent of disease. If surgical intervention is anticipated, a formal, open mediastinotomy may also be used.

Advanced disease. CT scanning of the brain is used primarily for small-cell, undifferentiated carcinomas and adenocarcinomas of the lung. Both of these have a high risk for central nervous system metastasis.

The use of formal thoracotomy for diagnosing and staging has generally been abandoned because of the availability of less-invasive interventional studies.

Hematological and serum chemical evaluations of the blood are important and should include a complete blood count (CBC) as well as an analysis of serum calcium, alkaline phosphatase, lactic dehydrogenase (LDH), and serum glutamic oxyloacetic transaminase (SGOT). Serum calcium elevation is indicative of osseous disease. Alkaline phosphatase, LDH, and SGOT may be indicative of liver or bone involvement.

Pathology

Histological cell types. The World Health Organization (WHO) has established a histological classification of lung cancer that includes 12 primary tumor types with additional subtypes (see the box to the right). Although little question exists whether these categories are distinct pathologically, they are somewhat cumbersome from a clinical perspective, and more frequently the nomenclature of small cell lung cancer (SCLC) and nonsmall cell lung cancers (NSCLC) are used. This breakdown is appropriate because of the distinct clinical differences between the small cell anaplastic carcinoma and the group of nonsmall cell lesions, including adenocarcinoma, large cell carcinoma, and epidermoid (squamous cell) carcinoma, which act in a similar fashion clinically. Mesothelioma of the lung remains a distinct, although less frequent, category.[14,27]

Location. Squamous cell (epidermoid) carcinoma is usually associated with tobacco consumption, occurs most frequently in men, and is often located centrally in proximal bronchi. This lesion represented the most common form of primary pulmonary malignancy until the recent rise in the incidence of adenocarcinomas, which now account for approximately 40% of lung cancers in North America.[38] Adenocarcinomas are less frequently associated with tobacco consumption, occur most often in women, and are frequently more peripheral in location, arising in bronchioles or alveolae. Small cell carcinomas and large cell carcinomas each represent approximately 20% of the remaining lesions, with small cell lesions tending to occur more centrally and large cell lesions appearing more peripherally. SCLC is prone to early spread, and fewer than 10% of these patients have diagnoses of limited stage disease.

Prognosis. Because of its predisposition for early metastasis, SCLC's prognosis is poor, with fewer than 10% of patients surviving 5 years. NSCLC has a better prognosis, with 5-year survival for 10% to 25% of patients and a higher survival time if the disease is completely resected. Evidence suggests that as the number of pathological specimens is increased in a tumor, a greater likelihood exists for a mixed-cell population to be found. This is most commonly a mixture of adenocarcinoma and squamous cell carcinoma.

Staging

The use of clinical and pathological staging represents an attempt to compare similar cases with regard to the effectiveness of treatment and the prognosis. Before the 1970s, conventional chest x-ray examinations, radioisotope scanning, and serum chemistry analyses were routinely used as the basis for clinical staging. Subsequent evidence has indicated the unreliability of these procedures for accurate evaluation of disease extent.

The advent of CT in the 1970s enhanced the ability to determine resectability before a formal thoracotomy by enabling greater definition of the mediastinum, lymph nodes, and chest-wall invasion. In many instances the presence of these factors was felt to be a contraindication to curative resection, and during the 1970s and 1980s the frequency of surgical intervention in lung cancer declined.

World Health Organization Histological Classification of Lung Cancer

I. Epidermoid carcinoma
II. Small cell anaplastic carcinoma
  1. Fusiform cell type
  2. Polygonal cell type
  3. Lymphocyte-like (oat cell) type
III. Adenocarcinoma
  1. Bronchogenic
    a. Acinar, with or without mucin formation
    b. Papillary
  2. Bronchoalveolar
IV. Large cell carcinoma
  1. Solid tumors with mucinlike content
  2. Solid tumors without mucinlike content
  3. Giant cell carcinoma
  4. Clear cell carcinoma
V. Combined epidermoid and adenocarcinoma
VI. Carcinoid tumors
VII. Bronchial gland tumors
  1. Cylindromas
  2. Mucoepidermoid tumors
  3. Others
VIII. Papillary tumors of the surface epithelium
  1. Epidermoid
  2. Epidermoid with goblet cells
  3. Others
IX. Mixed tumors and carcinomas
  1. Mixed tumors
  2. Carcinosarcoma of the enbryonal type (blastoma)
  3. Other carcinosarcomas
X. Sarcomas
XI. Unclassified
XII. Mesotheliomas
  1. Localized
  2. Diffuse

Modified from World Health Organization: *International histologic classification of tumors, NOS. 1-20,* Geneva, Switzerland, 1978, The Organization.

Improvements in local control and systemic chemotherapy have increased the interest in surgical intervention, even in the presence of mediastinal lymph node involvement. This intervention has necessitated a greater use of pathological staging. A frequently used system is the TNM system proposed by Mountain and Carr and accepted by the American Joint Committee on Cancer[3] (see the box on p. 123).

Routes of spread

Direct. As tumor cells continue to reproduce, the size of the mass increases. The mass itself may grow into surrounding structures. This is called *local extension.*[29] Tumors of the lungs are most likely to extend to the ribs, heart, esophagus, and vertebral column.[8] They may grow silently for long periods. Patients may seek medical attention for pain related to local extension.

Tumors that are not encapsulated have an ability to invade and attach themselves to local structures such as the chest wall, diaphragm, pleura, and pericardium. When tumors are continuous with local structures, they are called *fixed,* an ominous prognostic sign. In lung cancer, direct invasion constitutes a T3 tumor (i.e., a minimum of Stage III).[3]

Direct extension can occur through the visceral pleura into the pleural cavity. A malignant pleural effusion may occur as fluid in the pleural cavity accumulates. Another possible route of local extension is through the hila. A tumor at or near the midline may grow directly into the hilum of the opposite lung.

Lymphatic. Cancer cells break from the tumor mass and enter the lymphatics through two known routes. First, the cells can be trapped in the nodes as the lymphatic fluid is filtered. The cells continue to colonize in the nodes and eventually pass from one node to the next. This lymphatic spread is also called *regional extension.*[29] Second, cancer cells may grow through the lymph node and gain access to the circulatory system through blood vessels supplying the node.

The lymphatics that drain the lungs are the mediastinals and intrapulmonic channels (see the second box on p. 124).

The lymphatics of the other organs in the thoracic cavity play an important role in the spread of lung cancer. The diaphragm, esophagus, pleural cavity, and heart are all in intimate relationship to the lungs.

The drainage of the diaphragm runs through the muscle to the aorta, inferior vena cava, and esophagus. Periesophageal lymphatics connect to the cardiac lymphatics because the heart lymph flows in the direction of the periesophageal nodes. From there the flow is toward the thoracic duct. Some of the nodes of the diaphragm drain toward the stomach and pancreas.[17] From there the flow continues to the right lymphatic duct.

The pleural surfaces are rich in lymphatic channels. These superficial channels drain into the hilum and connect to the veins and arteries at the bronchioles. Also, the intercostal nodes (between the ribs) have many anastomoses. Drainage flows from the nodes between the ribs to the parasternal, paravertebral, and internal mammary nodes.[2] From there the drainage flows to the thoracic duct.

Lymphatics that drain the heart meet at the bifurcation of the trachea. Lymphatics from the left coronary and pulmonary arteries also connect to the cardiac nodes.[12] Thus, channels from the heart and lungs meet in the area of the carina.

Hematogenic. The circulatory system plays a major role in the distant spread of disease.[29] At the bifurcation of the trachea the lymphatic drainage from the lungs, diaphragm, esophagus, pleural cavity, heart, stomach, and pancreas converges.[17] The drainage then has access to the entire body through the circulatory system at the thoracic duct and aorta.

The thoracic duct drains the left side of the body. The lymph moves medially and superiorly from the lungs into the thoracic duct. After moving through the thoracic duct, the lymph enters the circulatory system at the brachiocephalic vein (Fig. 7-5). From the right side of the body the lymph moves superiorly and medially into the right lymphatic duct. From the right lymphatic duct the lymph flows into the subclavian vein[37] (Fig. 7-6).

Tumors also gain access to the circulatory system through blood vessels feeding the local lymphatic structures. In addition, spread occurs when malignant cells pass into blood vessels that supply the tumor.[17] Therefore lung cancer has access to the circulatory system from a variety of directions.

Common sites for metastasis. After gaining access to the circulatory system, tumors of the lung set up colonies in virtually any site. These metastases, or secondary growths, occur most commonly in the liver, brain, bones, adrenal glands, kidneys, and contralateral lung.[3]

Contralateral spread from hilum to hilum occurs as cells break away from the tumor and move to the area of the carina. Pressure changes as a result of respiration or gravity may transport the cell into the other hilum and then eventually into a resting place in the other lung. A "new" tumor may then begin to grow.

Treatment techniques

The primary purpose of clinical and pathological staging of lung cancer is to guide decision making regarding treatment goals. In the absence of demonstrable extrathoracic extension and despite poor long-term survival probability, patients should be considered as candidates for definitive-curative therapy. Individuals with extrathoracic metastasis, severe chronic obstructive pulmonary disease, or other limiting underlying medical problems may be candidates for palliative therapy or supportive care alone. After these decisions are made, despite the fact that lung cancer has been evaluated in clinical trials for decades, an extraordinary degree of controversy exists regarding appropriate management.

All conventional modalities (i.e., surgery, radiation, and chemotherapy) alone or in combination have been studied

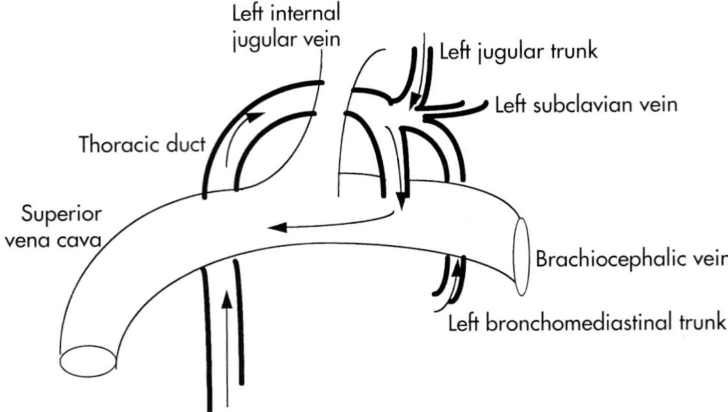

Fig. 7-5 The role of the thoracic duct in lymphatic drainage of the left chest. The lymph moves superiorly through the thoracic duct (left lymphatic duct) and joins the venous portion of the circulatory system at the level of the left brachiocephalic vein.

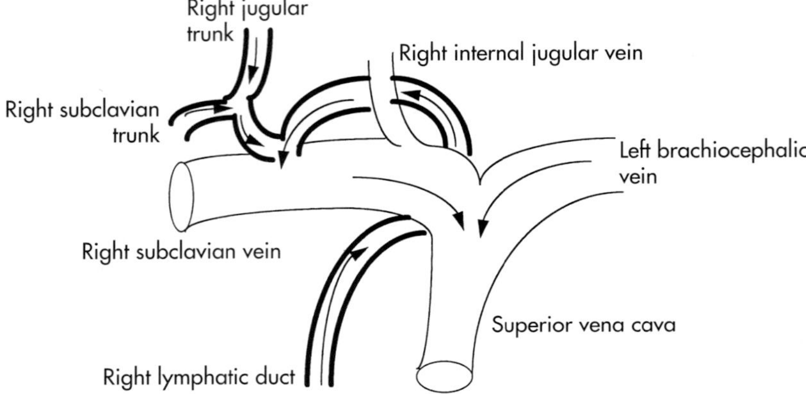

Fig. 7-6 The role of the right lymphatic duct in the drainage of the right chest. The lymph moves superiorly via the right lymphatic duct and enters the venous phase of the circulatory system at the level of the right subclavian vein.

extensively. Newer modalities such as immunotherapy and radiolabeled monoclonal antibodies are also being investigated. Even in circumstances in which combined modalities appear to be advantageous, uncertainty remains concerning the most appropriate tactics of sequencing and dose modifications.

Surgery. Patients who are clinically able to tolerate surgery and have intrathoracic disease of a limited nature without pleural effusion or evidence of mediastinal extension should be considered for definitive surgical intervention. With CT scanning and careful attention to the mediastinum and paramediastinal tissues, only approximately 20% of all patients with lung cancer may be considered candidates for surgery. Of those lung cancers, up to 90% may be resectable. Patients with complete resections (i.e., no evidence of a tumor at the resection margin and no evidence of regional lymphatic extension) have a 50% to 70% 5-year survival rate for clinical Stage I disease and a 45% to 55% 5-year survival rate for Stage II disease. The involvement of parahilar or mediastinal lymph nodes significantly and negatively affects survival.

In general, limited wedge resections of small portions of the lung have not been associated with a high probability for cure. If feasible, a lobectomy with regional lymph node sampling is the preferred procedure. Lesions that are central and involve a main-stem bronchus may require a total pneumonectomy. In this situation, careful attention must be given to preoperative and postoperative pulmonary function. Recently, video-assisted thoracoscopy has allowed for wedge and lobar resections, as well as occasional pneumonectomies, without the need for a formal, open thoracotomy. However, aside from some reduction in surgical morbidity, no evidence exists of improved local control or survival. Video-assisted thoracoscopy may play an important role in pathological staging in anticipation of a formal surgical resection.

If surgery is to be considered, there has been significant interest in the addition of radiation in a preoperative or postoperative setting. Although preoperative radiation is frequently used, especially for apical tumors, most studies have failed to show a significant improvement in survival or increased resectability.[22] Palliative indications for surgery include the control or prevention of pleural effusions, retardation of tumor growth, and control of pain.

Chemotherapy. Responses to chemotherapy alone have generally been poor, with a lack of effective drugs and difficulty in quantifying a response. The most effective single agents are cisplatin and doxorubicin, with approximately a 13% response (generally only partial) for 6 to 8 months at most. Additional studies using high-dose-rate methotrexate with leucovorin and vincristine, cisplatin plus mitomycin-C, and cisplatin and doxorubicin have demonstrated similar short-lived responses. Recent studies have suggested that concomitant chemotherapy consisting of cisplatin and 5-fluorouracil in combination with external radiation may improve the 3-year survival rate above that of radiation alone.[30]

Although chemotherapy has produced dramatic responses, the duration of response is generally short and an early site of recurrence is often in the primary lesion and central chest area. The addition of radiation has affected these local-regional control rates, with 75% to 80% failure centrally in patients treated with chemotherapy alone and 30% to 60% failure in patients treated with added radiation. Controversy continues regarding the precise sequencing of these modalities. However, the most dramatic prospective study indicates a 40% 2-year survival rate through the use of three cycles of systemic chemotherapy followed by a 4500 cGy dose to the mediastinum and primary lesion site and, with complete response, prophylactic radiation to the brain. The general use of prophylactic radiation to the brain has significantly reduced the percentage of patients having central nervous system failure but has not significantly affected long-term survival.

SCLC may respond dramatically to chemotherapy. Combinations such as cisplatin and VP-16 (etoposide) are used with limited-stage (intrathoracic) disease.

Radiation. No evidence suggests that postoperative radiation improves local control or survival in the absence of local residual disease or mediastinal-paramediastinal lymphadenopathy. Several studies have suggested an improvement in 3-year survival with postoperative radiation if lymph nodes are positive. In addition, studies have shown a reduction in local-regional failure.[5,15] Unfortunately, in many of these trials, no evidence has indicated a long-term survival benefit. In the absence of gross residual disease, standard postoperative radiation consists of 4500 to 5000 cGy through anterior and posterior or oblique parallel-opposed fields, with a limitation of the spinal cord dose to approximately 4500 cGy. Depending on the patient contour and primary tumor location, spinal cord protection may be accomplished through a posterior midline block, oblique parallel-opposed fields, anterior and two oblique posterior fields, or the addition of lateral fields.

Radiation alone has been used for clinically unresectable disease (i.e., mediastinal extension, chest-wall extension, and pleural effusion) or with more peripheral lesions in patients who are not candidates for surgery because of underlying medical problems or refusal. These patients rarely survive more than 2 years.

If radiation is used alone, there can be as much as a 30% to 35% 3-year survival rate for Stage I and a 20% to 25% 5-year survival rate. Evidence exists of a dose-response curve with the greatest evidence for control in the 6500- to 7500-cGy dose range. Lower doses increase the risk of local-regional failure significantly. For doses of 6000 cGy or below, the local control rate is less than 20%.[9,25]

Even in the radiation oncology community, controversy exists regarding optimal techniques. Based on criteria generally followed by the Radiation Therapy Oncology Group (RTOG), the standard practice has been to (1) allow a 2-cm normal tissue margin around known disease, (2) treat the entire width of the mediastinum and contralateral hilum, and (3) treat the ipsilateral supraclavicular lymph nodes for upper and middle lobe lesions. The addition of the supraclavicular region has improved local control but has not contributed to improved survival. For upper or middle lobe lesions the inferior margin of the field is usually 4 to 6 cm below the carina. Generally, parallel-opposed fields are used to 4000 to 4500 cGy to the spinal cord. After that, field sizes are frequently reduced and therapy is continued through alternate field arrangements to allow minimization of additional cord radiation. The use of inhomogeneity correction factors for various intrathoracic tissues is controversial and not universally applied for NSCLC.[24]

The RTOG has studied the use of hyperfractionated radiation with doses of 120 cGy delivered twice daily and separated by a 6-hour interval. With doses of 6000 and 6480 cGy, disease-free survival rates did not improve in patients having an unfavorable prognosis (i.e., greater than 5% weight loss or a Karnofsky score less than 70), but evidence of improved survival rates in patients treated with doses of 6960 cGy and above was apparent. Dose levels of 7440 and 7920 cGy produced similar responses but increased toxicity.

Mesotheliomas of the lung have not responded well to systemic chemotherapy or external radiation. The need to treat the entire pleural surface to doses of 4600 to 5500 cGy produces significant morbidity. This course is generally not followed. Some authors have suggested the routine use of radiation to treat biopsy-needle tracks or surgical-wound sites because of a high incidence of direct extension through these pathways.

Recent literature has suggested a potential role for new radiation modalities, such as the use of multileaf collimators, conformal radiation, proton beams, endobronchial brachytherapy, and stereotactic radiation. In the absence of a general agreement on standard treatment techniques, none of these new modalities are likely to show significant improvement in local control or survival in the foreseeable future.

Advanced disease. Palliative radiation is extremely effective and most commonly used for control of osseous and brain metastasis. Skeletal pain is relieved in up to 90% of patients treated. The probability of pain relief, however, is reduced as architectural bone disruption increases. Generally, doses up to 3500 cGy in 250- to 300-cGy daily dose fractions are sufficient for pain relief and bone healing. In instances in which a pathological fracture has occurred or evidence exists of an impending fracture based on the loss of bone calcium, consideration should be given to internal fixation before radiation. Because many patients treated for palliation of osseous pain have received previous systemic chemotherapy, careful attention must be paid to the stability of blood counts.

Brain metastases may occur as seizures, headaches, or focal motor or sensory deficits. Patients with seizure activity should receive antiseizure medication, such as Dilantin, and high-dose corticosteroids. In the absence of seizures, Dilantin therapy provides no benefit. Patients in whom significant intracranial edema is demonstrated may note the rapid relief of symptoms with the use of corticosteroids, but these generally provide only a short-term symptomatic response. Radiation must be used for tumor control. Doses of 3000 cGy in 10 fractions produce relief of symptoms in 35% to 75% of treated individuals.

Superior vena cava obstruction may be evident in 5% of all lung cancer patients and may be secondary to extrinsic compression of the vena cava or direct tumor extension into the vessel. Superior vena cava syndrome is considered an oncological emergency. Usual radiation techniques include three to four fractions of 300 to 400 cGy, followed by a reduction of the daily dose to a 180- to 250-cGy dose level. The total dose with this accelerated dose schema is usually 4500 to 5000 cGy. Approximately 85% of patients treated for vena cava obstruction experience some relief of symptoms within 3 weeks, but long-term survival rates are poor.

Radiation doses of approximately 3000 to 4000 cGy in 2 to 3 weeks through the use of small fields are generally sufficient to control hemoptysis if the site of bleeding can be well localized. Endobronchial hemoptysis or obstruction may be improved or relieved entirely through the use of endoscopic laser fulguration in conjunction with external radiation, conventional low-dose-rate brachytherapy, or high-dose-rate afterloading brachytherapy.[21]

Field design and critical structures

Parallel-opposed fields. The most simple fields used in the treatment of lung cancer are parallel-opposed mediastinal fields. The patient is treated with an anterior and a posterior field. This type of setup is sometimes called *AP/PA* or *POF* (parallel-opposed fields).

The anatomy included in basic mediastinal fields are structures located at or near the midline of the patient. These structures include the trachea, carina, primary bronchi, hilum of each lung, mediastinal vessels, esophagus, vertebral bodies, and spinal cord. Portions of the heart, diaphragm, and stomach may also be included. In the most basic type of fields, minimal or no blocking is used. Patients treated with mediastinal fields generally have disease limited to a midline structure, such as a hilum, or disease blocking an airway.

More commonly, fields are designed to encompass a nonmidline tumor and the mediastinum. In these situations the primary tumor plus the anticipated routes of extension are treated with parallel-opposed fields. If a lung tumor is found in a middle or lateral segment of the lung, the fields are similar to those in Fig. 7-7. Upper lobe tumors may spread to the supraclavicular nodes. Fields, therefore, are designed to cover the supraclavicular and lower cervical regions (Fig.7-8). Complex blocking is required.

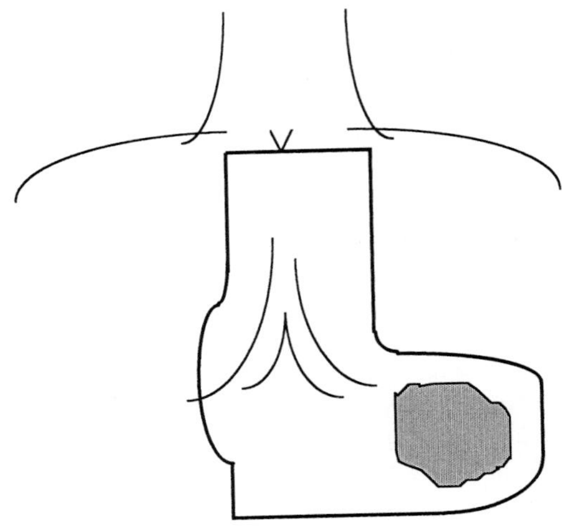

Fig. 7-7 The field shape for middle and lower lobe tumors includes the mediastinum, carina, bilateral hila, tumor mass, and adjacent routes of extension.

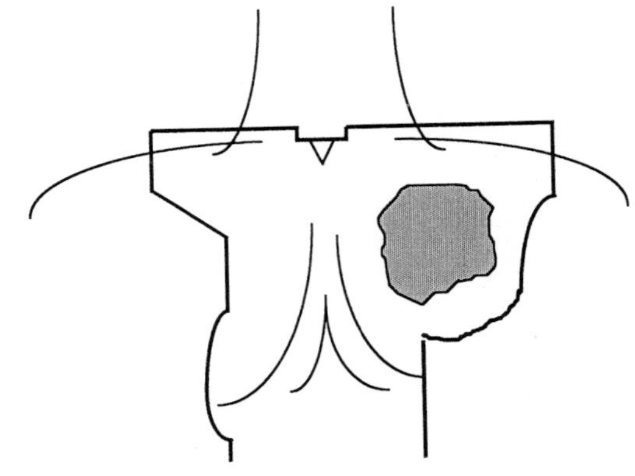

Fig. 7-8 The field shape for an upper lobe tumor includes the mediastinum, carina, bilateral hila, supraclavicular lymphatics, tumor mass, and adjacent routes of extension.

Depending on the location of the lung tumor, there are many variations of parallel-opposed fields. Generally, fields change throughout the treatment course in response to dose limitations, volume limitations, and the need to deliver a total dose that will eradicate the tumor.

Boosts fields. **Boost fields** are used to deliver a high dose to a small volume. With boost fields the radiation dose is directed to the gross tumor volume only.[10,13] The regional routes of spread are not included (Fig. 7-9). When the tumor is not near a radiosensitive structure, boost fields can be simply parallel-opposed with a small margin around the mass.

Frequently, boost fields must be designed to avoid the spinal cord. Many beam combinations will accomplish the goal of not exceeding spinal cord tolerance. Examples include, but are not limited to, parallel-opposed direct or oblique fields, paired wedges, weighted beams, and combinations of open and wedged fields (Fig. 7-10). The beam arrangements depend on the location of the primary tumor and its relationship to a critical structure.

Multiple field combinations. Generally, the treatment of lung cancer requires multiple field combinations that use combinations of different types of fields. More than one pair of parallel-opposed beams and/or off-cord obliques are common approaches used to achieve a tumoricidal dose. Boost fields are included in multiple field combinations. The **field-within-a-field** approach to therapy is a multiple field combination in which the larger field that covers the tumor and drainage routes is treated along with a concurrent boost field to the primary tumor.[10]

Often, **shrinking fields** are used in situations in which field sizes are reduced throughout treatment.[13] Reduced fields are used for two reasons. First, field sizes are made smaller as the size of the tumor decreases to improve the overall tolerance through the treatment of smaller volumes.[13,29] Second, and sometimes related to tumor reduction, the need exists to limit doses to normal structures such as the heart. This is accomplished by changing field sizes, adding shielding alloys, and/or using independent collimators (Fig. 7-11).

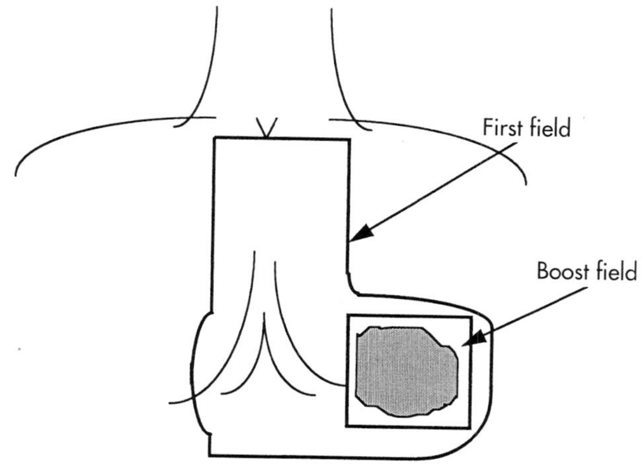

Fig. 7-9 A left lower lung tumor. The first field includes the left lung mass, mediastinum, and routes of extension. The boost field covers the mass plus a margin of 1 to 2 cm.

Accurate positioning of the patient is always important, and lasers should be used when possible. A sagittal laser and lasers aligned with marks on the sides of the patient increase the accuracy of the setup. Of critical importance is the arm position with off-cord boosts because the probability of the patient rolling to one side or the other increases if the arms are raised above the patient's head. In addition, the spinal cord can receive doses above tolerance if lasers are not aligned properly. Geographical misses can occur if the patient is not aligned accurately for every treatment. This goal of reproducibility is improved with the use of lasers for alignment.[36]

Critical structures. Three critical structures are frequently included in fields used to treat lung cancer: the spinal cord, heart, and normal lung.[29] Conceivably, the dose tolerances of these organs can be exceeded. Therefore, doses to these structures must be carefully documented during planning and throughout the treatment course. Fields are designed so that organ tolerance is not exceeded. Advance planning before organ tolerance is reached is critically important so that the optimal dose distributions can be achieved.[8]

The first critical structure considered is the spinal cord. Doses of radiation required to control lung cancer exceed the spinal cord tolerance of 4500 to 5500 cGy[34] (Table 7-1). Although higher spinal cord tolerance doses are discussed in the literature,[26,34] radiation oncologists generally take a conservative approach to the spinal cord dose by prescribing treatments that do not exceed the 4500-cGy limit.[23] Standard practice for radiation therapists is to require a written order for all cord doses greater than 4500 cGy. In charting daily treatments, radiation therapists should monitor a spinal cord dose column to ensure that tolerance is not exceeded. Frequently, the cord receives a daily dose that is higher than the prescribed dose to the tumor. The quality of a patient's life will be diminished and even death may result if these standards are not followed.

If cord tolerance is exceeded, neurological signals that normally move along the spinal cord will be blocked. Demyelination of the oligodendrocytes that conduct nerve impulses is responsible for some of the neurological complications. In addition, damages in the form of fibrosis and occlusion of capillaries and arterioles result in a reduced blood supply to the neurons and oligodendrocytes in the region treated. Because nervous system tissue has severely limited or no regenerative abilities, damage is irreparable.[33] Clinical manifestations of cord damage such as myelitis (inflammation of the spinal cord) can occur. Depending on the level of the cord affected, quadriplegia or paraplegia may follow. Necrosis and infarction of the cord can occur. When transection of the cord occurs, Brown-Séquard's syndrome results, with paralysis and loss of sensations such as pain and temperature.[29]

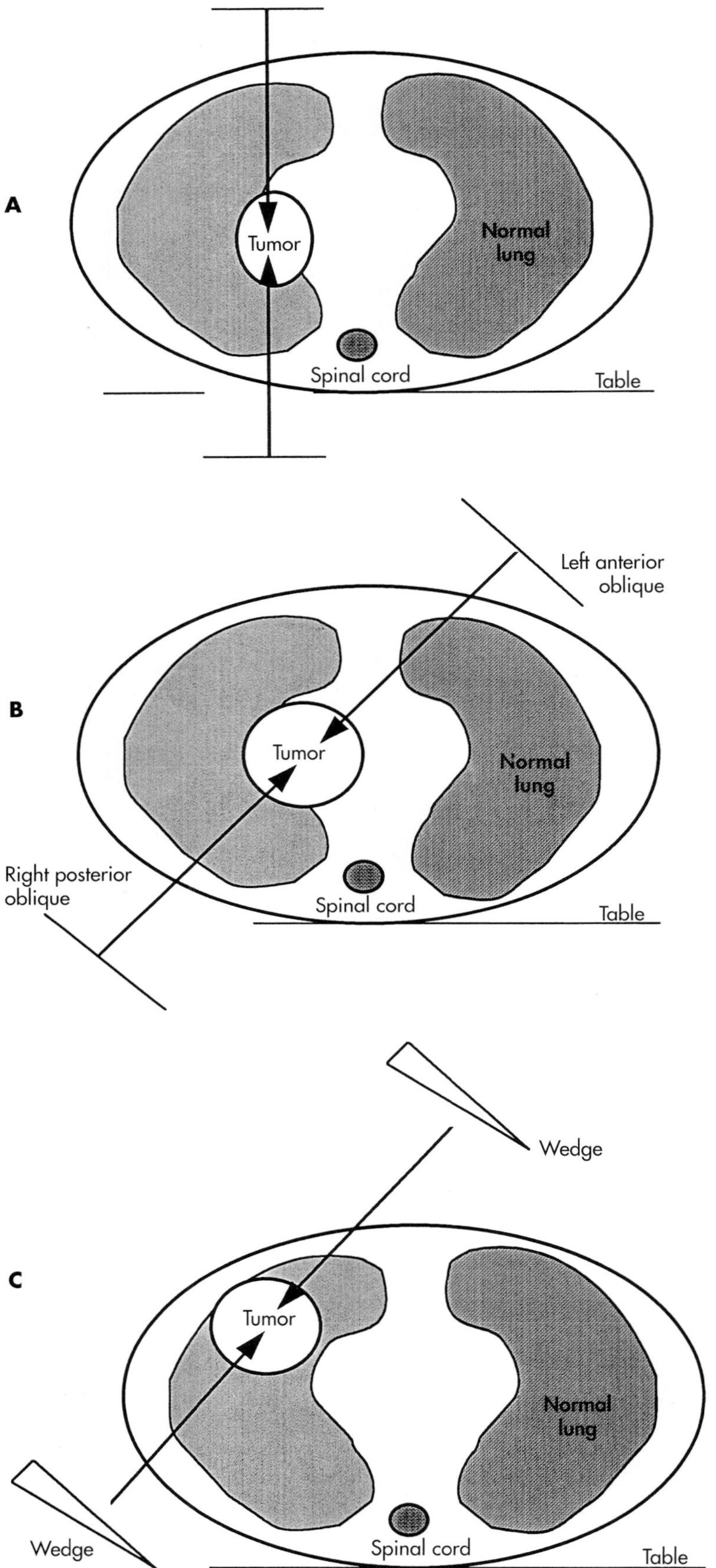

Fig. 7-10 Lung boosts. **A,** Off-cord, parallel-opposed fields. **B,** Off-cord, parallel-opposed oblique fields. **C,** Off-cord obliques with wedges.

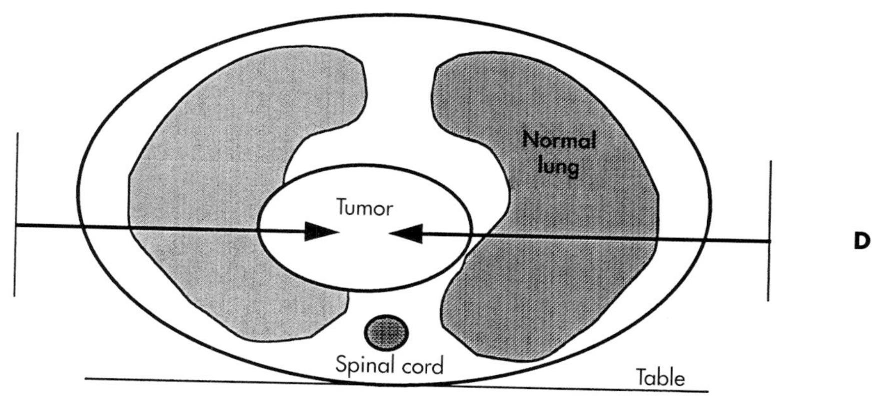

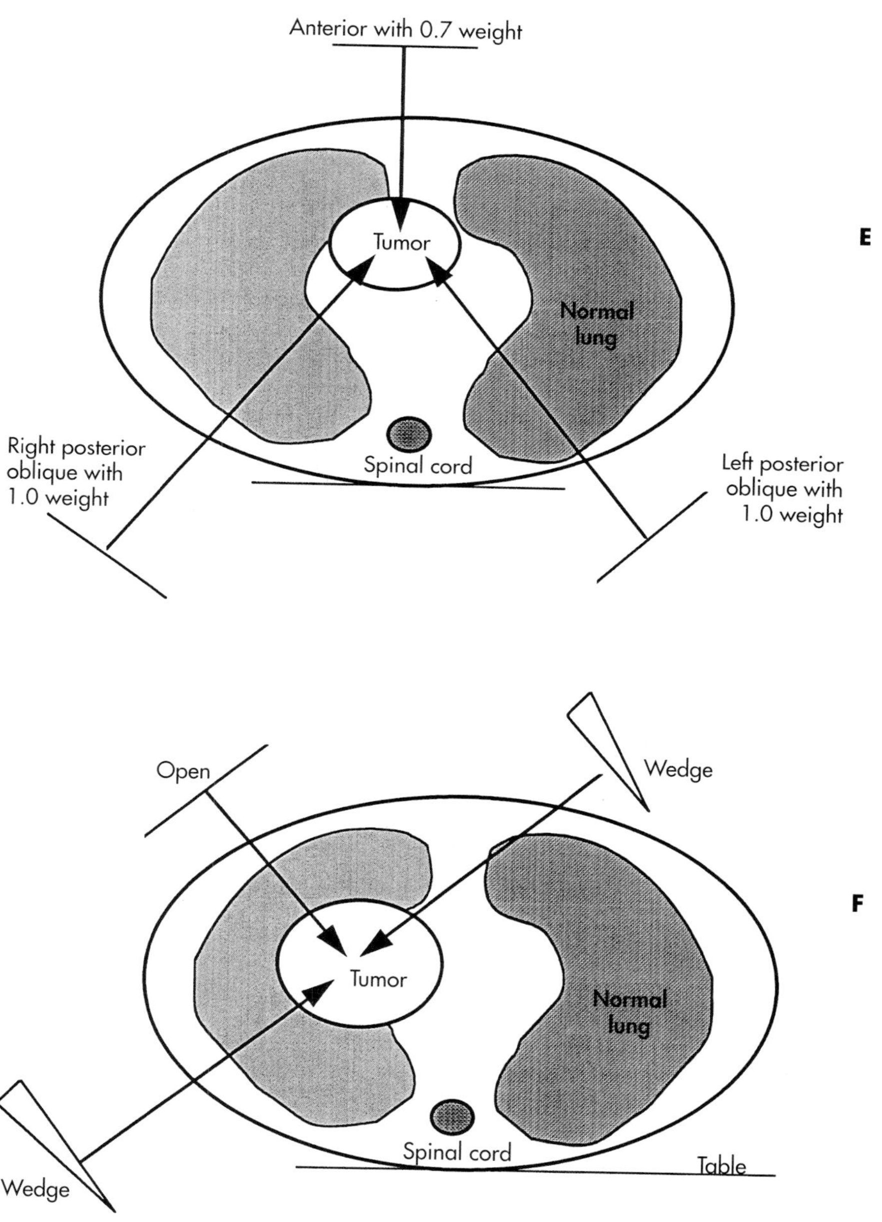

Fig. 7-10, cont'd. **D,** Parallel-opposed laterals. (Note the amount of uninvolved lung.) **E,** An open anterior field weighted 0.7 and two posterior obliques with equal weighting. **F,** Two off-cord obliques with wedges and an open field. (Note the position of the spinal cord in relation to the open

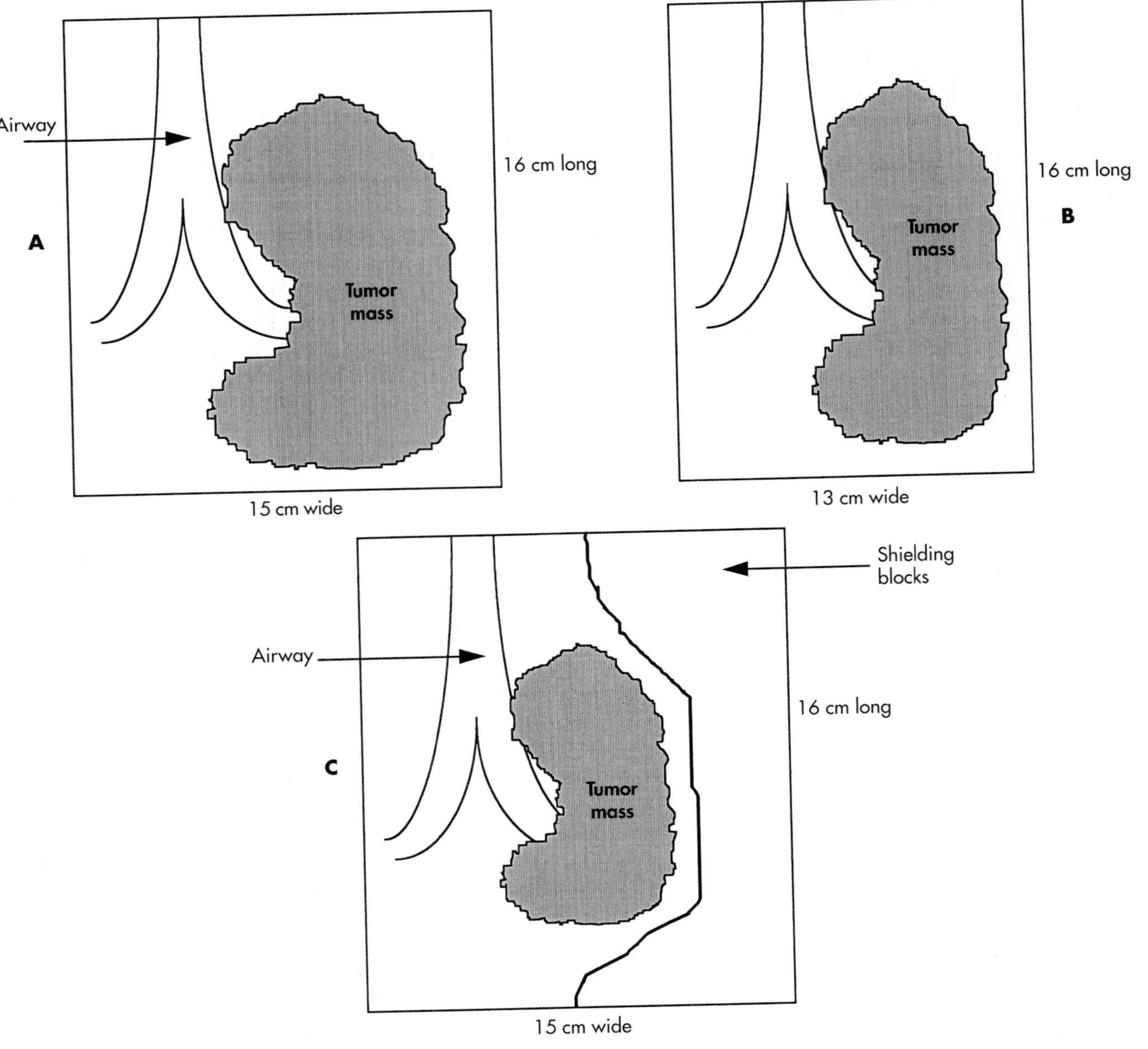

Fig. 7-11 Shrinking fields. **A,** The field size and tumor at the start of therapy. **B,** The tumor mass reduction during therapy and the field width reduction. **C,** Shielding blocks added to block uninvolved lung with smaller tumor mass.

During the planning process the depth of the spinal cord must be determined. If available, CT images are useful; the depth of the cord in the patient is determined from the images of the individual vertebral bodies in the field to be treated. In simulation, **orthogonal radiographs**[36] are taken to determine the cord depth. Generally, anterior and lateral films are taken at right angles. The physical depth of the cord in the patient is measured from the image through the use of a demagnification calculation.

The depth of the spinal cord is important for two reasons. First, tumoricidal doses exceed the tolerance of the spinal cord. Second, because the depth of the spinal cord varies along the vertebral column, the dose calculated to one point in the spinal cord is not the same for the remainder of the cord. For example, the depth of the cord in the lower cervical area may be 5 cm, whereas the depth in the lower thorax may be 8 cm. If the tumor is close to the midplane (approximately 10 cm), overdoses to both areas of the spinal cord can occur (Fig. 7-12). Even if cord tolerance is considered in the prescription, the dose the patient receives to the cord must be monitored closely because the dose along the length of the field varies as the depth of the cord changes.

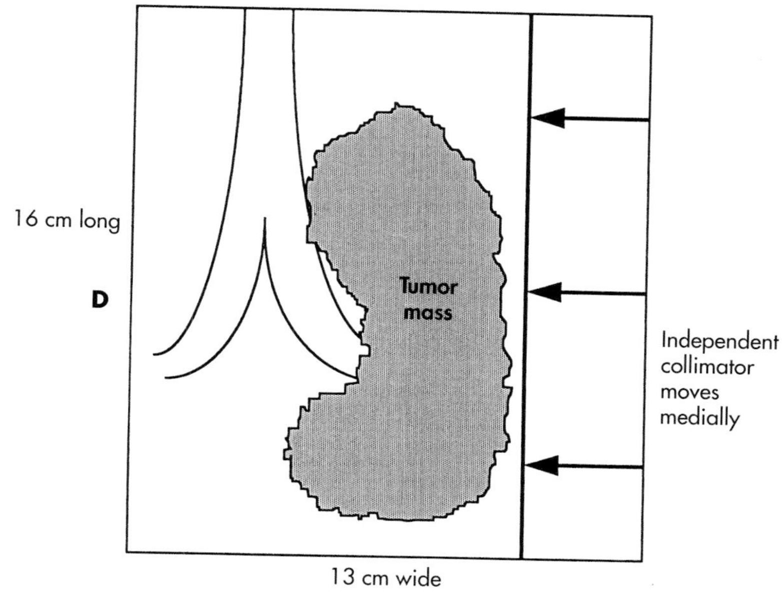

Fig. 7-11, cont'd. Shrinking fields. **D,** Width reduction to accommodate a smaller tumor size through the use of an independent collimator (beam off-sets).

Table 7-1 Organ tolerances

Organ	TD 5/5 (cGy)	TD 50/5 (cGy)
Spinal cord	4500	5500
Normal lung	1500-3000	2500-3500
Heart	4500	5500
Esophagus	6000	7500
Bone marrow	3000	4000
Skin	5500	7000
Liver	2500	4000

Modifed from Rubin P: *Radiation biology and radiation pathology syllabus,* Chicago, 1975, American College of Radiology.

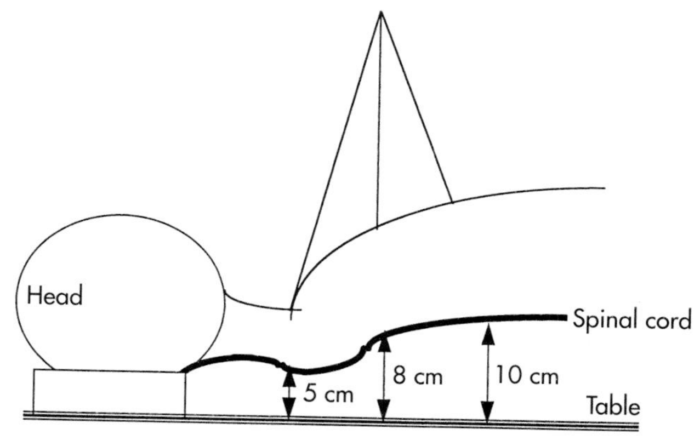

Fig. 7-12 Variations in spinal cord depths. The depth of the cervical spinal cord is closer to the posterior surface than that of the thoracic cord.

Avoiding the spinal cord with boost fields can be challenging, particularly considering the normal curvature of the vertebral column. With oblique and lateral fields, collimator rotations may be used to follow the curvature of the spinal column. The angle of rotation is calculated through the use of a geometrical slope formula. Blocking the cord may be useful, but the transmission of radiation through the block should be considered. Spinal cord tolerance can be exceeded with beam transmission through the block and with scatter radiation that occurs in the patient (under the shadow of the block projected on the skin).

When the spinal column is not midplane the image of the anterior field is different from that of the posterior field. This is caused by divergence. The effect of divergence can be seen through a comparison of the disc spaces on the anterior and posterior images. When fields are exactly parallel-opposed the images may not be identical.[4]

Magnification-measuring devices are used during simulation. Devices such as beaded trays are used so that comparisons can be made between the images and actual patient anatomy. Magnification-measuring devices are used for comparing objects of a predetermined size with objects of an undetermined size.[36] For example, fiducial trays containing the beads are placed above the patient in the head of the simulator. The spacing of the beads is such that the image projects a 2-cm (sometimes 1-cm) space between the beads at the axis of the machine. Through the use of a 100-cm isocentric unit the space between the beads is 2 cm at 100 cm. If the image is produced at a 140-cm source-film distance (SFD), a direct relationship exists between the space between the beads on the film and the space at the axis. With the use of a ratio the space is calculated to 2.8 cm. Other devices such as rulers, rings, or coins accomplish the same goal; a known dimension is used to find an unknown dimension.

In the planning of treatments for patients with lung cancer, magnification-measuring devices are particularly useful in finding the spinal cord depth. The cord depth can be determined from the lateral orthogonal film. The amount of the simulation table on the film causes a distortion because of the width of the table and the distance the beam travels. Tables can be marked with a radiopaque wire in the center to reduce distortion.[4] Alternatively, the therapist can palpate the spinous processes and carefully tape on the patient's back a piece of solder wire that will relate the vertebral column to the skin surface. During simulation in the supine position the wire will be in contact with the table, thereby indicating the table on the radiographic image.

The second critical structure in the treatment of lung cancer is the heart. When 60% or more of the heart is treated with 4500 to 5500 cGy, pericarditis (inflammation of the pericardium) and pancarditis (inflammation of all parts of the heart) may result[34] (Table 7-1). Long-term complications can follow because of damage of the interstitial components of cardiac tissue, and the resulting fibrosis may damage the valves.[29]

In the planning of fields for lung tumors near the heart, the volume of the heart treated should be considered. In particular, when parallel-opposed beams are weighted anteriorly to reduce the spinal cord dose, the dose to the heart should also be measured so that tolerance is not exceeded The use of chemotherapy should be monitored closely. Drugs such as doxorubicin (Adriamycin) have cardiac toxicity that has a synergistic effect when the drug is used in combination with radiation.[29]

The third critical structure to be considered in the treatment of lung cancer is the normal lung. The major complication that occurs is radiation pneumonitis, followed by fibrosis. Pneumonitis occurs from 1 to 3 months after radiation. Fibrosis occurs from 2 to 4 months after treatment.[29] Pneumonitis is the clinical manifestation of vascular, epithelial, and interstitial injuries. Patients exhibit dyspnea, fevers, night sweats, and/or cyanosis.[8] The chronic phase consists of severe dyspnea and coughing, clubbing of the fingers, and an abscess that can be followed by infection and sepsis.

The volume of lung treated and the total dose must be considered to avoid complications related to the lung. The dose tolerance to the lung generally ranges from 1500 to 3500 cGy[34] (Table 7-1). Large volumes of lung are projected to have at least a 50% complication rate at 4000 cGy (TD 50/5, or 50% of the patients in 5 years). Fraction sizes range from 180 to 200 cGy. Care is taken throughout the planning process to minimize the amount of noncancerous lung in the fields. Customized beams such as reduced and boost fields, shielding blocks, and off-cord arrangements are used to limit the beam transmission through unaffected lung. The nature of lung tissue itself is notable. Lung density is less than the density of other tissue because of the presence of air (oxygen and carbon dioxide) in the organs. Therefore the dose to the tumor and lung tissue is increased by 15% to 20%.[19,29] Heterogeneity corrections can be used to compensate for this phenomenon.

Other structures included in fields designed to treat lung cancers are important but not critical. The esophagus, bone marrow, skin, and sometimes the liver with right lower lobe tumors have dose tolerances identified in Table 7-1. Generally, however, tolerance of these organs is not exceeded.

Off-axis points. Typically, doses are calculated to the center of a field. With lung tumors, however, knowledge about the structures not in the center is important. For the calculation of doses to off-axis points, two measurements are needed: (1) the source-skin distance (SSD) to each point and (2) the corresponding patient thickness at each point. Depending on the institution, the physical measurement of the size of the patient may be referred to as the *patient thickness, separation,* or *diameter.* The physical measurement of a patient's size is determined through the use of calipers. SSDs are determined by reading and recording the distance that the optical distance indicator shows. Doses to the various points vary according to the inverse square law and attenuation.

Distances vary with patient size and anatomical variations. In Fig. 7-13, the SSD to the center is 90 cm, and the distance at the supraclavicular point is 93 cm. The patient measures 20 cm at the center and 14 cm at the supraclavicular point. Each anatomical point at which doses are needed will be measured. The SSDs and the corresponding patient diameters must be recorded. These distances and diameters work with each other. When the 90-cm SSD and 20-cm separation are accurate, the patient must measure 22 cm at the mediastinum if the 89-cm SSD to that point is correct (100 - 11 = 89) (Table 7-2). A patient with a left upper lobe tumor will have off-axis points to include the tumor, supraclavicular nodes, and mediastinum.

Customized beams. Optimal patient care frequently requires combinations of several types of field designs. For example, multiple fields with boosts, collimator rotations, and weighting may be needed to deliver the best dose distribution. Mixed beams, photons, and electrons may be used to meet specific clinical challenges, such as a mass extending through the chest wall. Also, dual-energy accelerators have the capacity to customize the beam to an effective energy level that is not possible with a single-energy conventional accelerator. Beam arrangements are selected to cover the tumor and simultaneously limit the dose to the normal tissue.

Specific anatomical features, such as a kyphosis (excessive curvature of the spine), need special attention. With curvatures of the spine the collimator can be rotated to follow

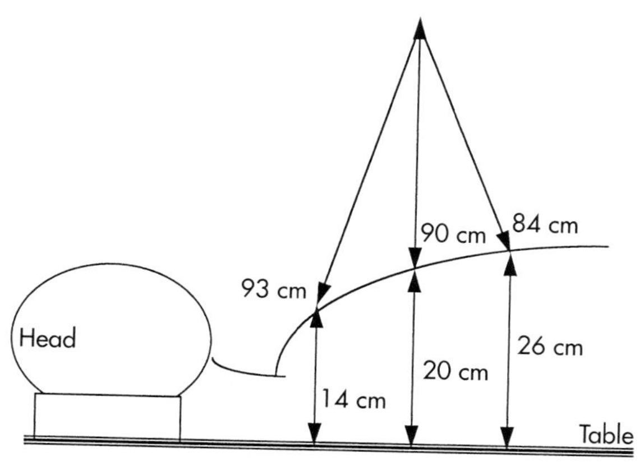

Fig. 7-13 Sloping chest. Superior, central, and inferior borders have different distances and corresponding patient measurements.

Table 7-2 Comparison of points and distances

Point	SSD (cm)	Diameter (cm)	Midplane depth
Center	90	20	10
Mediastinum	89	22	11
Supraclavicular	93	14	7
Mass	91	18	9

SSD, Source-skin distance.

the vertebral column. Another approach is the use of a customized shield (alloy) to tailor the field to meet the individual patient's anatomy without rotating the collimator.

If oblique fields are needed to boost the lung tumor and at the same time avoid treating the spinal cord, the varying depths of the spinal cord often present challenges. With the use of a collimator "twist," one section of the spine is included, whereas another section may be excluded in the fields. The use of alloys may solve this dilemma. However, if collimator rotations are used, care must be given to changing the rotation for the parallel-opposed field. With the clinical application of the concept of mirror images,[4] an anterior field with a 175-degree rotation off the 180 degrees requires a 5-degree twist in the opposite direction for the posterior field. The posterior collimator position, therefore, is 355 degrees so that the volume treated in these fields is truly parallel-opposed.

Compensators are used to adjust dose distributions for anatomical features such as a barrel-shaped chest. Either a customized device is made or a standard wedge, C-wedge (compensating wedge),[19] is used to improve the dose distribution. Compensators attenuate the beam. They are useful for correcting surface irregularities. Also, spinal cord dose variations resulting from spinal column curvature can be adjusted with the use of a compensator. A compensator is useful if the inferior thorax measures significantly more than the superior thorax.[23] Examples include C-wedges, conventional compensators (i.e., lead, brass, aluminum, plastic, or Lucite), and computerized custom compensators (Fig. 7-14). Bolus can be used to reduce surface irregularities, but the loss of a skin-sparing effect usually precludes its use in clinical practice.[19]

Wedges can be used to help shape dose distributions. In particular, wedges are useful for the delivery of boost doses with laterally located tumors. Multiple field arrangements that include a three- or four-field wedge and open field combinations are examples of the use of the wedges' beam-shaping characteristics (Figs. 7-10, *E* and *F*).

Doses. Total doses vary depending on the goal of the therapy. Definitive treatment, in which patients are treated with a long-term goal to control or cure the disease, typically requires high doses and complex field arrangements. Palliative treatment, in which patients are treated for the control of symptoms, generally has lower total doses with simple field arrangements.

Definitive doses to control or cure localized bronchogenic carcinomas range from 6000 to 7500 cGy[7,8,29] (Table 7-3). Initial field arrangements are generally prescribed between 4000 and 4500 cGy. Boost fields follow in various combinations until tumoricidal doses are achieved. Various fraction patterns can be used, depending on whether **conventional fractionation, hyperfractionation, accelerated fractionation,** or **accelerated hyperfractionation** is prescribed.[23,35] Conventional fractionation uses a 180- or 200-cGy dose given once per day. The other fraction patterns change the conventional approach by altering the fraction size, daily dose, number of treatment days, and/or total dose in an effort to improve patient tolerance and survival. Table 7-4 displays these different approaches to fractionation in a hypothetical patient.

Palliative treatment is given to relieve symptoms. For lung cancer, treatment can be given to relieve an airway obstruction. In these situations the total tumor dose ranges from 4000 to 5000 cGy,[29] depending on the patient's response.

For a patient with superior vena cava syndrome, initial doses are high for the first one to three treatments and range from 350 to 400 cGy.[7] Because of the large volume and high doses, the daily dose must be reduced after the initial treatments. Total prescribed doses are generally 350 to 1200 cGy, followed by 200-cGy fractions to a total dose of 4500 to 5000 cGy.

Brachytherapy can be used in the treatment of lung cancer. High-dose-rate remote afterloading (HDR) is used in the treatment of bronchial disease. For example, during a course of external beam radiation a supplemental dose of radiation can be given with HDR, using 500 cGy for two to four treatments. In the event of recurrent disease, HDR may also be useful, particularly if spinal cord tolerance has been reached or the airway is compromised.

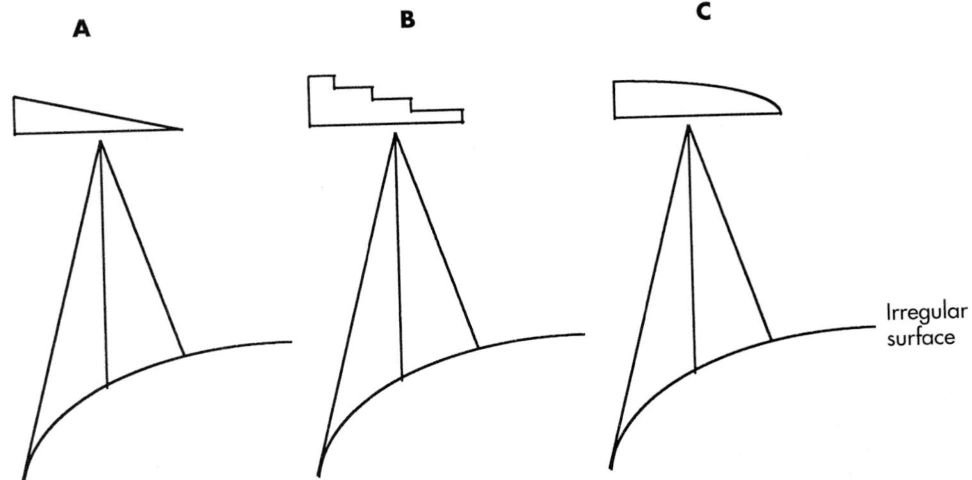

Fig. 7-14 Methods of compensation. **A,** C-wedge. **B,** Conventional compensator. **C,** Customized alloy compensator.

Side effects

Classification. During courses of radiation therapy, patients may experience side effects classified as acute or chronic. The short-term reactions that occur during treatment and subside after the course is completed are known as *acute side effects. Chronic side effects* are long-term effects of radiation treatments.

Clinical presentation. With lung cancer, common acute side effects are dermatitis, erythema, and esophagitis. Routine departmental skin care is recommended. Dysphagia associated with inflammation of the esophagus occurs at approximately 3000 cGy. Esophagitis can be relieved by medication or diet. Oral medications include liquid antacids and mucosal anesthetics such as lidocaine hydrochloride.[29] Nutritional suggestions include foods that are soft, moist, and nonspicy and liquids at room temperature or slightly chilled. Patients may also experience coughing, dry throat, and excessive mucous secretions.

A chronic side effect caused by irritation of the trachea and bronchi is a dry, nonproductive cough. Other chronic effects include fibrosis of the lung and subcutaneous fibrosis of the skin.

Complications are different from side effects because they are usually a result of doses that exceed organ tolerance. Complications are serious and, in the case of pneumonitis, may be life threatening. If spinal cord tolerance is exceeded, myelopathy may occur. With serious neurological complications the resulting infections can lead to fatalities.

Table 7-3 External beam treatment doses

Treatment approach	Total dose (cGy)
Primary radiation	6000-7500
Surgery + radiation (postoperative)	5000-6500
Chemotherapy + radiation	3000-5000
Palliation and/or recurrence	4000-5000
Preoperative (superior sulcus)	3000-4500

Modified from Cox JD, editor: *Moss' radiation oncology: rationale, technique, results,* ed 7, St. Louis, 1994, Mosby; DeVita V, Hellman S, Rosenburg S: *Principles and practice of oncology,* ed 4, Philadelphia, 1993, JB Lippincott; and Pancoast HK: Superior pulmonary sulcus tumor, *JAMA* 99:17, October 1932.

Role of radiation therapist

Education. Opportunities exist for the radiation therapist to evaluate the patient daily for needs related to education, communication, and assessment. Frequently, patients need education regarding testing procedures such as x-ray examinations and blood tests. The information should include the reason the tests are needed, the location and time to report, fasting, and other preparations. Procedures that seem uncomplicated to medical professionals may be overwhelming to patients and family members. Radiation therapists should take time to explain carefully and at the appropriate level the how, why, and when details of a particular study. Patient education is important from the time of consultation and continues to the last day of treatment. Education continues when patients return for follow-up visits. Patients have a right to this education as defined in the Patient's Bill of Rights supported by the American Hospital Association. At any point a patient can refuse care (i.e., refuse further treatment). When possible the therapist must try to ensure patient understanding. Sometimes questions can be one-sided; the patient is not given the opportunity to indicate an understanding of the information received. The therapist should use a questioning style permitting the patient to reflect an answer that indicates an understanding of the explanation. Because patient compliance is important to achieve the goal of therapy, whether definitive or palliative, education is critical.

Table 7-4 Fraction patterns and total doses for primary radiation

Type of fractionation	Fraction size	Daily dose	Treatment days	Total dose (cGy)
Conventional fractionation	180-200	180-200	30-34	6000-6120
Hyperfractionation	120	240	30	7200
Accelerated fractionation	160	320	19	6080
Accelerated hyperfractionation	160	320	23	7360

Communication. Communication with patients and family members is essential. Details related to daily treatments, appointment times, and the length of treatment require initial education followed by frequent reinforcement. Communication is almost continuous throughout the day. As related to the patient, the scheduling of daily treatments and other planning times throughout the course of therapy requires reinforcement. Also of concern to patients is the management of the other commitments in their lives. Radiation therapists need to be sensitive and responsive to the demands placed on the patient by competing forces. For example, the scheduling of a simulation appointment for off-cord boosts and subsequent patient notification should be done in advance. In this way the patient is given the opportunity to determine the best way to keep this appointment. If a problem arises, enough time should exist for the therapist and patient to collaborate in a positive manner on the way to work through the patient's special needs and concerns.

Assessment. Assessment is the process of evaluating a patient's condition. With lung cancer therapy, as with other types of treatment, the condition of a patient's skin should be assessed before daily treatment is given. Ongoing monitoring of dermatitis and erythema and appropriate skin care is necessary to prevent skin breakdown. If the skin is blistered, cracked or open, and oozing, treatment should be withheld until a physician's medical opinion is obtained. A nutritional evaluation of the ability to swallow solid foods, liquids, and medications should be done to determine whether dietary counseling or medical intervention is required. Adequate fluid intake is particularly important to prevent dehydration because patients may reduce or stop their fluid intake as a result of the discomfort associated with esophagitis. The status of blood counts should be reviewed. White blood cell counts ≤2000 and platelets ≤50,000 should not be treated without a written order. Patients receiving chemotherapy must be monitored closely.

Changes in a patient's condition can be observed during therapy. As described previously, lung cancer metastasizes to the central nervous system and skeletal system. Clinically, evidence of brain metastasis may be observed with personality changes, headaches, and visual disturbances. With spinal metastases, patients may complain of severe neck and/or back pain and they may describe bowel and/or bladder dysfunctions such as incontinence. In addition, patients may experience leg and/or motor weakness that the therapist may observe as an unsteady gait or limp. Symptoms related to pleural or pericardial effusion include dyspnea, increased respiratory effort, chest pain, a change in a cough, or a fever.[16] Such observations must be reported to the radiation oncologist for medical evaluation.

Medical problems unrelated to lung cancer and radiation therapy occur. If a patient has symptoms or describes a problem with which a therapist is unfamiliar, the therapist should refer the patient to the radiation oncologist. For cardiac or respiratory arrest, therapists should respond appropriately. Knowledge of living wills is important. In particular, if a patient having a cardiac arrest has a do-not-resuscitate (DNR) or similar order, that request should be honored.

Accessory medical equipment. Accessory medical equipment used with lung cancer may include oxygen tanks, respirators, and intravenous (IV) bottles. This equipment must be maneuvered cautiously to avoid collision hazards. Oxygen tanks must be maneuvered close to the treatment tables, and the catheter must be kept free from table and gantry motions. IV bottles should remain above a patient's head to allow the fluid to move with gravity and prevent backflow or clotting. Because fluid moves from areas of high pressure to low pressure, the IV fluid flows from the bottle above the head (high pressure) into the vein (low pressure). When the bottle is placed at a level below the head, the pressure gradient changes and blood flows into the IV tubing because the pressure in the vein is greater than the bottle pressure. In the case of chest tubes the bottle must remain below the patient. The pressure in the chest cavity is greater than the pressure in the bottle. Because of this pressure difference, the fluid flows from higher pressure (chest) to lower pressure (bottle). When the table is raised, the bottle should not be placed on the table because the pressure gradient change forces the fluid from the bottle into the chest. Caution must be observed to ensure that the attached lines are long enough to reach to adjacent stretchers and/or poles.

Patients with superior vena cava syndrome are transported to the treatment units on stretchers with respirators, oxygen tanks, IV lines, and cardiac and other monitoring equipment. A team approach is needed to safely move the patient and accessory equipment to and from the treatment table.

Case Studies

CASE I

A 61-year-old woman had increasingly severe right-arm pain and hypersensitivity for approximately 2 years. She complained of sharp pains that radiated down the arm to the hand. She also described numbness in the fingers and episodes of arm weakness. She had a long smoking history of approximately 40 years. During the past 3 years, she smoked approximately two packs per day.

A chest radiograph demonstrated an ill-defined density in the apex of the right lung. A CT scan demonstrated a right apical mass with destruction of the second rib posteriorly and extension into the muscular tissues of the posterior thoracic wall. An MRI scan demonstrated right paraspinal disease at T_1, T_2, and T_3. A percutaneous, CT-directed needle biopsy was done, and a histological evaluation revealed a mixed adenocarcinoma and squamous cell carcinoma consistent with bronchogenic carcinoma.

The patient consulted a surgeon, who felt the lesion was resectable and advised that she receive preoperative radiation therapy. A second surgical opinion was more doubtful about the resectability of the tumor, even after radiation therapy, and recommended that the patient be treated with definitive radiation therapy only.

A course of anticipated preoperative radiation therapy began with anterior and posterior parallel-opposed-shaped portals measuring 18.5 × 15 cm on the 4-Mv linear accelerator (Figs. 7-15 and 7-16). A conventional fraction pattern of 180 cGy each day was used. Shrinking fields were used, and at 3780 cGy the field size was reduced to 13.5 × 9 cm through the use of an isocentric technique. Treatment to the right upper mediastinum, apex of the right lung, and supraclavicular region continued to a dose of 5544 cGy (Fig. 7-17).

A repeat MRI scan failed to reveal significant tumor resolution in the paravertebral region. Therefore surgical intervention was not recommended. The radiation volumes were reduced again, and radiation to the tumor was boosted through the use of 13.5 × 6 cm oblique fields to 7358 cGy (Fig. 7-18).

The patient tolerated the course of radiation therapy satisfactorily, with increasing weight and stable blood counts. During the initial portion of therapy, she complained of minimal dysphagia and later of mild pruritis of the skin secondary to a dry skin reaction. She also noted complete resolution of the shoulder and arm pain, with cessation of the need for analgesics and improved strength in the right arm.

A

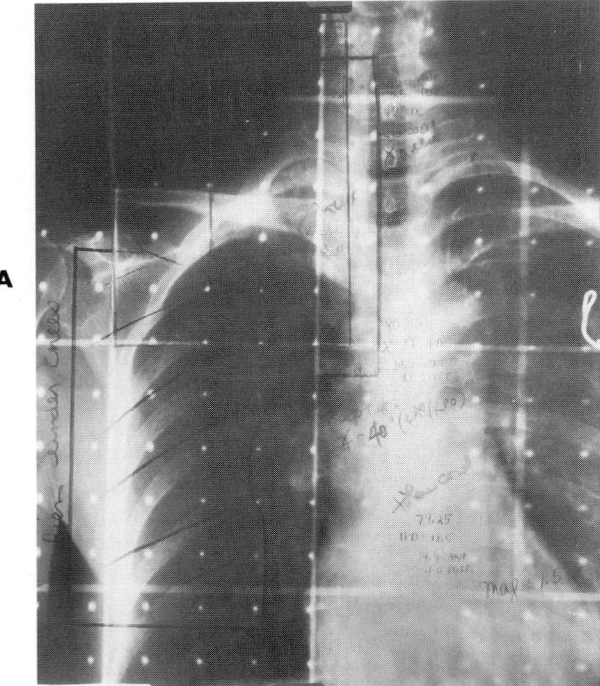

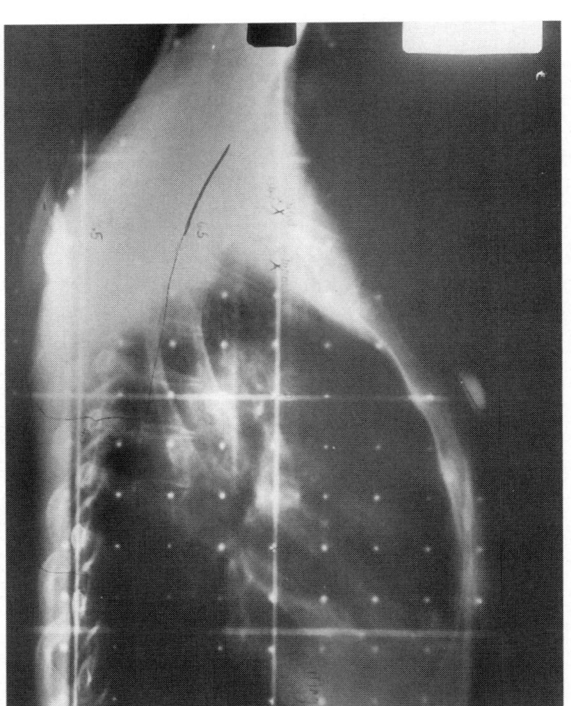

B

Fig. 7-15 Anterior (**A**) and lateral (**B**) simulation films with planning information for blocks, measurements, and boost fields.

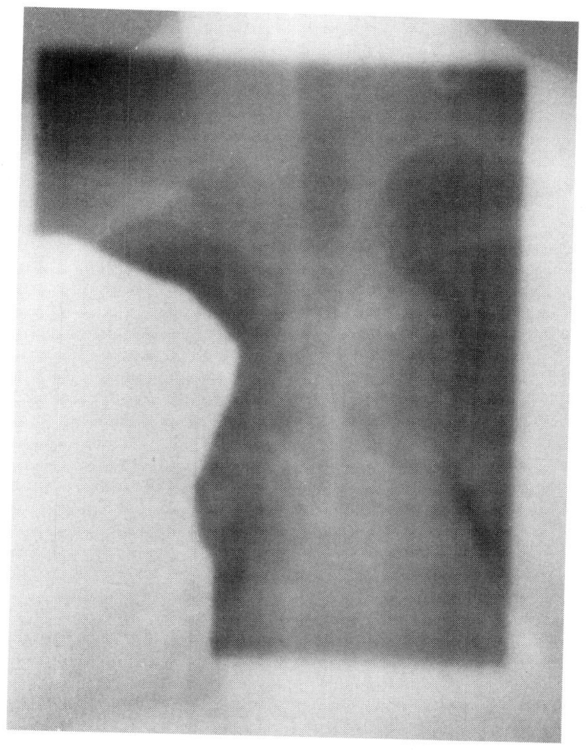

Fig. 7-16 Anterior portal film for 18.5 × 15 cm fields treated to 3780 cGy.

A

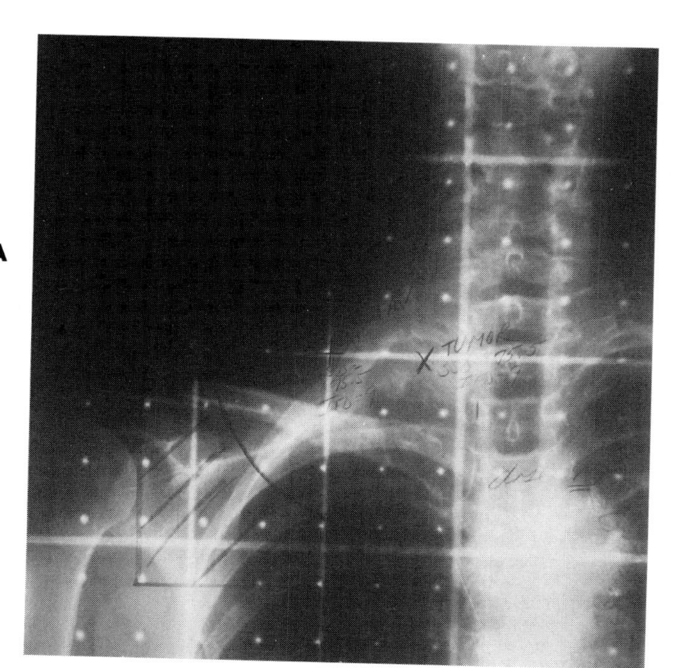

B

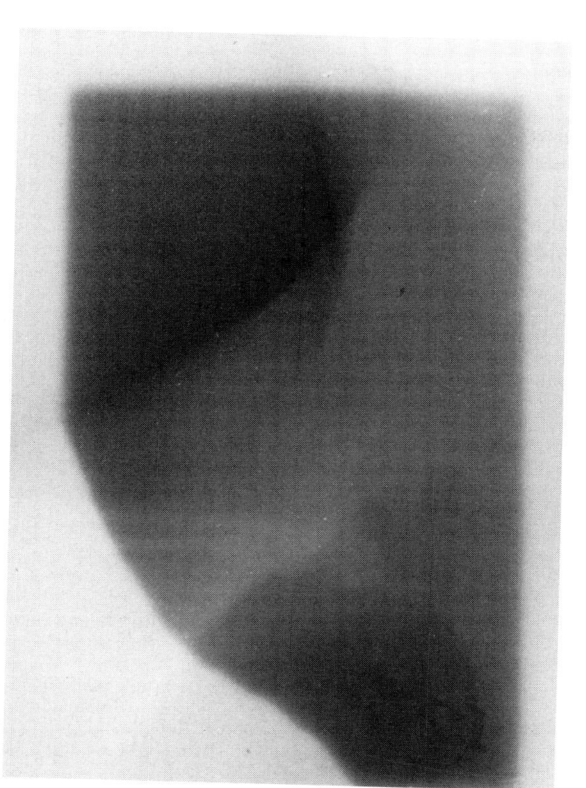

Fig. 7-17 Simulation (**A**) and portal (**B**) films for 13.5 × 9 cm right upper lobe fields treated to 5544 cGy.

A

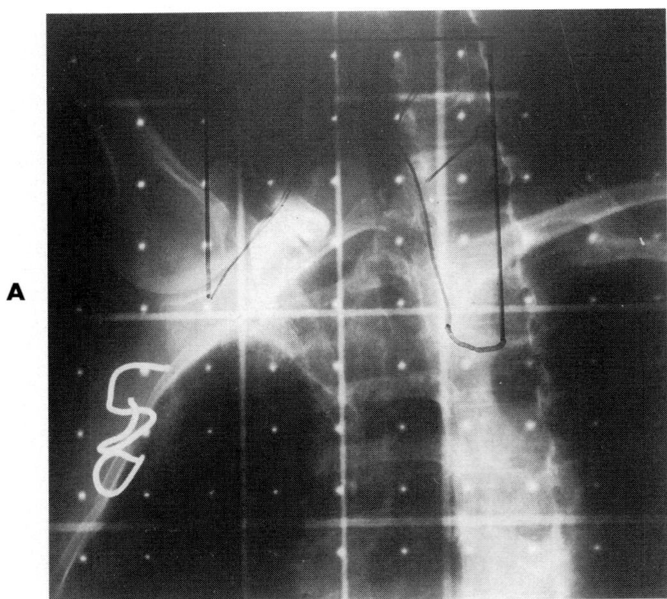

B

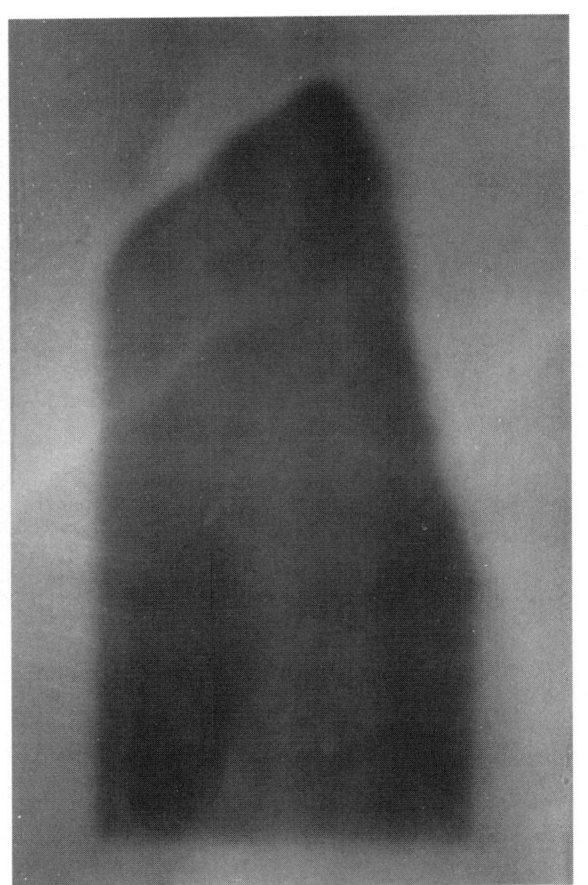

Fig. 7-18 Simulation (**A**) and portal (**B**) films for 13.5 × 6 cm oblique boost fields treated to 7358 cGy.

CASE II

A 52-year-old man suffered from carcinoma of the right lung. A routine chest x-ray examination revealed that he had a right hilar mass. A CT scan of the chest revealed a 3-cm mass in the posterior aspect of the right upper lobe and a soft tissue mass surrounding the right main-stem bronchus with narrowing (Fig. 7-3). Significant adenopathy was present in the middle mediastinum, the anterior mediastinum anterior to the aortic arch, the aortic pulmonary window, the subcarinal region, and the right hilum. A bronchoscopy demonstrated diffuse submucosal tumor involvement of the right main-stem bronchus with associated narrowing. Bronchial brushings were positive for poorly differentiated large cell carcinoma. Because of complaints of headaches, a CT scan was done that was negative for metastasis.

He described shortness of breath and wheezing when laying flat, and his best position was on his left side. He had a 7-pound weight loss over the past few months. His medical history was significant for hypertension and congestive heart failure as a result of a cardiomyopathy of unknown etiology diagnosed 11 years ago. His last episode of heart failure was 1 year ago. He had a significant smoking history of one to two packs per day for 25 years, but he quit 10 years ago. He was staged T_1 N_3 M_O, with poorly differentiated large cell carcinoma. His tumor was surgically unresectable.

The plan was to start chemotherapy for three cycles and follow with radiation therapy. He began radiation therapy on the week after the last cycle of chemotherapy. The long-term risks because of his cardiomyopathy were explained. These risks included heart damage possibly leading to myocardial infarction, pericardial effusion, and arrhythmia. The total dose planned was 6000 cGy through the use of conventional fractionation, with two dose evaluation points at 3600 and 5000 cGy to the carina. The initial fields were parallel-opposed, 19.5 × 15.5 cm with alloys, and 4 MV. They used 80-cm SSD (Fig. 7-19). At 3600 cGy to the carina the fields were changed to a three-field isocentric technique consisting of two obliques with wedges, shielding blocks, and an open field (right posterior oblique, left anterior oblique, and right anterior oblique) (Figs. 7-20 and 7-21). After eight treatments in this manner, the fields were changed again at 5040 cGy. The tumor was boosted to a total dose of 5940 cGy through the use of 11 × 6.5 cm parallel-opposed fields (AP/PA) (Figs. 7-22 and 7-23). The treatment was given in 33 fractions over 46 days. The patient had a significant loss of appetite and esophagitis, which were treated with oral Megace and viscous Xylocaine, respectively. A local skin reaction occurred in the treated field, and the patient was given routine skin care instructions.

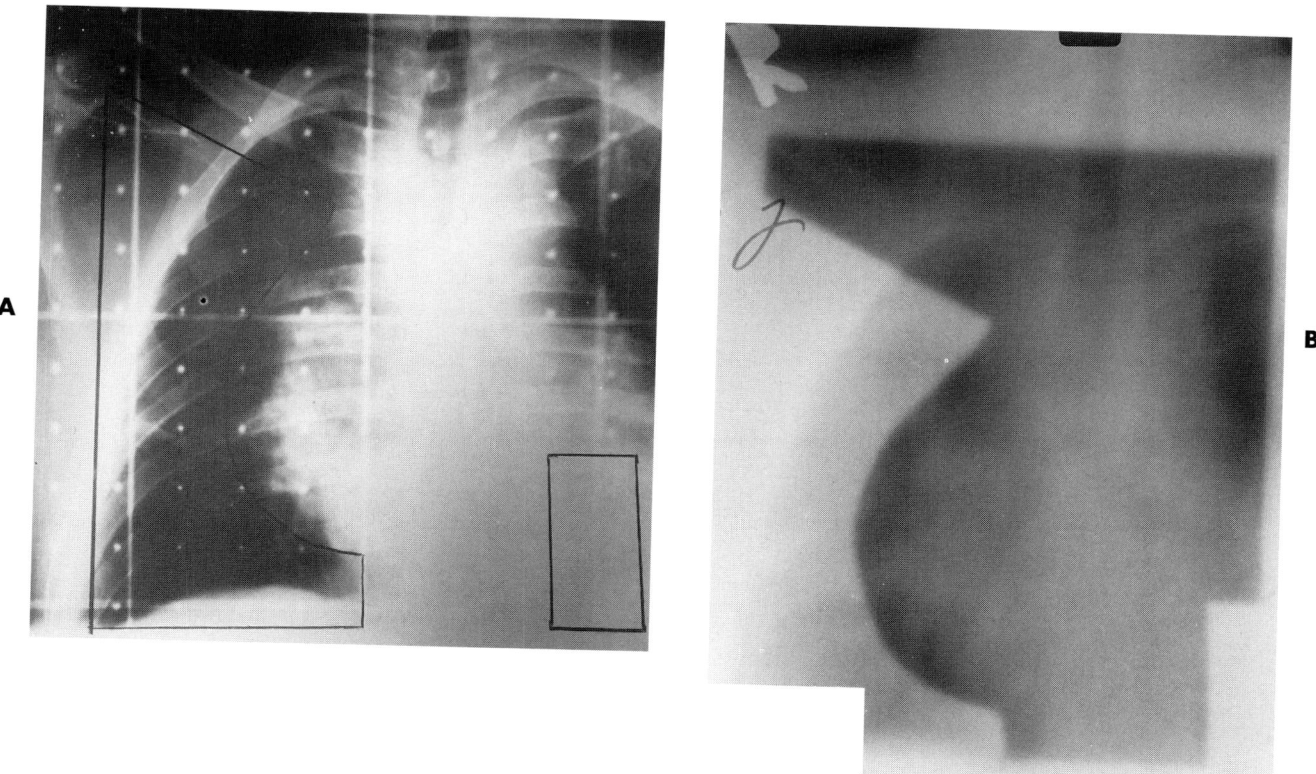

Fig. 7-19 Anterior simulation (**A**) and portal (**B**) films for 19.5 × 15.5 cm fields treated to 3600 cGy.

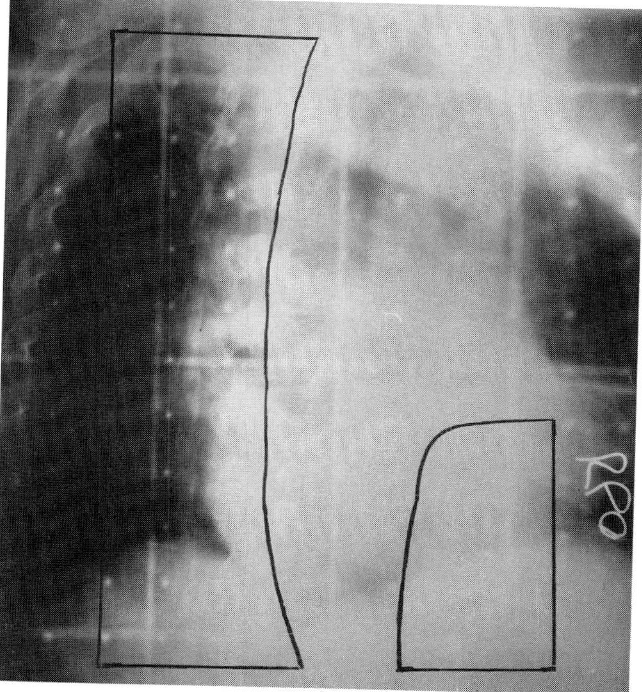

Fig. 7-20 Oblique simulation film of a three-field technique treated to 5040 cGy.

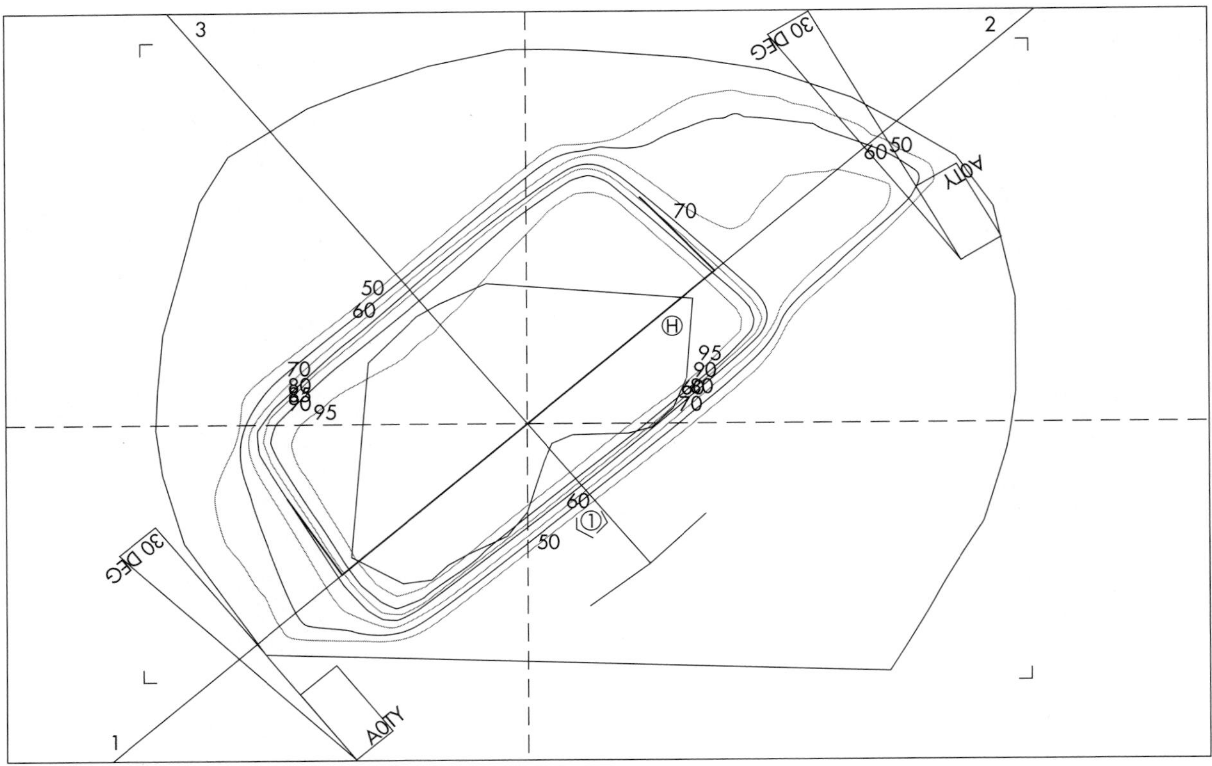

Fig. 7-21 Dose distribution of a three-field technique for RPO, LAO and RAO fields.

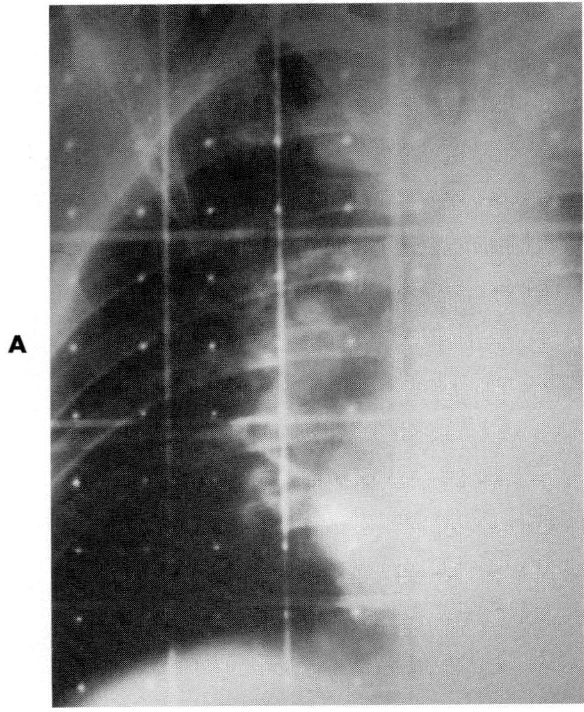

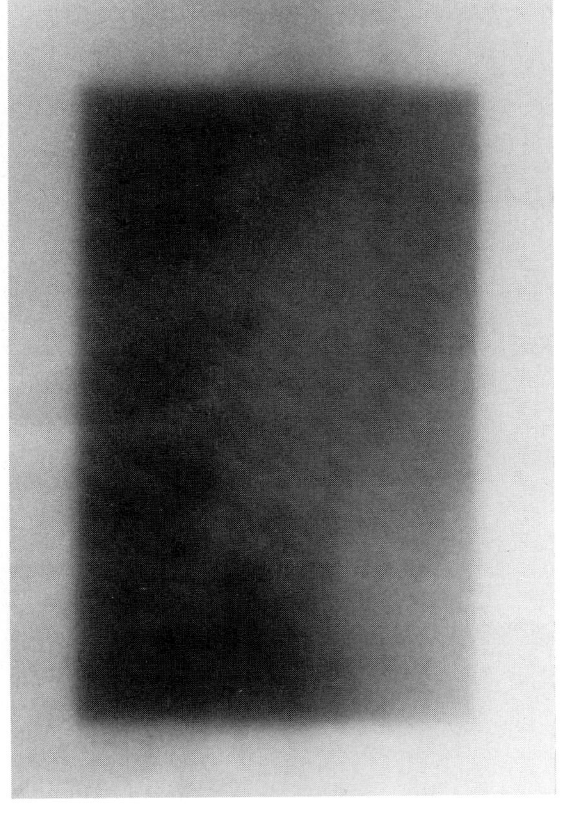

A

B

Fig. 7-22 Anterior simulation (**A**) and portal (**B**) films for boost fields treated to 6080 cGy.

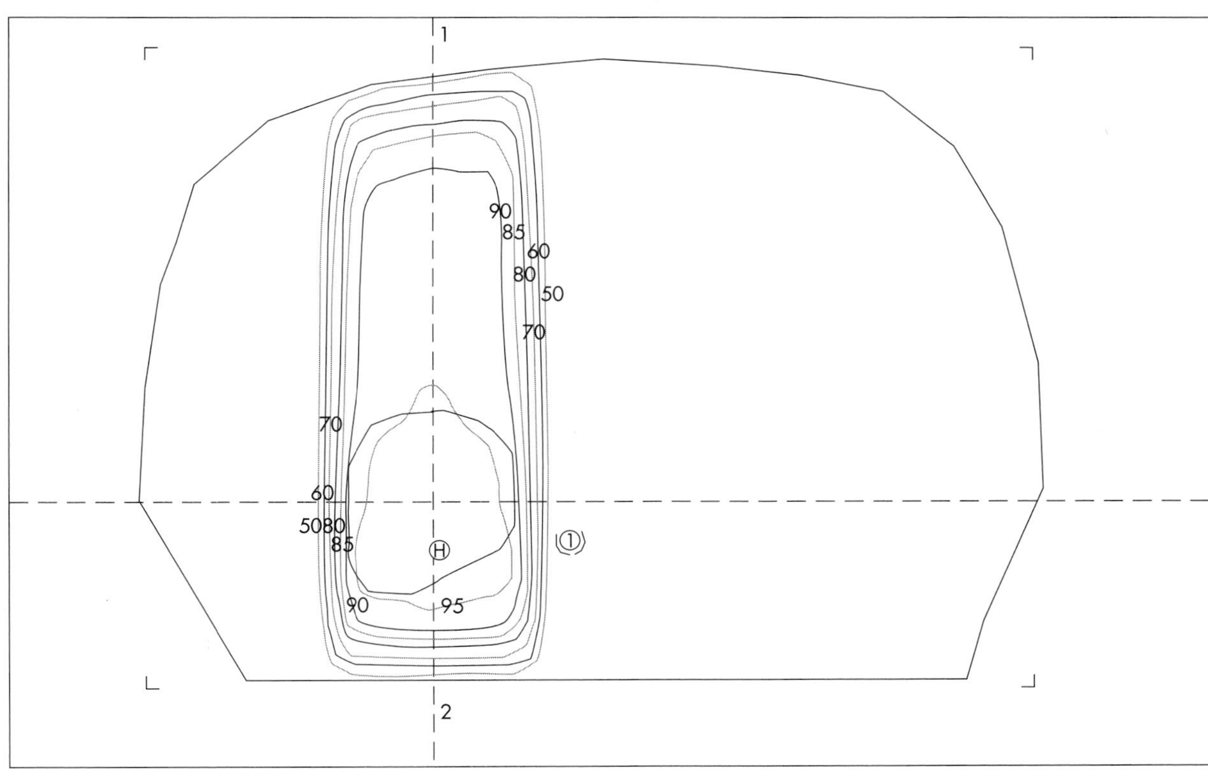

Fig. 7-23 Dose distribution of parallel-opposed boost fields for 11 × 6.5 cm fields.

Review Questions

Essay

1. Describe three criteria related to an individual's tobacco exposure that appear to increase the risk of developing lung cancer.
2. What are three variables that appear to affect significantly the prognosis of patients with lung cancer?
3. Name the two groups of lymphatics that are primarily responsible for the regional spread of bronchogenic carcinoma.
4. With conventional fractionation, what is the commonly accepted definitive dose range for localized bronchogenic carcinomas?
5. List at least three common acute side effects a patient may experience during the course of treatment.

Multiple Choice

6. Microscopically, diffusion of oxygen and carbon dioxide takes place at which of the following:
   a. Bifurcation of the trachea
   b. Right and left primary bronchi
   c. Bronchiolar ducts
   d. Alveolar-capillary membranes
7. Symptoms associated with local disease include which of the following?
   I. Hemoptysis
   II. Dyspnea
   III. Orthopnea
   a. I only
   b. II only
   c. I and II only
   d. I, II and III
8. Symptoms associated with regional disease include which of the following?
   I. Dysphagia
   II. Superior vena cava syndrome
   III. Orthopnea
   a. I only
   b. II only
   c. I and II only
   d. I, II and III
9. In what part of the lung are primary squamous cell carcinomas usually found?
   a. Superiorly
   b. Centrally
   c. Laterally
   d. Peripherally
10. Critical structures frequently located in the treatment fields for lung cancer include which of the following?
    a. Normal lung and trachea
    b. Esophagus and trachea
    c. Spinal cord and heart
    d. Heart and esophagus

Questions to Ponder

1. Discuss reasons that the incidence of lung cancer is rising.
2. Compare and contrast the various issues related to radiosensitivity and radiocurability of lung cancer.
3. What are common signs and symptoms of bronchogenic carcinomas? What are uncommon signs and symptoms?
4. Discuss the nonrespiratory signs and symptoms of lung cancer (i.e., neurological findings).
5. Analyze the anatomical considerations in treatment field design.

REFERENCES

1. Bauer M et al: Prognostic factors in cancer of the lung. In Cox JD, editor: *Syllabus: a categorical course in radiation therapy: lung cancer,* Oak Brook, Illinois, 1985, Radiological Society of North America.
2. Baum GL, Wolinski E: *Textbook of pulmonary diseases,* ed 5, New York, 1994, Little, Brown, and Co.
3. Beahrs OH et al: *AJCC Manual for staging of cancer,* ed 4, Philadelphia, 1988, JB Lippincott.
4. Bentel GC, Nelson CE, Noell KT: *Treatment planning and dose calculation in radiation oncology,* ed 4, New York, 1989, Pergamon Press.
5. Chung CK et al: Evaluation of adjuvant postoperative radiotherapy for lung cancer, *Int J Radiat Oncol Biol Phys* 8:1877-1880, 1982.
6. Cohen MH: Signs and symptoms of bronchogenic carcinoma. In Straus MJ, editor: *Lung cancer clinical diagnosis and treatment,* New York, 1977, Grune & Stratton.
7. Cox JD, editor: *Moss' radiation oncology: rationale, technique, results,* ed 7, St. Louis, 1994, Mosby.
8. DeVita, V Hellman S, Rosenberg S, editors: *Principles and practice of oncology,* ed 4, Philadelphia, 1993, JB Lippincott.
9. Eisert DR, Cox JD, Komaki R: Irradiation for bronchial carcinoma: reasons for failure. I. Analysis as a function of dose-time-fractionations, *Cancer* 37:2655-2670, 1976.
10. Emami B et al: Phase I/II study of treatment of locally advanced (T3T4) non-oat ell lung cancer with high dose radiotherapy (rapid fractionation): radiation therapy oncology group study, *Int J Radiat Oncol Biol Phys* 15:1021-1025, October 1988.
11. Erozan YS, Frost JK: Cytopathological diagnosis of lung cancer, *Semin Oncol* 1(3):191-198, 1974.
12. Fishman AP: *Pulmonary diseases and disorders,* ed 2, New York, 1988, McGraw-Hill.
13. Fletcher GH, editor: *Textbook of radiotherapy,* ed 3, Philadelphia, 1980, Lea & Febiger.
14. Gazdar AF: Pathology's impact on lung cancer management, *Contemp Oncol* 3(11):22-31, November 1993.
15. Green N et al: Postresection irradiation for primary lung cancer, *Radiology* 116:405-407, 1975.
16. Groenwald SL et al: *Manifestations of cancer and cancer treatment,* Boston, 1992, Jones & Bartlett.
17. Haagensen CD et al: *The lymphatics in cancer,* Philadelphia, 1972, WB Saunders.
18. Hall TC, editor: Paraneoplastic syndromes, *Ann NY Acad Sci* 230:1-577, 1974.
19. Kahn FM: *The physics of radiation therapy,* ed 2, Baltimore, 1994, Williams & Wilkins.
20. Karnofsky DA, Burchenal JH: The clinical evaluation of chemotherapeutic agents in cancer. In Macleod CM, editor: *Evaluation of chemotherapeutic agents,* New York, 1949, Columbia University Press.
21. Komaki R: Preoperative radiation therapy for superior sulcus lesions, *Chest Surg Clin North Am* 1:13-35, 1991.
22. Komaki R, Garden AS, Cundiff JH: Endobronchial radiotherapy. In Roth HA, Cox JD, Hong WK, editors: *Advances in diagnosis and therapy of lung cancer,* Cambridge, Massachusetts, 1993, Blackwell.
23. Levitt SH, Kahn FM, Potish RA: *Levitt and Tapley's technological basis of radiation therapy practical clinical applications,* ed 2, Philadelphia, 1992, Lea & Febiger.
24. Mah K, van Dyk J: On the impact of tissue inhomogeneity corrections in clinical thoracic radiation therapy, *Int J Radiat Oncol Biol Phys* 21:1257-1267, 1991.
25. Mantravadi RVP et al: Unresectable non-oat cell carcinoma of the lung: definitive radiation therapy, *Radiology* 172:851-855, 1989.
26. Marcus RB, Million RR: The incidence of myelitis after irradiation of the cervical spinal cord, *Int J Radiat Oncol Biol Phys* 19:3-8, July 1990.
27. Mew D, Pass H: Malignant mesotheliomas: a clinical challenge, *Contemp Oncol* 3(12):50-67, December 1993.
28. Pancoast HK: Superior pulmonary sulcus tumor, *JAMA* 99:17, October 1932.
29. Perez CA, Brady LW, editors: *Principles and practice of radiation oncology,* ed 2, Philadelphia, 1992, JB Lippincott.
30. Rapp E et al: Chemotherapy can prolong survival in patients with advanced non-small-cell lung cancer: report of a Canadian multicenter randomized trial, *J Clin Oncol* 6:633-641, 1988.
31. Richardson RH et al: The use of fiberoptic bronchoscopy and brush biopsy in the diagnosis of suspected pulmonary malignance, *Am Rev Respir Dis* 109:63-66, 1974.
32. Rigler LG: The earliest roentgenographic signs of carcinoma of the lung, *JAMA* 195:655, 1966.
33. Rubin P, editor: *Radiation biology and radiation pathology syllabus,* Reston, Virginia, 1975, American College of Radiology.
34. Rubin P, Casarett GW: *Clinical radiation pathology,* Philadelphia, 1968, WB Saunders.
35. Seydel HG et al: Hyperfractionation in the radiation therapy of unresectable non-oat cell carcinoma of the lung: preliminary report of a RTOG pilot study, *Int J Radiat Oncol Biol Phys* 11:1841-1847, 1985.
36. Stanton R, Stinson D: *An introduction to radiation oncology physics,* Madison, Wisconsin, 1992, Medical Physics Publishing.
37. Tortora GJ, Grabowski SR: *Principles of anatomy and physiology,* ed 7, New York, 1993, HarperCollins College Publishers.
38. World Health Organization: *International histologic classification of tumors,* NOS. 1-20, Geneva, Switzerland, 1978, The Organization.
39. Wynder EL, Hoffmann D: *Tobacco and tobacco smoke: studies in experimental carcinogenesis,* New York, 1967, Academic Press

BIBLIOGRAPHY

American Cancer Society: *Cancer facts and figures*—Atlanta, 1996, The Society.

Nakhashi H et al: Results of surgical treatment of patients with T3 non-small cell lung cancer, *Ann Thorac Surg* 46:178-181, 1988.

Schultheiss TE: Spinal cord radiation "tolerance": doctrine versus data, *Int J Radiat Oncol Biol Phys* 19:219-221, July 1990.

Valley JF, Mirimanoff RO: Comparison of treatment techniques for lung cancer, *Radiother Oncol* 28:168-173, 1993.

CHAPTER

8

Head and Neck Cancers

Dan Strahan

Outline

Key terms

Accelerated fractionation
Cryotherapy
Digestive tubes
External auditory meatus (EAM)
Electrocautery
Endophytic
Erythroplasia
Exophytic
Hemiglossectomy
Heterogeneity
Hyperfractionation
Jugulo-digastric
Keratosis
Leukoplakia
Multicentric
Shine over
Synergistic

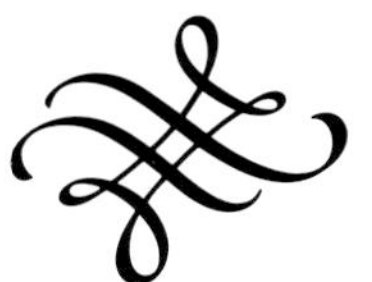

Although head and neck cancer comprises a small proportion of all malignancies encountered, this disease presents the cancer care team with multifaceted problems, complicated by the complex arrangement and location of the respiratory and digestive systems. Compounding the situation are the number of radiation-sensitive organs located in this area and the large number of lymphatic chains that can harbor microscopic disease. Lesions located in one type of tissue may directly or indirectly influence another anatomical region functionally or even cause some structural morbidity. Lesions tend to be **multicentric** (having multiple origins) and can arise sequentially or simultaneously.

The management of head and neck malignancies requires a multidisciplinary team approach, with an understanding that this disease can produce significant morbidity and survival cannot be measured only in terms of mortality. Reducing the deformity, maintaining the reduction, and restoring the function are essential to the management of head and neck cancer. From a structural standpoint, mutilation is no longer an acceptable goal for cure because of its psychosocial stresses. Treatment that causes the permanent loss of vision, smell, taste, or hearing should be evaluated concerning its effect on quality of life and survival. Maintaining food paths and airways is vital, but the treatment decision should also preserve the patient's ability to interact as a human. The eradication of head and neck cancer involves the close cooperation of the radiation oncologists, medical oncologists, dentist, nutritionist, surgeon, nurse, radiologist, social worker, and radiation therapists.

CANCER OF THE HEAD AND NECK

Epidemiology

Head and neck cancers account for 5% of all malignancies. Approximately 58,980 cases were reported in 1996.[1] The American Cancer Society reports that 68% of these cancers are found in males and 32% in females. The incidence rate in females is on the rise, notably because more women are smoking. The highest incidence occurs over the age of 50. Increased frequency is seen in textile, furniture, and mining regions. India and China have particularly high incidence rates. The overall survival rate is expected to be 65%, with females exhibiting a better survival rate. Anatomically, the most common sites, in order, are the larynx, oral cavity, pharynx, and salivary glands.

Etiology

Combined alcohol and tobacco use is a leading factor in the development of head and neck cancer. The use of smokeless tobacco is associated with squamous cell cancer of the cheek and gum in the oral cavity. Other implicated high-risk factors are as follows: previous radiation exposure, poor oral hygiene, asbestos, wood mill workers, betel nut chewers in India, the Epstein-Barr virus for nasopharyngeal cancer, Plummer-Vinson syndrome (iron deficiency in women), textile-processing workers, plastic fabrication workers, and environmental pollutants in China.

Some conditions occurring in the epithelium of the buccal mucosa suggest or are visible markers for a dysplastic change. **Leukoplakia** (white patches), if raised and thickened, should be removed. **Keratosis** (lesions on the epidermis characterized by overgrowth of the horny layer) is an indication of cellular atypia and should be excised and examined. **Erythroplasia** (red velvet patches) in 80% of patients contains carcinoma in situ and requires an excisional biopsy. A biopsy should be done for any mouth or throat ulcer that persists for 2 weeks or more. Finally, any change in or near the gum line of denture wearers should be watched for any reactionary keratosis caused by trauma.

Prognostic indicators

In general, the morbidity of treatments increases and the prognosis decreases as the affected area progresses backward from the lips to the hypopharynx, excluding the larynx. Lesions that cross the midline, exhibit endophytic growth (invasion of the lamina propria and submucosa), have cranial nerve involvement, have fixed nodes or a fixed lesion in the anatomical compartments, are poorly differentiated, and are nonsquamous cell cancers represent advanced growth and have an unfavorable prognosis.

Anatomy

The organs comprising the head and neck region serve dual purposes in that respiratory *and* digestive activities take place. For a better appreciation of this complex system, a brief anatomical review is necessary.

The staging and classification of head and neck tumors are based on subsite involvement, which concerns nearly 50% of the patients. Understanding the physiological relationships of adjacent structures in the head and neck region is of paramount importance. The opening of the nasal cavities into the nasopharynx (Fig. 8-1) provides a natural pathway for tumor spread. During the act of swallowing the soft palate elevates and prevents food from entering the nasopharynx. Tumors in this location do not allow this activity to occur. An enlargement of the pharyngeal tonsil can obstruct the upper air passage and allow breathing only through the mouth, resulting in the passing of unfiltered, cool, dry air to the lungs. Collectively, the tonsils are bands of lymphoid tissue that provide protection against airway infections and form a barrier between the respiratory tubes (nasopharynx) and **digestive tubes** (oropharynx and hypopharynx). In addition, knowing the location of a cervical vertebral body provides boundary locations of the soft tissue aspects of the head and neck region. The first cervical vertebra (C-1) lies at the inferior margin of the nasopharynx, whereas the second and third cervical vertebrae (C-2/C-3) contain the oropharynx. The epiglottis is in line with C-3, whereas the true vocal cords lie along the fourth cervical vertebra (C-4) (Fig. 8-1).* Any tumor of the salivary glands (Fig.8-2) can involve major cranial nerves and arterial neck blood flow. Tumors in this area can cause facial paralysis, nerve pain, and interruption of the neck muscles' blood supply.

As mentioned, tumors can damage the cranial nerves, which control our major senses. The involvement of the cranial nerves leads to signs and symptoms that can point to a possible location of a tumor. Table 8-1 lists the 12 cranial nerves and their associated functions.

Lymphatics. The lymphatics of the head and neck and their involvement exhibit a direct correlation to the prognosis. Nearly one third of the body's lymph nodes are located in the head and neck area. Fig. 8-3 depicts the major chains of the head and neck. Some nodes have two names. For example, the **jugulo-digastric** node is called the *subdigastric node,* the node of Rouvière is also called the *lateral retropharyngeal node,* the spinal accessory chain is also called the *posterior cervical lymph node,* and the mastoid node is also called the *retroauricular node.*

Because a metastatic cervical node is clinically present in many of the tumors found in the head and neck area, an assessment of node involvement dictates the size of the radiation portal and the treatment plan. For example, in Fig. 8-4 the jugulo-digastric group (the group of neck nodes below the mastoid tip) receives nearly all the lymph from the head area and is usually treated, whereas the Rouvière node is included as the minimum target volume for nasopharyngeal cancer. This node is inaccessible to the surgeon, and because of its proximity to the carotid artery, it can be a problem if not treated.

*Throughout this chapter, refer to Fig. 8-1 when descriptions of the tumor location and routes of spread are given.

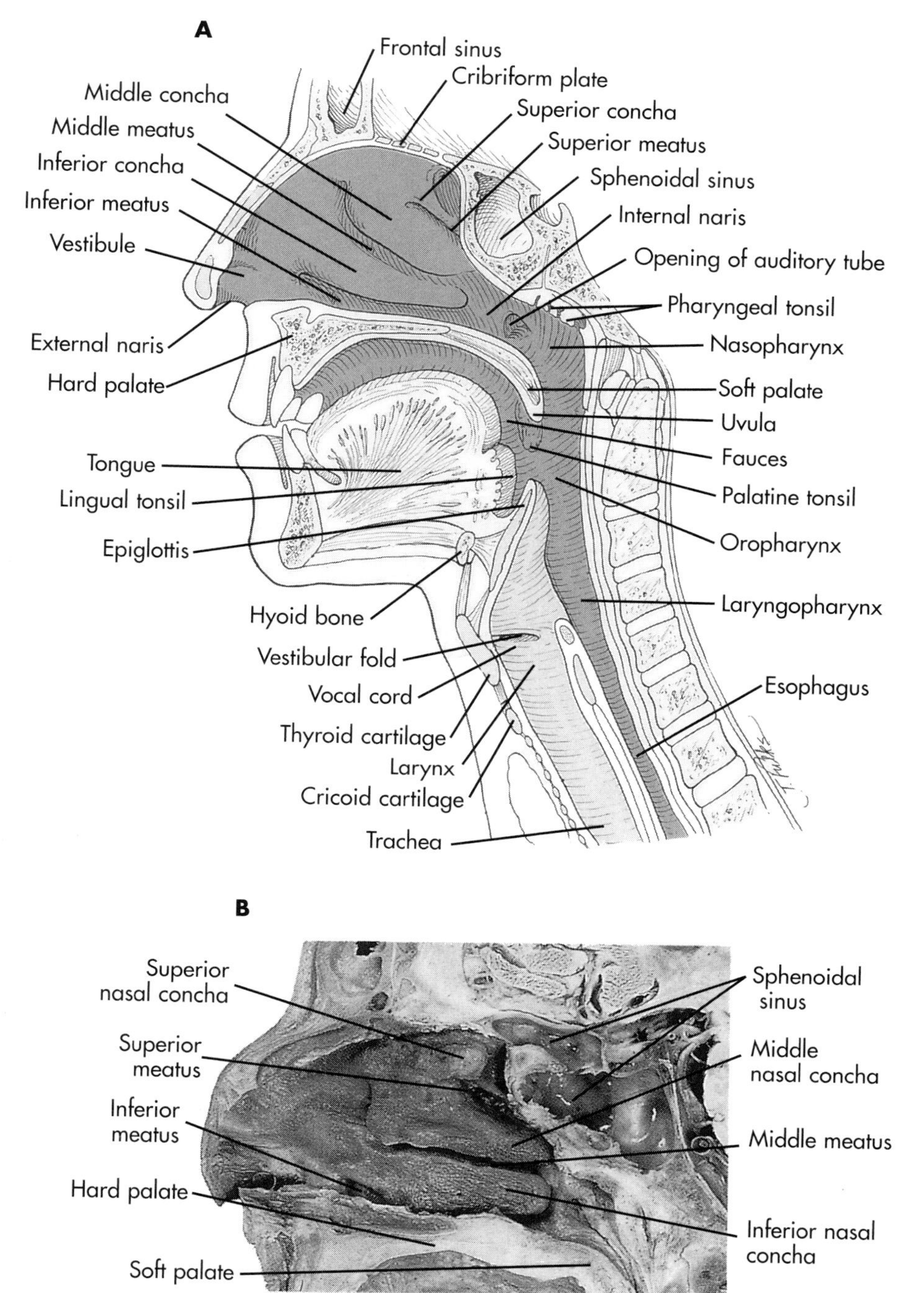

Fig. 8-1 **A,** A sagittal section through the nasal cavity and pharynx. **B,** A photograph of a sagittal section of the nasal cavity. (From Seeley RR, Stephens TD, Tate P, editors: *Essentials of anatomy and physiology,* ed 3, St Louis, 1996, Mosby.)

The port size of the irradiated fields in the head and neck area are quite large because of the risk of nodal spread. As shown in Fig. 8-5 the inferior cervical nodes are clinically positive in 6% to 23% of the cases for nasopharyngeal cancer. For this reason the supraclavicular area requires treatment, which an anterior port can accomplish. Generally, hematogenous spread below the neck is rare, except in nasopharyngeal carcinoma (NPC) or in the parotid gland. Over 75% of all head and neck cancers recur locally or regionally above the clavicle.[10]

NPC disease with known bilateral cervical node involvement has shown a 25% chance of blood-borne distant spread first to the bone and then to the lung.[10] In addition, for non-NPC disease the development of a second primary has a higher risk than distant spread.

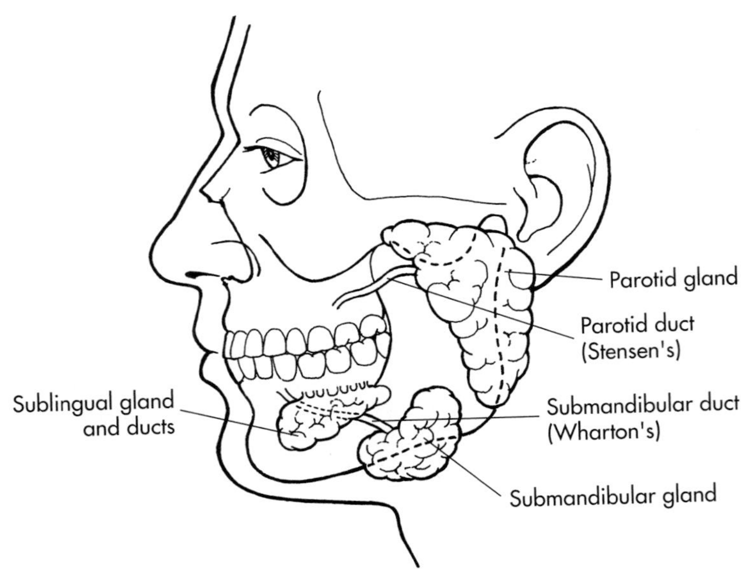

Fig. 8-2 The salivary glands and ducts. (From Chaffee EE, Griescheimer EM: *Basic physiology and anatomy,* ed 3, Philadelphia, 1974, JB Lippincott.)

Table 8-1 Cranial nerves and their functions

Name (number)	Function
Olfactory I	Smell
Optic II	Sight
Oculomotor III	Eye movement (up and down)
Trochlear IV	Eye movement (rotation)
Trigeminal V	Sensory (facial) and motor (jaw)
Abducens VI	Eye movement (lateral)
Facial (masticator) VII	Expressions, muscle contractions, and mouthing
Acoustic VIII	Hearing
Glossopharyngeal IX	Tongue and throat movement
Vagus X	Talking and sounds
Spinal accessory XI	Movement of shoulders and head
Hypoglossal XII	Movement of tongue and chewing

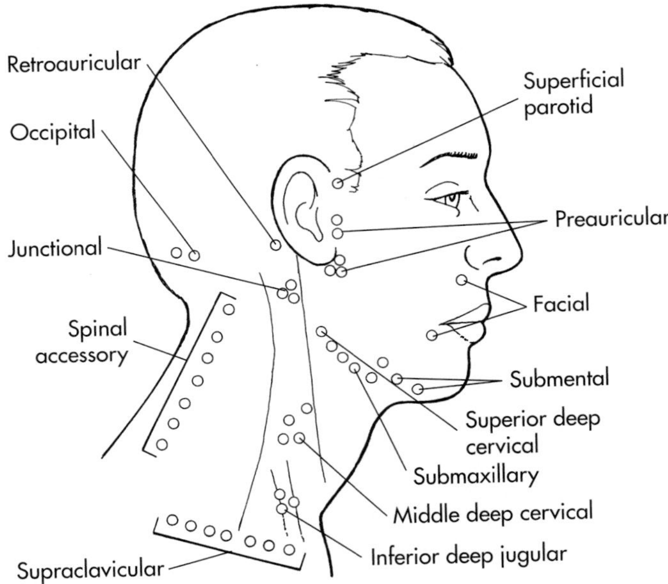

Fig. 8-3 Lateral view of the head and neck. (From Moss WT, Cox JD: *Radiation oncology: rationale, technique, results,* St Louis, 1987, Mosby.)

The normal lymphatic drainage by site is listed in the first box on p. 154.

Clinical presentation

Most head and neck cancers are infiltrative lesions found in the epithelial lining. They can be raised or indurated (hard and firm). These growths are sometimes classified as **endophytic** tumors, which are more aggressive in spread and harder to control locally. **Exophytic** tumors are noninvasive neoplasms characterized by raised, elevated borders. Specific signs and symptoms correlate with anatomical sites. The second box on p. 154 provides a list of the common symptoms by site. A cervical lymph node mass can be present clinically from any of these sites. In an adult, any enlarged cervical node that persists for 1 week or more should be regarded as suspicious and should be evaluated for a malignancy.[10]

Detection and diagnosis

Careful examination and inspection of the head and neck via indirect laryngoscopy, palpation, and fiber-optic endoscopy

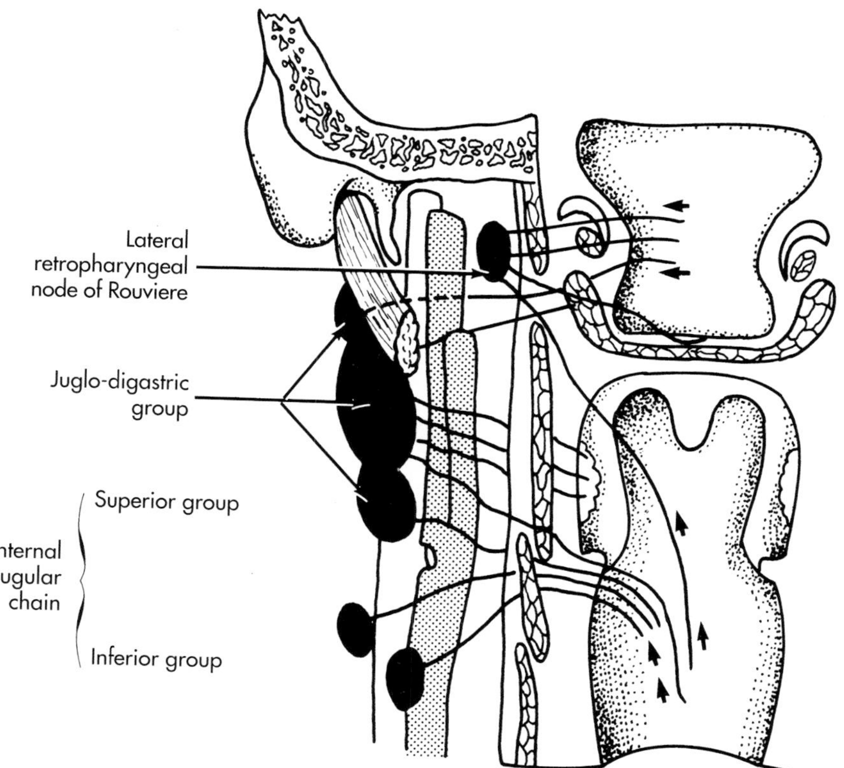

Fig. 8-4 An oblique view of the neck showing the base of the skull and a cross-section through the sphenoid sinus-hyophysis. (From Cox JD: *Moss' radiation oncology: rationale, technique, results,* ed 7, St Louis, 1994, Mosby.)

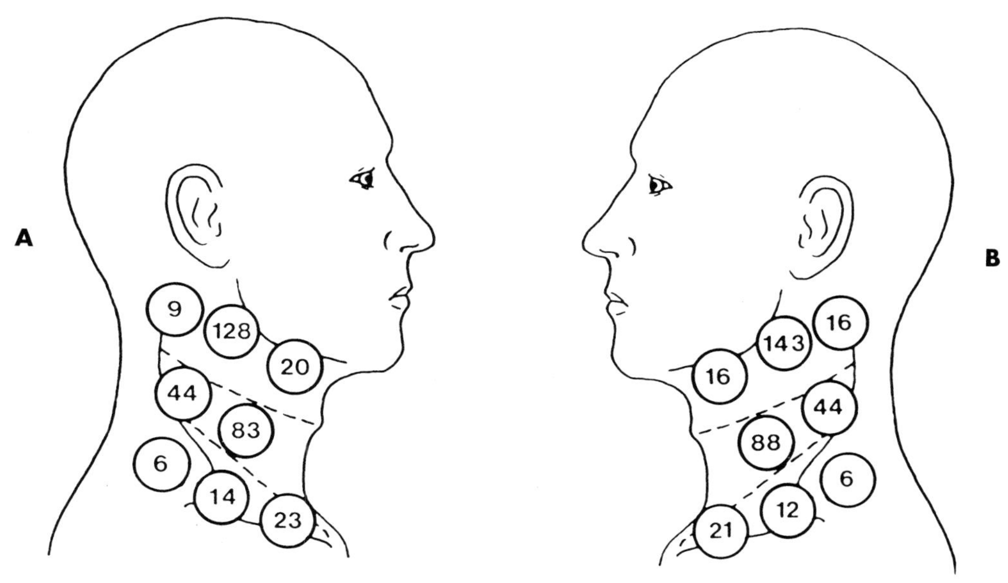

Fig. 8-5 Distribution of lymphadenopathy in 204 of 271 patients who presented with enlarged nodes. **A,** Right cervical region. **B,** Left cervical region. (From Cox JD: *Moss' radiation oncology: rationale, technique, results,* ed 7, St Louis, 1994, Mosby.)

Lymphatic Drainage by Site

Oral cavity

1. Lips into the submandibular, preauricular, and facial nodes
2. Buccal mucosa into the submaxillary and submental nodes
3. Gingiva into the submaxillary and jugulo-digastric nodes
4. Retromolar trigone into the submaxillary and jugulo-digastric nodes
5. Hard palate into the submaxillary and upper jugular nodes
6. Floor of mouth into the submaxillary and jugular (middle and upper) nodes
7. Anterior two thirds of the tongue into the submaxillary and upper jugular nodes

Oropharynx

1. Base of the tongue into the jugulo-digastric, low cervical, and retropharyngeal nodes
2. Tonsillar fossa into the jugulo-digastric and submaxillary nodes
3. Soft palate into the jugulo-digastric, submaxillary, and spinal accessory nodes
4. Pharyngeal walls into the retropharyngeal nodes, pharyngeal nodes, and jugulo-digastric nodes

Nasopharynx

1. Retropharyngeal nodes into the superior jugular and posterior cervical nodes

Sinuses

1. Retropharyngeal and superior cervical nodes

Larynx

1. Glottis—extremely rare nodal involvement
2. Subglottis into the peritracheal and low cervical nodes
3. Supraglottis into the peritracheal, cervical submental, and submaxillary nodes

are of paramount importance. A systemic, step-by-step examination of all the anatomical compartments for any suspicious growths or nodes is needed. Nodes that are hard, greater than 1 cm, nontender, nonmobile, and raised are probably metastatic. The number of nodes should also be assessed. The location of neck masses can often suggest the site of the primary tumor. The third box on this page lists some indications of the origin of head and neck cancers.

Biopsies are performed on all suspicious lesions to determine a precursor benign condition or to evaluate the predominate malignant growth pattern (grading). A fine-needle aspiration biopsy (FNAB) is performed for neck masses.

Radiographic studies performed routinely include computed tomography (CT), magnetic resonance imaging (MRI), and x-ray examinations of the skull, sinuses, and soft tissue.

Common Symptoms by Site

Oral cavity—swelling or an ulcer that fails to heal
Oropharynx—painful swallowing and referred otalgia
Nasopharynx—bloody discharge and difficulty hearing
Larynx—hoarseness and stridor
Hypopharynx—dysphagia and painful neck node
Nose and sinuses—obstruction, discharge, facial pain, diplopia, and local swelling

Common Clinical Presentations by Site

1. A high cervical neck mass often represents metastases from the nasopharynx.
2. Positive subdigastric nodes are often the site of metastases from the oral cavity, oropharynx, or hypopharynx.
3. Positive submandibular triangle nodes arise from the oral cavity.
4. Midcervical neck masses are associated with tumors of the hypopharynx, base of tongue, and larynx.
5. Preauricular nodes frequently arise from tumors found in the salivary glands.

For symptomatic patients, barium swallow is recommended, along with chest films and bone scans to rule out metastases.

Pathology

Over 80% of head and neck cancers arise from the surface epithelium of the mucosal linings of the upper digestive tract. These cancers are mostly squamous cell carcinomas. Adenocarcinomas are found to a lesser extent in the salivary glands. Squamous cell carcinomas seen in the head and neck region include lymphoepithelioma, spindle cell carcinoma, verrucous carcinoma, and undifferentiated carcinoma.

Lymphoepithelioma occurs in places of abundant lymphoid tissue (i.e., the nasopharynx, tonsil, and base of the tongue). This type of histology exhibits a better cure rate than squamous cell carcinoma via radiation therapy.

Spindle cell carcinoma has a nonneoplastic background and responds to radiation therapy in much the same manner as squamous cell carcinoma.

Verrucous carcinoma is most often found in the gingiva and buccal mucosa. This type of carcinoma has an indolent pattern of growth and is associated with chewing tobacco or snuff. Verrucous carcinomas tend to be exophytic, have distinct margins, and look like warts. They are often hyperkeratotic, treated according to their appearance alone, and watched for further growth.

Undifferentiated lymphomas are similar histopathologically to undifferentiated carcinomas and should be treated as

Head and Neck Cancer Cell Types

Squamous cell carcinoma

- Lymphoepithelioma
- Spindle cell carcinoma
- Verrucous carcinoma
- Undifferentiated carcinoma
- Transitional cell carcinoma
- Keratinized carcinoma
- Nonkeratinized carcinoma

Adenocarcinoma

- Malignant mixed carcinoma
- Adenocystic carcinoma
- Mucoepidermoid carcinoma
- Acinic cell carcinoma

carcinomas if doubt exists after a microscopic evaluation. The box above lists some cell types found in the head and neck region. Tumor grading is classified as G-1 (well differentiated), G-2 (moderately well differentiated), or G-3 (poorly differentiated). A variety of nonepithelial malignancies, melanomas, soft tissue sarcomas, and plasmacytomas, can also occur in the head and neck region.

Staging

The staging system for head and neck cancers is based mostly on clinical diagnostic information that determines the size, extent, and presence of positive nodes. The surgical-pathological classification is crucial for determining the need or type of adjuvant therapy.

The box on p. 156 contains a developed version of the American Joint Committee on Cancer (AJCC) TNM (tumor, node, metastasis) Classification System by site and the stage groupings.[8] This system does not relate to the site-specific **heterogeneity** (variation in tissue density) of tumors in the head and neck, nor does it take into account the depth of invasion of small lesions.

The T system used varies with each anatomical site. Cancers found in the lip, oral cavity, oropharynx, salivary gland, or thyroid gland are size oriented. Designations are as follows*:

T_1 < 2 cm
T_2 > 2 cm or = 4 cm
T_3 > 4 cm
T_4 > 4 cm, with muscle or bone involvement

The nasopharynx, hypopharynx, larynx, and maxillary antrum are classified according to the involvement of the anatomical subsite by the depth of extension. The *N* classifications are uniform for all sites, except for the thyroid. The sizes and locations of nodes determine the *N* designation.

*The thyroid gland uses 1- to 4-cm criteria.

Stage groupings can exhibit a wide spectrum of diseases. Stage IV disease is always distant metastasis. However, in the head and neck region, M_O as N_2 or N_3 with any T disease (which is usually curable) is quite possible. The TNM classification alone is not adequate for choosing the best method of treatment. The staging work-up should include evaluation of the primary lesion size, examination of the depth of invasion into surrounding anatomical subsites, and mapping and measurement of the cervical or at-risk nodal stations. Careful attention is given to the mobility of the nodes. Fixed nodes result in a poor prognosis. Contrast-enhanced CT and MRI scans can define the size and shape of the tumor better than a clinical evaluation.

Three-dimensional multiplanar imaging has made staging much more precise and accurate for deeply invading disease or in the assessment of inaccessible neck nodes.

Routes of Spread

Physiologically, the head and neck region has rather distinct anatomical compartments. As a malignant lesion starts to grow, it exhibits a somewhat unique tendency of direct invasion. Figs. 8-6 and 8-7 depict open-mouth views that demonstrate a tumor's expected location of infiltration and thus determine the size of the target volume during irradiation. Fig. 8-8 is a lateral view of the anatomical subdivision of the head that shows the underlying or adjacent structures. (See also Fig. 8-1 for anatomical locations.)

The box on p. 158 lists areas of the head and neck region and the expected direct spread of a tumor in each area.*

Treatment techniques

Radiation and surgery are the major curative modalities. The eradication of the disease, maintenance of physiological function, and preservation of social cosmesis determine the best modality. The ability to cure and eradicate the disease without severe complications necessitates extremely selective treatment criteria. Radiation therapy is indicated in the majority of head and neck cancers because the tumors located in this region are often inaccessible to the surgeon's knife.

The use of surgery as a curative modality is correlated to the possibility of an en-block resection. Partial resections involve a high risk of recurrence. Wide margins (> 2 cm) are usually necessary. A biopsy of the cervical nodes and lesion is mandatory and should be performed by experienced oncologic surgeons. Surgery is the mode of treatment for early-stage lesions of the oral cavity and floor of the mouth if no clinically positive nodes are present or if the risk of deep cervical node involvement is low. Surgery reduces the risk of dental or salivary deficiencies, which radiation therapy routinely produces. Laser therapy, **cryotherapy** (the use of cold temperatures to treat a disease), and **electrocautery** (the application of an electric current for the destruction of tissue) are conventional curative surgical modalities.

*The order shown is not necessarily sequential.

AJCC Staging System for Head and Neck Cancer

Primary tumor (T)

(General—for all sites)

TX No available information on primary tumor

T_0 No evidence of primary tumor

TIS Carcinoma in situ

Oral cavity and oropharynx

T_1 Greatest diameter of primary tumor < or = 2 cm

T_2 >2 cm or = 4 cm

T_3 > 4 cm

T_4 Massive tumor, with deep invasion into maxilla, mandible, pterygoid muscles, deep tongue muscle, skin, and soft tissues of neck

Hypopharynx

T_1 Tumor confined to region of origin

T_2 Extension into adjacent region or site, without fixation of hemilarynx

T_3 Extension into adjacent region or site, with fixation of hemilarynx

T_4 Massive tumor invading bone or soft tissues of neck

Nasopharynx

T_1 Tumor confined to one site or identified during biopsy only (no tumor visible)

T_2 Involvement of two sites within nasopharynx

T_3 Extension into nasal cavity or oropharynx

T_4 Invasion into skull and/or cranial nerve involvement

Larynx

GLOTTIC

T_1 Confinement to true vocal cords; normal mobility; includes anterior or posterior commissure

T_2 Supra- or subglottic extension; normal or impaired mobility

T_3 Confinement to larynx proper; cord fixation

T_4 Cartilage destruction and/or extension out of larynx

SUPRAGLOTTIC

T_1 Confinement to site of origin; normal mobility

T_2 Extension to glottis or adjacent supraglottic site; normal or impaired mobility

T_3 Confinement to larynx proper; cord fixation and/or extension into hypopharnyx or preepiglottic space

T_4 Massive tumor; cartilage destruction and/or extension out of larynx

SUBGLOTTIC

T_1 Confinement to subglottic region

T_2 Glottic extension; normal or impaired mobility

T_3 Confinement to larynx proper; cord fixation

T_4 Massive tumor; cartilage destruction and/or extension out of larynx

Nodal metastasis (N)

NX Nodes cannot be assessed

N_o No clinically positive nodes

N_1 Single, clinically positive, ipsilateral node; < or = 3 cm

N_{2a} Single, clinically positive, ipsilateral node; >3 or = 6 cm

N_{2b} Multiple, clinically positive, ipsilateral nodes; all < or = 6 cm

N_{3a} Clinically positive, ipsilateral node(s); one > 6 cm

N_{3c} Contralateral, clinically positive node(s) only

Distant metastasis (M)

MX Not assessed

M_0 No distant metastases identified

M_1 Distant metastasis present

Site specification

PUL—pulmonary

OSS—osseous

BRA—brain

LYM—lymph nodes (noncervical)

MAR—bone marrow

PLE—pleura

SKI—skin

OTH—other

Stage grouping

Stage I $T_1\ N_0\ M_0$

Stage II $T_2\ N_0\ M_0$

Stage III $T_3\ N_0\ M_0,\ T_1\ T_2$, or $T_3\ N_1\ M_0$

Stage IV $T_4\ N_0$ or $N_1\ M_0$

Any T N_2 or $N_3\ M_0$

Modified from Holleb AI, Fink DJ, Murphy GP: *American Cancer Society textbook of clinical oncology,* Atlanta, 1991, The Society.

Surgery has a higher success rate for palliative salvage therapy in the event of failure after radiation therapy. Surgery offers better local control of disease that has invaded bone because curative radiation therapy doses have shown a high risk of necrosis.[4]

The role of chemotherapy in head and neck cancer is standard for metastatic disease, locally recurrent disease, or salvage therapy, for which surgery and radiation therapy can no longer be used. Chemotherapy's role is limited, but it is evolving. Single-agent therapy with methotrexate, cisplatin, bleomycin, and vinblastine[10] has shown significant clinical responses. However, these responses last just a few months. Combination drug therapy has produced higher response rates, but the prognosis has not improved, and the toxicity to the patient is higher. Adjuvant chemotherapy has been disappointing at best.[10] Because of the poor health and nutritional

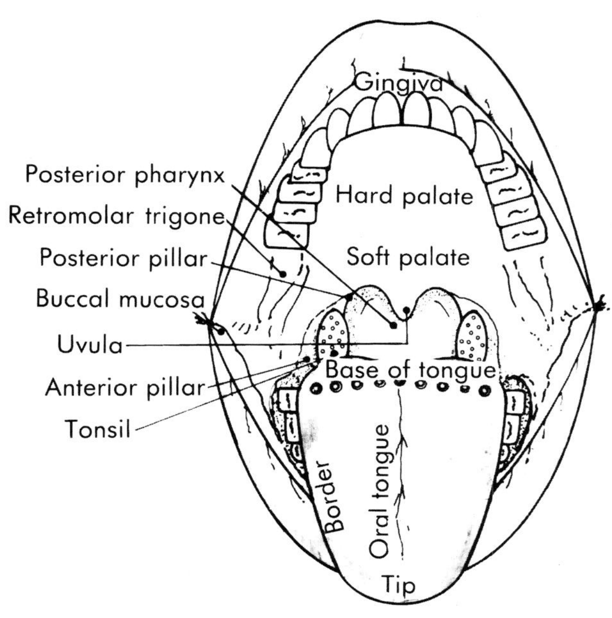

Fig. 8-6 A front open-mouth view of the oral cavity. (From Cox JD: *Moss' radiation oncology: rationale, technique, results,* ed; 7, St Louis, 1994, Mosby.)

Fig. 8-7 A front open-mouth view of the floor of the mouth with the tongue raised. (From Cox JD: *Moss' radiation oncology: rationale, technique, results,* ed 7, St Louis, 1994, Mosby.)

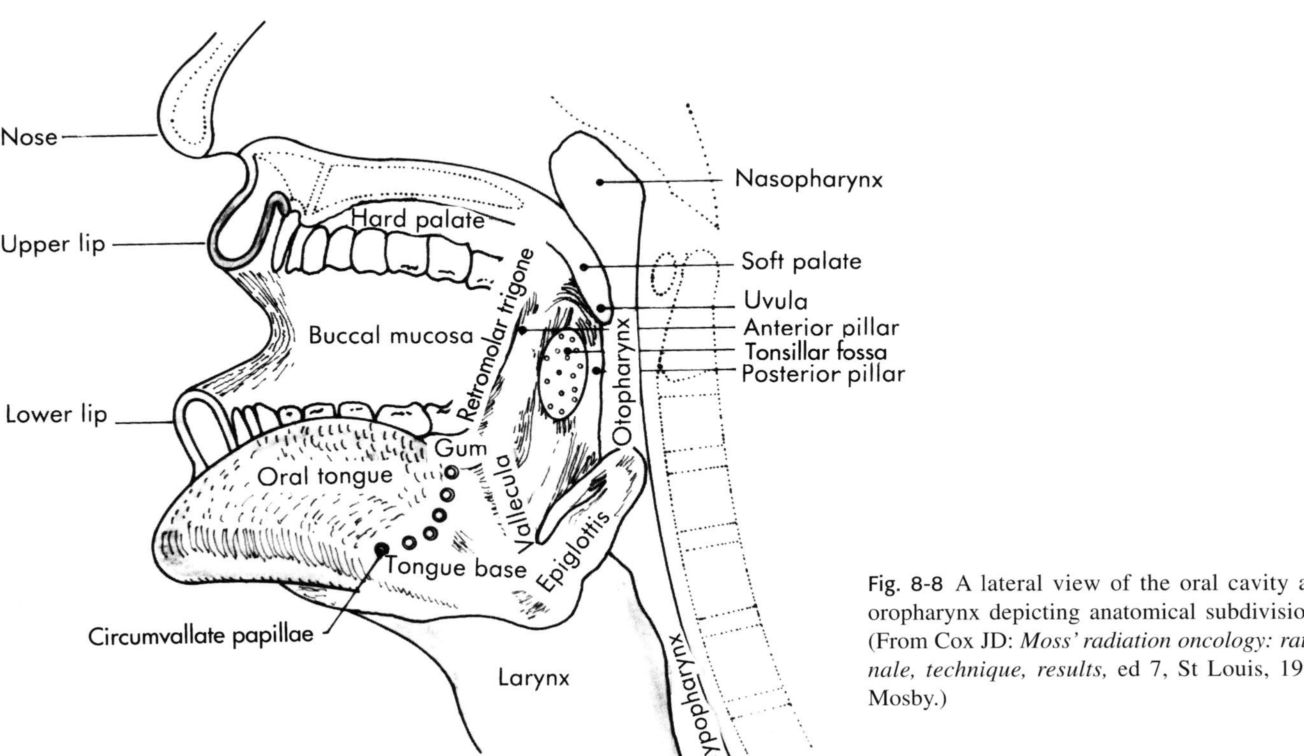

Fig. 8-8 A lateral view of the oral cavity and oropharynx depicting anatomical subdivisions. (From Cox JD: *Moss' radiation oncology: rationale, technique, results,* ed 7, St Louis, 1994, Mosby.)

status of head and neck cancer patients, the use of chemotherapy as a front line modality has not been favorable.

The use of radiation is considered the mainstay of cancer management for the treatment of cancer in the head and neck region. The choice of external beam therapy and/or brachytherapy depends on the individual and location of the tumor. Customization of the treatment technique is essential.

Brachytherapy (interstitial methods) is often used as a boost to get higher curative doses to areas that cannot tolerate the large ports encompassed by external beam therapy.

The addition of electron beam therapy has decreased the use of implants, and intraoral orthovoltage cone therapy has practically disappeared because of the increased incidence of radiation-induced osteonecrosis to the mandible.

The energy used depends on the depth and isodose distribution needed to encompass the target volume. Some examples of the radiation type used are as follows:

External beam therapy

1. Cobalt 60 (limited use, high morbidity)
2. 4 MV
3. 6 to 10 MV
4. Electron beams, 4 to 18 MeV

Brachytherapy

1. Iridium
2. Gold
3. Cesium
4. Iodine 125

Generally, palliative doses are 4500 cGy in $4^1/_2$ weeks. Curative doses are given via a shrinking-field technique. In general, doses follow the scheme shown in the box on p. 159.[10]

The delivery of radiation to areas in which the dose will exceed 7000 cGy is usually accomplished with brachytherapy or electrons. Implant therapy is administered via seeds, ribbons, or needles that allow high-concentration doses to a small volume (e.g., 1000 cGy in 1 day). The daily delivery of 180 to 200 cGy determines the number of fractions. A conventional treatment plan lasts from 5 to $7^1/_2$ weeks. Recently, **hyperfractionation** has gained favor with Radiation Therapy Oncology Group (RTOG) protocols. Daily doses of 230 cGy (115 cGy in the morning and 115 cGy in the evening) to a total dose of 7000 to 8000 cGy are used. Survival rates have improved by 15%. Salvage surgical therapy should be delayed 2 to 3 months after a therapy follow-

Expected Direct Spread of a Tumor

1. Lips (Fig. 8-8)
   a. Skin
   b. Commissure
   c. Mucosa
   d. Muscle
2. Gingiva (Fig. 8-8)
   a. Soft tissue and buccal mucosa
   b. Periosteum
   c. Bone and maxillary antrum
   d. Dental nerves
3. Buccal mucosa (Fig. 8-8)
   a. Side walls of the oral cavity
   b. Lips
   c. Retromolar trigone
   d. Muscles
4. Hard palate (Fig. 8-8)
   a. Soft palate
   b. Bone and maxillary antrum
   c. Nasal cavity
5. Trigone (Figs. 8-6 and 8-8)
   a. Buccal mucosa
   b. Anterior pillar
   c. Gingiva
   d. Pterygoid muscle
6. Floor of mouth (Figs. 8-6 and 8-7)
   a. Soft tissue, tonsils, and salivary glands
   b. Root of tongue
   c. Base of tongue
   d. Geniohyoid-mylohyoid muscles
7. Tongue (Figs. 8-6 and 8-7)
   a. Anterior two thirds of tongue
   b. Lateral borders
   c. Base and underside of tongue
   d. Floor of mouth
8. Soft palate (Figs. 8-1 and 8-8)
   a. Tonsillar pillars
   b. Pharyngeal walls
   c. Hard palate
   d. Nasopharynx
9. Larynx (Figs. 8-21 and 8-22)
   a. True cords
   b. False cords
   c. Arytenoid muscles
   d. Epiglottis
   e. Hypopharynx
   f. Aryepiglottic folds
   g. Ventricles
10. Pharynx (Figs. 8-1, 8-6, and 8-8)
   a. Anterior walls
   b. Posterior tongue
   c. Base of tongue
   d. Lateral walls
   e. Tonsillar pillars
   f. Uvula
   g. Soft palate
   h. Posterior walls
   i. Muscles and epiglottis
11. Tonsils (Figs. 8-1 and 8-6)
   a. Palatine-linguinal tonsil
   b. Tonsillar pillars
   c. Base of tongue
   d. Soft palate
   e. Pharyngeal wall

up for nodes <6 cm and a longer time if the disease is large and bulky.[10]

Clinically positive anatomy and suspicious microscopic findings in the margins determine the port size and shape. Positive neck nodes and any nodes believed to harbor subclinical disease (15% risk probability) are included. Normal tissue will be included in the ports. Therefore the dose to critical organs in the treatment field must be calculated. Adherence to the TD $_{5/5}$ is required for irradiation of the total volume to a tumoricidal dose. Table 8-2 gives the tolerance doses for special organs found in the head and neck area.[3]

Treatment consideration and principles

Oral cavity. The oral cavity consists of the lips, gingiva, floor of the mouth, tongue, buccal mucosa, and hard palate, including the retromolar trigone. Oral cavity cancers, the most common aerodigestive tract carcinomas, occur mostly (80%) in men between the ages of 55 and 65. Alcohol and tobacco have a **synergistic** (a combined effect greater than the individual effect) etiological history. Patients who have oral cavity cancer often demonstrate poor oral and dental hygiene. In females, Plummer-Vinson syndrome (iron deficiency anemia) is considered an important etiological factor. Because premalignant conditions are usually asymptomatic, the general practitioner or dentist is responsible for clinical detection.

Typical Curative Radiation Doses for Head and Neck Lesions

5000 cGy = Nodes
5000 cGy = Any subclinical disease
6000-6500 cGy = T_1 lesions
6500-7000 cGy = T_2 lesions
7000-7500 cGy = T_3-T_4 lesions

As previously stated, leukoplakia and erythroplasia represent severe dysplastic changes and should be regarded as serious pathological problems. Most often, oral cavity cancers appear as nonhealing ulcers with little pain. Localized pain is considered a symptom of advanced disease. Cervical lymph node involvement at the time of presentation is uncommon, and oral cavity cancer demonstrates the lowest incidence (except glottic cancer) of nodal metastasis in the head and neck region. Blood-borne spread occurs in fewer than 20% of patients. Of those patients, most have cervical node involvement at the time of presentation and advanced-stage disease.

Squamous cell carcinoma accounts for 90% to 95% of the histopathological types, either well or moderately well differentiated.[10] Early-stage (<1 to 1.5 cm) and premalignant lesions are candidates for surgery alone. If inadequate surgical margins and neck node involvement are present, combination radiation therapy and surgery is indicated. The sequence of the therapy is usually dictated by the first treatment's design. If radical surgery is planned, the radiation therapy should not be given before surgery. Elective irradiation of the lymph nodes is included if a lesion demonstrates a high rate of spread or has a history of bilateral movement (anatomically) via the lymphatics. A 5-year follow-up plan is recommended because lesions in most sites recur within 2 years and rarely after 4 years. The expected 5-year survival rates are listed in the box on p. 160.

Lips and gums. Lip cancer (Fig. 8-9, *A*) is treated with radiation in the same manner as skin cancer. Successful control is achievable by external beam therapy, interstitial implants, or both. Single, anterior source-skin distance (SSD) ports, given 100- to 200-kVp x-rays or 3- to 7-MeV electrons at the 100% isodose line is a common regimen. Protracted treatment schedules (4 to 6 weeks) with deliveries of 200 to 300 cGy per day can be given for lesions less than 2 cm. Larger, bulkier lesions require doses of 5000 to 6000 cGy. Regional (submental) lymphatics are rarely treated, whereas patients with advanced-stage or recurrent

Table 8-2 Doses allowed for special organs in the head and neck region

Organ	TD $_{5/5}$ (in cGy)	TD $_{5/50}$ (in cGy)	Whole or partial organ
Muscles (adult)	6000	8000	Whole
Oral cavity	6000	8000	50 cm^2
Spinal cord	4500	5500	Whole or partial
Lens of eye	500	1200	Whole
Brain	6000	7000	Whole
Retina	5500	7000	Whole
Cornea	5000	>6000	Whole
Ear	5000	7000	Whole
Thyroid gland	4500	15000	Whole
Pituitary gland	4500	20000	Whole

Modified from Bentel GC: *Treatment planning and dose calculation,* ed 4, New York, 1989, Pergamon Press.

disease should have neck irradiation. Face shielding must be constructed to delineate the target volume and thus only expose 1 to 2 cm of normal tissue. Fig. 8-9, *B* shows a lead shield in place for a lip lesion. Fig. 8-9, *C* demonstrates a patient being treated with 100-KVP x-rays through a cone. To reduce complications to teeth and gums, a stent coated with wax or a low-atomic-number compound (tissue equivalent) can be made to fit over the teeth. The face-mask shielding should also be coated with wax to reduce the electron scatter to the adjacent tissues. Exit radiation to the bone and gums needs to be controlled at safe levels to prevent progressive, long-term physiological changes. With megavoltage electron energies a tissue compensator is sometimes used to make the dose more uniform (Fig. 8-10). The expected 5-year survival rate is 90%.[6]

Floor of the mouth. Cancers in this area arise on the anterior surface on either side of the midline. They can spread to the bone and tongue. About 30% of these cancers have positive submaxillary and subdigastric nodes. Therefore opposed lateral ports are used.[7] The entire width of the mandibular arch is included in the port (Fig. 8-11). The superior border is designed to spare the maxillary antrum. If the lesion is small and does not involve the tongue, the tip of the tongue is pushed out of the treatment field (Fig. 8-11). Large, bulky lesions usually require that the tongue be flattened and included in the port. An off-cord boost via opposed laterals occurs at 4500 cGy. If the neck nodes are clinically positive, the lateral ports are enlarged to include all the upper cervical nodes, and an anterior, bilateral, supraclavicular neck field is added (Fig. 8-12). The midline cord block is included up to the thyroid notch so that the tumor is not shielded.

The lateral borders of the anterior supraclavicular field extend to the coracoid process. The inferior borders extend horizontally 1 to 2 cm below the suprasternal notch, and the superior borders abut via (megavoltage x-ray) the lateral borders at the thyroid notch. The supraclavicular field is taken to 5000 cGy. The bilateral neck fields receive a minimum of 5000 cGy, with boost fields added to bring the dose between 6000 and 7000 cGy.[9] The reduced boost fields can be treated with an intraoral cone (limited use now), needle implants, or small external photon beams. The expected 5-year survival rate is approximately 50%.[10]

Five-Year Survival Rates for Head and Neck Cancer

Stage I—75%-90%
Stage II—40%-70%
Stage III—20%-30%
Stage IV—10%-30%

Modified from Rubin P: *Clinical oncology*, ed 7, Philadelphia, 1993, WB Saunders.

Tongue. Lesions of the tongue usually appear on the lateral borders near the middle and posterior third section. The lesions can be quite large and still confined to the tongue. Only a limited number of tongue cancers can be excised. Therefore, external beam irradiation can achieve the best control with interstitial boost fields.

Lesions on the tip of the tongue are seen first and are commonly in an early stage, whereas lesions at the base and

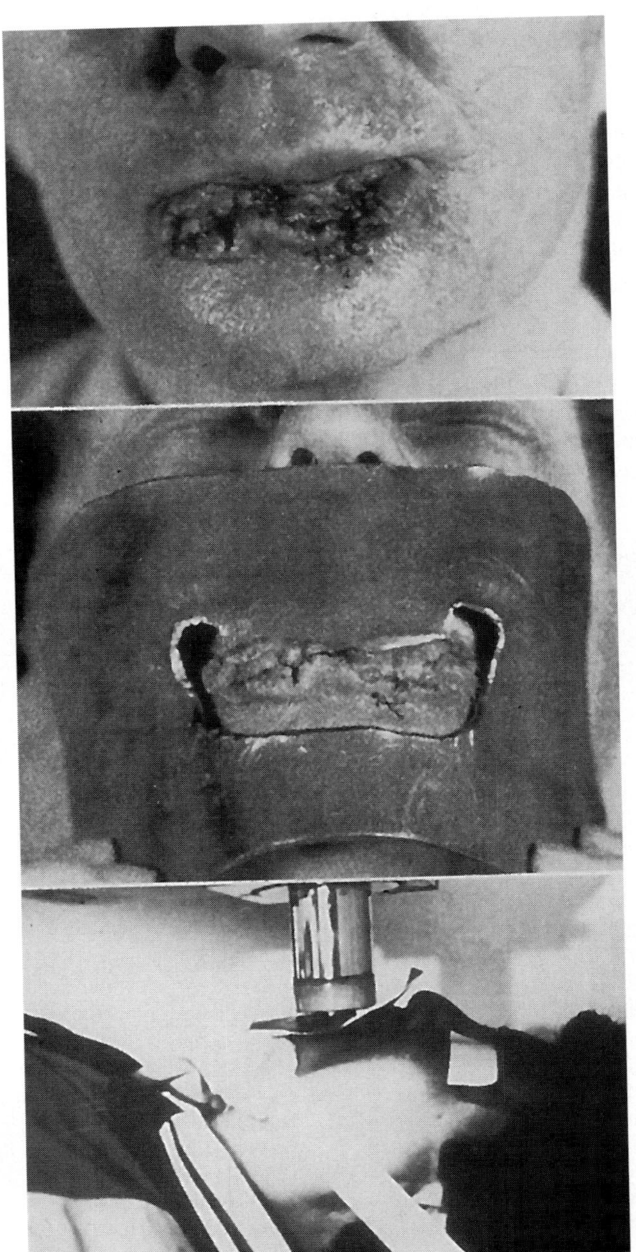

Fig. 8-9 **A,** Deep, infiltrative lip cancer. **B,** An anterior view of a lead shield in place for a lip cancer. (From Moss WT, Cox JD: *Radiation oncology: rationale, technique, results,* St Louis, 1987, Mosby.) **C,** A lateral view of a patient receiving superfacial x-ray treatment.

posterior one third of the tongue invade the floor of the mouth, the tonsils, or the muscles; are advanced; and have a higher incidence of nodal metastasis. About 35% of patients with tongue cancer demonstrate clinically positive nodes and have a 25% risk of developing contralateral nodal disease with an N_1-N_2 ipsilateral classification.[6] An early-stage lesion of the tongue can be cured with a local excision or **hemiglossectomy** (surgical removal of half the tongue). For the preservation of speech and swallowing functions, external beam irradiation is the best choice for large T_3-T_4 lesions. Iridium 192 implants follow the external beam. Fig. 8-12 depicts radiation ports for the base of a tongue. A depressor is sometimes inserted to push the tongue back and keep as much of the mandible out of the field as possible. The subdigastric and submaxillary nodes must always be included in the port. Opposed lateral fields are used, with the posterior borders encompassing the upper cervical nodes and the superior border aligned to miss the maxillary

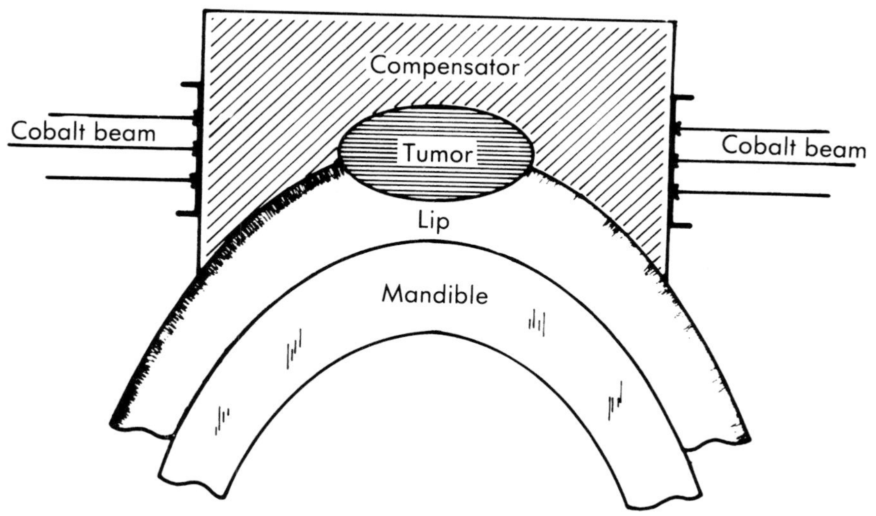

Fig. 8-10 A cross-sectional view of a lip lesion and the placement of a tissue compensator to achieve dose uniformity. (From Cox JD: *Moss' radiation oncology: rationale, technique, results,* ed 7, St Louis, 1994, Mosby.)

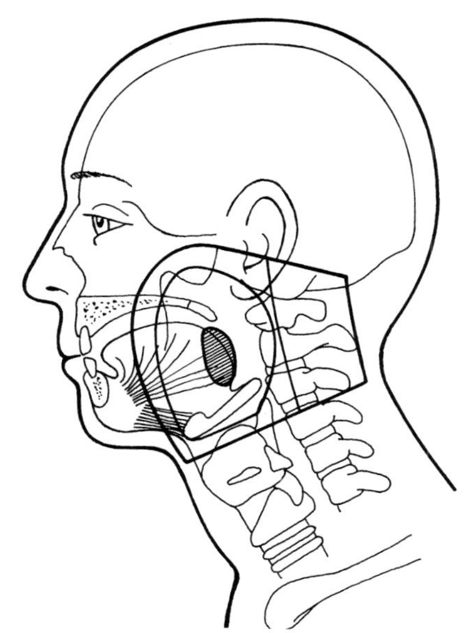

Fig. 8-11 A lateral view of the base of the tongue. Boost fields are indicated. (From Thawley SE, Panje WR, Lindgerg RD: *Comprehensive management of head and neck tumors,* 1987, WB Saunders.)

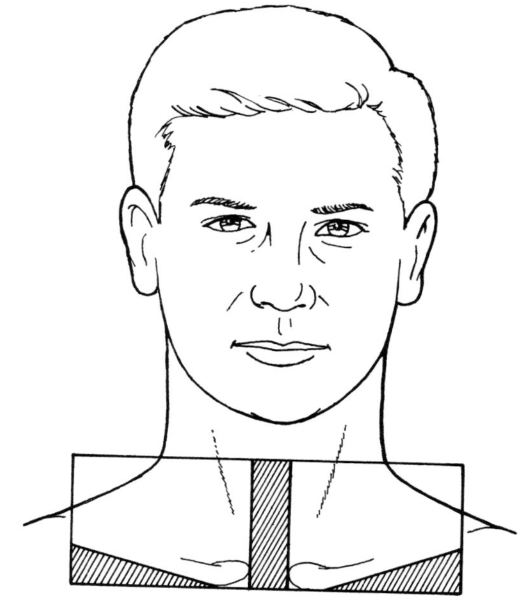

Fig. 8-12 An anterior view of a bilateral supraclavicular port with a 5-HVL spinal cord block. (From Bentel, GC: *Treatment planning and dose calculation in radiation oncology,* ed 4, New York, 1989, McGraw-Hill.)

antrum. Conventional fractionation (180 cGy/day) is used to deliver 6500 to 7500 cGy to the tumor volume. Clinically positive nodes need 6000 cGy. An off-cord boost is delivered through opposed lateral fields, with a posterior electron-boost field added to increase the dose to 6000 cGy. With the 80% to 90% depth dose line, 3- to 7-MeV electron beams can safely be used to avoid spinal cord damage. If the lesion is not midlined, weighting of the daily dose at a ratio of 3:2 or 2:1 (involved versus noninvolved side) can be indicated. Large, bulky tumors with neck nodes will most likely need a supraclavicular field that matches the borders of the lateral fields. If not at risk for involvement, the larynx, trachea, and spinal cord must be shielded. The expected 5-year survival rate is 50%.[11]

Buccal mucosa. The buccal mucosa is the mucous membrane lining the inner surface of the cheeks and lips. Most lesions originate on the lateral walls, have a history of leukoplakia, and appear as a raised, exophytic growth. As it grows, the lesion invades the skin and bone. Usually, the patient notices a bump with the tip of the tongue. Pain is not associated with this lesion unless the nerves to the tongue or ear become involved. Advanced lesions bleed. Early lesions often appear as an inflammatory process, so care should be taken during a biopsy to obtain a differential diagnosis.

Stensen's duct can become obstructed. This enlarges the parotid gland, thereby necessitating surgical intervention. Small (1 cm) lesions can be excised, whereas larger lesions are treatable with combination surgery and radiation therapy, radical surgery, or radical radiation therapy alone. If radiation therapy is chosen as a treatment modality, a single-plane photon or electron beam that spares contralateral tissues can be used. The submaxillary and subdigastric nodes are at risk. If positive, these nodes require a controlling dose. Depending on the lesion size, a tumor dose of 5000 to 6000 cGy is needed for control. The expected 5-year survival rate is 58%.[11]

Hard palate and retromolar trigone. Hard palate carcinomas are quite rare and are mostly adenocarcinomas. They tend to spread to the bone and invade the maxillary antrum. Surgical resection is the usual treatment, with postoperative radiation therapy given as needed. Extensive disease requires radiation therapy. Most cancers in this area are the result of secondary spread from the upper gum. A history of ill-fitting dentures or trauma is common.

The retromolar trigone is the triangular space behind the last molar tooth. Lesions in this area (Fig. 8-3) can cause tongue pain, ear-canal pain, or if the muscles become involved, trismus. X-ray examinations are needed to detect bone invasion. Lymphatic spread occurs to the submaxillary and subdigastric nodes. Moderately advanced lesions are usually managed with resection and postoperative radiation therapy. For disease confined to one side of the head, ipsilateral mixed beams (electrons-photons or intraoral cones) with stents in place are used to standardize doses. Surgery is preferred unless the patient does not accept the functional and cosmetic effect. A 5-year survival rate of 60% is expected. Figs. 8-13, 8-14, 8-15, and 8-16 are pictorial evidence of head and neck cancer management.

As will be discussed in later sections, the precise delivery of radiation to the head and neck requires strict attention to positioning and immobilization of the area targeted for treatment. The use of the Aquaplast mask system provides more than adequate stabilization to the anatomical site. The bite-block system is also used to keep the tongue in the desired position. Whichever method is used in the clinic, it must be individualized to suit the patient.

Pharynx. The pharynx is subdivided into three anatomical divisions: the oropharynx, nasopharynx, and hypopharynx (Fig. 8-17). Diseases in these regions have a pronounced functional and structural effect on the aerodigestive tract.

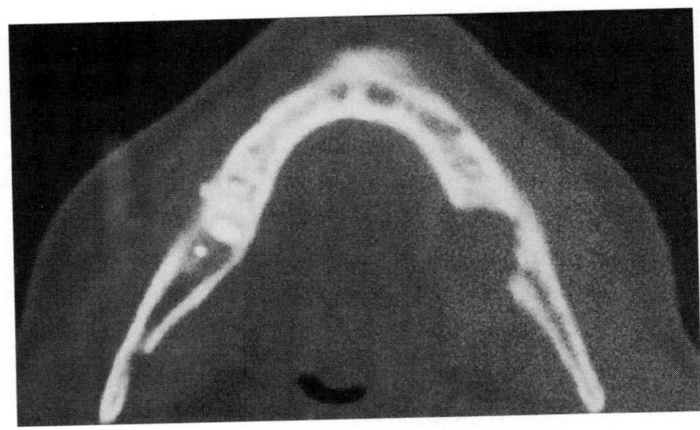

Fig. 8-13 An axial CT image at the level of the mandible demonstrates a destructive lesion predominantly involving the lingual cortex. (From Cox JD: *Moss' radiation oncology: rationale, technique, results,* ed 7, St Louis, 1994, Mosby.)

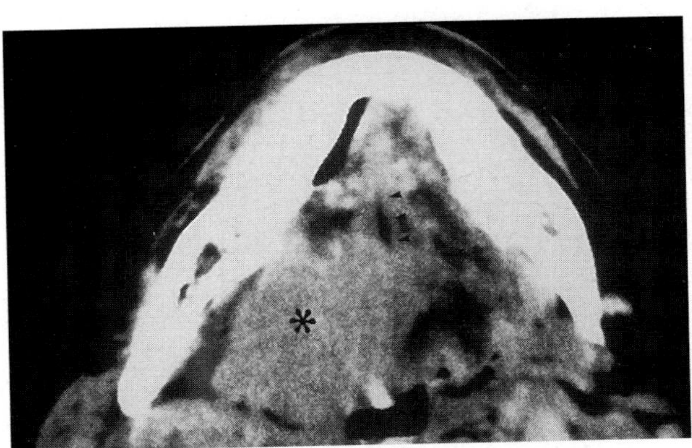

Fig. 8-14 An axial contrast-enhanced CT scan demonstrates a pathological appearing enhancing mass involving the oropharyngeal and oral portions of the right side of the tongue. Note the obliteration of the normal fatty lingual septum *(arrows)*, indicating extension across the midline. (From Cox JD: *Moss' radiation oncology: rationale, technique, results,* ed 7, St Louis, 1994, Mosby.)

Surgical intervention is quite a task for the excision of any lesion without some functional loss in speech, chewing, or swallowing. This inaccessibility of the surgeon's knife leads to radiation therapy as the predominant modality for therapeutic control of cancers in this region.

The oropharynx consists of the base of the tongue, the tonsils (fossa and pillars), the soft palate, and the pharyngeal walls. The oropharynx is situated between the axis and C-3 vertebral bodies. The soft tissue regions include the anterior tonsillary pillars, the soft palate, the uvula, the base of the tongue, and the lateral-posterior pharyngeal walls (Fig. 8-8). The tonsils are the most common site of disease. Clinically, a sore throat and pain during swallowing are the most common presenting symptoms. Upper spinal accessory nodes are involved bilaterally in 50% to 70% of the patients.

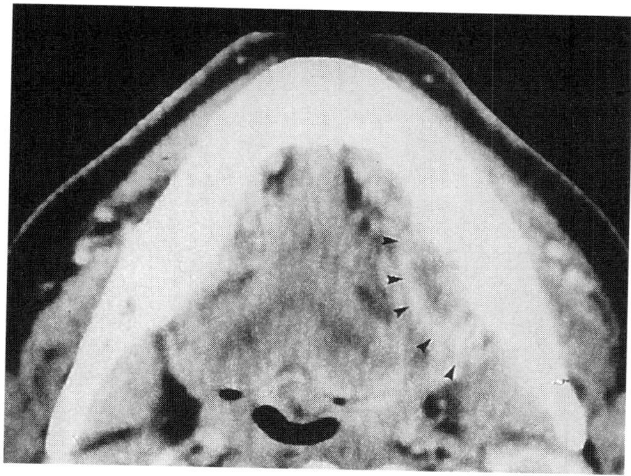

Fig. 8-15 A contrast-enhanced CT scan (same patient as in Fig. 8-13) demonstrating an enhancing mass in the posterior left side of the floor of the mouth extending to the retromolar trigone *(arrows)*.

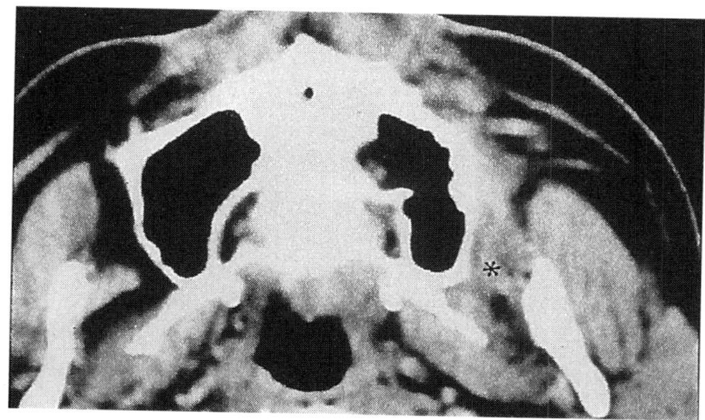

Fig. 8-16 A contrast-enhanced CT scan (same patient as in Fig. 8-14) at the level of the maxilla demonstrating submucosal infiltration along the pterygomandibular raphe to the posterior aspect of the normally fat-filled buccinator space. This was a clinically occult disease identified only by imaging. (From Cox JD: *Moss' Radiation oncology: rationale, technique, results,* St Louis, 1994, Mosby.)

Early T_1-T_2 lesions are treatable with external beam irradiation alone. Large ports are required for T_3-T_4 lesions that encompass the cervical and supraclavicular neck nodes. Fig. 8-18 depicts a small-field technique for a lesion of the soft palate. The field is reduced at 5000 cGy, and then the primary receives a boost of 1500 to 2500 cGy, depending on the lesion size. Positive clinical nodes receive at least 6000 cGy. The bilateral supraclavicular field, if needed, requires at least 5000 cGy for local control.[10]

Acute mucosa reactions are common, and complications from the radiation pose a significant medical problem. The total treatment time schedule runs from 6 to 9 weeks.

The soft palate and tonsils have the best prognosis (50% and 45%, respectively). The overall 5-year survival rate is only 35%.[6]

Hypopharynx. The hypopharynx (Fig. 8-8) is composed of the pyriform sinuses, postcricoid, and lower posterior pharyngeal walls. It is anatomically situated between the vertebral bodies C3-C6. The cricoid cartilage represents the inferior border, and the epiglottis is the superior border.

Typically, disease of the hypopharynx is advanced. Nodal metastasis has a high rate (70%) and is highly infiltrative. Treatment can also be debilitating. The rare T_1-T_2 lesions are controllable through radiation or surgery, and the expected survival rate is 70%.[7] The pyriform sinus is the site of highest incidence of hypopharyngeal cancer. The majority of patients receive combined radical surgery and radiation therapy for curative purposes. Large radiation ports are common. The radiation ports for tonsillar, pharyngeal-wall, and poste-

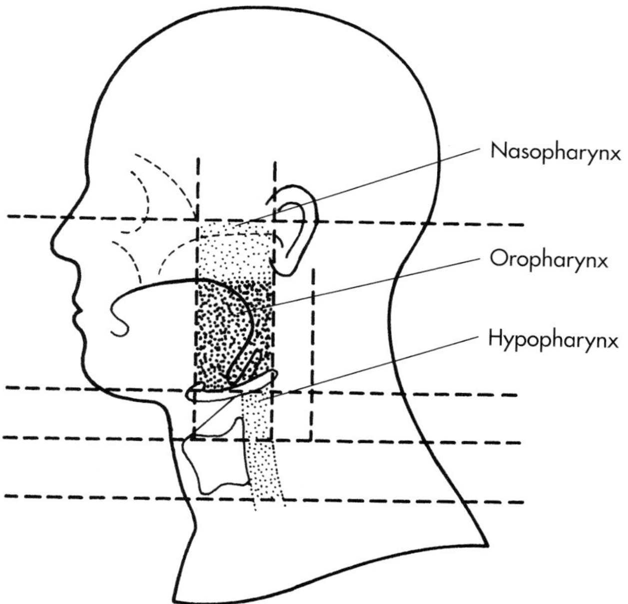

Fig. 8-17 Subdivisions of the pharynx. The dotted lines represent palpable anatomical structures: the zygomatic arch, EAM, mastoid process, hyoid bone, and thyroid cartilage. (From Rubin P: *Clinical oncology: multidisciplinary approach for physicians and students,* 1993, WB Saunders.)

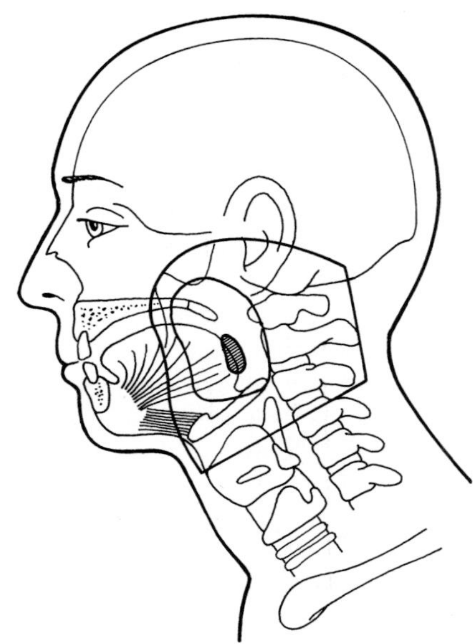

Fig. 8-18 A lateral view of the head. Initial and reduced lateral fields for an early-stage soft-palate lesion. (From Thawley SE, Panje WR, Lindgerg RD: *Comprehensive management of head and neck tumors,* vol 1, Philadelphia, 1987, WB Saunders.)

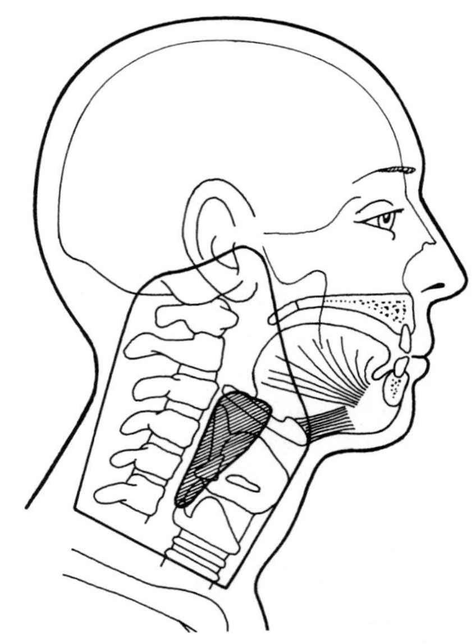

Fig. 8-19 A lateral view of the head and neck, depicting opposing lateral radiation ports for a pyriform sinus. (From Levitt SH, Tapley N: *Technological basis of radiation therapy: practical clinical applications*, ed 2, 1992, St Louis, Lea & Febiger.)

rior cricoid are quite similar stage for stage. Fig. 8-19 depicts a typical field alignment.

Postoperative doses to 6500 cGy are planned, with an additional boost of 500 cGy. Opposed laterals are matched with an anterior bilateral supraclavicular field. The inferior border of the lateral port is difficult to treat because of interference of the shoulders. Care must be taken to ensure that the shoulders are pulled down toward the feet and remain that way during treatment.

An off-cord boost to the cervical nodal chain can be delivered via electron beam therapy. The lateral retropharyngeal and jugular chain nodes are treated, even if they are clinically negative. Anterior **shine over** (falloff) is usually not necessary from the laterals unless the larynx is involved.

Substantial soft tissue, cord damage, airway damage, or fibrosis is possible with these fields if the radiation dose to the critical organs is not carefully monitored. Full-course therapy can last 7 to 8 weeks.

Nasopharynx. The nasopharynx is a cuboidal structure lying on a line from the zygomatic arch to the **external auditory meatus (EAM)**, extending inferiorly to the mastoid tip. The nasopharynx lies behind the nasal cavities and above the level of the soft palate (Fig. 8-1).

The nasal cavity drains into the nasopharynx via the two posterior nares and also has on its lateral walls the two eustachian tubes, which connect to the middle ear. Disease in the nasopharynx can mimic an inflammatory process and cause considerable respiratory or auditory dysfunction.

Cranial nerve involvement occurs frequently. The ninth to the twelfth cranial nerves can be affected by enlargement of the retropharyngeal nodes (Fig. 8-4), as can the external carotid artery. Because of its proximity to the base of the brain, a lesion can directly invade the third through sixth nerves. Any cranial nerve involvement signifies advanced, widespread disease.

Surgical intervention in the nasopharynx is extremely difficult. This disease is not associated with tobacco consumption. The Epstein-Barr Virus is associated with NPC. Nasopharyngeal cancer is uncommon in whites and demonstrates a bimodal peak incidence of 30 years and 50 to 70 years, with nearly 20% of all cases (rare in the U.S.—2% of 43,000 total head and neck cancers) occurring in the younger age group.[7]

Because 70% to 85% of NPC patients have clinically positive cervical nodes, radiation ports are quite large to encompass all the nodes and at-risk tissue. The lateral retropharyngeal and jugulo-digastric are nearly always treated as tumor volume during any cone down procedure. Bilateral involvement occurs in 50% of all patients.[5]

NPC disease demonstrates a 25% to 40% risk of blood borne metastasis, primarily to the bone and then the lung to a lesser extent.[5] NPC disease spreads to adjacent subsites rather quickly and demonstrates a 30% to 40% local recurrence rate. For these reasons, aggressive, large-volume radical radiation therapy is necessary.

Fig. 8-20 depicts a three-field setup. Opposing laterals with a matching anterior supraclavicular field are used to deliver a minimum of 5000 cGy to all areas. Subsequent cone down fields boost the dose to 6500 cGy, with careful consideration of the dose to the spinal cord, optic nerve,

A

B

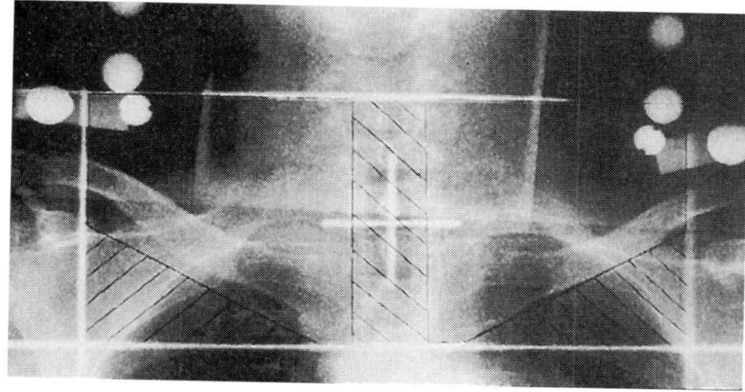

Fig. 8-20 A simulation film of a nasopharynx treatment. **A,** Opposed laterals. **B,** An anterior supraclavicular port. (Lateral borders, superiorly, base of brain; inferiorly, below the angle of the jaw; anteriorly, posterior one third of the orbit; posteriorly, 2 cm posterior to the spinous process. (From Bentel GC, Nelson CE: *Treatment planning and dose calculation,* New York, 1989, McGraw-Hill.)

pituitary, and brain stem. An electron boost of 7000 cGy to bulky disease or positive nodes is warranted if lymphadenopathy is present. Recurrences are treatable with small, multiple ports; arcs; or brachytherapy. Any external beam reirradiation should avoid the same surface-entrance points.

This disease has an overall 45% survival rate. Generally, nonpalpable nodes exhibit a 50% to 70% survival rate, but this drops to 20% to 40% if palpable nodal disease is present.[10] Unfortunately, 40% of all failures result in a relapse at the primary site, whereas 60% of the failures occur distally, thus making chemotherapy an added treatment modality.

Larynx. Cancer of the larynx is the most common malignant tumor encountered in the head and neck region. Fig. 8-21 depicts a posterior view of the larynx and surrounding structures. Carcinomas of the glottis (true vocal cord) are not considered life threatening, and the choice of therapy is based on the preservation of speech and maintenance of the airway. Larynx cancer is mostly (90%) a male-dominated disease, with a peak incidence in the 50- to 60-year age group.[10]

The larynx is subdivided into three sites (Fig. 8-22): the glottis, supraglottis, and subglottis region. Glottic cancer accounts for roughly 65% of the cases, with a 30% site incidence in the supraglottic region. The remainder of the larynx cancers appear in the subglottic area.[10]

Laryngeal carcinomas display an extremely high etiology toward smoking. A persistent sore throat and hoarseness are classic presenting symptoms. Cervical lymph node involvement, if present, is seen in supraglottic lesions but not in glottic lesions. Carcinoma in situ (Tis) is rather common on the vocal cords. Glottic lesions are well to moderately differentiated, with supraglottic lesions being less differentiated and more aggressive. About 65% to 75% of glottic lesions appear on the anterior two thirds of one cord. Cord mobility is a factor in the classification (see the box on p. 159) of the lesions. Radiation therapy is the primary choice of treatment for nonfixed surface lesions that have not extensively infiltrated muscle, bone, or cartilage.

Glottic cancer is treated with opposing lateral fields, 4 × 4 cm to 6 × 6 cm. Wedges are indicated if the tissue inhomogeneities produce unacceptable hot spots in the posterior margins. Daily doses can be 200 to 220 cGy, up to a total dose of 6000 to 7000 cGy, depending on the size of the lesion and mobility of the cord. Large, fixed lesions need more aggressive therapy.

The radiation port's borders can be clinically determined before simulation. Fig. 8-23 depicts a typical lateral port.

The typical radiation field borders are as follows:

- Superior—top of hyoid
- Inferior—cricoid cartilage
- Anterior—1- to $1\frac{1}{2}$-cm shine over (flash)
- Posterior—just anterior to the vertebral body

Large T_3-T_4, transglottic lesions are treated with radiation alone. In the event of a recurrence, salvage surgery is an option. However, the voice is usually sacrificed. Radiation therapy offers the best method of voice preservation.

Supraglottic lesions are frequently large and bulky but (despite appearances) do not usually invade the inferior false cord or the ventricles. These lesions tend to spread superiorly to the epiglottis.

Lymph node metastasis is expected in 40% to 50% of the patients. Therefore the radiation ports are much larger than the glottic ports. Posteriorly, the spinal accessory chain is included in the lateral treatment fields. Superiorly, the field border extends along the mandible. If necessary, an anterior bilateral supraclavicular field (Fig. 8-12) is matched to the laterals. The midline block, placed below the cricoid, should only shield the trachea and cord. Because of the risk of blocking tumor, no midline block is used in some instances,

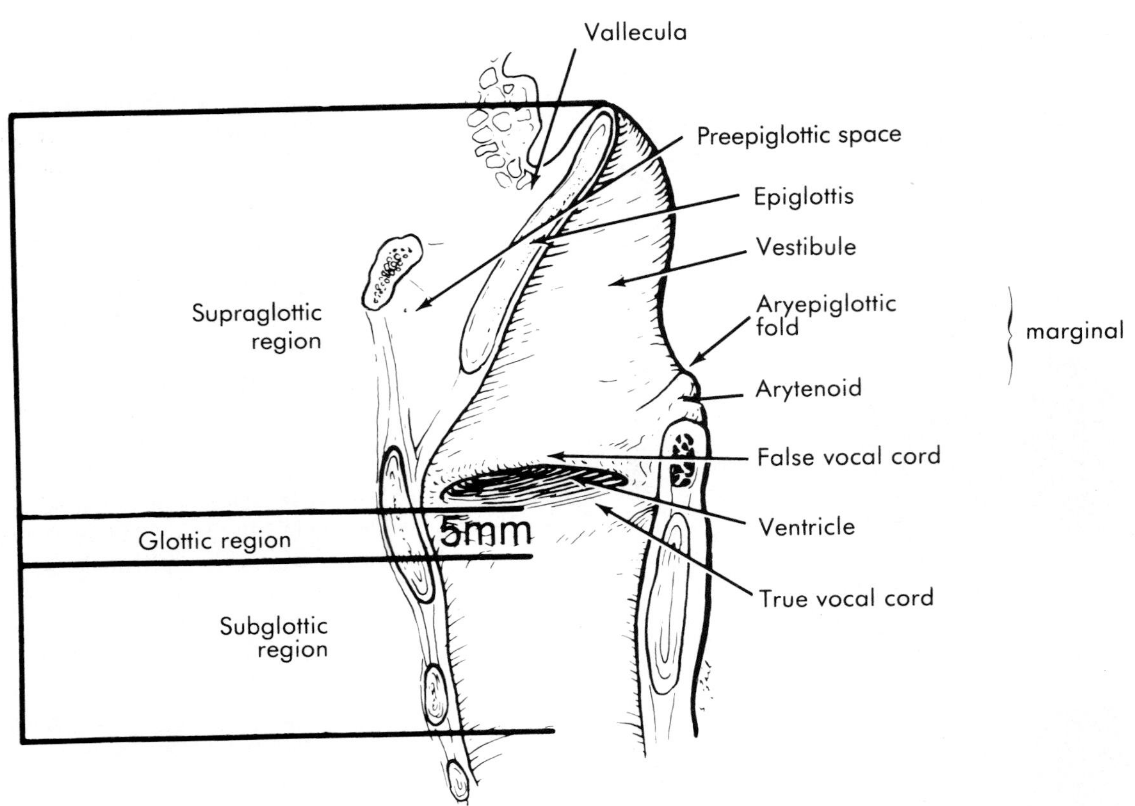

Fig. 8-21 A posterior view of the base of the tongue, larynx, and hypopharynx. (From Cox JD: *Moss' radiation oncology: rationale, technique, results,* ed 7, St Louis, 1994, Mosby.)

thereby requiring that a safety block be placed in the lateral fields at the match line junction. Positioning and immobilizing the head is critical for this type of treatment port. No movement of the head is allowed.

Surgery can control 80% of supraglottic T_1-T_2 lesions, whereas radiation therapy offers 75% local control. Radiation therapy alone for T_3-T_4 supraglottic lesions is contraindicated. Relapses are treated with surgery.

The tumor dose needed to achieve control is 6600 to 7000 cGy. Electron beam boosts are needed for the cervical lymph nodes.

Subglottic cancers are treated with a total laryngectomy, with postoperative radiation therapy given for any residual disease.

Survival rates are good for glottic cancer: 80% to 90% without cord fixation, 50% to 60% if fixation exists. Patients with supraglottic cancers have a 60% to 70% 5-year survival rate with negative nodes, but this rate drops to 30% to 50% if positive clinical nodes are present.[10]

Salivary glands. Carcinoma of the salivary gland constitutes less than 1% of all cancers of the head and neck region. The parotid is the site of highest incidence of salivary glands tumors (80%). Of these tumors, nearly two thirds are benign.[5] The submandibular gland is involved in about 10% of all instances. Histologically, the more common cell types are the adenoid cystic, mucoepidermoid, and adenocarcinoma. Risk factors include previous irradiation to the face and facial skin cancer. Presenting symptoms are localized swelling and pain, facial palsy, and rapid growth. Facial nerve involvement is highly suggestive of a malignancy.

Incisional biopsies are not routinely performed. A diagnosis via a lobectomy is done. Submandibular lesions are excised for a frozen section.

The AJCC clinical TNM staging system[2] is given in the box on p. 168. The incidence of cervical node involvement varies according to the histological subtype. High-grade mucoepidermoid tumors display a 50% to 60% metastatic behavior. The rate for this behavior in adenoid cystic tumors is 15%, and for malignant mixed tumors it is 25%.[10]

Although tumors in this area are mostly benign, the risk of local recurrence is high. They are treated as low-grade cancer and are optimally treated via total resection, with generous margins for sparing facial nerves.

Radiation therapy is given postoperatively for residual, recurrent, or inoperable lesions. Tumor doses of 5000 to 7000 rads are delivered depending on the T stage. Neck nodes should receive 5000 to 6000 cGy.[5]

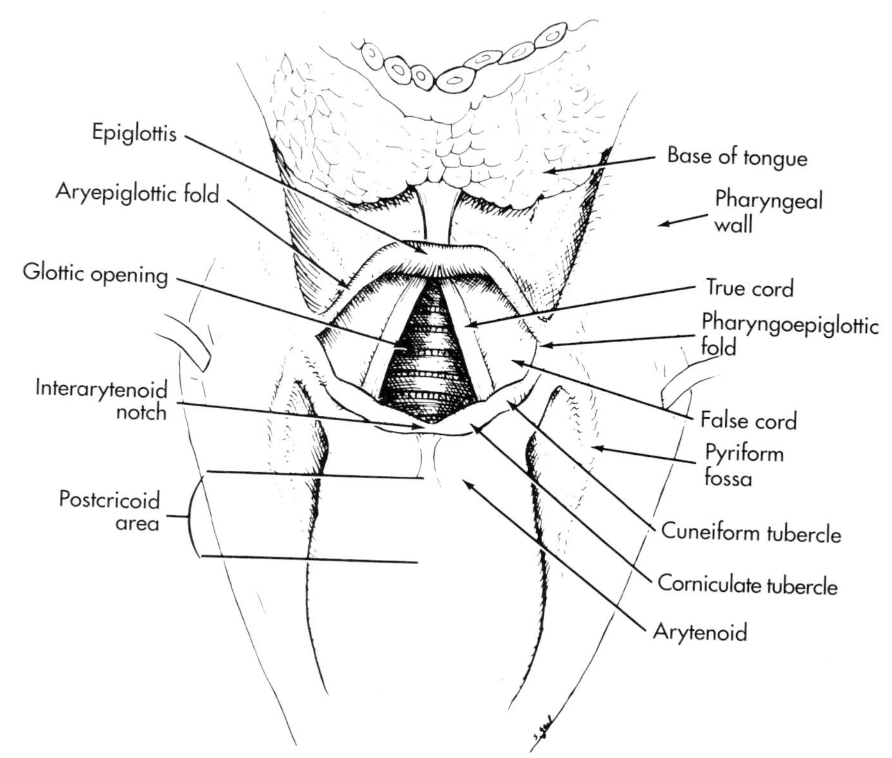

Fig. 8-22 A saggital cross-section of the larynx. (From Cox JD: *Moss' radiation oncology: rationale, technique, results,* ed 7, St Louis, 1994, Mosby.)

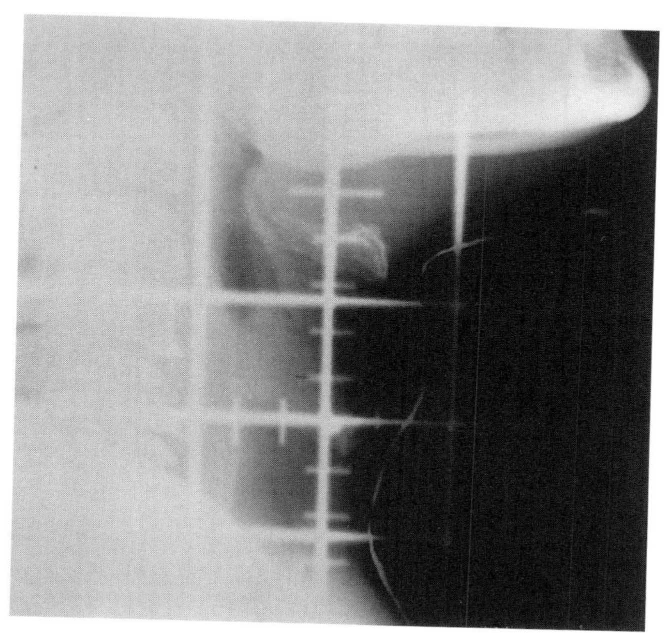

Fig. 8-23 A simulation film of a lateral port, T_1 N_0, glottic cancer. (From Cox JD: *Moss' radiation oncology: rationale, technique, results*, ed 7, St Louis, 1994, Mosby.)

The radiation is delivered through a single lateral port (Fig. 8-24) with a mixed beam of photons and electrons. The electron field is 1 to 1 1/2 cm larger than the photon field because of the way electron beam isodose lines constrict on the peripheral edges. The electron beam allows for sparing of the contralateral tissues of the face.

In addition, treatment of the parotid with a wedged pair is possible, blocking the orbit and oral cavity. Care should be taken to monitor the dose to the base of the brain and contralateral maxillary antrum with this technique. Neutron therapy is being investigated and practiced at some institutions.[5] Control rates and survival seem to favor neutron therapy over photon therapy. However, more serious complications have been associated with neutrons, and the trials have apparently involved low-grade, early-stage diseases so that favorable results might be expected.

The overall survival rate is 50% to 70%. In 1991 Wang and Goodman reported a 100% control rate for parotid tumors and a 65% 5-year survival rate. They used cobalt 60 and 6 MV, a wedged pair with an electron boost, and 160 cGy twice per day to a total dose of 6000 to 7800 cGy.[5]

Maxillary sinuses. Maxillary sinus disease accounts for 80% of all sinus cancers. Patients with this type of cancer have a history of long-standing sinusitis, nasal obstructions, and bloody discharge. These cancers are mostly squamous cell carcinomas and tend to invade the floor of the orbit, eth-

AJCC Clinical Staging System for Carcinomas of the Salivary Glands

Primary tumor (T)

Tx	Primary tumor cannot be assessed
T_0	No evidence of primary tumor
T_1	Tumor 2 cm or less in greatest dimension
T_2	Tumor more than 2 cm but not more than 4 cm in greatest dimension
T_3	Tumor more than 4 cm but not more than 6 cm in greatest dimension
T_4	Tumor more than 6 cm in greatest dimension

Regional lymph nodes (N)

Nx	Regional lymph nodes cannot be assessed
N_0	No regional lymph node metastasis
N_1	Metastasis in a single ipsilateral lymph node, 3 cm or less in greatest dimension
N_2	Metastasis in a single ipsilateral lymph node, more than 3 cm but not more than 6 cm in greatest dimension; or in multiple ipsilateral lymph nodes, none more than 6 cm in greatest dimension; or in bilateral or contralateral lymph nodes, none more than 6 cm in greatest dimension
N_{2a}	Metastasis in a single ipsilateral lymph node more than 3 cm but not more than 6 cm in greatest dimension
N_{2b}	Metastasis in multiple ipsilateral lymph nodes, none more than 6 cm in greatest dimension
N_{2c}	Metastasis in bilateral or contralateral lymph nodes, none more than 6 cm in greatest dimension
N_3	Metastasis in a lymph node more than 6 cm in greatest dimension

Distant metastasis (M)

Mx	Presence of distant metastasis cannot be assessed
M_0	No distant metastasis
M_1	Distant metastasis

Stage grouping

Stage I	T_{1a}	N_0	M_0
	T_{2a}	N_0	M_0
Stage II	T_{1b}	N_0	M_0
	T_{2b}	N_0	M_0
	T_{3b}	N_0	M_0
Stage III	T_{3b}	N_0	M_0
	T_{4a}	N_0	M_0
	Any T	N_1	M_0 (except T_{4b})
Stage IV	T_{4b}	Any N	M_0
	Any T	N_2	M_0
	Any T	N_3	M_0
	Any T	Any N	M_1

From Beahrs OH et al, editors: *AJCC manual for staging of cancer,* ed 4, Philadelphia, 1992, JB Lippincott.

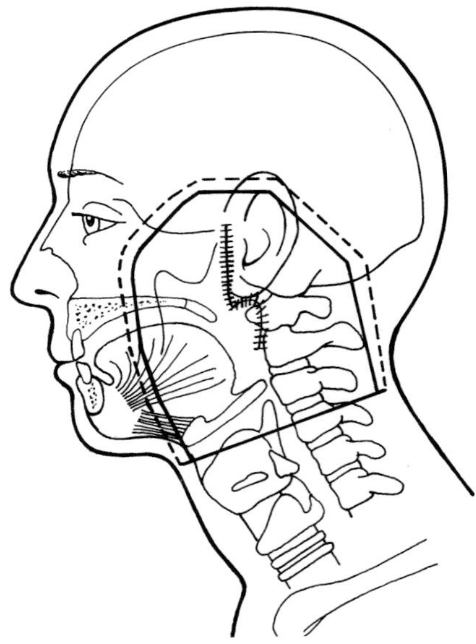

Fig. 8-24 A portal arrangement for a postoperative parotid gland. The solid line represents the photon field. The dashed line represents an electron field with a 1-cm overlap (From Levitt SH, Tapley N: *Technological basis of radiation therapy,* Philadelphia, 1992, Lea & Febiger.)

moid sinuses, hard palate, and zygomatic arch. Displacement of the eye is common. The box on p. 169 gives the AJCC TNM classification.[5]

Conventional tomography provides good detail of bony destruction, soft tissue damage, and brain or orbital spread. However, it is not used for diagnostic staging. CT and MRI are reserved for staging. Cervical nodal spread is uncommon, but if it is present, the submandibular node is the first station involved and will be treated.

The principle method of treatment is combined surgery and radiation therapy. Preoperative doses of 6000 cGy are delivered via an external beam, wedged-pair technique. Lateral and anterior ports are custom designed to follow the expected route of spread. If the orbit is involved, eye blocking should not be used. Care should be taken to miss the cord and contralateral lens. Angling the anterior beam a few degrees off the vertical spares brain tissue.

If the nasal cavity is at risk, bolus material should be inserted to improve dose homogeneity. Angling the lateral port a few degrees off the horizontal plane spares the contralateral optic nerve and lens.

The 5-year survival rate is poor because of the patient's history of recurrent disease and invasion of the brain and skull. An overall survival rate of 20% to 30% is expected.[10] Fortunately, this is a rare type of head and neck cancer.

Role of radiation therapist

The extent of radiation therapy side effects varies from patient to patient. During the initial consultation the radiation therapist should inform the patient of all possible

AJCC Staging System for Cancer of the Maxillary Antrum

Primary tumor (T)

Tx Primary tumor cannot be assessed
T_0 No evidence of primary tumor
Tis Carcinoma in situ
T_1 Tumor limited to the antral mucosa, with no erosion or destruction of bone
T_2 Tumor with erosion or destruction of the infrastructure,* including the hard palate and/or middle nasal meatus
T_3 Tumor invasion of any of the following: skin of cheek, posterior wall of maxillary sinus, floor or medial wall of orbit, or anterior ethmoid sinus
T_4 Tumor invasion of orbital contents and/or any of the following: cribriform plate, posterior ethmoid or sphenoid sinuses, nasopharynx, soft palate, pterygomaxillary or temporal fossae, or base of skull

Regional lymph nodes (N)

NX Regional lymph nodes cannot be assessed
N_0 No regional lymph node metastasis
N_1 Metastasis in a single ipsilateral lymph node, 3 cm or less in greatest dimension
N_2 Metastasis in a single ipsilateral lymph node, more than 3 cm but not more than 6 cm in greatest dimension; or in bilateral or contralateral lymph nodes, none more than 6 cm in greatest dimension
N_{2a} Metastasis in a single ipsilateral lymph node more than 3 cm but not more than 6 cm in greatest dimension
N_{2b} Metastasis in multiple ipsilateral lymph nodes, none more than 6 cm in greatest dimension
N_{2c} Metastasis in bilateral or contralateral lymph nodes, none more than 6 cm in greatest dimension
N_3 Metastasis in a lymph node more than 6 cm in greatest dimension

Distant metastasis (M)

MX Presence of distant metastasis cannot be assessed
M_0 No distant metastasis
M_1 Distant metastasis

Stage grouping

Stage 0	Tis	N_0	M_0
Stage I	T_1	N_0	M_0
Stage II	T_2	N_1	M_0
Stage III	T_3	N_0	M_0
	T_1	N_1	M_0
	T_2	N_1	M_0
	T_3	N_1	M_0
Stage IV	T_4	N_0	M_0
	T_4	N_1	M_0
	Any T	N_2	M_0
	Any T	N_3	M_0
	Any T	any N	M_1

Modified from Beahrs OH et al, editors: *AJCC manual for staging of cancer,* ed 4, Philadelphia, 1992, JB Lippincott.
*Ohngren's line joins the medial canthus of the eye with the angle of the mandible denoting the position of an imaginary plane that divides the maxillary antrum into the anteroinferior portion (infrastructure) and superoposterior portion (suprastructure).

complications that can arise from the treatment or disease process. The entire oncology team is responsible for assessing the efficiency of the treatment in terms of the health and well-being of the patient. Head and neck cancer patients need to know that the side effects encountered are site specific and related to dose dependency. Patients also need to understand that communicating any discomfort they are experiencing to the radiation therapists or other team members is vital to good cancer treatment management of the head and neck region.

Radiation therapists should encourage patients to express any fears they have about the side effects, disease outcomes, or procedures that can alter speech, food intake, or breathing. Patients should also be informed that follow-up after treatment is an important aspect of head and neck cancer because they are at risk for a recurrence and the development of a second primary within 2 years. Radiation therapists should give patients explicit instructions regarding physical changes to look for in tissue color, texture, new growths, or unexplained pain. Patients should be instructed to seek medical advice as soon as possible.

Some patients undergoing treatment to the head and neck region have redness and irritation in the mouth, a dry mouth, difficulty swallowing, and changes in tastes and sensation. The therapist should instruct the patient to try and not let these conditions interfere with their eating habits.

Earaches (caused by hardened ear wax), jaw stiffness, hoarseness, and loss of facial and scalp hair are also possible side effects. Gums and teeth are especially at a high risk for problems from external beam irradiation. Radiation therapists should introduce head and neck cancer patients to a dental-hygiene program that helps prevent tooth caries and infection. Radiation increases the chance of getting cavities. Bad teeth are usually extracted before radiation therapy. The box on the left side of p. 170 contains a representative oral program.

Soreness of the throat and mouth is expected to appear in the second or third week of standard fractionated external beam therapy. Minor irritations often remain for about a month after treatments end. Xylocain viscus or dyclonine are good liquid pain relievers. Over-the-counter medication (approved by a physician) such as Ora-gel for babies and ambersol can provide temporary relief.

Denture wearers probably notice that the dentures no longer fit as a result of swelling of the gums. If in the way, dentures usually should be removed during therapy. The patient cannot risk getting any infection in the oral cavity.

Loss of saliva is a common side effect of radiation to the oral cavity. Sipping cool carbonated drinks during the day may alleviate some of this. Lemon drops (sugar free) help promote saliva production and taste.

The radiation therapist should instruct the patient to choose foods that are easy to eat. As chewing and swallowing become more difficult, the therapist should recommend more liquid, semisolid meals moistened with sauces, and gravies to make eating easier. Artificial saliva is a possible remedy; a physician should be consulted.

The therapist should instruct the patient about wound care, cleaning of tracheostomies, and speech-rehabilitation options. The therapist should be mindful of any weeping surgical sites or a change in the healing process that can indicate an infection. To better facilitate communication with a speech-impaired patient, the therapist should provide a pad and pencil. Hand signals should be arranged with the patient in the event something goes wrong in the treatment room during beam-on conditions. The radiation therapist must understand that the head and neck cancer patient will undergo some structural and functional losses; the therapist should be ready to answer any questions or provide for the specific needs of the patient.

Skin care during treatment is also an important tool of patient care management. The box below gives some general recommendations for skin care during external beam irradiation of the head and neck region.

Finally, the radiation therapist needs to know the dose limitations to the specific tissues included in the typical head and neck port. Table 8-3 gives an approximate dose-tissue response schedule for a conventional fractionation scheme.[2] **Accelerated fractionation** (fractional doses [smaller than conventional] given two to three times daily, increasing the total dose in the same overall time), or hyperfractionation, schemes make the side effects appear much earlier. Therefore the total dose received to the normal tissue is reduced.

Recommended Oral-Hygiene Program

- Clean teeth and gums daily with a soft brush after meals.
- Use fluoride toothpaste or fluoride rinses daily.
- Floss daily.
- Rinse the mouth with salt and a baking-soda solution (1 qt water, 1/2 Tsp salt, 1/2 Tsp baking soda).
- See a dentist regularly during treatment for a teeth and gum examination.

To reduce the severity of any head and neck complication, the patient should be encouraged to avoid the following:

- Spicy hot foods, course or raw vegetables, dry crackers, chips, and nuts
- Smoking, chewing tobacco, and alcohol
- Sugary snacks
- Commercial mouthwash that contains alcohol because it drys the mouth
- Cold foods and drinks

Recommended Skin-Care Program

- Wash the skin with luke-warm water, pat dry, and do not wash off marks.
- Use mild soaps (e.g., Basis, Neutrogena).
- Use water-based lotions or creams (e.g., Aquaphor, Eucerin).
- Avoid lotions with perfume and deodorants.
- Avoid direct sunlight.
- Do not use straight razors.
- Avoid tight-fitting collars and hat brims.
- Do not use aftershave lotions or perfumes.
- Apply only nonadherent, hydrophilic dressings to wounds.

Table 8-3 Approximate dose-tissue response schedule for a conventional fractionation scheme

Response	Dose (cGy)
Dry mouth	2000
Erythema	2000
Brachial plexus	5500
Spinal cord	4500
Lhermitte's sign	2000-3000
Mandible, teeth and gums	5000-6000
Mucositis	3000
Ears	4000
Cataracts	500-1000
Dry eye	4000+
Optic nerve	5000
Retina	5000
Trismus	6000
Laryngitis	5000

Review Questions

Fill in the Blank

1. Identify the signs and symptoms associated with a primary of each of the following:
   a. Oral cavity________________________
   b. Larynx________________________
   c. Nasopharynx________________________
2. Most cancers of the tongue are found anatomically ________________________.

Essay

3. Describe the TNM classification for laryngeal cancer.
4. Identify the four major anatomical borders of the nasopharynx for treatment with external beam irradiation.
5. Identify the head and neck cancer that demonstrates the highest incidence of nodal metastases.
6. At what vertebral level does the epiglottis lie?
7. Name four treatment complications that are expected from radiation therapy of the head and neck region.
8. Identify two precancerous lesions associated with malignant head and neck cancers.
9. Identify three major nodal chains of the head and neck region. Which chain drains the majority of this region?
10. Identify the 12 cranial nerves and their functions.

Questions to Ponder

1. A majority of head and neck cancers are grouped together by anatomical site. Why then is there such diverse difference in biological and clinical behavior between the same cell type and structures that are only a few millimeters apart?
2. What is the reason for the high incidence of a second primary for patients with early-stage squamous cell disease that was cured?
3. Are there biological markers that can be identified early and will decrease the toxicity and morbidity from treatments?
4. Will nonstandard radiation therapy fractionation schemes improve survivability at the expense of second malignancies?
5. Does chemotherapy have a role in the elective treatment of premalignant conditions seen in head and neck disease?

REFERENCES

1. American Cancer Society: *Cancer manual,* Atlanta, 1996, The Society.
2. Beahrs OH et al, editors: *AJCC manual for staging of cancer,* ed 4, Philadelphia, 1992, JB Lippincott.
3. Bentel GC: *Treatment planning and dose calculation in radiation oncology,* ed 4, New York, 1989, Pergamon.
4. Bragg DG, Rubin P: *Oncologic imaging,* Elms Ford, New York, 1985, Pergamon.
5. Cox JD: *Moss' radiation oncology: rationale, technique, and results,* ed 6, St Louis, 1989, Mosby.
6. Devita VT: *Cancer principles and practice of oncology,* ed 3, Philadelphia, 1989, JB Lippincott.
7. Devita VT Jr, Hellman S, Rosenberg SA: *Cancer principles and practice of oncology,* Philadelphia, 1982, JB Lippincott.
8. Holleb A, Fink D, Murphy GP: *American Cancer Society textbook of clinical oncology,* Atlanta, 1993, The American Cancer Society.
9. Levitt, SH, Tapley N: *Technological basis of radiation therapy: practical clinical applications,* ed 2, Philadelphia, 1992, Lea & Febiger.
10. Rubin P: *Clinical oncology,* ed 7, Philadelphia, 1993, WB Saunders.
11. Stryker JA: *Clinical oncology for students of radiation therapy technology,* St Louis, 1992, Green.

BIBLIOGRAPHY

Al-Sarraf M: Head and neck cancer: chemotherapy concepts, *Semin Oncol* 15, 1988.

Brady-Davis LW: Treatment of head and cancer by radiation therapy, *Semin Oncol* 15, 1988.

Chaffee EE: *Basic physiology and anatomy,* ed 3, Philadelphia, 1974, JB Lippincott.

Del Regato JA: *Cancer: diagnosis, treatment and prognosis,* ed 6, St Louis, 1985, Mosby.

Fletcher GH: Basic principles of combination or irradiation and surgery, *Intl J Radiat Oncol Bio Phys* 19, 1972.

Fletcher GH: *Textbook of radiotherapy,* ed 3, Philadelphia, 1980, Lea & Febiger.

Perez CA: *Principles and practice of radiation oncology,* ed 2, Philadelphia, 1992, Lippincott.

Sheldon H: *Boyd's introduction to the study of disease,* ed 10, Philadelphia, 1988, Lea & Febiger.

Strauss MB: *Familiar medical quotations,* Boston, 1968, Little, Brown.

Walter J, Miller H, Bomford CK: *A short textbook of radiotherapy,* ed 4, New York, Churchill L ivingstone.

Wang CC: *Clinical radiation oncology: indication, techniques, and results,* Boston, 1988, PSG.

CHAPTER

9

Central Nervous System

Linda Langlin

Outline

Key terms

Blood-brain barrier (BBB)
Cerebrospinal fluid (CSF)
Debulking surgery
Drop metastases
Friable tumors
Gadolinium
Karnofsky Performance Scale (KPS)
Radiation necrosis
Radiosensitizers
Regeneration

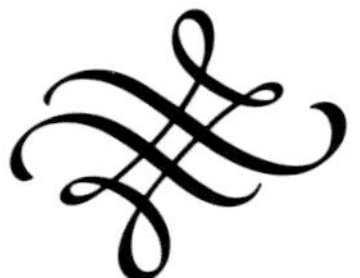

Central nervous system (CNS) tumors include brain and spinal cord tumors. The tumors can be primary or secondary (metastatic) and benign or malignant. Some are regarded as benign because of slow growth rates and the way they respond to therapy.[20]

In recent years, radiation therapy has played a significant part in the treatment of CNS tumors. Radiation therapy has provided a means of increased survival time, resulted in a regression of the effects of neurological deficit, and enhanced the quality of life.[15]

Although CNS tumors rarely metastasize, they are often locally invasive and create significant problems. Structures that become involved with these neoplasms are not capable of **regeneration** (repair or regrowth). Tumors of the CNS, even if benign histologically, are considered malignant in part because of their inaccessible location.[16] As shown in Table 9-1, 14 different cell types are believed to produce CNS and spinal axis tumors. Because CNS tumors arise in different areas of the cranium and spinal axis, the belief is that different molecular and genetic mechanisms are at work during various times of life.

Currently, combined modality treatment (including surgery, radiation therapy, and chemotherapy) offers the most hope for patients afflicted with CNS tumors.

CANCER OF THE CNS

Epidemiology

Approximately 15,000 cases of primary brain tumors and 4,000 cases of spinal cord tumors are diagnosed annually in the United States. Brain tumors account for 1.5% of all malignan-

Table 9-1 Classification of primary intracranial tumors by cell of origin

Normal cell	Tumor
Astrocyte	Astrocytoma, glioblastoma multiforme
Ependymocyte	Ependymoma, ependymoblastoma
Oligodendrocyte	Oligodendroglioma
Arachnoidal fibroblasts	Meningioma
Nerve cell or neuroblast	Ganglioneuroma, neuroblastoma, retinoblastoma
External granular cell or neuroblast	Medulloblastoma
Schwann's cell	Schwannoma (neurinoma)
Melanocyte	Melanotic carcinoma
Choroid epithelial cell	Choroid plexus papilloma or carcinoma
Pituitary	Adenoma
Endothelial or stromal cell	Hemangioblastoma
Primitive germ cells	Germinoma, pinealoma, teratoma, cholesteatoma
Pineal parenchymal cell	Pineocytoma
Notochordal remnant	Chordoma

Modified from Levins V, Guten P, Leibel S: Neoplasms of CNS. In DeVita VT, Hellman S, Rosenberg SA: *Cancer: principles and practice of oncology,* ed 4, Philadelphia, 1993, JB Lippincott.

cies. About 80% of CNS tumors involve the brain, whereas 20% involve the spinal cord. CNS neoplasms result in 11,000 deaths annually. This number is 20% of all cancer deaths.

The incidence rate is 5 per 100,000 people and varies according to race, gender, and age. Brain tumors are the second leading cause of death in children (behind leukemia). The mortality associated with these tumors is due in part to a poor prognosis after the diagnosis.[22] Males are affected more often than females. Astrocytomas occur more frequently in males, whereas meningiomas are more common in females. Incidence rates are also higher among whites than among blacks.

Age is a dominant variable, with the incidence of CNS tumors in older patients appearing to rise. Most CNS tumors occur in persons between the ages of 50 and 80. The incidence is above 20 per 100,000 for older men and fewer than 2 per 100,000 for children under age 15.[15] The majority of brain tumors occur in two age peaks: childhood (3 to 12 years) and later in life, as previously mentioned.[10,25]

Approximately 20% of all pediatric malignancies are brain tumors. Pediatric tumors differ in histology and behavior from those of adults. An increase in the frequency of adult tumors may be the result of improved diagnostic methods. Because the rise began around the time of the introduction of computed tomography (CT) scanning, some think the increase may be largely the result of this new diagnostic tool. Whether this increase is due to primary disease or metastatic disease is the question. The increase may be the result of metastatic brain lesions with primary cancers that remain undiagnosed.[13]

Sampling errors also affect these numbers. Many variables are involved in reporting CNS neoplasms. Stumbling blocks to accurate reporting include geographical and ethnic variations and discrepancies among institutions in the way cases are reported. Worldwide, patterns due to geography or ethnicity are difficult to recognize because of different recording methods and the lack of a single pathological classification system.

Multiple tumors are included in the CNS category. However, gliomas comprise 50% of all primary brain tumors in adults.[18] The most common location of these tumors is the cerebrum, which is the largest part of the brain and consists of two hemispheres. The functions of the cerebrum include interpretation of sensory impulses and voluntary muscular activities; it is the center for memory, learning, reasoning, judgment, intelligence, and emotions. Gliomas commonly occur in persons between the ages of 40 and 74.[19]

Approximately 45% of childhood tumors are astrocytomas, with the majority involving the cerebellum and to a lesser degree, the brain stem. The cerebellum is the part of the brain that controls skeletal muscles and plays a role in the coordination of voluntary muscular movements. It forms the largest portion of the rhombencephalon, or the primary division of the embryonic brain.

Long-term survival for patients with CNS tumors is uncommon. Factors such as the patient's age, Karnofsky status, and neurological signs and symptoms at the time of diagnosis are important in the chances for survival.

Most spinal-axis tumors are extradural (on the outside of or unconnected to the dura mater). They are predominantly metastatic carcinomas, lymphomas, or sarcomas; they are rarely chordomas. Most primary spinal-axis tumors are intradural (within or enclosed by the dura mater).

Etiology

Little is known concerning the etiology, development, and growth mechanisms of CNS tumors. Increasingly, a genetic link is thought to exist. Weingart and Brem[24] have noted recent reports implicating several growth factors, protein kinase C, and the p53 gene with tumor growth and progression. However, absolute proof of a genetic predisposition for all CNS tumors in unavailable. According to Filippini and Artuso,[11] fewer than 1% of patients are known to have inherited disorders, although certain genetic disorders have been associated with CNS tumors.

Tuberous sclerosis (a disease involving the CNS and cutaneous sites) is associated with astrocytomas, glioblastomas, ependymomas, and ganglioneuromas. Von Recklinghausen's disease is associated with meningiomas, multiple ependymomas, and optic gliomas. It is marked by the occurrence of multiple neurofibromata on the skin along the course of the nerves. Von Hippel-Lindau disease is associated with hemangioblastomas and characterized by lesions involving the retina, the cerebellum, and sometimes the spinal cord. Brain tumors are also associated with polyposis coli in Turcot's syndrome.

Because gliomas are the most common type of CNS tumors, they have received the most attention in studies focusing on the identification of amplified genes. The first gene shown to be amplified was the epidermal growth factor receptor (EGFR) gene.[8] Cytogenic observation provided the first evidence that gene amplification may be occurring in glioblastomas. Studies have now shown that gene amplification occurs in up to 50% of glioblastomas.[3,4]

The p53 gene on chromosome 17 encodes a nuclear phosphoprotein that may be a suppressor gene. Gliomas have been associated with mutations and deletions of chromosome 17. Studies indicate that this occurs more often in high-grade than low-grade gliomas. These mutations and deletions are also involved in tumor progression from low- to high-grade gliomas.[24]

Chromosome abnormalities have been identified in high-grade and low-grade tumors. Studies to date suggest that low-grade tumors tend to have fewer chromosome abnormalities than high-grade tumors.[19]

Protein kinase C has also been associated with the growth of gliomas. Activity rates of protein kinase C are increased in malignant gliomas, compared with normal brain, and are associated with proliferation rates.

Environmental factors also may play a role in the etiology of CNS tumors. The association between chemical exposure and brain tumors is limited to a few occupations. Exposure to pesticides, herbicides, fertilizers, petrochemical industries, and health professions result in a higher incidence rate than normal. The only documented link associates gliomas with vinyl chloride and rubber manufacturing industries. The incidence of increased brain tumors has been the same for both genders in most countries; therefore occupational exposure is not a likely explanation for the increases.[13] Studies revealing potential links to N-nitroso compounds, power magnetic fields, dental amalgrams, x-rays, and passive smoking have generated considerable interest.[1] Occupational exposure to metals, paints, and some hydrocarbons is associated with excess risks that contribute to parental exposure as an added risk for the later development of CNS tumors. The prenatal environment may influence subsequent carcinogenesis if exposure to N-nitroso compounds is involved. This has been demonstrated in animals through brain tumors that are experimentally induced by transplacental exposure to these compounds.[11] Cell change may appear years later through the production of tumors in offspring. Excessive numbers of tumors have resulted from postnatal exposure to high doses of irradiation for tinea capitis, which is a fungus skin disease of the scalp similar to ringworm.

Viral infections have recently been associated with the development of CNS neoplasia in animals. Patients who have CNS lymphomas also seem to have a high incidence of the Epstein-Barr virus. Trauma does not seem to influence the incidence to CNS neoplasia. However, trauma to the brain can cause a breakdown of the **blood-brain barrier (BBB)**. After such a breakdown, normally restricted substances are allowed to pass into the brain tissue.

Only a small incidence of CNS tumors occurring after treatment for another malignancy has been documented. Patients with acquired immunodeficiency syndrome (AIDS) and those receiving transplants have an increased risk for primary CNS lymphoma, but not for gliomas. Because these patients are immunologically compromised, whether this problem is a cause or an effect needs further investigation.

The oncogene theory remains unproved in relation to intracranial tumors.[17] The oncogene theory offers an explanation for the neoplastic transformation of the host cell.

Prognostic indicators

Several factors have been identified as prognostic indicators for CNS disorders. The three most important factors are age, the Karnofsky score, and the size of the remaining tumor after debulking surgery.

The prognosis tends to be better in younger patients, with one exception. Children under the age of 4 present a particular problem with respect to a treatment regimen. Therapy must be modified because of the developing brain, which is more sensitive to radiation; therefore treatment in children less than 4 years old needs to be avoided. By age 4 the child's brain development and growth is basically completed.

Doses must be modified to prevent later learning difficulties. Late effects after CNS treatment in children is an area of concern. A study by Avizonis et al. [2] focused on several areas of interest. Mean IQ scores after treatment indicated slightly decreased scores as whole-brain dose radiation increased. However, learning disabilities can be overcome so that the children can go on to lead productive lives. Another area monitored in the study, the regrowth of hair, appeared to be dose related, with diminished regrowth as the dose increased. The measured late effects after radiation did not seem to vary with regard to age at the time of treatment, gender, tumor type, or tumor location.

Chemotherapy or a routine follow-up after surgery is the preferred manner of treatment. More aggressive treatment is reserved until the child reaches age 4 or the tumor progresses.

A higher age is generally indicative of a worse prognosis because of two factors. With advanced age the rate of incidence increases, and an older patient with a CNS disorder lacks the ability to adapt.

The mortality rate for both genders and for blacks and whites has increased since 1950, and that trend seems to be continuing. The mortality rate for adolescents and young adults remains unchanged or has decreased slightly over the past 30 years.

Histopathology is more important than anatomical staging in determining the outcome, behavior, prognosis, and treatment plan. Of critical importance in staging is the tumor grade, as opposed to the tumor size. The location of the tumor is of great importance, serving as a natural prognostic indicator for survival time and neurological deficits.

Benign tumors cause effects by pressure, whereas malignant or invasive tumors affect the patient by causing pressure and functional destruction.

The **Karnofsky Performance Scale (KPS)** measures the neurological and functional status, allowing for measurements of the quantity and quality of neurological defects. The KPS ranges from 0 to 100 and is measured in decades. Patients who are able to work have scores in the 80, 90, or 100 range. Patients who are unable to work but can still care for themselves have scores in the 50 to 70 range (see the box to the right). Patients who are chronically ill from the disease process have scores of 40 or below.

Tumor grade rather than size is the primary factor involved with staging. The tumors are normally grouped into benign or low-grade and malignant or high-grade categories. The presence or absence of necrosis in a tumor has prognostic significance.

Necrosis is the death of a cell or cell group resulting from disease or injury. The process is caused by the action of enzymes and can also affect part of a structure or an organ. Low-grade tumors have cellularity patterns that look similar to those found in reactive hyperplasia, whereas marked cellularity has been recognized in high-grade tumors, with necrosis being the most important factor. Tumor grade is also an indicator of survival rates; the higher the grade, the shorter the survival time.

A biopsy is indicated if a lesion is deep seated, is probably malignant, and occurs in older or debilitated patients who cannot tolerate a surgical procedure. The risks of a biopsy include approximately a 30% rate of inadequate diagnosis.[16] Other risks include hemorrhage in the area of the biopsy and postoperative swelling. A simple biopsy alone has no therapeutic value and therefore offers a worse prognosis than a partial or total surgical resection. Debulking procedures are performed if the tumor location is accessible and the tumor volume is large. Debulking accomplishes a reduction in tumor size and the opportunity to obtain a pathological diagnosis. A stereotactic biopsy allows all areas of the tumor and its borders to be studied before surgery causes changes in the appearance of the tumor.

Symptoms of long duration are thought to represent a slow-growing tumor; therefore the survival time is lengthened. **Friable tumors** (those easily broken or pulverized) indicate a worse prognosis. If a tumor is friable, a higher grade is indicated. Postoperative residual tumor is considered a poor prognostic indicator for survival. Complete resection is associated with a longer survival time. Partial removal of the tumor does not seem to enhance the patient's chances for survival. The survival time is longer in patients who do not exhibit postoperative performance deficits. Although CT and magnetic resonance imaging (MRI) scans done after an operation can show an apparently normal study, residual tumors have been found in those areas. Almost all patients experience a recurrence (with high-grade tumors) postoperatively, and 80% of all recurrences are within a 2-cm margin.[5]

Karnofsky Performance Scale

Performance criteria

Able to carry on normal activity; no special care needed	100	Normal; no complaints; no evidence of disease
	90	Ability to carry on normal activity; minor signs or symptoms of disease
	80	Normal activity with effort; some signs or symptoms of disease
Unable to work; able to live at home and care for most personal needs; a varying amount of assistance needed	70	Self-care; inability to carry on normal activity or do active work
	60	Occasional care for most needs required
	50	Considerable assistance and frequent medical care required
	40	Disabled; special care and assistance required
Unable to care for self; required equivalent of institutional or hospital care; disease may be progressing rapidly	30	Severely disabled; hospitalization indicated, although death not imminent
	20	Extremely sick; hospitalization necessary; active supportive treatment necessary
	10	Moribund; fatal processes progressing rapidly
	0	Dead

Performance scale (Eastern Cooperative Oncology Group)

Grade	
0	Fully active; able to carry on all predisease activities without restriction (Karnofsky score of 90 to 100)
1	Restricted in physically strenuous activity, but ambulatory and able to carry out work of a light or sedentary nature, such as light housework or office work (Karnofsky score of 70 to 80)
3	Capable of only limited self-care; confined to bed or chair 50% or more of waking hours (Karnofsky score of 30 to 40)
4	Completely disabled; Unable to carry on any self-care; totally confined to bed or chair (Karnofsky score of 10 to 20)

Modified from Carter S et al: *Principles of cancer treatment,* New York, 1992, McGraw-Hill.

Radiation therapy provides an effective form of treatment for CNS tumors. This treatment can cure certain tumors and is associated with longer survival times for patients with other tumors.

Chemotherapy produces a response in about one third of the patients. However, chemotherapeutic options are limited in CNS tumors. The blood-brain barrier is a limiting factor in the delivery of chemotherapeutic drugs.

Anatomy and lymphatics

The brain, a mushroom-shaped organ, is one of the largest organs in the body (Fig. 9-1), weighing approximately 3 pounds. It is composed of two hemispheres contained in the brain case, or cranium. The cranial bones, meninges, and **cerebrospinal fluid (CSF)** provide protection for the brain. The principal parts of the brain are the brain stem, diencephalon, cerebrum, and cerebellum. Brain vesicles are formed during the embryonic-growth period and serve as the beginnings of various parts of the brain.

The ventricles are four cavities that form the communication network with each other, the center canal of the spinal cord, and the subarachnoid space. They are filled with CSF. These cavities are the right and left lateral ventricles and the third and fourth ventricles. The lateral ventricles are located below the corpus callosum and extend from front to back. Each opens into the third ventricle. The lateral ventricles are able to communicate with the third ventricle via the interventricular foramen, which is a small oval opening. The third ventricle is located in the diencephalon, or afterbrain. The diencephalon is a slit between and inferior to the right and left halves of the thalmus. The hypothalmus forms its floor. The cerebral aquaduct is a canal that passes between the third and fourth ventricles. The fourth ventricle lies between the cerebellum and inferior brain stem. Three small openings also allow the CSF to pass into the subarachnoid space. The openings also allow communication with the cord and subarachnoid space.

The supratentorial and infratentorial regions comprise the two major intracranial compartments. The tentorium (a fold of dura mater, or the outer covering of the brain) separates these compartments. It passes transversely across the posterior cranial fossa in the transverse fissure and acts as a line of separation between the occipital lobe of the cerebrum and the upper cerebellum. The cerebral hemispheres and the sella, pineal, and upper brain-stem regions are located in the supratentorial region. The infratentorial region, which leads to the upper spinal cord, houses the brain stem, pons, medulla, and cerebellum. The brain is surrounded by the pia mater, arachnoid, and dura mater.

The CNS is composed of 40% gray matter and 60% white matter. The gray matter contains the nerve cells and related processes. It forms the cortex, or outer part of the cerebrum, and surrounds the white matter. The white matter is composed of bundles of nerve fibers, axons carrying impulses away from the cell body, and dendrites carrying impulses toward the cell body. The nerve cells are the control centers. The spinal cord is also composed of a gray substance that forms the inner core, which contains the nerve cells. The outer layer, or white substance, is the location of the nerve fibers. The gray matter varies at different levels of the spinal cord. The blood supply for the brain comes from the internal carotid arteries and vertebral arteries via the circle of Willis. The blood that enters the brain contains glucose, which is the primary source of energy for the brain cells. If the blood supply to the brain

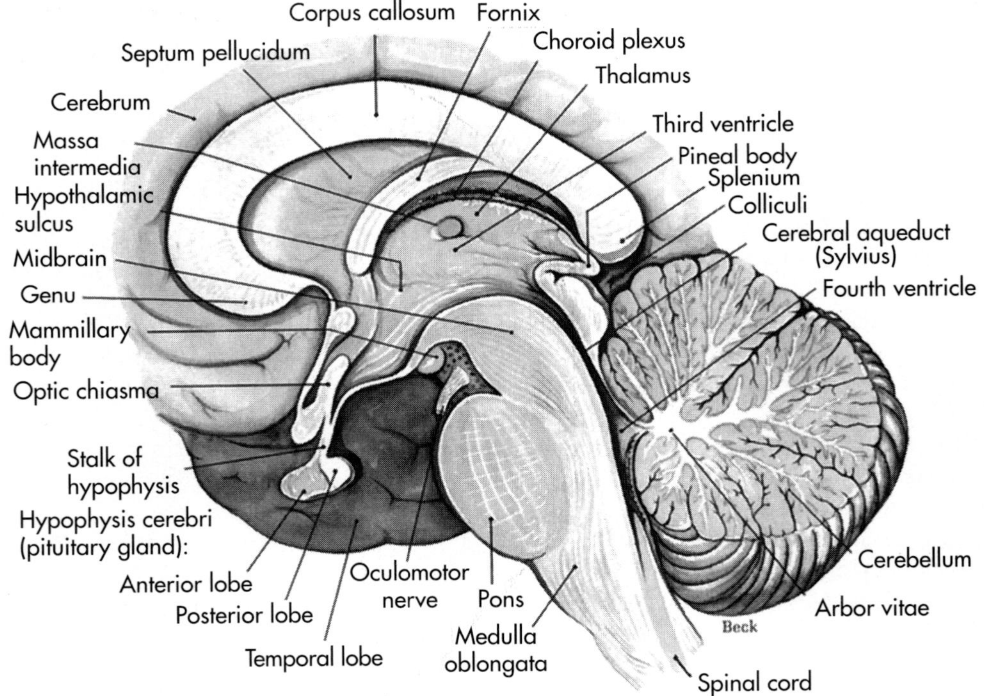

Fig. 9-1 Sagittal section through the midline of the brain. (From Ackerman and del Regato's *Cancer: diagnosis, treatment, and prognosis,* ed 6, St Louis, 1985, Mosby.)

is not continuous, dizziness, convulsions, or mental confusion may result.

The spinal cord is the continuation of the medulla oblongata and forms the inferior portion of the brain stem. The anterior and lateral portions contain motor neurons and tracts, whereas the posterior portions contain the sensory tracts. The motor neurons are nerve cells that convey impulses from the brain to the cord. This system allows communication between the spinal cord and various parts of the brain. The cord continues down to the level of the first and second lumbar vertebrae. From the spinal cord come 31 pairs of nerves. The spinal cord is surrounded by the same material that surrounds the brain. The CSF flows between the arachnoid and pia arachnoid. Blood is supplied to the cord from the vertebral arteries and radicular branches of the cervical, intercostal, lumbar, and sacral arteries (Fig. 9-2). No lymphatic channels exist in the brain substance.

The BBB, which hinders the penetration of some substances into the brain and CSF, exists between the vascular system and brain. Its purpose is to protect the brain from potentially toxic compounds. Substances that can pass through the BBB must be lipid or water soluble. These substances require a carrier molecule to cross the barrier by active transport. Lipid-soluble substances include alcohol, nicotine, and heroin. Examples of water-soluble substances are glucose, some amino acids, and sodium. Various drugs pass the barrier with varying degrees of difficulty, (but never easily). Tumor cells infiltrating normal tissue cannot be reached by drugs that do not cross the BBB (Fig. 9-3).

Local invasion and CSF seeding provide the major patterns of spread for CNS tumors. These tumors tend to have cells that can invade normal brain. **Drop metastases** occur via the CSF and can form secondary tumors. The confines of the brain itself limit the spread of disease, but local recurrence is a major concern. Secondary seedings may grow along nerve roots, causing pain or cord compression. Although the lumbosacral area is the most frequent site of CSF seeding, any area along the spinal axis can become involved. Hematogenous spread is rare.

Natural history of disease

Primary CNS neoplasms tend to spread invasively because they do not form a natural capsule that inhibits growth. These neoplasms are unique because they do not metastasize through a lymphatic drainage system and rarely metastasize outside the CNS. Two possible explanations for this have been offered: (1) The CNS has a "relatively immunologically privileged status," and (2) the life expectancy after the diagnosis of highly malignant tumors is so short that systemic metastases do not have time to occur.[16]

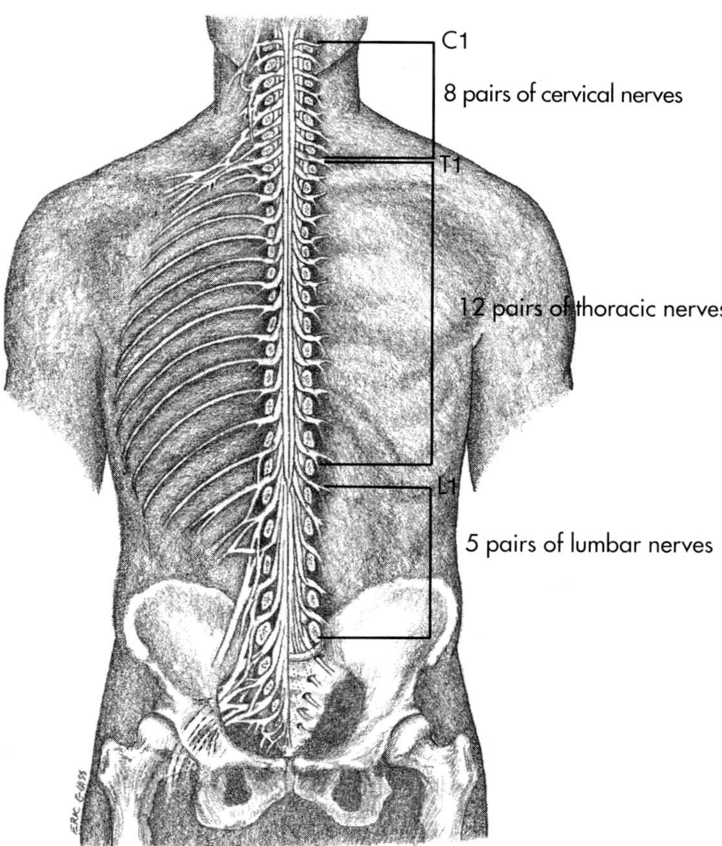

Fig. 9-2 Spinal cord and nerves.

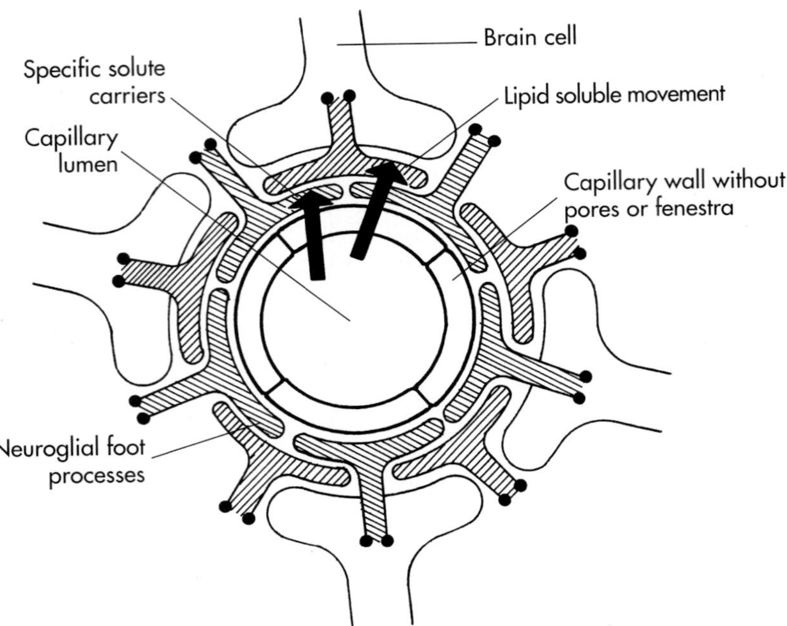

Fig. 9-3 Blood-brain barrier. (Redrawn from Maisey M, Britton KE, Gilday DL: *Clinical nuclear medicine,* ed 2, New York, 1992, Chapman and Hall.)

Occasionally, surgical intervention causes seeding to extracranial sites. After seeding, tumors such as medulloblastomas grow rapidly in extracerebral tissues.[20] The more common route of spread is via CSF to points in the CNS. The CSF is a clear, colorless fluid resembling water. The entire CNS contains 3 to 5 ounces of this fluid, which is composed of proteins, glucose, urea (a compound formed in the liver and excreted by the kidney), and salts. The CSF performs several functional roles, including buoyancy to protect the brain, a link in the control of the chemical environment of the CNS, a means of exchanging nutrients and waste products with the CNS, and a channel for intracerebral transport. High-grade tumors of the brain and meninges are able to seed into the subarachnoid and ventricular spaces by gravity of the CSF flow and cause metastasis to the spinal canal. Causes for seeding are a lack of intercellular cohesiveness and close proximity to CSF channels.

CNS tumors are characterized by their heterogeneity, which makes understanding their biology difficult. With an imroved understanding of the reason and way CNS tumors develop, grow, and progress, new treatment approaches can be developed and implemented.

Clinical presentation

As stated, the location of the tumor correlates with the presenting symptoms (Table 9-2). The initial symptom is often a headache, which is usually worse in the morning. This is due to the differences in the CSF drainage from the recumbent to upright positions. Seizures occur as a result of irritation of the CNS tissue. Difficulties with balance, gait, and ambulation are also common presenting signs. Focal signs are usually unilateral. Lobar signs can include aphasia, hemiplagia, and paresis. Ocular symptoms may result in decreased vision, oculomotor defects, proptosis, and ophthalmic defects. Other presenting signs may be expressive dysphasia, sensory dysphasia, mental and personality changes, short-term memory loss, hallucinations, and changes in intellectual functions. Increased intracranial pressure can result from the obstruction of CSF flow. The symptoms can result from direct invasion of the tissue by the tumor, destruction of brain tissue and bone, and increased pressure.

Patients with spinal cord tumors have pain, weakness, loss of sensation, and bowel- and bladder-control problems. Although pain may be an early symptom, additional symptoms may signal a cord compression or vascular problems. Weakness usually occurs in the distal part of the extremity first and progresses proximally. Rapid deterioration of motor and sensory functions soon follows. Immediate treatment is required for patients who have a sudden onset of symptoms so that permanent paralysis may be prevented (Table 9-3).

Detection and diagnosis

The composition and importance of the initial work-up are critical to a definitive diagnosis, and a complete history and physical examination are necessary. Because some CNS tumors are genetic, associated with exposure to chemicals, or related to infection, previous medical, family, and social histories are extremely important.

Information gathered from people other than the patient may also be beneficial in making a diagnosis. Mental changes, personality changes, and changes in behavior are not often noticed by the patient, but by other individuals.

Table 9-2 Symptoms, signs, and diagnostic characteristics of various intracranial tumors

Tumor	Common symptoms	Common signs	Diagnostic characteristics*
Primary			
Malignant astrocytoma	Headache, seizure, unilateral weakness, mental changes	Focal presentation related to tumor location	Enhancing CT lesion, tumor blush on angiography
Glioblastoma multiforme (GM)			Hypodense interior of enhanced CT lesion
Astrocytoma with anaplastic foci (AAF)			No hypodense interior enhanced CT lesion
Brain stem or thalamus	Nausea, vomiting, ataxia	Increased intracranial pressure (papilledema), abducens and oculomotor nerve defects	May not enhance on CT scan, biopsy may not be appropriate
Meningioma (B, M)	Localized headache, seizure	Focal presentation related to tumor location	Enhancing CT lesion associated with dura
Astrocytoma (B, M)	Headache, seizure, unilateral weakness, mental changes	Focal presentation related to tumor location	May not enhance on CT
Cerebral	Headache, seizure, unilateral weakness, mental changes	Focal presentation related to tumor location	
Cerebellar	Occipital headache	Increased intracranial pressure (papilledema), abducens and oculomotor nerve defects, coordination	
Brain stem or thalamus	Nausea, vomiting, ataxia	Increased intracranial pressure (papilledema), abducens and oculomotor nerve defects, coordination	May be seen only on MR image biopsy may not be appropriate
Optic nerve	Ocular changes	Ocular changes	Detailed CT scan
Pituitary (B, M)	Vertex headache, ocular changes	Ocular and endocrine abnormalities	Hormone analysis, resection histopathology
Medulloblastoma (M)	Morning headaches, nausea, vomiting	Coordination, increased intracranial pressure (papilledema), abducens and oculomotor nerve defects	CT scan, careful lumbar puncture recommended
Ependymoma (B, M)	Morning headaches, nausea, vomiting	Coordination, increased intracranial pressure (papilledema), abducens and oculomotor nerve defects	CT scan, careful lumbar puncture recommended
Hemangioma, arteriovenous malformation (B, M)	Migrainous headache	Focal presentation related to tumor location	Angiography, biopsy may not be appropriate
Neurilemoma, schwannoma, neurinoma (B, M)	Unilateral deafness, vertigo	Ipsilateral acoustic and facial or trigeminal nerve defects	CT scan, resection gives histopathology
Oligodendroglioma (B, M)	Insidious headache, mental changes	Focal presentation related to tumor location	Radiographic calcification
Sarcoma (M), neurofibroma (B)	Focal presentation related to tumor location	Focal presentation related to tumor location	
Pinealoma (B, M), dysgerminoma	Various (ocular, vestibular, endocrine)	Parinaud's syndrome, endocrine changes, ocular changes, increased intracranial pressure (papilledema), abducens and oculomotor nerve defects	Biopsy or resection may not be obtained, markers in CSF misinformative
Lymphoma (M), reticulum cell sarcoma, microglioma	Focal presentation related to tumor location	Focal presentation related to tumor location	Soft CT enhancement
Unspecified (B, M)	Focal presentation related to tumor location	Focal presentation related to tumor location	
Other			
Craniopharyngioma	Headache, mental changes, hemiplegia, seizure, vomiting (and ocular changes)	Cranial nerve defects (II-VII)	Bone erosion, mass effective for base of skull
Syringomyelia, syringobulbia	Pain, weakness	Sensory level, paresis	MR imaging, CT scan, myelogram, biopsy not appropriate
Midline granuloma syndrome, lymphoid granulomatosis	Various (ocular, vestibular, endocrine)	Various (ocular, vestibular, endocrine)	Diagnosis presumed
Arachnoiditis		Fasciculations	

Modified from Nelson D et al: *Clinical oncology: a multidisciplinary approach for physicians and students,* ed 7, Philadelphia, 1993, WB Saunders.
*Unless noted, a biopsy is assumed.
B, benign; *M,* malignant; *CT,* computed tomography; *MR,* Magnetic resonance.

Table 9-3 Clinical manifestations of spinal cord tumors

Location	Findings
Foramen magnum	Eleventh and twelfth cranial nerve palsies; ipsilateral arm weakness early; cerebellar ataxia; neck pain
Cervical spine	Ipsilateral arm weakness with leg and opposite arm in time; wasting and fibrillation of ipsilateral neck, shoulder girdle, and arm; decreased pain and temperature sensation in upper cervical regions early; pain in cervical distribution
Thoracic spine	Weakness of abdominal muscles; sparing of arms; unilateral root pains; sensory level with ipsilateral changes early and bilateral with time
Lumbosacral spine	Root pain in groin region and sciatic distribution; weakened proximal pelvic muscles; impotence; bladder paralysis; decreased knee jerk and brisk ankle jerks
Cauda equina	Unilateral pain in back and leg, becoming bilateral when the tumor is large; bladder and bowel paralysis

Modified from Levins V, Guten P, Leibel S: Neoplasms of CNS. In DeVita VT, Hellman S, Rosenberg SA: *Cancer: principles and practice of oncology,* ed 4, Philadelphia, 1993, JB Lippincott.

Symptoms of long duration may indicate a slow-growing tumor, whereas the sudden onset of symptoms may point toward a tumor of higher grade and size.

A neurological workup includes an evaluation in several key areas. The patient's mental condition at the time of the diagnosis often reflects changes in behavior, mood, thought, and speech patterns, and intelligence. Intellectual function is crucial, and the level of consciousness must be evaluated quickly. One test for intellectual function includes orientation to person, place, and time as well as the quickness of the responses to these questions. Further intellectual functions are determined by studying speech, memory, and logical thought processes.

Coordination skills (including walking, balance, and gait), sensations, reflexes, and motor skills are also examined. Lesions that inhibit motor function tend to affect fine motor skills first and produce a spastic paralysis. Sensory functions can be tested with a pin, temperature, and vibrations. These functions can be affected before motor skills. Reflexes may be hyperactive with intracranial tumors early but may become hypoactive in later stages.

If spinal cord tumors are suspected, the evaluation of motor, sensory, and reflex functions is also important. Sensory testing is helpful in determining the level of the lesion. Motor testing may reveal some paralysis.

An ophthalmoscopy is a test designed to check for papilledema (edema of the optic disk), which results from increased intracranial pressure. Visual fields may decrease and blind spots increase as the disease progresses. An increase in intracranial pressure is usually the result of the flow of CSF becoming obstructed. This can indicate an increase in the tumor mass. If CSF flow is obstructed or production of the fluid is changed, hydrocephalus may appear on CT scans. Infection, edema, or hemorrhage may also cause rising pressure. Edema may cause hemioparesis.

Invasion, irritation, and compression of the brain by the tumor cause symptoms. Seizures result from irritation of CNS tissue. The initial presentation of symptoms depends on edema in different locations and the room available for the tumor to expand. Benign tumors generally cause symptoms produced by pressure, whereas malignant tumors can cause pressure *and* destruction of CNS tissue. The involvement of specific regions of the brain generally produces symptoms specific to the areas controlled by those regions, thereby making tumor localization possible (Table 9-4). Therefore patients typically have symptoms that reflect the site of involvement. For example, if a tumor occurs in the frontal portion of the brain, symptoms likely to be identified include personality changes, memory defects, gait disorders, and speech difficulties. Lesions occurring in the parietal regions of the brain can produce symptoms such as loss of vision, spatial disorientation, and seizures.

Skull x-rays may show several changes that have occurred as a result of an ongoing tumor process. The pineal body may be calcified and deviated, increasing pressure may show erosion of the posterior clinoid process, or calcification of certain tumors may be seen. Calcifications, which represent slow tumor growth, occur mostly in oligodendrogliomas. Because astrocytomas occur more frequently, however, calcifications occur in about 20% of them. Radiographs may show a hammered-metal appearance, which results from chronic pressure on the inner table of the skull. This condition is seen more often in skull films of children. Erosive changes also may occur if the tumor invades the skull by eroding through the dura or outermost, toughest, and most fibrous membranes covering the brain and spinal cord.

The CT scan can distinguish the CSF, blood, edema, and tumor from normal brain tissue. The risks to the patient are minimal with CT. The use of iodine-based contrast to enhance the study increases the risk of an allergic reaction. Localization of the tumor is achievable through the use of a contrast-enhanced study. This also provides information regarding tumor extension, grade, and growth patterns. An area of higher or lower x-ray scattering power differentiates between necrosis or edema and calcification. Contrast-enhanced volume is indicative of a tumor. If used in conjunction with MRI, CT can confirm calcification or verify hemorrhage (Fig. 9-4).

MRI is useful for showing the normal anatomical structure and changes in the parenchyma. Having several advantages over CT scanning, MRI is the best noninvasive procedure. After radiation therapy or surgery, MRI provides a method of evaluating tumor response or recurrence. Iodine contrast is not necessary to perform the procedure, reducing the risk for a patient's reaction. Tumors smaller than 1 cm can be detected. With MRI, three-dimensional imaging is

Table 9-4 Brain tumor localization chart

	Frontal	Parietal	Temporal	Occipital
Symptoms	Often asymptomatic until late Symptoms of increased ICP Bradyphrenia Personality changes Libido changes Impetuous behavior Excessive jocularity Defective memory Urinary incontinence Seizures (generalized, becoming focal) Gait disorders Weakness Loss of smell Speech disorder Tonic spasms of fingers and toes	Symptomatic earlier than frontal lobes Symptoms of increased ICP Loss of vision Spatial disorientation Tingling sensation Dressing apraxia Loss of memory Seizures (focal sensory epilepsy) Weakness (anterior extension)	Speech disorders (left hemisphere dominant; not only for right-handed, but for most left-handed persons) Loss of smell (superior lesion) Disturbance in hearing, tinnitus, etc. Speech disturbance Uncinate fits Seizures with vocal phenomena in aura, including speech arrest Hallucinations, dreams, déja vu Space-perception disturbances Dysarthria Dysnomia Disturbance of comprehension	Seizures (relatively less common, but with auras including flashing lights and unformed hallucinations) Loss of vision Tingling (early) Weakness (late)
Specific cerebral functions	Behavioral problems (anterior location) Labile personality Mental lethargy Defective memory Motor aphasia	Anosognosia Autotopagnosis Visual agnosia Graphesthesia (X) Loss of memory Proprioceptive agnosia	Dysarthria Sensory asphasia Defective hearing Defective memory	Visual agnosia Visual impulses
Cranial nerve functions	Anosmia (inferior lesion) Nerve VI palsy with increased ICP Papilledema with increased ICP Foster Kennedy's syndrome Proptosis	Hemianopsia Papilledema (with increased ICP)	Superior quadrantanopsia (X) (could be homonymous hemianopsia with tumor extension) Central weakness of the cranial nerve VI Papilledema with increased ICP	Macular-sparing hemianopsia Horizontal nystagmus
Motor system	Contralateral weakness (late) Paresis (flaccid spastic) Disturbed gait (midline lesion) Automatism Persistence of induced movement (Kral's phenomenon) Diagonal rigidity [arm (X); leg (-)] Loss of skilled movement (X) Urinary incontinence (superior lesion)	Weakness Atrophy Clumsiness Dysdiadochokinesia Independent movements (unrecognized by patient)	Dysdiadochokinesia (early) Drift (secondary in later stages, involving arm more than leg)	Late appearance of motor signs, manifested by drift or dysdiadochokinesia
Sensory functions	Rare involvement initially, unless invasion of sensory area (posterior lesion)	Dysesthesias (tingling)(X) Pallesthesia (loss of vibratory sense)(X) Loss of touch, press, and position sense (X), but pain and temperative usually unaffected	Initially minimal	Somatosensory disturbances earlier than motor changes as adjacent structures are involved Visual phenomena, such as persisting images, unformed hallucinations, and aura
Reflex changes	Tonic plantar reflex Hoffmann's sign Grasp reflex Babinski's sign	Babinski's sign Hoffmann's sign	May occur contralateral to tumor	No effect in early stages

Modified from Karlsson UL et al: *Principles and practice of radiation oncology,* Philadelphia, 1992, JB Lippincott.
ICP, Intracranial pressure; *(X),* contralateral; *(-),* ipsilateral.

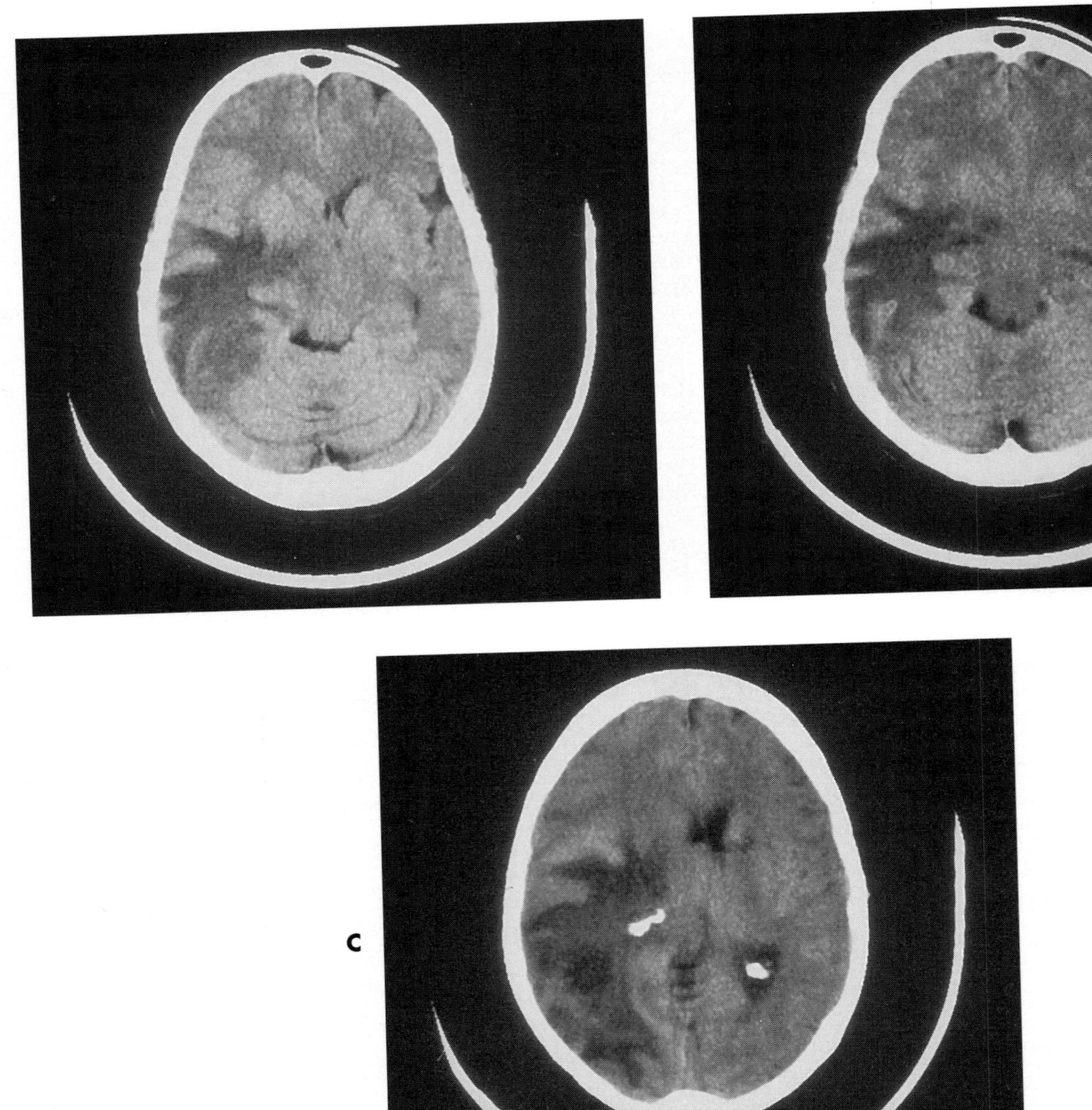

Fig. 9-4 **A** and **B,** Noncontrast CT scans of the head. Extensive edema can be seen through the white matter of the right temporal, parietal, and occipital lobes. A relatively well-circumscribed central area of low density appears to represent necrotic debris in the nidus (nucleus) of a tumor. This is strongly suggestive of a glioblastoma multiforme. **B** and **C,** Edema results in a midline shift approaching 1 cm to the left. **C,** Calcifications in the choroid plexus.

possible and bone artifacts are absent. Contrast-enhanced studies can be performed through the use of **gadolinium**, which is a noniodine-based intravenous (IV) contrast agent. Gadolinium helps differentiate between edema and the tumor and can detect surface seeding. MRI may not be able to detect treatment-related changes from recurrent disease. CT is more cost effective, allowing for more economical use in follow-up post treatment (Fig. 9-5).

Brain scans using technetium 99m (^{99m}Tc) provide information concerning blood flow and demonstrate vascular lesions and those altering the BBB. These studies are no longer widely in use because of the availability of better diagnostic tools.

A funduscopic examination should be done. The test involves an examination of the optic nerve and retina without the use of drugs called *mydriatics,* which cause pupillary

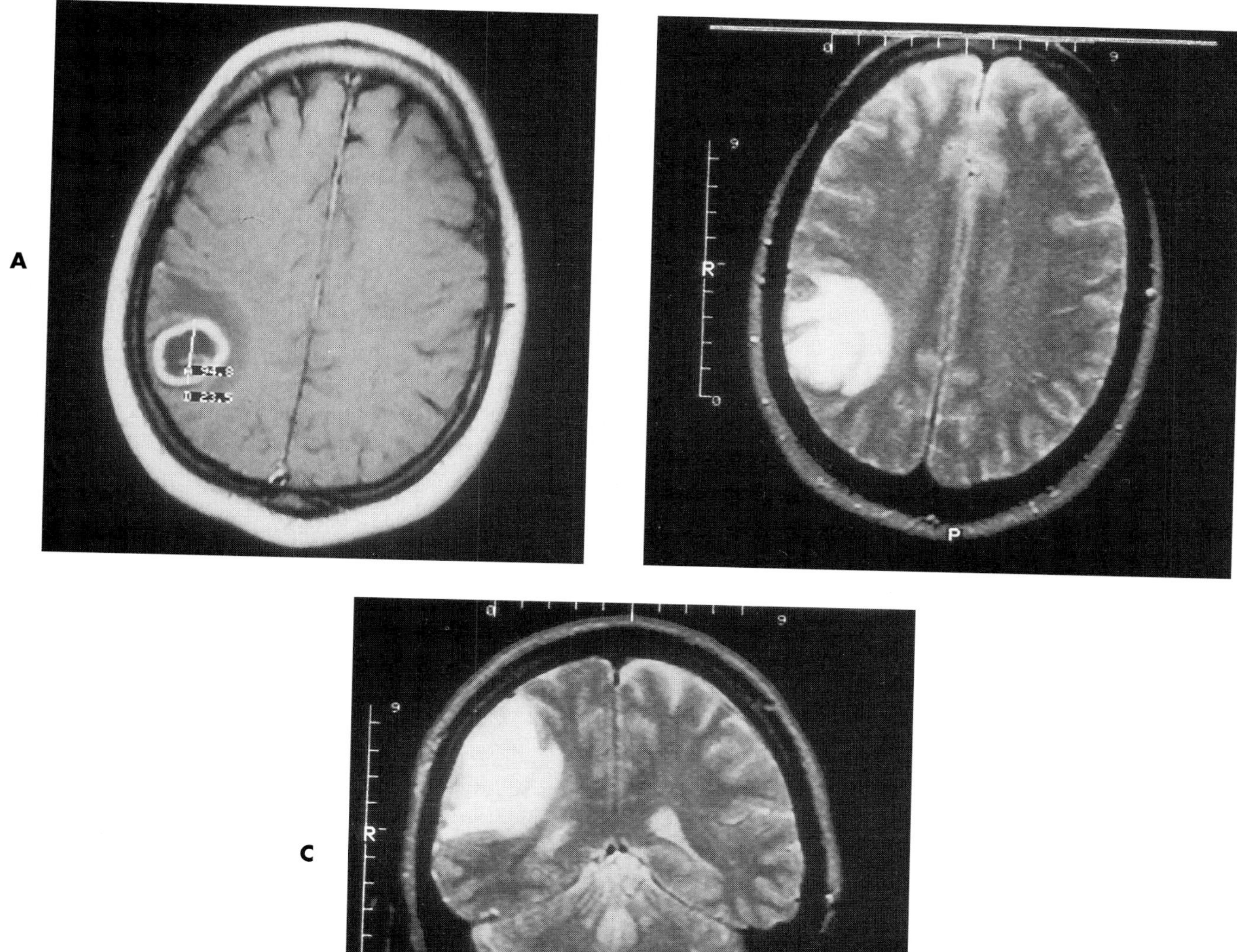

Fig. 9-5 A 3-cm mass located in the right posterior parietal lobe with surrounding edema. The peripheral aspect of the lesion exhibits gadolinium enhancement. **A,** an axial MRI cut showing a lesion with a necrotic center. **B,** The mass is enhanced by gadolinium and shows surrounding edema. **C,** A coronal cut.

dilatation. These types of drugs may suggest nerve involvement where it does not exist and may obscure possible involvement.

Positron emission tomography (PET) is a new diagnostic tool that can be useful in determining differences between necrosis and malignancy, which are associated with areas of high metabolism. PET uses radionuclides and CT to help detect lesions. PET incorporates the localizing ability of CT scanning with the ability of the isotopic agent to concentrate in lesions and help differentiate between various types of CNS lesions, infections, and degenerative processes.[16]

Deoxyribonucleic acid (DNA) measurements can be used in conjunction with cytological and histological diagnoses to provide additional information in distinguishing between benign and malignant lesions. This can be accomplished because benign lesions usually exhibit a euploid DNA-distribution pattern and malignant tumors more frequently exhibit an aneuploid pattern. However, the diagnostic usefulness of DNA measuring is not conclusive because some subsets of tumors may show normal or only slight deviations in DNA. This makes distinguishing normal tissue from benign tissue difficult. Aneuploidy is associated with better survival rates for patients who have neuroblastoma compared with patients who have diploid or near diploid with the same disease.[21]

Continued investigation and interest is being given to gene alterations and molecular genetics. This includes the involvement of oncogenes, tumor-suppressor genes, growth factors, and receptors. The correlation of these alterations with clinical and histological parameters points to the potential use by clinicians and neuropathologists in terms of classification and predictions for response and survival. The types of changes seen include gene amplification, messenger ribonucleic acid (RNA) protein overexpression, allelic loss or recombination, and the loss of entire chromosomes.[6] Altered genes may produce proteins that are tumor specific and significantly affect biology and function. Testing methods using DNA have revealed that patients with gene amplification have shorter survival times than those without amplification.

Protein Kinase C is an enzyme associated with cell proliferation and differentiation. An analysis of this enzyme may be useful as a biological marker of malignancy and in grading astrocytomas. Levels of protein kinase C have been shown to decrease as the tumor grade increases. A nuclear marker, Ki-67, is the most commonly used marker in studying cell proliferation. An association seems to exist between the proliferation rate and biological aggressiveness of the tumor.

Monoclonal antibodies can also be used during the synthesis of DNA to determine the S phase in cell cycles. Investigation of the antibodies as carriers of chemotherapeutic drugs or radioactive agents continues.

DNA flow cytometry is used to study ploidy (the status of the chromosome sets in the cell nucleus) and cells in the S phase. Flow cytometry can offer new insight into the diagnosis and prognosis of solid tumors. It can also aid in the study of hematological tumors by defining the cell of origin. The use of DNA flow cytometry is controversial because results include vascular cells, hematogenous elements, and adjacent reactive elements.

Several diagnostic tools have become outdated in the detection of CNS tumors. Cerebral angiography has value for planning surgical intervention as a means for surgeons to study the intrinsic vasculature (blood supply) of the tumor and surrounding blood vessels. This tool is of little value in establishing a definitive diagnosis.

A lumbar puncture should be avoided in the presence of increased intracranial pressure (ICP) because the risk of herniation is too great. If CSF is withdrawn or leaks through the puncture site, the intracranial contents can shift, thus causing or worsening the herniation. A lumbar puncture can be used to determine an elevation of ICP.

Because electroencephalography is imprecise and not specific for brain tumors, it is of little diagnostic value. Pneumoencephalography and ventriculography are now obsolete.

Pathology

The most important prognostic factor for CNS tumors is the histopathological diagnosis. Benign lesions are indicative of a better prognosis, and the potential for a cure with the use of surgery and/or radiation therapy exists. Intracranial tumors are considered locally malignant based on the limited space for expansion in the cranium. Treatment of the neuraxis is indicated for some histopathologically malignant lesions because of the risk of metastatic seedings.

Tumor growth is not hindered because CNS tumors do not form a natural capsule to contain them. Although seeding occurs in the CNS, extracranial metastases rarely occur, in part because no lymphatic drainage system exists. Growth kinetics are variable, with slow growth expected for low-grade tumors and a more rapid growth with decreased survival rates for high-grade tumors. Cellularity patterns differ according to the tumor grade. Low-grade tumors exhibit reactive hyperplasia, whereas marked cellularity is common in high-grade tumors. Necrosis is an important feature in high-grade tumors. Survival rates, with or without treatment, are clearly associated with tumor grade.

Staging

No universal staging system is currently in use. The expected problems result because of the lack of a standardized method of staging. The American Joint Committee on Cancer uses a system based on the GTM (grade, tumor, metastasis) classification (see the boxes on p. 185). Grade (G) has prognostic significance, ranging from well differentiated to poorly differentiated (G1 to G3). Glioblastoma multiforme is equal to G4. The histopathological features of pleomorphism* and necrosis are included in G4. The tumor (T) stage identifies the size and location of the tumor. Infratentorial and supratentorial tumor locations are included, with the sizes being 3 cm and 5 cm, respectively. T_1 tumors are less than 3 cm (or 5 cm) and have only unilateral extension. T_2 tumors are greater than 3 cm (or 5 cm) and also have only unilateral extension. T_3 tumors show ventricular encroachment, whereas T_4 tumors cross the midline with extension beyond the tentorium. Five staging groups are also represented in this system: (1) clinical-diagnostic, (2) surgical-evaluative, (3) postsurgical resection, (4) pathological retreatment, and (5) autopsy. Because the brain does not contain lymph-draining channels, an N stage (lymph node metastatic) does not exist.

*Pleomorphism means to occur in various forms.

TN Classification and Stage Grouping for Supratentorial Tumors and Malignant Gliomas

TN classification

T_1	Diameter <5 cm; confined to one side
T_2	Diameter >5 cm; confined to one side
T_3	Diameter may be <5 cm; invades or encroaches ventricular system
T_4	Crosses midline; invades opposite hemisphere; extends infratentorially
N	Does not apply in this site

Stage grouping

		Grade	Tumor	Metastases
Stage I				
	IA	G1	T_1	M_0
	IB	G1	$T_{2,\ 3}$	M_0
Stage II				
	IIA	G2	T_1	M_0
	IIB	G2	$T_{2,\ 3}$	M_0
Stage III				
	IIIA	G3	T_1	M_0
	IIIB	G3	$T_{2,\ 3}$	M_0
Stage IV				
		G4	$T_{1\text{-}4}$	M_0
		G1-3	T_4	M_0
		Any G	any T	Any M

Modified from Beahrs OH et al, editors: *AJCC manual for staging of cancer,* ed 4, Philadelphia, 1992, JB Lippincott; Rubin P: *Clinical oncology,* ed 7, Philadelphia, 1993, WB Saunders.
T, Tumor; *N,* node; *M,* metastasis; *G,* grade

TNM Staging System for Infratentorial Tumors and Malignant Gliomas

T_1	Tumor <3 cm in diameter and limited to the classic midline position in the vermis, the roof of the fourth ventricle, and less frequently to the cerebellar hemisphere
T_2	Tumor ≥3 cm in diameter, further invading one adjacent structure or partially filling the fourth ventricle
$T_{3\text{-}A}$	Tumor further invading two adjacent structures or completely filling the fourth ventricle with extension into the aqueduct of Sylvius, foramen of Magendie, or foramen of Luschka, thus producing marked interal hydrocephalus
$T_{3\text{-}B}$	Tumor arising from the floor of the fourth ventricle of the brain stem and filling the fourth ventricle
T_4	Tumor further spreading through the aqueduct of Sylvius to involve the third ventricle or midbrain, or tumor extending to the upper cervical cord
N	Does not apply to this site
M_0	No evidence of gross subarachnoid or hematogenous metastasis
M_1	Microscopic tumor cells found in cerebrospinal fluid
M_2	Gross nodular seedings demonstrated in the cerebellar or cerebral subarachnoid space or in the third or lateral ventricles
M_3	Gross nodular seeding in spinal subarachnoid space
M_4	Metastasis outside the cerebrospinal axis

Modified from Beahrs OH et al, editors: *AJCC manual for staging of cancer,* ed 4, Philadelphia, 1992, JB Lippincott.
T, Tumor; *N,* node; *M,* metastasis.

The Kernohan grading system has also been used. It is also a four-grade system, but it is difficult to use. The Kernohan system considers cellularity, anaplasia, mitotic figures, giant cells, necrosis, blood vessels, and proliferation.

Treatment techniques

A multidisciplinary approach is necessary for the treatment of CNS tumors (Table 9-5). A biopsy is extremely important for diagnostic purposes and essential for therapeutic decision making. Because it allows deep tumors and borders to be studied before the tumor becomes deformed by surgery, stereotactic biopsy may be better than a surgical biopsy. **Debulking surgery** (surgery done to reduce a large tumor) followed by radiation therapy to a residual tumor is often recommended. Interstitial brachytherapy can be used for small tumors that are surgically unresectable, and external beam radiation therapy is warranted for tumors that are surgically inaccessible. Steroids should be administered to reduce the risks of radiation-induced edema, and slow withdrawal from steroids is advisable to reduce adverse side effects. The use of chemotherapeutic agents is limited by the BBB. Patient support is important during any form of treatment to monitor side effects and medications, analyze improvements, and be alert for signs of recurrence.

Surgery. With the development of new surgical techniques, preoperative evaluation is even more important to further aid the surgeon. The tumor size and extent should be determined before surgery. The introduction of microsurgery, the ultrasonic aspirator, the laser, and perioperative ultrasound have made the surgeon's job easier. Computer-assisted stereotactic neuronavigation provides a new tool with the potential for great medical value.

When possible, surgery should be performed on tumors that are symptomatic and offer a chance for complete resection. Debulking is indicated with a large tumor volume and if a complete resection is not possible. Surgery can range from a debulking procedure to complete microsurgical removal. The primary goal for surgery is the radical removal of the tumor and the obtaining of a histological diagnosis. Surgery can be limited by the tumor location and extent, patient status, and risk of causing debilitating neurological deficits. The patient's chances for survival are not enhanced by partial removal of the tumor. Tumor recurrence occurs from residual tumor that invades healthy brain tissue. Decreases in morbidity and mortality rates result from an earlier diagnosis, the use of steroid therapy, improvements in anesthetic techniques, and improved surgical methods. Aggressive surgery is needed, but a lobectomy has become obsolete. Surgical approaches to tumors depend on anatomical pathways, the tumor size, and the tumor location. According to Fransen and de Tribolet,[12] general opinion in the surgical world is that early and radical excision provide the best chance for a good outcome because of an accurate histological diagnosis, control of a mass effect, and cytoreduction, which allow or enhance adjuvant therapy.

Surgery also plays a crucial role in the management of some spinal cord tumors. Surgery can establish a diagnosis and make possible the removal of the tumor. Because of the location of the cord, a surgical resection is difficult at best to perform and impossible in some instances. Serious neurological deficits are always a risk.

Radiation therapy. Radiation therapy is indicated for malignant tumors that are incompletely excised, those inaccessible from a surgical approach, and those with metastatic lesions.

Several factors are considered in determining the doses for treatment. Tumor type, tumor grade, and patterns of recurrence are particularly important. The radioresponsiveness of the tumor must also be considered. The total dose must be limited by normal tissue tolerance because radiation necrosis develops if tissue tolerance is exceeded. The risk of tumor progression must be balanced against the potential risk of necrosis when the dose is determined. In addition, consideration should be given to the side effects that may be induced. These side effects include acute reactions (or those encountered during the course of treatment), early delayed reactions occurring from a few weeks until up to 3 months after treatment, and late delayed reactions occurring months to years later. Threshold doses and the therapeutic ratio also must be considered.

Several approaches are available for treating tumors of the brain, depending on the type of disease, tumor location and extent, and whether the spinal axis requires treatment. Because brain malignancies can result from primary brain tumors, metastases from another site, or meningeal involvement, each type of malignancy needs to be handled appropriately.

The total surgical resection of a brain tumor for cure is an extremely difficult task to accomplish, partly because of the difficulty in obtaining generous enough resection margins in brain tissue. Radiation therapy usually follows surgery in an attempt to prevent tumor regrowth or recurrence. In the past, whole-brain irradiation has been used via lateral portals with a boost to the tumor bed after initial treatment. With the advent of CT and MRI, more accurate tumor localization allows smaller fields to be simulated and treated. Smaller field designs and unique configurations through the use of specialized blocking make simulation and daily reproducibility of the setup an even more important part of the treatment process.

If brain metastases are present from another primary site of involvement, whole-brain irradiation is the preferred treatment. Even with a solitary mass, occult disease is often present, although undetected. Therefore the whole brain should

Table 9-5 Multidisciplinary treatment decisions for various brain tumors

Tumor	Surgery		Radiation therapy	Chemotherapy
Low-grade glioma	Complete resection if possible	and/or	For residual and recurrent tumor: ART/CRT 50-60 Gy	NR
Malignant glioma (AAF + GBM)	Partial resection and decompression	and/or	DRT high doses are used 60-80 Gy with implants 100-120 Gy	CCR/IC* III
Medulloblastoma and ependymoblastoma	Complete resection if feasible	and/or	CRT 45-55 Gy, depending on age	CCR/IC III
Meningioma	Complete resection if feasible	and/or	For residual and recurrent tumor: ART/CRT 60 Gy	NR
Pituitary adenoma	Complete resection if possible	and/or	ART/CRT 45-55 Gy	Bromocriptine is used to lower prolactin level
Craniopharyngioma	Complete resection	and/or	ART/CRT 55-60 Gy	NR
Pinealomas	Stereotactic only	and/or	CRT 50 Gy	NR
Midbrain and brain stem	Stereotactic biopsy at most, unless tumor is exophytic		DRT 50-60 Gy	NR

From Nelson D, et al: Central nervous system tumors. In Rubin P, editor: *Clinical oncology-multidisciplinary approach for physicians and students,* ed 7, Philadelphia, 1993, Saunders.
RT, radiation therapy; *ART,* adjuvant; *CRT,* curative; *DRT,* definitive; *NR,* not recommended; *RCT,* recommended chemotherapy; *AAF,* astrocytoma with foci of anaplasia; *GBM,* glioblastoma multiforme; *CCR,* concurrent chemotherapy and radiation; *IC III,* investigational chemotherapy, phase II/III clinical trials.
PDQ RCT*CCN = BCNU + RT for glioblastoma.

be treated. Treatment of meningeal disease should also include whole-brain irradiation. The meninges encompass the entire brain, optic nerve to the orbit, and cervical spinal cord. Therefore the orbit, tip of the temporal lobe, and first two segments of the cervical spinal cord need to be treated. Special blocking is necessary for protecting the eyes.

Simulation provides the foundation for treatment. The simulation procedure should be carefully explained to the patient before it begins. The patient's understanding of the complexity of the procedure and the necessity for daily reproducibility of the treatment setup should be stressed. Patients should be aware of the importance of their compliance and cooperation in relation to the outcome of the treatment. Accurate reproducibility is a must. Head rotation and tilting create the potential for smeared borders. Immobilization is extremely important and can be achieved through the use of head-holding devices. The use of the Aquaplast system is beneficial for treating patients via lateral ports to a limited brain field with the patient in the supine position. The mask greatly reduces errors in the reproducibility of the setup.

Lateral portal fields are used for treating the whole brain. The inferior margin of the field intersects the superior orbital ridge and EAM. In selecting the field size, 1 cm of flash or shine over should be seen at the anterior, posterior, and superior borders of the field. The flash reduces the chances of clipping any of the anatomy as a result of the field size being too small. The fields may be treated isocentrically or with a fixed source-skin distance (SSD). Isocentric setups are quicker to set up and carry out because the patient and table are not moved between lateral fields. This approach reduces error rates. If a cone down field is required, lateral portals are used again. For treatment to the craniospinal axis the patient is simulated and treated in the prone position (Fig. 9-6). Lateral fields are used for treatment of the whole brain, whereas a gapped posterior field is used for treatment of the spinal cord. Care must be taken to match the beam divergence, allowing no overlap. Hot or cold spots can be avoided by feathering the gap. This can be accomplished by shifting the gap by 1 cm every 1000 cGy. Other methods of feathering the gap can be used. Moving junctions can be used to accomplish the same goal. This approach allows a 1-cm gap

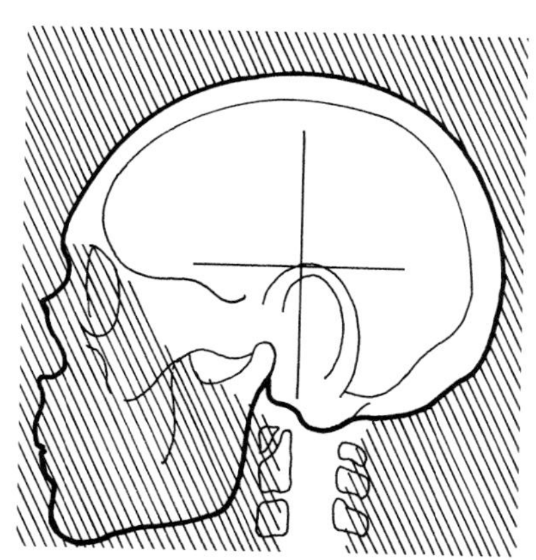

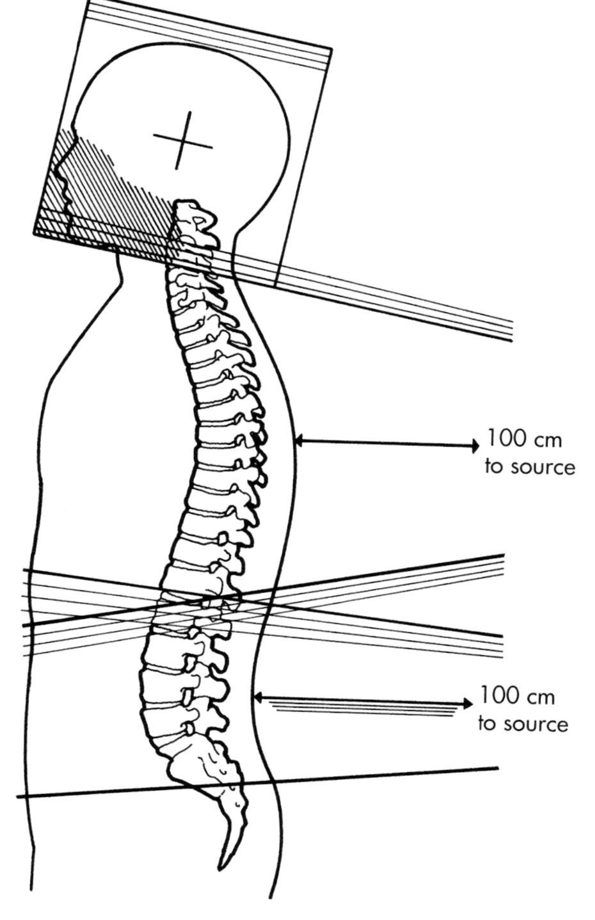

Fig. 9-6 Helmet field and craniospinal field setup. (Redrawn from Perez CA, Brady LW: *Principles and practice of radiation oncology,* ed 2, Philadelphia, 1992, JB Lippincott.)

between fields daily. With this technique the length of the brain and spine fields change daily. The central axis of the spine fields is shifted superiorly to accommodate the gap. The central axis of the brain field remains constant, whereas the field size changes. Limiting the field size to the whole brain may be warranted if the entire tumor plus a margin can be encompassed in a smaller volume. This avoids treating tissue whose injury may cause additional morbidity, loss of function, or death.

The treatment volume is determined by the tumor's extent, which (as shown by CT and MRI) includes the gross tumor volume and related tumor edema. Because tumor cells have been found in edema, this area must be included in the treatment field with a margin. A 2.5-cm margin for malignant tumors and a 1.0 to 2.0-cm margin for benign tumors is recommended. This margin should be treated to the total tumor dose.

Radiation therapy is the most important form of treatment. Most tumors respond to irradiation. In some instances, tumors can be cured; in other instances, prolonged survival can be achieved.

Temporary hair loss occurs with doses ranging from 2000 to 4000 cGy. With doses of greater than 4000 cGy, hair loss is usually permanent. Erythema, tanning, dry and moist desquamation, and edema are also side effects of the treatments. Early delayed reactions include drowsiness, lethargy, dysphasia, a decreased mental status, and a worsening of symptoms. These reactions can occur up to 3 months after treatment, are usually temporary, and disappear without therapy. Recognition of early delayed symptoms is extremely important. The occurrence of apparently new symptoms at this time is not necessarily indicative of treatment failure or the need for any change in therapy. **Radiation necrosis** (tissue death resulting from the effects of radiation) is a classic complication and can occur from 6 months to many years after irradiation. Late reactions are usually irreversible and progressive. Radiation cataracts can be avoided by shielding or keeping the eyes out of the field.

Local control continues to be a challenge. Hypoxia contributes to the local failure of radiation therapy. The impaired immunological status of the patient may be another explanation for local failure. The BBB hinders the work of killer T cells and phagocytes, enabling them to eliminate remaining tumor cells after treatment, whether the treatment is radiation therapy, surgery, or chemotherapy.

Local recurrence occurs within a 2-cm margin of the primary tumor 90% of the time. Most patients die within 2 years because of recurrence.

Conventional fractionation administers external beam radiation once daily for a period of 5 to 6 weeks. Doses vary from 180 to 200 cGy, to a total dose of 5000 to 6000 cGy.

Accelerated fractionation reduces the overall treatment time and reduces the likelihood of tumor repopulation during treatment. Standard-sized fractions are used with treatments delivered two or three times per day. Accelerated fractionation has not shown any increase in survival rates. However, it is well tolerated and has not shown any increase in late reactions.

Hyperfractionation uses a larger number of smaller-sized fractions to a total dose higher than that of conventional therapy but delivered in the same overall time. In theory, the improved repair of sublethal damage at lower-sized fractions may enable a higher total dose with the same late side effects.

Chemicals that enhance the lethal effects of radiation are known as **radiosensitizers**. Hypoxic cell sensitizers and halogenated pyrimidines are under investigation. Hypoxic cells are more radioresistant than oxic cells to radiation. The use of sensitizers makes the cells more susceptible to the radiation without increasing the radiation effects to the normal tissue, which is well oxygenated. Halogenated pyrimidines are used with DNA to increase the sensitivity of the cells to radiation and ultraviolet light. Mitotically active tumor cells use these compounds more than replicating normal glial cells and vascular cells.

Interstitial implants are done with the use of radioactive seeds that are temporarily placed in tumors. Adjacent normal tissue is spared from excessively high doses because of the rapid decrease outside the high-dose volume. Normal tissue can better tolerate the low-dose rate, so a higher dose can be delivered. The effectiveness of the radiation is enhanced by continuous low-dose radiation. Interstitial implants provide a less invasive treatment modality than surgery if recurrence occurs. Interstitial irradiation (IIR) may provide an alternative in the treatment of infants and children. Because large-volume brain irradiation may produce unacceptable late neurological deficits, IIR can be used if local control is necessary, despite the patient's age and long-term effects to be avoided. Brachytherapy may be beneficial to patients suffering from recurrent disease, but it does not play a major role in the management of the disease.

Particle therapy uses subatomic particles to treat in place of photons. The particles can include neutrons, protons, helium ions, heavy nuclei, and pions. Better dose localization to the tumor volume and greater biological effects compared with photons can be achieved.

Hyperthermia is based on the following considerations: (1) Heat is cytotoxic as a single modality, (2) cells in S phase are sensitive to heat, (3) hypoxic cells are sensitive to heat, (4) heat inhibits the repair of sublethal damage from radiation, and (5) heat enhances the effects of some chemotherapeutic drugs.[14] Radiation effects are complemented by the use of heat. The inhomogeneity of the tumor volume heating is currently a problem to its use.

Stereotactic radiosurgery is an important new treatment option for patients with CNS tumors. The process combines stereotactic localization techniques with a sharply collimated beam to direct the dose of radiation to a specific, well-defined lesion. The patient is positioned in a halo device that is used as an immobilization device to ensure the accuracy and reproducibility of the treatment setup. The target volume should be spherical and only up to 3 cm at its maximum dimension. Accuracy approaches 1 mm. A necrosing dose of radiation can be given in a single-fraction treatment or in multiple fractionations. A local dose to the tumor can be increased while sparing surrounding tissue. The process can be accomplished with the use of different sources of radiation. Heavy charged particles, a gamma knife with cobalt 60 sources, and linear-accelerator-based systems can be used with comparable results. The role of radiosurgery in the management of primary, metastatic, and recurrent disease is still under investigation. Some discomfort can be anticipated from the procedure. The patient should not eat before the procedure to reduce the risk of vomiting. Reactions include a headache, an elevated temperature, and seizures. Alopecia may result adjacent to the treatment volume. Radiosurgery is also useful in treating benign lesions.

Conventional therapy has been enhanced through the use of three-dimensional treatment planning, portal imaging, and multileaf collimators. Irregularly shaped fields can be created in seconds through the use of these collimators, eliminating the need to construct blocks. Checking patients' setups before treatment is now possible because of portal imaging. Three-dimensional treatment planning allows the use of multiple noncoplaner fields to a well-defined target volume.

Primary brain tumors are relatively uncommon. However, cerebral metastases occur in approximately 30% of patients with cancer and are the most common brain lesions. The most common primary site of disease responsible for producing brain metastases is the lung. Most metastatic lesions occur in the cerebral hemispheres. Single metastases occur 40% to 45% of the time. Brain metastases may be the only indication of malignant disease. These metastases can occur early in the disease process or may not appear until years later.

Palliative doses of radiation to these types of lesions vary from the curative doses administered to primary lesions. For brain metastases the whole brain is treated via lateral portals to a dose of 3000 cGy in 10 to 12 treatments delivered in daily fractionations of 300 cGy or 250 cGy. Radiation therapy for brain metastases can lengthen the survival time from 1 to 6 months. Patients with solitary lesions can be treated with radiosurgery, but this remains a controversial form of treatment. Surgery may be indicated if the primary tumor site is not known, if doubt exists about the nature of the intracranial mass, or if only a single lesion exists.

Chemotherapy. Three general principles must be considered in planning treatment with chemotherapeutic agents. These include the prompt delivery of drugs before metastatic disease occurs, the use of a multiple-drug approach that provides different mechanisms of action without overlapping toxicities, and the use of the highest possible safe doses of drugs. The disease stage and histology are noted for determining dosages and drug combinations.

Progress has been slow in the area of chemotherapeutic drugs. Several reasons account for this. According to Chatel, Lebrun, and Freny,[7] the number of effective drugs is limited, adjuvant therapy has not changed the time to progression, adjuvant chemotherapy only slightly increases the percentage of survival at 18 and 24 months, a 20% to 25% response rate exists when drugs are given at recurrence, and multidrug therapy does not seem to be more efficient than single-agent chemotherapy. Other reasons for the difficulty in finding useful drugs include the small number of patients with CNS tumors for use in clinical trials compared with more prevalent diseases, difficulties measuring the tumor response, and the fact that one measurement of response is survival time. Effective chemotherapy for CNS tumors is furthered hindered by the BBB, which impedes the penetration of the drugs into the brain. "High concentration in cerebral tumors can nevertheless be reached due to the frequent extensive disruption of the BBB, but tumor cells infiltrating normal tissue are theoretically inaccessible to drugs that do not cross the BBB."[9]

Chemotherapeutic drugs can be administered orally, intravenously, and by direct carotid perfusion. Most chemotherapeutic drugs cause cytotoxic effects by disrupting DNA synthesis in rapidly dividing cells.

Interstitial chemotherapy provides a new method of increasing the tumor concentration of the drugs. No systemic toxicity is achievable if the tumor bed is implanted with high local concentrations of chemotherapeutic agents.

Intraarterial routes and bone marrow transplantation have been used to improve drug delivery. Regardless of whether drugs are given neoadjuvantly (before), adjuvantly (during), or at the time of recurrence in relation to other forms of treatment, response rates range only from 27% to 60%.[7]

The designing of new drugs that allow better penetration of the BBB and can exhibit better distribution and lower toxicity has become extremely important. Limited studies suggest that the drug concentrations in the area around the tumor or in normal brain may be lower than those in the tumor itself, where the BBB is inefficient. The concentrations of drugs in the normal brain tissue decreases as the distance from the tumor increases. Therefore drug concentrations in the brain surrounding the tumor may be too low to eliminate infiltrating tumor cells. This can be a reason for therapeutic failures.[9] The nitrosourea drugs are lipid soluble, allowing them to cross the BBB. Because of this ability, these drugs can work against brain tumors. These drugs include BCNU (carmustine), CCNU (lomustine), methylCCNU, and streptozotocin. The toxicities of these agents include nausea and vomiting, delayed myelosuppresion (bone marrow depression), and delayed nephrotoxicity. BCNU can cause pulmonary fibrosis. Streptozotocin can also cause hyperglycemia (an increase in blood sugar). These drugs are cell cycle phase nonspecific.

Drugs of choice for CNS neoplasms include carmustine, procarbazine, vincristine, and 5-fluorouracil (5-FU). Carmustine (BCNU) is used alone, whereas procarbazine is used in combination with other drugs (Table 9-6).

Table 9-6 Response rates to single-agent chemotherapy in recurrent or malignant gliomas

Drug	Response rate (%)
Effective therapy	
Single-agent regimens	
Procarbazine	27-50
Teniposide	63
Carmustine	48-51
Lomustine	43-47
Semustine	56
Multiagent regimens	
Carmustine + vincristine	25-41
Carmustine + 5-FU	31-39
Procarbazine, lomustine, vincristine	60
Teniposide + lomustine	18-75
Teniposide, lomustine, doxorubicin	72
Methotrexate, lomustine, vincristine	36-40
Cyclophosphamide, lomustine, vincristine	38
Ineffective therapy (response rate <30%, duration <35 weeks)	
Doxorubicin	
AZQ	
Chlorozotacin	
Cisplatin	
DDP	
Hydroxyurea	
Imidazole	
Carboxamide	
Methotrexate	
Mithramycin	
Thiotepa	
Triazinate	

Modified from Rubin P: *Clinical oncology: multidisciplinary approach for physicians and students,* ed 7, Philadelphia, 1993, WB Saunders.
5-FU, 5 fluorouracil; *AZQ*, diaziquane *DDP*, cisplatin.

Carmustine can cause pulmonary and renal toxicity. Demyelination or white matter necrosis occurs with some chemotherapeutic drugs and more commonly if used in combination with radiation therapy. Leukoencephalopathy (dysfunction of the white matter) becomes a risk after radiation has induced alterations in the BBB. This allows increased drug penetration, resulting in increased drug concentration in the brain. The risks of CNS toxicity can be reduced when chemotherapy is given before radiation therapy.

Experimental approaches for the use of chemotherapy are being investigated. These include interferon, infusional therapy, tumor implants, disruption of the BBB, and lymphocyte-activated killer cells with interleukin-2. Immunotoxins and biological response modifiers have been studied and developed since 1977.

CNS tumors (especially high-grade tumors) result in a grim prognosis. Survival rates have not changed significantly in the last 35 years. Long-term survival is uncommon. Combined-modality treatment offers the best chance for survival. First, the patients that will benefit from this approach must be determined. Consideration must be given to the maintenance of the quality of life, not the quantity. Long-term survivors are usually young and have minimal deficits at the time of the diagnosis. The mean KPS score of survivors is 76. Death from recurrent disease is unusual in glioma patients who survive more than 4 or 5 years.[23] Left untreated, patients can expect a survival time of about 17 weeks. If a complete resection of the tumor can be accomplished, the survival time is about 70 weeks. However, for patients who undergo a biopsy only, the median survival time is approximately 19 weeks. For patients under age 65 and in good neurological condition, the best approach to maintain the quality of life and extend the survival time includes maximal surgical resections followed by radiation therapy, with a boost to the resection margin and adjuvant chemotherapy.

Role of radiation therapist

Patient education is a primary goal of the physician, oncology nurse, and radiation therapist. Although the physician and nurse initially discuss treatment procedures, side effects, skin care, nutrition, and psychosocial issues with the patient and family members, the emotional state of those persons at that time is generally not conducive to remembering and complying with all the information they are given. It becomes the responsibility of the therapist, who sees the patient daily, to reiterate and reinforce all these issues with the patient.

Daily contact allows the therapist to build a professional bond of trust, understanding, and communication with the patient. The therapist must be ready to step in and provide patients with emotional support, answers to their questions and concerns, and referrals to persons they may need to see (e.g., social worker, pastor, nutritionist, business office personnel, and support groups).

The therapist's daily contact also allows monitoring of the patient's mental and physical well-being. Some patients still feel overwhelmed, angry, and vulnerable and are in denial at the beginning of treatments. It is far better for patients and for their families if the patients can vent some of those feelings with or toward the therapist than it is for those feelings to be directed toward family members, who are already coping with so much.

A separate patient-waiting area allows patients to talk and share their thoughts with other persons who have the same concerns. This area allows discussions regarding issues the patient may not be able to discuss with family members.

Patients undergoing treatment for CNS neoplasms can expect specific side effects. Most commonly, patients complain of fatigue. Reassuring patients that this is not unusual helps them a great deal to cope with the situation. Explaining to patients that the body requires plenty of rest while it tries to heal itself from the disease and effects of daily treatment eliminates some concern. Suggesting that patients pamper themselves and take a nap when they feel tired, rather than fight the fatigue, is an option.

A proper diet is a must for the healing process and well-being of the patient. If food becomes unappealing in looks, taste, and smell, the patient will not want to eat. The patient can try eating smaller portions several times a day rather than sitting down to a large meal. Large portions are sometimes quite discouraging to someone with no appetite. A change in the location of eating can sometimes help, as well as having someone else cook. Nutritional supplements should be available to patients, including different kinds of supplements so patients can then purchase the brand that appeals to them most.

Frequent blood tests may be required. The white cell count and platelet counts may decrease in patients treated with craniospinal irradiation. These counts require close monitoring in the event the patient requires a break in treatment until the situation corrects itself.

Permanent hair loss for persons being treated for primary brain tumors occurs. A loan closet with wigs, turbans, and kerchiefs ranging in a wide variety of colors and styles should be available to patients. Shops specializing in these items should also be suggested. Therapists should caution patients to use a mild shampoo to prevent skin irritation. Moisturizing creams can be prescribed for dry desquamation and other products for moist desquamation. Therapists can also recommend skin conditioners if erythema tanning occurs.

The patient should be cautioned against exposing to direct sunlight areas of the body being treated. The radiation from the sun in combination with the radiation from treatment enhances the adverse side effects. Because cataracts can develop if the eye is treated, cerrobend block shielding is required or the eye should be kept out of the treatment field.

Most patients begin to feel a sense of security that develops over the course of treatment from the daily contact with the therapy team. When treatment ends, patients feels a sense of loss and abandonment after weeks of daily attention being focused on them and their needs. Patients should be called 1 week to 10 days after the completion of treatment (before the first follow-up visit) just to check on them and evaluate their physical and mental condition. This provides the patient with a sense of ongoing care.

The therapist must also be watchful for signs of medical complications that may arise as a result of the treatment. Early intervention of potential problems can prevent unnecessary suffering later in the course of treatment. Attention to detail regarding treatment setups and parameters is a must, and providing professional, competent, efficient, and accurate treatment in a relaxed and friendly atmosphere completes the role of the therapist.

Case Study

A 31-year-old white male noted a change in vision and headaches. An initial work-up included an MRI scan about 4 months later that revealed gadolinium enhancement in the region of the hypothalmus. Separate disease was noted in the corpus callosom. The pineal gland was enlarged but not enhanced.

A spinal MRI showed no evidence of spinal tumors. An additional workup included serum alpha-fetoprotein (AFP) and human chorionic gonadotropin (HCG), which were within normal limits. A lumbar puncture for cytology was performed. CSF was negative for malignant cells. The patient's history revealed that, at the age of 15, the patient was treated for failure to grow and diabetes insipidus. Diabetes insipidus sometimes occurs for years before other symptoms develop. A CT scan performed at that time (1977), which revealed a questionable suggestion of an abnormality in the hypothalmic region, apparently was not pursued. The patient was treated at the time with growth hormones, thyroid supplements, and vasopressin with response.

A biopsy was performed via a right frontotemporal craniotomy 5 months after the onset of symptoms. A preoperative diagnosis considering the patient's long history indicated a glioma. A postoperative diagnosis was probable hypothalmic glioma. A pathology report was positive for hypothalmic germinoma with metastasis to the corpus callosom. Several special stains were used to confirm this diagnosis, and several pathologists reviewed the slides because the patient's history was unusual for a diagnosis of germinoma.

The patient's visual-field deficits were unchanged postoperatively. The craniotomy incision healed well.

The patient presented himself for radiation therapy consultation shortly after surgery. His history revealed panhypopituitarism manifested by hypothyroidism, high prolactin levels, adrenal insufficiency, diabetes insipidus, and abnormal testosterone levels. The family history was unremarkable. The patient's mental status was intact. A neurological review was within normal limits. Vision testing revealed greater deficits on the right. The patient had blurred vision on the right and denied having a headache.

Because the patient had metastasis to the corpus callosom, he was a candidate for curative radiation therapy to the cranial spinal axis. Risks and benefits of the treatment were explained to the patient. Side effects during treatment can include skin irritation, hair loss, and fatigue. The white cell count and platelet counts tend to become lower in adults who are treated with craniospinal irradiation. The patient's blood counts were monitored weekly. Long-term risks included radiation damage to the brain, lens with cataract formation, and spinal cord.

Because there was no seeding to the spinal cord, the plan was to administer 2550 cGy in 17 fractions to the craniospinal axis. After this a conedown boost of 2500 cGy was given to the gross disease, as seen on an MRI scan. The craniospinal axis was treated with 6-MV photons. The boost to the conedown used 10-MV photons. If seeding to the spinal column had been present, those areas would also have been boosted.

The patient was simulated in the prone position with an alpha cradle to ensure reproducibility. Lateral fields to the whole brain and a PA spinal field were planned. Customized blocks were made for the portals.

The patient experienced minimal nausea after his first treatment. Compazine spansules given before further treatments helped relieve this problem. The patients blood counts dropped after receiving 750 cGy. Because the white count was below 1000, the patient was given time off with orders for a stat complete blood count to be done before resuming treatment. A 1-week break resolved this problem. He was cautioned not to use a toothbrush because of his decreased platelet count. He was told to sponge his teeth or gargle. The patient's visual deficits remained unchanged since the beginning of treatment.

Shifting of the fields to incorporate a gap began at 2100 cGy. A cone down began after 2500 cGy. At 3090 cGy the patient experienced less nausea but had complaints of altered taste with salty taste buds. At 3990 cGy he was doing well but had flulike symptoms. He continued to have poor visual acuity but had improved visual-field changes with a decrease in bilateral hemianopsia. The patient finished treatment at a total dose of 5070 cGy. He had only a 1-week break because of falling blood counts. The patient was suffering from severe fatigue and had complaints of indigestion and reflux. He lost a total of 10 pounds during treatment.

The patient was feeling well and eating better at the time of his 1-month follow-up visit. He continued to have some fatigue, which the oncologist felt would resolve itself after a little more time. The patient was able to regain some of the weight he had lost. Vision testing revealed no papilledema. The patient's vision was still poor, and he was unable to read a page in a book. Visual fields revealed marked improvement in the inferior aspect fields. Cranial nerves III to XII were intact. No motor or sensory abnormalities were present, and cerebellar findings were intact. There was epilation over his skull consistent with the treatment portal. No evidence existed of skin changes along his spine or cranium. A recent MRI scan showed no evidence of remaining germinoma.

At a follow-up 3 months later, the patient had a good appetite with his energy level improving, although he was still having problems gaining weight. An ophthalmologist examined the patient for his poor vision. Other than magnifying glasses, nothing could be done to help him. Optic nerve deficits were again noted with greater difficulty on the right than left. The patient had moderate alopecia with patchy regrowth. His blood counts had improved and were expected to continue to do so.

Approximately 1 year has now passed since the completion of treatment, and the patient appears to be doing well. An MRI scan done recently shows no evidence of disease. A repeat MRI scan will be done in 2 years. The long-term survival prognosis for patients who have germinomas is 85% at 5 years. However, because this patient had metastases, his chances for long-term survival are reduced.

Review Questions

Multiple Choice

1. Multiple tumor types are included in the CNS category. Which type of primary brain tumor is most common?
   a. Ependymoma
   b. Medulloblastoma
   c. Glioma
   d. Meningioma
2. What is the purpose of the blood-brain barrier?
   I. To hinder the penetration of some substances into the brain and CSF
   II. To protect the brain from potentially toxic substances
   III. To protect the brain from radiation
   IV. To prevent the passage of lipid- or water-soluble substances into the brain
   a. I and III
   b. II and III
   c. I and II
   d. II and IV
3. Which of the following are important factors to consider in the initial work-up for a definitive diagnosis of CNS neoplasms?
   a. Family and social histories
   b. Changes in behavior or personality
   c. Difficulties with speech, memory, or logical thought processes
   d. Walking, gait, or balance problems
   e. All of the above
4. What is the best approach to treating CNS neoplasms?
   a. Surgery and radiation
   b. Surgery and chemotherapy
   c. Radiation and chemotherapy
   d. A multidisciplinary approach
5. Surgery for CNS neoplasms can be limited by which of the following?
   a. Tumor location and extent
   b. Patient status
   c. Risk of causing neurological deficits
   d. All of the above

6. What is the most common brain lesion?
   a. Astrocytoma
   b. Glioma
   c. Metastatic
   d. Medulloblastoma

True or False

7. Little is known concerning the etiology, development, and growth mechanisms of CNS tumors.
   True____________ False ____________
8. Prognosis tends to be better in younger patients.
   True____________ False ____________
9. Tumor grade rather than size is the primary factor involved with staging.
   True____________ False ____________
10. Side effects from radiation treatment include erythema, dry and moist desquamation, edema, and hair loss.
   True____________ False ____________

Questions to Ponder

1. Explain the benefits and risks involved in treating patients who have CNS neoplasms with surgery, radiation therapy, and chemotherapy.
2. What are some of the presenting signs and symptoms you would anticipate with patients who have CNS tumors?
3. What is the purpose of the feathered-gap technique for treating patients to the craniospinal axis?
4. Why is radiation therapy not the treatment of choice for children less than 4 years old?
5. Analyze the expected side effects from radiation therapy to the CNS?
6. What are the long-term risks of radiation therapy treatment to the craniospinal axis?
7. Describe some of the unique characteristics of CNS tumors.

REFERENCES

1. Ahlbom A: A review of the epidemiologic literature on magnetic fields and cancer, *Scand J Work Environ Health* 14:337-343, 1991.
2. Avizonis, VN et al: Late effects following central nervous system radiation in a pediatric population, *Neuropediatrics* 23:228-234, 1992.
3. Bigner SH et al: Gene amplification in malignant human gliomas, *J Neuropathol Exp Neurol* 47:191-205, 1988.
4. Bigner SH et al: Characterization of the epidermal growth factor receptor in human gliomas, cell lines, and xenografts, *Cancer Res* 50:8017-8022, 1990.
5. Black KL, Ciacci M: The limits of treatment of malignant gliomas, *West J Med* 158:65-66, January 1993.
6. Bruner J: Neuropathology, cell biology, and new diagnostic methods, *Curr Opin Oncol* 5:441-449, 1993.
7. Chatel M, Lebrun C, and Freny M: Chemotherapy and immunotherapy in adult malignant gliomas, *Curr Opin Oncol* 5:464-473, 1993.
8. Collins VP: Amplified genes in human gliomas, *Semin Cancer Biol* 4:27-32, 1993.
9. Donnelli MG, Zucchetti M, D'Incali M: Do anticancer agents reach the tumor target in the human brain? *Cancer Chemother Pharmacol* 30:251-260, 1992.
10. Farwell J, Dohrmann GJ, Flannery JT: Central nervous system tumors in children *Cancer* 40:3123-3132, 1977.
11. Filippini G, Artuso A: International incidence of CNS tumors in children, *Ital J Neurol Sci* 13:395-400,1992.
12. Fransen P, de Tribolet N: Surgery for supratentorial tumors, *Curr Opin Oncol* 1993 5:450-457, 1993.
13. Frelich R, Huang P, Topham A: Cancer current—brain and CNS tumors Delaware 1980-1989, *Del Med J* 64(9):571-573, 1992.
14. Hall EJ: *Radiobiology for the radiologist,* ed 2, New York, 1978, Harper & Row.
15. Karlsson U et al: The brain. In Perez C, Brady L, editors: *Principles and practice of radiation oncology,* ed 2, Philadelphia, 1992, JB Lippincott.
16. Kornblith PL, Walker MD, Cassady, JR: Neoplasms of the central nervous system. In Devita VT, Hellman S, Rosenberg SA, editors: *Cancer principles and practice of oncology,* Philadelphia, 1982, JB Lippincott.
17. Laem OD, Mork SJ, DeRidder L: The transformation process. In Rosenblum ML , Wilson CB, editors: *Brain tumor biology: progress in experimental research,* 1984, Basel S. Karger .
18. Levin VA, Sheline GE, Gutin PH: Neoplasms of the central nervous system. In Devita VT, Hellman S, and Rosenberg SA, editors: *Cancer principles and practice of oncology,* ed 3, Philadelphia, 1989, JB Lippincott.
19. Myers MH, Gloechler Ries LA: Cancer patients survival ratio: SEER program results for 10 years of follow-up, *CA Cancer J Clin* 39:21-32, 1989.
20. Ranskoff J, Koslow M, Cooper P: Cancer of the CNS and pituitary. In Holleb A, Fink D, Murphy G, editors: *A.C.S. textbook of clinical oncology,* Atlanta, 1991, American Cancer Society.
21. Salmon I et al: DNA histogram typing in a series of 707 tumors of the central and peripheral nervous system, *Am J Surg Pathol* 17 (10):1020-1028, 1993.
22. Silverberg E: Cancer statistics, *CA Cancer J Clin* 32:1, 1982.
23. Vertosich F Jr, Selker RG: Long term survival after the diagnosis of malignant glioma: a series of 22 patients survive more than 4 years after diagnosis, *Surg Neurol* 38: 359-363, 1992.
24. Weingart J, Brem H: Biology and therapy of glial tumors, *Curr Opin Neurol Neurosurg,* 5:808-812, 1992.
25. Youmans JR: *Neurological surgery,* vol 3, Philadelphia, 1973, WB Saunders.

BIBLIOGRAPHY

del Regato JA, Spjut HJ, Cox JD: *Ackerman and del Regato's: Cancer: diagnosis, treatment, and prognosis,* ed 6, St Louis, 1985, Mosby.

Griffin C et al: Chromosome abnormalities in low grade CNS tumors, *Cancer Genet Cytogenet* 60:67-73, 1992.

Nelson D et al: Central nervous system tumors. In Rubin P, editor: *Clinical oncology—a multidisciplinary approach for physicians and students,* ed 7, Philadelphia, 1993, WB Saunders.

CHAPTER

10

Digestive System

Leila A. Bussman
James A. Martenson

Outline

Key terms

Abdominoperineal resection
Achalasia
Anterior resection
Barrett's esophagus
Chronic ulcerative colitis
Endocavitary radiation therapy
Esophagitis
Familial adenomatous polyposis
Gardner's syndrome
Hereditary nonpolyposis colorectal syndrome
Intraoperative radiation therapy (IORT)
Leukopenia
Odynophagia
Orthogonal radiographs
Peritoneal seeding
Plummer-Vinson syndrome
Tenesmus
Three-point setup
Thrombocytopenia

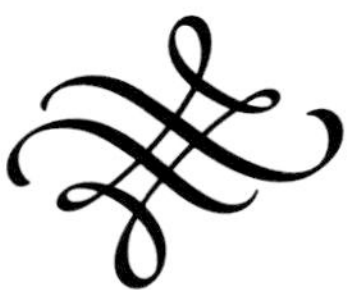

This chapter discusses the three major malignancies of the gastrointestinal system that are managed with radiation therapy (i.e., cancers of the rectum, esophagus, and pancreas). Colorectal cancer is the most common gastroinstestinal malignancy and is associated with the best prognosis. Cancers of the esophagus and pancreas are usually diagnosed with advanced-staged disease and do not have many long-term survivors.

COLORECTAL CANCER

Epidemiology and etiology

The incidence of colorectal cancer has been steadily declining since 1980. However, in 1994 149,000 new cases were projected in the United States. The disease affects men and women equally. Cancer of the colon is ranked third in incidence in comparing men and women separately. The risk of developing cancer of the large bowel increases with age. The incidence rate for persons under 65 years of age is 19.2 cases per 100,000, compared with 337 cases per 100,000 for persons over 65.[12] Cancer of the large bowel more commonly affects the rectum or distal colon. However, an increase has occurred in right (proximal) colon lesions, especially in older women. The reason for this is unclear, but the increase may be the result of earlier detection of precancerous lesions in the distal colon. Colorectal cancer is the second leading cause of cancer death in the United States, accounting for approximately 56,000 deaths in 1994.[3,8,12,36]

The cause of colorectal cancer has largely been attributed to a diet high in animal fat and low in fiber. The excess fat in a person's diet may act as a promoter of the development of colon cancer. The intake of fiber into diets may act as an inhibitor, diluting fecal contents and increasing fecal bulk, resulting in quicker elimination and therefore minimizing the exposure of the bowel epithelial lining to the carcinogens.[12,36,47] Some authors suggest that the type of fiber consumed determines the effectiveness of reducing or neutralizing mutagens in the diet. Cellulose and wheat bran have been considered more effective than alternate forms of fiber in reducing the mutagen formation.[8,47] A diet high in fiber is considered an effective means of preventing the development of colon cancer. However, further studies are needed to determine the effectiveness of different types of fiber sources.

Other principle factors in the development of colon cancer include the following: **chronic ulcerative colitis,** carcinomas arising in preexisting adenomatous polyps, and the hereditary cancer syndromes. These syndromes are **familial adenomatous polyposis** (FAP) and **hereditary nonpolyposis colorectal syndrome.**[12,36,40,47]

Chronic ulcerative colitis usually occurs in the rectum and sigmoid area of the bowel but may spread to the rest of the colon. This condition is characterized by extensive inflammation of the bowel wall and ulceration. A patient experiences attacks of bloody mucoid diarrhea up to 20 times a day. These attacks persist for days or weeks and then subside, only to recur.[43] The risk of developing colon cancer depends on the extent of bowel involvement, age of onset, and severity and duration of the active disease.[8,12,43] The earlier the age at onset and the longer the duration of the active disease, the higher the risk of developing cancer. Studies have shown the risk to be 3% at 15 years duration, increasing to 5% at 20 years.[8,12,43] Only 1% of patients with a diagnosis of colorectal cancer have a history of chronic ulcerative colitis.

Adenomatous polyps are growths that arise from the mucosal lining and protrude into the lumen of the bowel. They are classified as tubular or villous, based on their growth pattern and microscopic characteristics. Polyps are considered a precursor to the development of a malignancy.[8,12,40,43,47] The larger the size of the polyp, the greater the risk of malignant transformation.[8,12,40] Villous adenomas are 8 to 10 times more likely than tubular adenomas to be malignant.[8,40,43]

Virtually all patients with the hereditary condition FAP, if left untreated, develop colon cancer.[8,12,36,43] FAP is characterized by the studding of the entire large bowel wall by thousands of polyps. Persons affected with this disease do not have polyps at birth. Progression to extensive involvement of the colon usually occurs by late adolescence. FAP is treated by the complete removal of the colon and rectum. **Gardner's syndrome** is another inherited disorder similar to FAP. Patients with Gardner's syndrome have adenomatous polyposis of the large bowel as well as other abnormal growths, such as upper gastrointestinal polyps, periampullary tumors, lipomas, and fibromas.[8,12,43]

The frequent occurrence of colorectal cancer in families without polyposis has been termed *hereditary nonpolyposis colorectal syndrome.*[3,8,12] Patients with this family history of colon cancer usually develop right-sided colon cancers at a much younger age than the general population. These patients are also at an increased risk for the development of a second cancer of the colon and adenocarcinomas of the breast, ovary, endometrium, and pancreas.[8,12] Individuals with this family history should undergo physical examinations regularly.

Anatomy and lymphatics

Cancer of the large bowel is usually divided into cancer of the colon or rectum because the symptoms, diagnosis, and treatment are different based on the anatomical area involved. A major factor determining the treatment and prognosis is whether a lesion occurs in a segment of bowel that is located retroperitoneally or intraperitoneally. This is discussed further in the section on the anatomy and lymphatic drainage of these areas.

The colon is divided into eight regions: the cecum, ascending colon, descending colon, splenic flexures, hepatic flexures, transverse colon, sigmoid, and rectum. Located intraperitoneally, the cecum, transverse colon, and sigmoid have a complete mesentery and serosa and are freely mobile (Fig. 10-1).[8,25,36,39] Lesions occurring in these regions can usually be surgically removed with an adequate margin unless the tumor is adherent or invades adjacent structures.[8,25,36] Treatment failure or recurrence is most likely attributed to peritoneal seeding.

Located retroperitoneally, the ascending and descending colon and the hepatic and splenic flexures are considered immobile. They lack a true mesentery and a serosal covering on the posterior and lateral aspect. Because of the retroperitoneal location and lack of a mesentery for these regions, early spread outside the bowel wall and invasion of the adjacent soft tissues, kidney, and pancreas are common. Thus adequate surgical margins are more difficult to achieve and may result in a local recurrence.[8,25,36]

The rectum is continuous with the sigmoid and begins at the level of the third sacral vertebra. Like the sigmoid, the upper rectum is covered by the peritoneum, but only on its lateral and anterior surfaces. The peritoneum is then reflected over the anterior wall of the rectum onto the seminal vesicles and bladder in males or the vagina and uterus in females, forming a cul de sac termed the *rectovesical pouch* or *rectouterine pouch,* respectively. The lower half to two thirds of the rectum is located retroperitoneally. Three transverse folds divide the rectum into areas known as the *upper valve, middle valve,* and *lower valve,* or *ampulla* (Fig. 10-2). The middle valve is located 11 cm superior from the anal verge and represents the approximate location of the peritoneal reflection.[36,39] Because of the retroperitoneal location, tumors of the rectum can invade adjacent structures of the pelvis, such as the prostate, bladder, vagina, and sacrum. Treatment options depend on the location of the lesion. As mentioned earlier, retroperitoneally located lesions are more

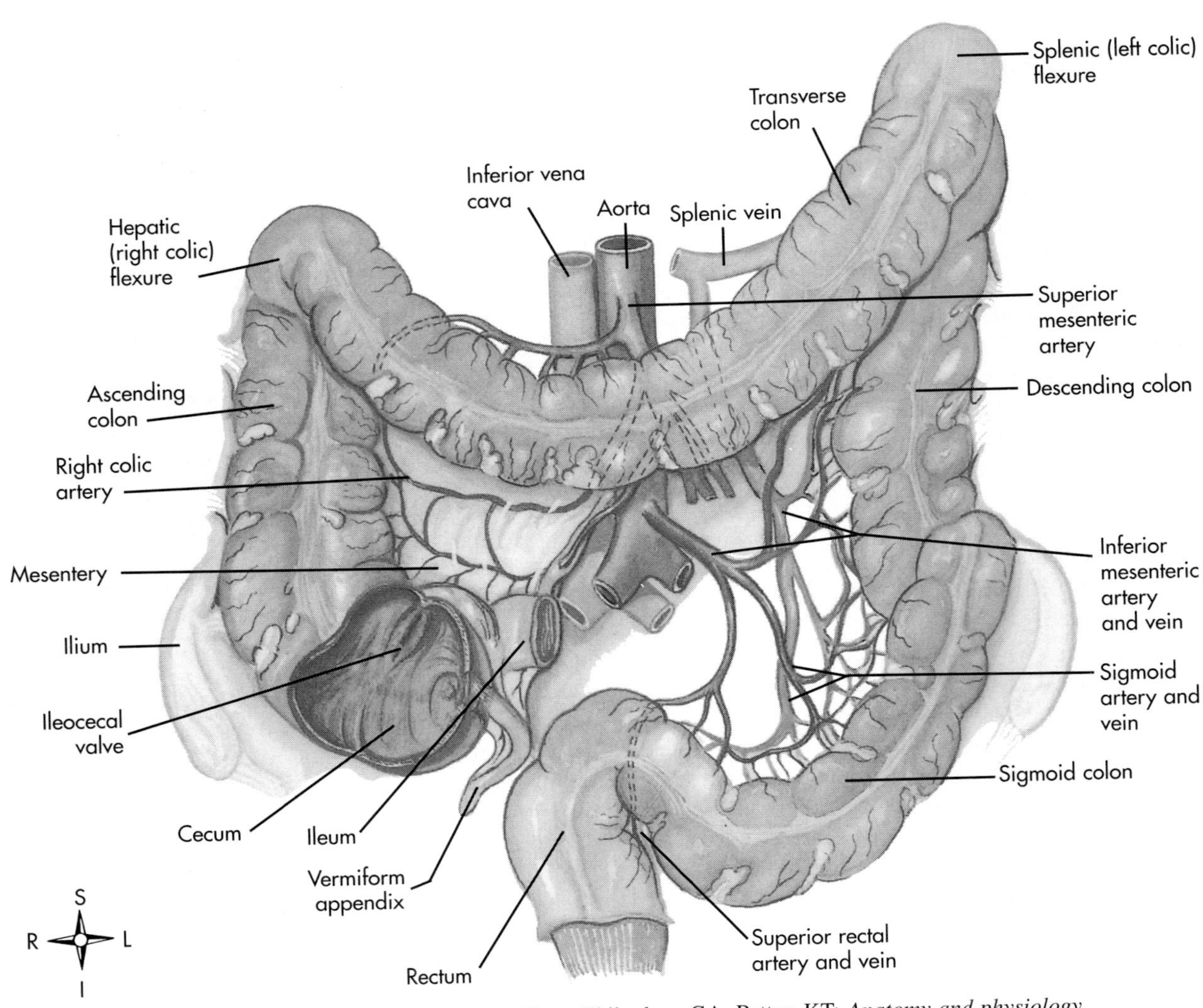

Fig. 10-1 Anatomy of the large bowel. (From Thibodeau GA, Patton KT: *Anatomy and physiology,* ed 3, St Louis, 1996, Mosby.)

apt to fail locally because of close surgical margins and may require adjuvant treatment subsequent to a complete surgical resection.[25]

A cross section through a segment of large bowel reveals four main layers: the mucosa, submucosa, muscularis propria, and serosa (Fig 10-3).[1,36] These layers are used in the staging system to define the amount of involvement through the bowel wall. The mucosa, or innermost layer, forms the lumen of the bowel and consists of two supporting layers: the lamina propria and muscularis mucosa. The next layer, the submucosa, is rich in blood vessels and lymphatics. The muscularis propria contains two muscle layers, one circular and one longitudinal, which are responsible for peristalsis. Beneath the muscularis layer is a lining of fat termed the *subserosal layer.* The outermost layer is the serosa. Not all segments of the colon have a serosal layer. This layer is provided by the visceral peritoneum.[8]

The lymphatic drainage of the colon follows the mesenteric vessels. The right colon follows the superior mesenteric vessels and includes the ileocolic and right colic nodes (Fig. 10-3). The left colon follows the inferior mesenteric vessels and includes the regional nodes termed the *midcolic, inferior mesenteric,* and *left colic.* The sigmoid region drains into the inferior mesenteric system but also includes the nodes along the superior rectal, sigmoidal, and sigmoidal mesenteric vessels.[1] Lymphatic drainage of the upper rectum follows the superior rectal vessels into the inferior mesenteric system. Middle and lower rectum lymphatic drainage is along the middle rectal vessels, with the principal nodal group being the internal iliac nodes.[13,25,36] Other nodal groups at risk for involvement with rectal cancer are the perirectal, lateral sacral, and presacral nodes.[1,13] Low rectal lesions that extend into the anal canal can drain to the inguinal nodes (Fig. 10-4)

With any of these regions, other nodal groups may be involved or at risk for involvement if the tumor has invaded an adjacent structure. For example, if a rectal cancer has invaded the vagina or prostate, the external iliac nodes may be involved with disease. For a lesion in the ascending colon

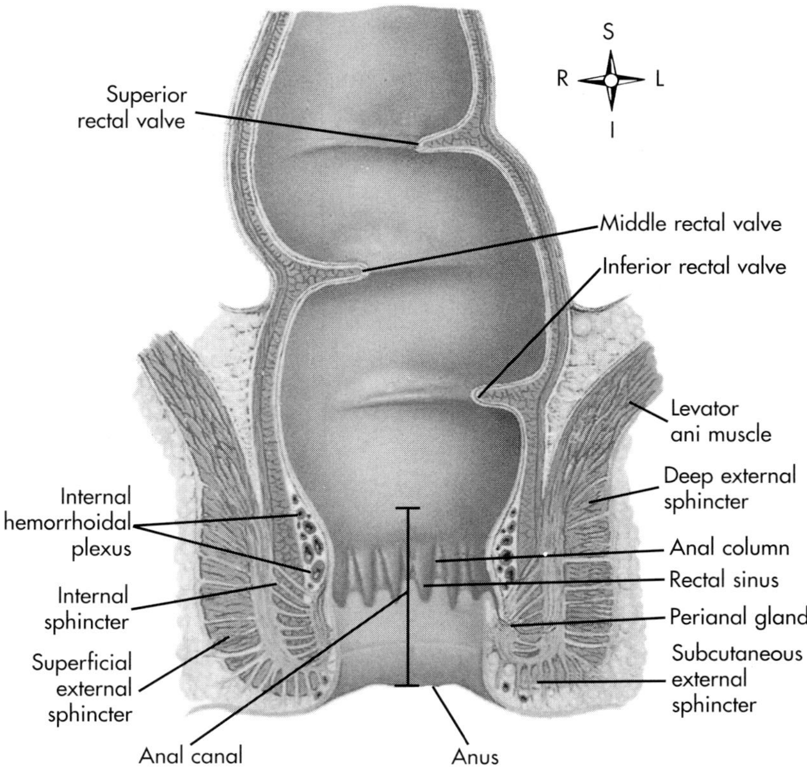

Fig. 10-2 A coronal section through the rectum. (From Thibodeau GA, Patton KT: *Anatomy and physiology,* ed 3, St Louis, 1996, Mosby.)

that has invaded the posterior abdominal wall, the paraaortic nodes may be positive for disease.[25,36]

Clinical presentation

Patients with rectal cancer usually have rectal bleeding. This may be bright red blood on the toilet paper or mixed in or on the stool.[7,36] Other symptoms include a change in bowel habits, diarrhea versus constipation, or a change in the stool caliber.[7,21,36] Pencil-thin stools, constipation, or diarrhea may be indicative of a tumor filling the rectal valve area and causing an obstructive type process. **Tenesmus** may be a patient's complaint with locally advanced rectal cancer. Pain in the buttock or perineal area may occur from tumor extension posteriorly.[7]

Presenting symptoms of patients with lesions in the left colon are similar to those of rectal cancer. Blood in the stool, a change in stool caliber, obstructive symptoms, and abdominal pain are the most common complaints.[8,42] In contrast, patients with right-sided colon lesions usually have abdominal pain, which is often accompanied by an abdominal mass. Nausea and vomiting are other possible symptoms. Occult blood in the stool and microcytic anemia are two other symptoms of colon cancer.[8,36]

Detection and diagnosis

In general, a cancer in the large bowel is diagnosed via findings of the physical examination and radiographic and endoscopic studies. Together, these findings provide crucial information in the detection and extent of the disease process.

The initial procedure for any patient with a malignancy is a thorough history and physical examination. For all colorectal cancer patients, a digital rectal examination should be performed and attention should be given to the approximate size of the lesion, the mobility, the location from the anal verge, and the rectal wall involved.[36] Enlarged perirectal nodes may also be detected during the digital examination.

A proctosigmoidoscopy is performed as a complementary procedure and allows a more accurate depiction of the size and location of the lesion. This procedure also determines whether the mass is exophytic or ulcerative. A tissue diagnosis is obtained from a biopsy during the endoscopic procedure. A pelvic examination should be performed for colon or rectal cancer to rule out any other pelvic masses. An anterior extrarectal mass (a lesion in the cul de sac) may be indicative of peritoneal seeding. In women an anterior rectal mass may invade the vaginal wall, putting the external iliac nodes at risk for involvement. The left supraclavicular and inguinal lymph nodes should also be palpated,

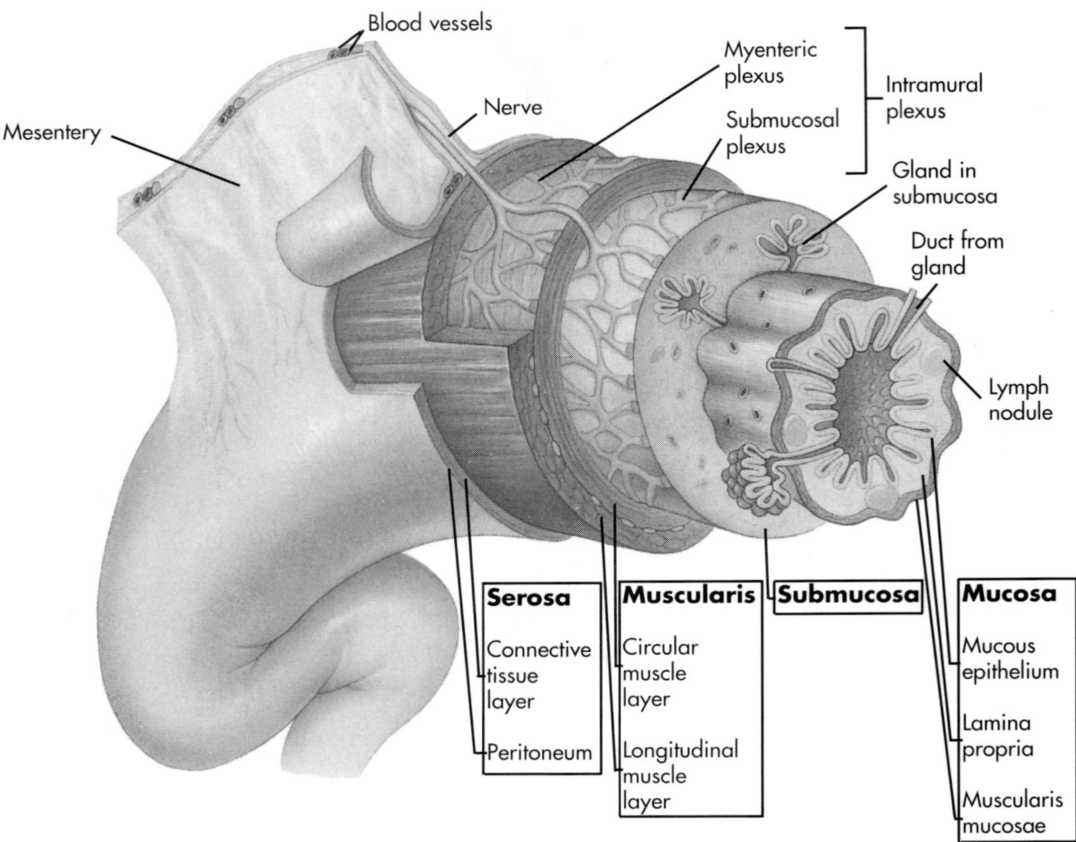

Fig. 10-3 A cross section of the bowel wall. (From Thibodeau GA, Patton KT: *Anatomy and physiology,* ed 3, St Louis, 1996, Mosby.)

especially in patients with low rectal lesions nearing the dentate line.[36] Supraclavicular lymph node involvement indicates extensive incurable disease and generally occurs as a result of spread from metastatically involved paraaortic nodes via the thoracic duct. The physical examination should also assess potential sites of distant spread. Palpation of the abdomen should be performed to check for masses in the abdomen, liver, and ascites.

An air-contrast or regular barium-enema study, especially a cross-table lateral view for rectal tumors, is particularly helpful for the radiation oncologist in reconstructing the tumor volume three dimensionally and facilitating treatment planning. This study is not always conclusive for small lesions in the rectum. Therefore an endoscopic procedure should be obtained for a more definitive picture of activity in the bowel.[25,36]

Endoscopic procedures, colonoscopies, and proctosigmoidoscopies can assess the size and location of lesions. They are also used for obtaining biopsies of lesions or removing polyps for histological confirmation of malignancy.[36]

After a diagnosis is established, a patient undergoes a staging work-up to determine the extent or amount of spread of the disease. A chest radiograph is usually obtained to detect metastasis to the lungs.

Laboratory studies used in the diagnosis and work-up of colon cancer include a complete blood count and blood-chemistry profile. Elevated liver function tests indicate the need for imaging of the liver by computed tomography (CT) or sonography.

Pathology and staging

Adenocarcinoma is the most common malignancy of the large bowel, accounting for 90% to 95% of all tumors.[7,42] Other histologies include mucinous adenocarcinoma, signet-ring cell carcinoma, and squamous cell carcinoma.[42]

Three principal staging systems exist. Two of the systems, Dukes' classification and the modified Astler-Coller (MAC) system, are postoperative, whereas the American Joint Committee on Cancer (AJCC) TNM (tumor, node, metastases) system may be used clinically (preoperatively) or postoperatively.

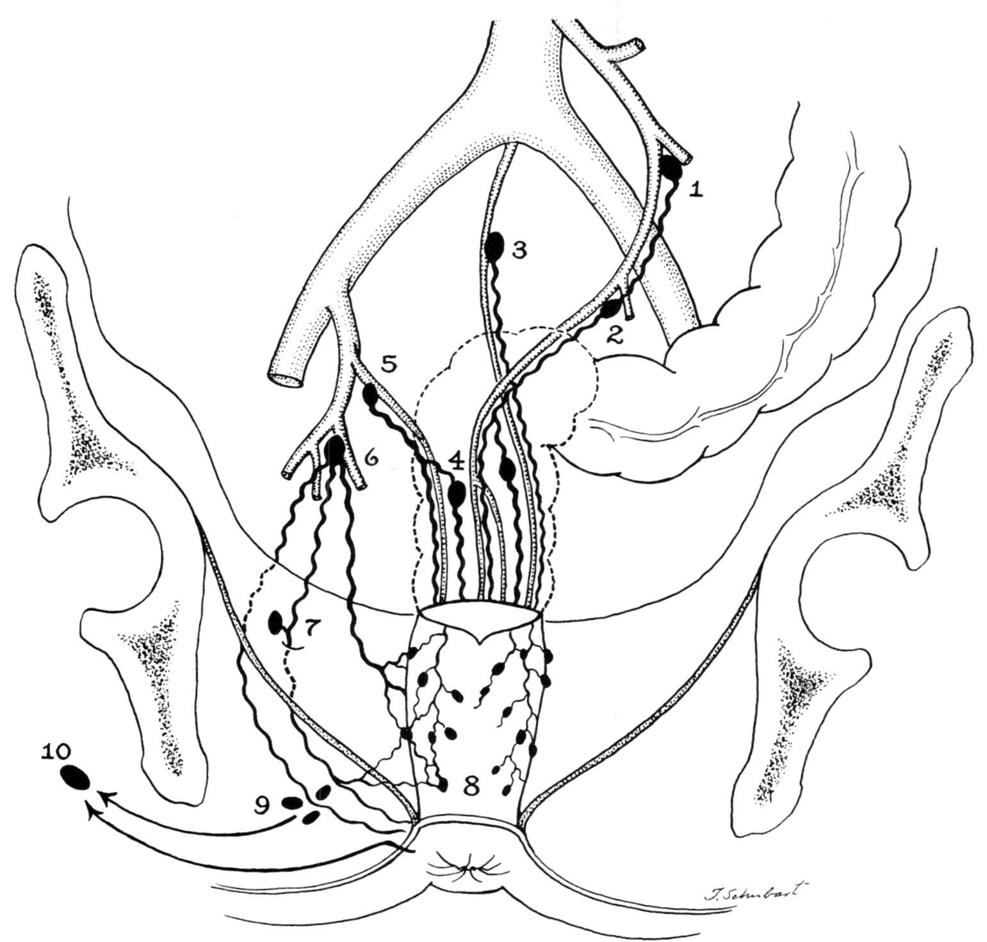

Fig. 10-4 Lymphatic drainage of the rectum: nodes at the origin of the inferior mesenteric artery and origin of the sigmoid vessels (*1* and *2*); nodes of the sacral promontory (*3*); sacral nodes (*4*); internal iliac nodes, hypogastric (*5* and *6*); external iliac nodes may be involved in low rectal lesions (*7*); nodes located at the rectal wall (*8*); ischiorectal nodes (*9*); and inguinal nodes (*10*). (From Del Regato JA, Spjut HJ, Cox JD: *Ackerman and del Regato's cancer: diagnosis, treatment, and prognosis,* ed 6, St Louis. 1985, Mosby.)

The staging system devised by Duke in the 1930s was the first useful system. Tumors of the rectum are classified according to the level of invasion into the bowel wall and the absence or presence of positive nodes. The tumors are given a letter designation from A to C. Duke's A designation indicates a lesion that has not penetrated through the bowel wall. The B designation indicates a lesion that has penetrated the bowel wall with negative nodes, and the C designation indicates a lesion with positive nodes.

Astler-Coller expanded Duke's system, making it more specific regarding the level of penetration through the bowel wall and nodal status. These modifications in the staging system were based on studies showing that penetration through the bowel wall, the number of positive nodes, and tumor adherence to adjacent structures were important predictors of survival (Table 10-1).[8,36] In the MAC system, Gunderson and Sosin created separate categories for tumors that microscopically or grossly ($B2_m$ or $B2_g$) involved surrounding organs or structures.[8]

The TNM system incorporated these changes into the current system, which is similar to the MAC system.[2,8] The revisions in the staging systems reflect that the two most important prognostic indicators of survival are the number of positive nodes and depth of penetration through the bowel wall.[8,25]

Routes of spread

As implied in the staging system, malignancies of the large bowel usually spread via direct extension, lymphatics, and hematogenous spread. Direct extension of the tumor is typically in a radial fashion, penetrating into the bowel wall rather than longitudinally.[8]

Lymphatic spread occurs if the tumor has invaded the submucosal layer of the bowel. The initial lymphatic and venous channels of the bowel wall are found in the submucosal

Table 10-1 Colorectal staging systems

Duke	Astler-Coller	Modified Astler-Coller	TNM	Description
A	A	A	T_1, N_0	Nodes negative; limited to mucosa
	B1	B1	T_2, N_0	Nodes negative; penetration into submucosa but not through bowel wall
		B2	T_3, M_0	Nodes negative; penetration through muscularis propria (bowel wall)
B	B2			
		B3	T_4, N_0	Nodes positive; penetration through muscularis propria and invasion or adherence to other structures
	C1	C1	$T_{1\text{-}2}$, $N_{1\text{-}3}$	Nodes positive; limited to bowel wall
C		C2	T_3, $N_{1\text{-}3}$	Nodes positive; penetration through wall
	C2	C3	T_4, $N_{1\text{-}3}$	Nodes positive; extension through bowel wall and invasion or adherence to adjacent organs

Modified from Martenson JA, Gunderson LL: Colon and rectum. In Perez CA, Brady LW: *Principles and practices of radiation oncology,* Philadelphia, 1992, JB Lippincott.

layer. Lymphatic spread is orderly. The initial nodes involved for rectal cancer are the perirectal nodes.[8,25] Approximately 50% of patients have positive nodes.[25]

Blood-borne spread to the liver is the most common type of distant metastasis. The mechanism of spread involves the venous drainage of the gastrointestinal system (the portal circulation). The second most common site of distant spread is the lung. This spread results from tumor embolus into the inferior vena cava.[8]

Lesions may also spread within the peritoneal cavity. The growth of a tumor through the bowel wall onto the peritoneal surface of the colon can result in tumor cells shedding into the abdominal cavity. These shedded cells then take up residence on another surface (i.e., peritoneal lining, cul de sac) and begin to grow. This process is called **peritoneal seeding.** The implantation of tumor cells onto a surface at the time of surgery is another mechanism of spread.[8,25]

Treatment techniques

Surgery is considered the treatment of choice. The tumor, an adequate margin, and draining lymphatics are removed. The type of procedure depends on the location of the tumor. For colon tumors the removal of a large segment of bowel, adjacent lymph nodes, and the immediate vascular supply by procedures such as a right hemicolectomy or left hemicolectomy is common. For rectal cancer the two most common procedures are the anterior and abdominoperineal (AP) resection.

The **anterior resection** involves the removal of the tumor plus a margin (an en bloc excision) and immediately adjacent lymph nodes.[16] The bowel is then reanastamosed. Therefore a colostomy is not required. This procedure is used in the treatment of colon cancers and select rectal cancers.[7,8] Patients with disease in the upper third or middle third of the rectum (6 to 12 cm above the verge) are usually candidates for this sphincter-preserving surgery.[7,16,34]

An **abdominoperineal resection** is used in patients with rectal cancer in the lower third (distal 5 cm) of the rectum.[7] An anterior incision is made into the abdominal wall to construct a colostomy. Then a perineal incision is made to resect the rectum, anus, and draining lymphatics, pulling the entire en bloc specimen out through the perineal opening. Because of the narrow, bony configuration of the pelvis and closeness of adjacent structures (i.e., prostate and vagina), adequate margins laterally, anteriorly, and posteriorly are difficult.[34,36] Surgical clips placed to outline the tumor area assist the radiation oncologist in the design of treatment portals.[7,36] The final phase of the procedure involves the reconstruction or reperitonealization of the pelvic floor through the use of an absorbable mesh, omentum, or peritoneum. This is extremely important for the patient who needs postoperative radiation therapy. Reperitonealization allows the small bowel to be displaced superiorly, reducing the amount of small bowel in the treatment field and minimizing the treatment toxicity from radiation therapy.[7,16,36]

Radiation therapy. Radiation therapy is most commonly used as an adjuvant treatment postoperatively for rectal cancer. However, preoperative radiation therapy and radiation alone may also be used in selected patients.[7,25,26,28,36]

Postoperative adjuvant radiation therapy and concurrent chemotherapy is advocated based on the high local failure rate of surgery alone in rectal cancer patients who have positive nodes or tumor extension beyond the wall. Postoperative radiation therapy and chemotherapy is the only adjuvant treatment approach consistently shown to improve survival rates in rectal cancer patients and is preferred over other adjuvant approaches such as preoperative radiation therapy. A major advantage of postoperative adjuvant treatment is that the physician has pathological confirmation of the extent of the tumor spread through the wall to nodes or distant sites. This information is critical in determining whether adjuvant treatment is necessary.[35] Studies have shown that patients with positive nodes but with a tumor confined to the bowel wall (C1) have a 20% to 40% recurrence rate.[8,25,36] A similar local recurrence rate (20% to 35%) is found with B2 and B3 lesions, tumors that extend through the bowel wall with or without adherence and negative nodes. A patient with both poor prognostic factors (extension through the wall and positive nodes [C2 and C3]) has almost twice the risk for local recurrence. Various studies have reported recurrence rates in these patients of 40% to 65% in a clinical series and up to 70% in a reoperative series.[25,26]

Endocavitary radiation therapy is a sphincter-preserving procedure done for curative intent in a select group of patients with low- to middle-third rectal cancers that are confined to the bowel wall. Papillon established the following characteristics for patients eligible for this procedure: no extension of the tumor beyond the bowel wall, a maximum tumor size of 3 × 5 cm, a mobile lesion with no significant extension into the anal canal, a well- to moderately well-differentiated exophytic tumor that is accessible by the treatment proctoscope (≤ 10 cm from the anal verge).[21,41] Patients receive four doses of 3000 cGy each, separated by a 2-week interval. This is done on an outpatient basis through the use of a 50-kVp contact unit (4 cm source-skin distance [SSD]), with 0.5- to 1.0-mm aluminum filtration at a dose rate of 1000 cGy per minute. Treatments are delivered directly to the rectal tumor through an applicator inserted into the rectum and held in place by the radiation oncologist (Fig. 10-5). If the size of the lesion exceeds the diameter of the applicator (3 cm), overlapping fields are necessary. Treatment results have been excellent with this technique. Papillon reported only a 11% locoregional failure rate with a 5-year follow-up out of 207 patients treated.[36,41]

Radiation alone has also been used in patients who are medically inoperable or who have locally advanced rectal cancer and are deemed unresectable.[7,36] In this setting, radiation provides palliation and is rarely curative. Radiation combined with chemotherapy (5-fluorouracil [5-FU]) has proved more effective than radiation alone in relieving symptoms, decreasing tumor progression, and increasing overall survival. Preoperative radiation (≥ 45 Gy) has resulted in 50% to 75% of patients becoming resectable, but 35% to 45% of the patients still experience local recurrence, necessitating additional treatment.[36]

Chemotherapy. The addition of adjuvant chemotherapy combined with radiation therapy in the postoperative setting in high-risk rectal and colon cancer patients (MAC B2-C3) has demonstrated an increase in overall survival rates (Fig. 10-6).[10,26,28,35,36] The Gastrointestinal Tumor Study Group (GTSG) and Mayo Clinic/North Central Cancer Treatment Group (NCCTG) have performed many randomized trials of adjuvant therapy for rectal cancer. These studies have demonstrated a decreased disease recurrence and improved survival rates with a combination of 5-FU and pelvic radiation therapy. The most recently completed study indicated that the best result is obtained with two cycles of 5-FU before and after pelvic radiation therapy and continuous infusion 5-FU during radiation therapy (Fig. 10-7).[33]

Field design and critical structures. Patients receiving postoperative adjuvant radiation therapy for rectal cancer are at a high risk for local recurrence. These patients include those with extension beyond the bowel wall, tumor adherence (MAC B2-3), or positive lymph nodes (MAC C1-3). The treatment fields are typically designed to encompass the primary tumor volume and pelvic lymph nodes, shrinking the field to treat the primary target volume to a higher dose. Anatomical boundaries of the portals depend on whether the patient underwent an anterior resection or abdominoperineal

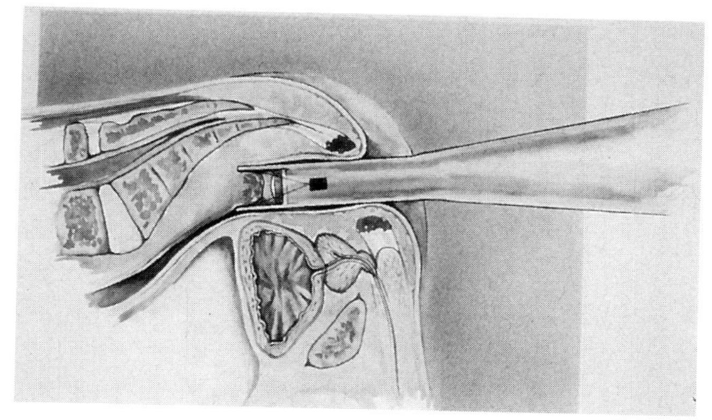

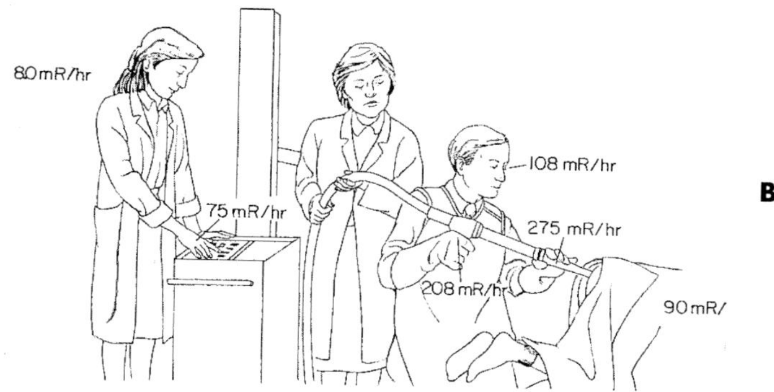

Fig. 10-5 **A** and **B**, Sphincter-preserving endocavitary radiation therapy of the low rectal tumor. (Courtesy Dr. Alan J. Stark.)

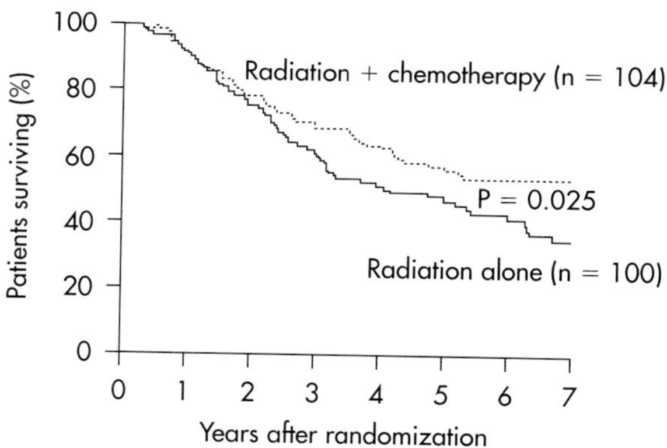

Fig. 10-6 Improved survival rates with postoperative radiation and chemotherapy versus radiation alone. (Modified from Krook et al: *N Engl J Med* 324(11):713, 1991.)

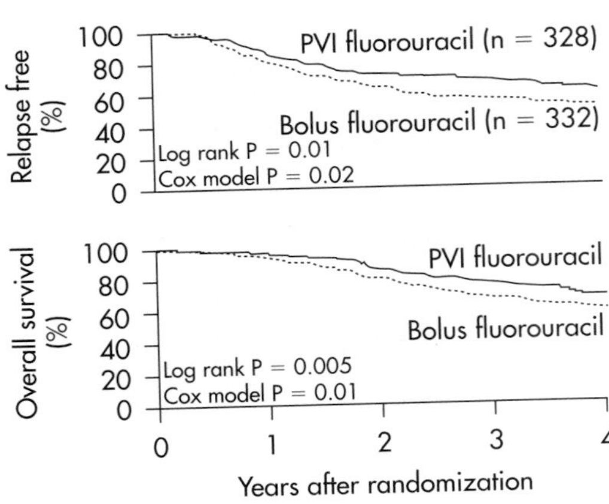

Fig. 10-7 A comparison of protracted venous infusion (PVI) fluorouracil and bolus fluorouracil. Improved relapse-free and overall survival rates occur with PVI. (Modified from O'Connell et al: Improving adjuvant therapy for rectal cancer by combining protracted-infusion fluorouracil with radiation therapy after curative surgery, *N Engl J Med,* 331:502, 1994.)

resection directly relating to the areas at risk for recurrence. For patients with rectal cancer, most recurrences occur in the posterior aspect of the pelvis, including metastasis to the internal iliac and presacral lymph nodes.[25,36] These two nodal groups are not included in a standard surgical resection for rectal cancer and need to be encompassed in radiation portals.[36] For irradiation of the pelvis the dose-limiting structure is the small bowel. Radiation treatment techniques and the field design must take into consideration the amount of small bowel in the field to minimize treatment-related toxicities. The reduction of the small-bowel dose is achieved through patient positioning and positioning devices, bladder distention, multiple-shaped fields, and dosimetric weighting.[8,25,36] The dose delivered to the large volume (tumor plus regional nodes) is 4500 cGy, with the coned down volume (primary tumor bed) receiving 5000 cGy to 5500 cGy in 6 to $6^1/_2$ weeks. Doses in excess of 5000 cGy are not achievable unless the small bowel can be excluded from the field.[7,25,36]

Usually, a four-field (anterior-posterior [AP/PA] and opposed laterals) or three-field technique (PA and opposed laterals wedged) is used, allowing a homogenous dose to the tumor bed while sparing anterior structures, including the small bowel. For patients who have undergone an anterior resection the superior extent of the field is placed 1.5 cm superior to the sacral promontory, which correlates to L_5-S_1 innerspace.[7,25,36] Depending on the superior extent of the lesion and clinical indications, the field may need to be placed at the L_4-L_5 interspace or extend superiorly to include the paraaortic lymph node chain.[25] The more superiorly the field extends, the more precautions are necessary to avoid small-bowel injury and complications. The width of the AP/PA fields is designed to provide adequate coverage of the iliac lymph nodes. This border is placed 2 cm lateral to the pelvic brim and inlet. The inferior border generally includes the entire obturator foramina, although this may vary depending on the location of the lesion. The recommended inferior margin is 3 to 5 cm on the gross tumor preoperatively or below the most distal extent of dissection postoperatively (Fig. 10-8).[25] A rectal tube is inserted at the time of simulation. Barium or Gastrografin contrast (30 to 40 cubic centimeters) is injected into the rectum to facilitate the localization of critical structures and design of treatment fields. Lead shot or a BB is placed on the anal verge to reference the perineal surface on simulation films.

Lateral treatment portals and prone positioning with full bladder distention allows the small bowel to be excluded from the treatment volume. This position also assists in the localization of critical posterior structures. Anatomically, the rectum and perirectal tissues are extremely close to the sacrum and coccyx. In locally advanced disease the tumor may spread along the sacral nerve roots, resulting in tumor recurrence in the sacrum. Therefore the posterior field edge is placed 1.5 to 2.0 cm behind the anterior bony sacral margin. In advanced situations the entire sacral canal plus a 1.5-cm margin is recommended.[25,36] This margin allows day-to-day variances in the patient setup caused by movement. Anteriorly, the field border is placed at the anterior edge of the femoral heads to ensure coverage of the internal iliac nodes. The lower third of the rectum lies immediately posterior to the vaginal wall and prostate, placing these organs and their draining lymphatics at risk for involvement. If the rectal lesion has invaded anterior structures (prostate or vagina), the anterior border is placed on pubic symphysis for inclusion of the external iliac nodes (Fig. 10-8, *C*).[7,25,36] In female patients a tampon soaked with iodinated contrast is inserted into the vagina to ensure adequate coverage of the vagina in the radiation portals.

In patients having an abdominoperineal resection the field design is similar, except the posterior and inferior borders are extended to include the entire perineal incision. The perineal region is included in the treatment volume to decrease the risk of tumor recurrence in the scar from implantation of tumor cells at the time of surgery. The entire perineal scar is outlined at the time of simulation with solder wire or lead BBs. The posterior and inferior margins are established by placing the field edge 1.5 to 2.0 cm beyond the radiopaque perineal markers. This corresponds to flashing the posterior and inferior perineal skin surfaces (Fig. 10-8).[25,36] The perineal scar is then bolused (thickness/energy dependent) during the PA treatment. The buttocks are taped apart, and bolus is placed on the entire perineal scar to have a controlled measurable bolusing effect. Because of the tangential radiation beam, the perineal tissue and thinner upper thigh tissue may exhibit acute skin reactions, requiring interruption of the planned treatment course. In male patients the penis and scrotum are shifted superiorly under the pubic region to lessen this reaction. Alternatively, the reaction to male genitalia can be reduced by the use of a three-field technique (PA and laterals).

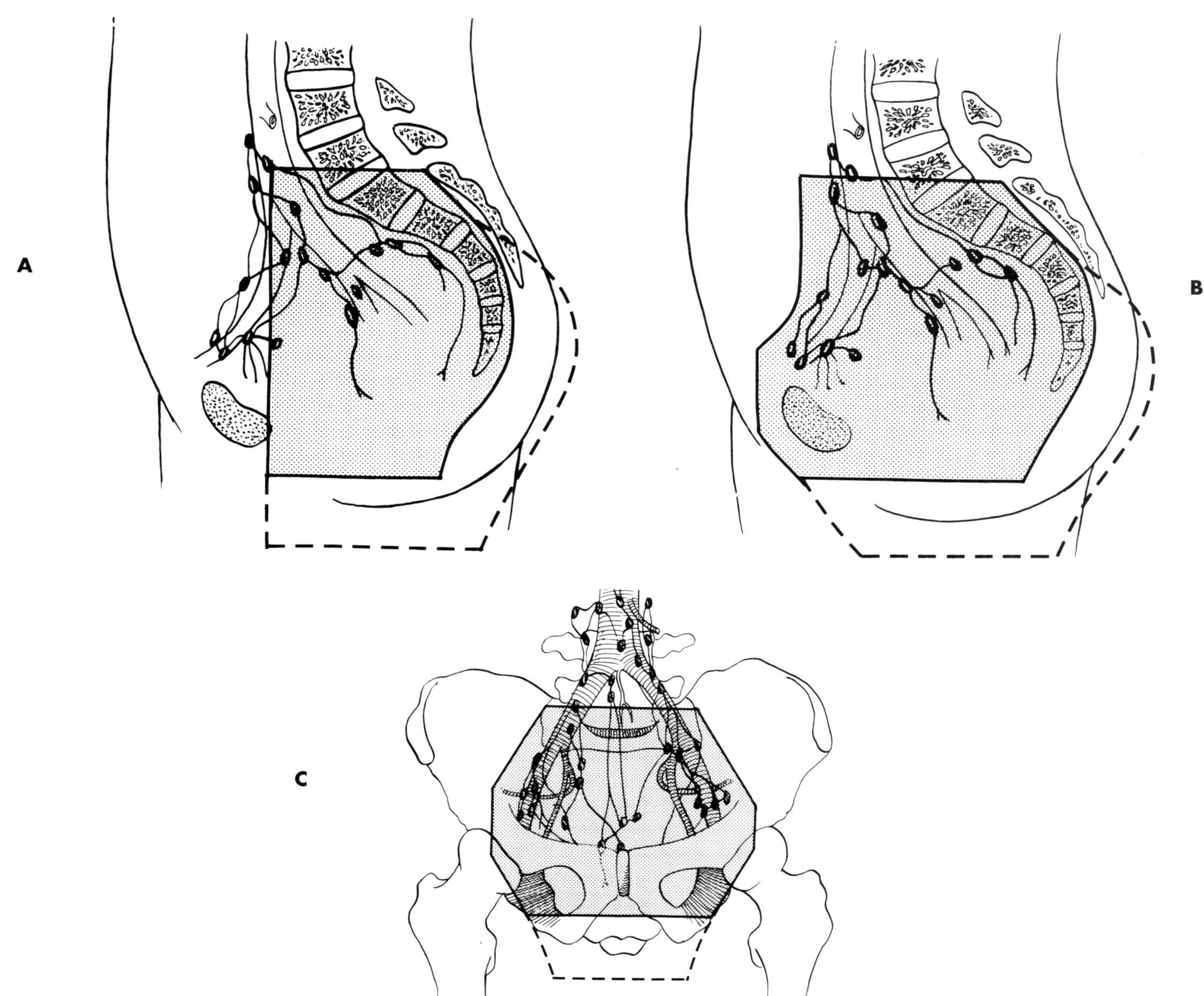

Fig. 10-8 Radiation treatment fields. In all figures the dotted line indicates the field extension to be used after an abdominal-perineal resection. **A,** A standard AP/PA field. **B,** A standard lateral field. **C,** A lateral field to include external iliacs in patients who have involvement of structures with external iliac lymph node drainage.

An extrapelvic colon cancer field design should include an initial margin of 3 to 5 cm beyond the tumor plus high-risk nodal groups and adjacent structures. If the tumor invaded or was adherent to an organ such as the ovary or stomach, the majority of the organ and its draining lymphatics should be encompassed in the treatment portal unless the organ was completely resected. Adherent structures should be included with a 3- to 5-cm margin. Usually, an AP/PA technique is used. However, CT treatment planning and clip placement may determine that a multifield approach more optimally spares normal tissue. The initial large volume is treated to 4500 cGy with a shrinking-field technique used to boost the tumor bed (with a 2- to 3-cm margin) an additional 540 to 900 cGy.[25,36]

Dose-limiting structures for treating an ascending or descending colon cancer include the kidney and small bowel. Contrast studies for assessing renal function and kidney localization films should be performed before treatment or at the time of simulation to ensure the adequate sparing of at least one kidney. For example, when treating a right-sided colon lesion, 50% or more of the right kidney may be in the field; therefore the left kidney must be spared.[25,36] For limiting the dose to the small bowel the patient can be treated in the decubitis position, resulting in a shift of the bowel away from the treated area and reducing the volume of the small bowel in the field. For a right-sided colon lesion the patient is simulated by lying on the left side, outlining the field based on surgical clips and preoperative imaging studies. A special tabletop device can be used that supports the patient's upper back and buttock-thigh region to aid in stability and reproducibility of the setup. Contrast in the small bowel at the time of simulation demonstrates whether an adequate shift of the small bowel takes place to make these fields feasible.

In patients with locally advanced colorectal cancer or recurrent disease, local control is difficult to achieve. This is due to the limited surgical options because of fixation of the tumor to pelvic organs (prostate, uterus) or unresectable structures such as the presacrum or pelvic sidewall. If microscopic residual disease exists, an external beam dose of ≥6000 cGy is necessary to provide a reasonable chance for control. This dose is even higher (≥7000 cGy) if gross residual disease exists.[22,24] These doses exceed the normal tissue-tolerance dose of abdominal or pelvic structures and cannot be safely delivered with conventional external beam irradiation.[24,27]

Intraoperative radiation therapy. **Intraoperative radiation therapy (IORT)** is a mechanism for supplementing the external beam dose to assist in obtaining local control of the tumor while sparing dose-limiting normal structures. IORT is a specialized boost technique similar to brachytherapy. As the name implies, IORT involves an operative procedure requiring general anesthesia. The radiation oncologist and surgeon must work closely with one another to determine whether IORT is appropriate and which diagnostic tests would be helpful in planning the IORT and external beam radiation treatments. A contraindication for IORT is the presence of distant metastasis. The surgeon and radiation oncologist also determine the optimal sequence of surgery and external radiation by discussing the benefits and side effects of each.[22,24]

Patients undergoing an IORT procedure receive a dose of 1000 to 2000 cGy of electrons in a single fraction directly to the tumor bed. Critical dose-limiting structures (i.e., kidney, bowel) are shielded or surgically displaced out of the radiation portal so that these normal tissues receive little or no radiation. This dose, delivered in a single fraction, is two to three times the dose if delivered at conventional fractionation of 180 to 200 cGy/fx. For example, an IORT single dose of 1500 cGy equals 3000- to 4500-cGy fractionated external radiation. When adding the effective IORT dose to the 4500 to 5000 cGy, delivered with conventional external beam radiation, the total effective dose equals 7500 to 9500 cGy.[22,24] A dose this high cannot be safely given with standard external irradiation.

The IORT dose is calculated at the 90% isodose line, with the energy and dose being delivered depending on the depth or amount of residual disease. Electron energies of 9 to 12 MeV are used after a gross total resection or minimal residual and high energies of 15 to 18 MeV are used for patients who have recurrent disease with gross residual or unresectable disease.[22,24] The target volume is encompassed in a lucite cylinder that projects from the patient and is docked to the treatment head of the linear accelerator. The beam of electrons travel through the lucite cylinder directly onto the tumor bed (Fig. 10-9).

The precise role of IORT in the treatment of large bowel cancer has not been definitively documented. Although some data suggest better local control and survival rates with this form of treatment, this improvement is quite possibly due to the selection of the most favorable patients for this form of treatment rather than an effect of the treatment itself. Moreover, toxicity can be significant. Further study is needed before IORT becomes a widely accepted tool in the treatment of colorectal cancer.

Side effects. The acute and chronic side effects of irradiation to the pelvis or abdomen are directly related to the volume and type of tissue irradiated, as well as the dose. The larger the area treated, the greater the associated toxicities. The toxicities of treatment increase with escalating doses and depend on the normal tissue tolerances of the structures in the irradiated volume. For patients with colorectal cancer the main dose-limiting structure for acute and chronic side effects is the small bowel. Acute toxicities of treatment include diarrhea, abdominal cramps and bloating, proctitis, bloody or mucus discharge, and dysuria. Patients may also experience **leukopenia** (an abnormal decrease in the white blood cell count) and **thrombocytopenia** (an abnormal decrease in the platelet count). Gastrointestinal and hematological toxicities are increased if chemotherapy is used with radiation therapy.[7,29,33,36] In patients who have their perineum treated, a brisk skin reaction (moist desquamation) may result, sometimes requiring a treatment break.[25]

Chronic effects occur less often than acute side effects but are more serious. Persistent diarrhea, increased bowel frequency, proctitis, urinary incontinence, and bladder atrophy have occurred in patients after radiation therapy. The most common long-term complication is damage to the small bowel, resulting in enteritis, adhesions, and obstruction.[7] The incidence of small-bowel obstruction requiring surgery may be decreased by radiation oncologists and surgeons working together to determine methods for minimizing the amount of small bowel in the radiation field.

As mentioned earlier, treatment techniques and fields are designed to limit the dose to the small bowel. These include surgical and radiation therapy interventions. For example, the surgeon can reconstruct the pelvis to minimize the amount of small bowel in the pelvis after an AP resection. The surgeon can help limit the volume of tissue irradiated by placing clips to demarcate the tumor bed, allowing the radi-

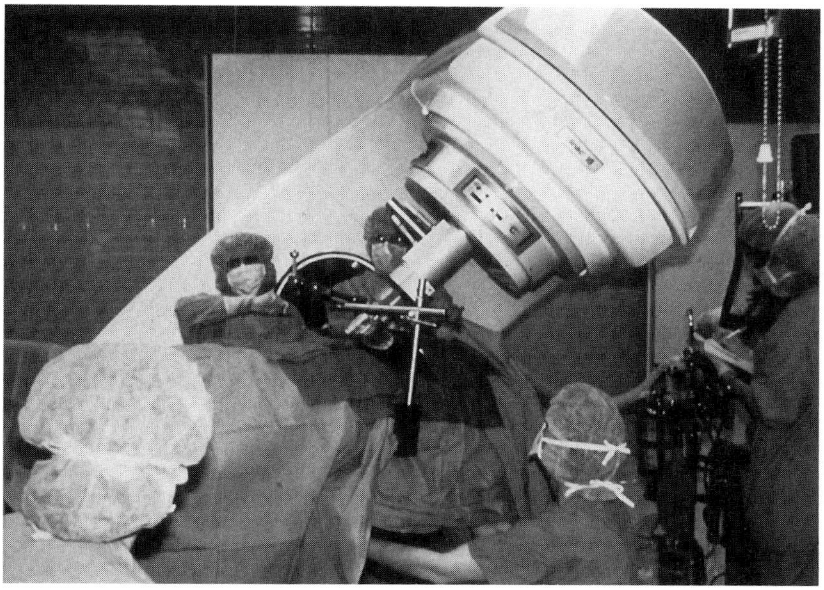

Fig. 10-9 Intraoperative radiation therapy with a linear accelerator. Direct irradiation of the tumor bed with a single dose of megavoltage electrons.

ation oncologist to more precisely outline the area at risk instead of requiring a more generous treatment volume.[7]

Radiation therapy techniques for limiting the small-bowel dose are numerous and involve the efforts of the radiation oncologist, radiation therapists, and dosimetrists. During simulation the physician uses previous imaging studies, such as CT and barium studies, to determine the tumor-small bowel relationship. After the radiation portals are established, a small-bowel series of radiographs is obtained in the simulator to document the mobility and amount of small bowel in the radiation portal. The patient is placed in a prone position, and films are taken with and without the patient having a full bladder to demonstrate the amount of small-bowel shift superiorly out of the treatment field (Fig. 10-10). Other devices used to minimize the small-bowel dosage are a false tabletop (FTT), or belly board, and an external compression device. The FTT fits over the treatment couch and has an opening to allow the bowel to shift anteriorly as a result of gravity when the patient is in the prone position . An FTT is used with bladder distention or an external compression device to shift the small bowel superiorly.[4,7,36] Care must be taken to ensure reproducibility of the setup if using any positioning device.

The radiation oncologist and dosimetrist work together to further reduce the small-bowel dose by carefully planning the initial and boost-field volumes through the use of intricate blocking. High-energy beams ($\geq$6 MV) are preferable because of the depth-dose characteristics that deliver a homogenous dose to the target volume while allowing the more anterior normal structures to be spared. A multiple-field approach (three or four fields) coupled with weighting of the fields to the posterior in rectal cancer patients further reduces the dose to the anteriorly located small bowel (Fig. 10-11).[7,21,27]

Role of radiation therapist

The radiation therapist plays a major role in the education of patients and their families. Communication is the key factor in making a patient's experience with a cancer diagnosis and treatment less traumatic and anxiety ridden. The therapist's first major role with the patient is in simulation. The therapist should inform the patient that the simulation is not a treatment but a planning session to locate and outline the area requiring treatment. The therapist should describe the procedure to the patient, indicating the length of time it will take and pointing out that the treatments themselves do not require the same amount of time. The patient's position during the treatment should also be discussed. The therapist should inform the patient about the contrast materials that will be used during the procedure, the skin marks to be used to outline radiation portals, and the importance of maintaining those marks. Most patients are treated in the prone position; therefore the therapist should explain the procedure before the patient is positioned. After the simulation begins, the therapist should continually update the patient on what is happening throughout the procedure. Keeping patients informed reduces the anxiety they may be experiencing.

At the time of the first treatment therapists should familiarize patients with the treatment room, then the location of the camera and audio equipment and explain what to do if

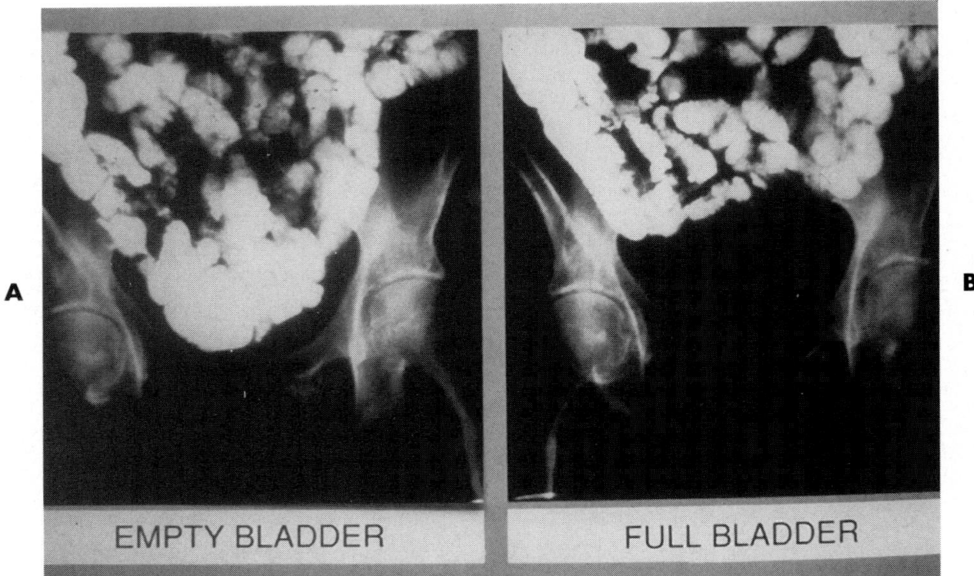

Fig. 10-10 Radiographs of the small bowel demonstrating a superior shift of bowel with bladder distention. **A**, Empty bladder. **B,** Full bladder.

they need something (e.g., raising their right hand). A common fear of patients is being alone in the room. Therapists should discuss the actual length of time the machine is on per treatment and explain that they will be in the room after treatment to each area. Therapists should also inform the patients about the types of noises that will be heard as the machine is programmed and treatment is initiated. If the patient's family members are also present, the therapist may offer to show them the treatment room and control area so they may see the videocamera; however, the family should not be in the control area during the initiation of treatment so that the therapist's performance is not hindered.

The therapist should assess the information given to the patient regarding treatment instructions (e.g., full bladder) and potential side effects. At many centers the oncology nurse sees the patient to discuss such issues. If this is the situation, the patient's appointment should be confirmed with the nurse. Written materials regarding bladder distention, a low-residue diet, and available support services should be distributed during the first week of treatment.

As treatments progress, the therapist is responsible for inquiring about how the patient is feeling, monitoring any treatment-related side effects, and checking on the patient's emotional well-being. If the patient complains of abdominal cramping and diarrhea, the therapist should determine whether the patient is following a low-residue diet or has a prescription for an antidiarrheal agent, such as Lomotil or Imodium. The therapist should ask the patient about the physician's instructions regarding the prescription. In some instances the patient may not be taking the medication correctly. The therapist can refer the patient to seek clarification regarding the correct administration of the antidiarrheal agent.

Table 10-2 Dietary guidelines for patients receiving pelvic irradiation

Recommended foods	Foods to avoid
White bread	Whole-grain breads or cereals
Meat baked, broiled, or roasted until tender	Fried or fatty foods
Macaroni	Milk and milk products
Cooked vegetables	Raw vegetables
Peeled apples and bananas	Fresh fruit

Dietary suggestions regarding which foods to avoid or recommendations for a low-residue diet are the therapist's responsibility. If the patient is experiencing diarrhea, instructions to avoid whole-grain breads or cereals, fresh fruits, raw vegetables, fried or fatty foods, milk, and milk products may be helpful. Recommended foods include white bread; meats that are baked, broiled, or roasted until tender; peeled apples; bananas; macaroni and noodles; and cooked vegetables (Table 10-2).[49] If the patient still complains of diarrhea after a diet and medications have been discussed, the patient may need to be referred back to the physician or dietitian for further evaluation.

Skin reactions on the perineum are quite common, especially in patients who have had a combined abdominoperineal resection (AP resection) in which the entire perineal

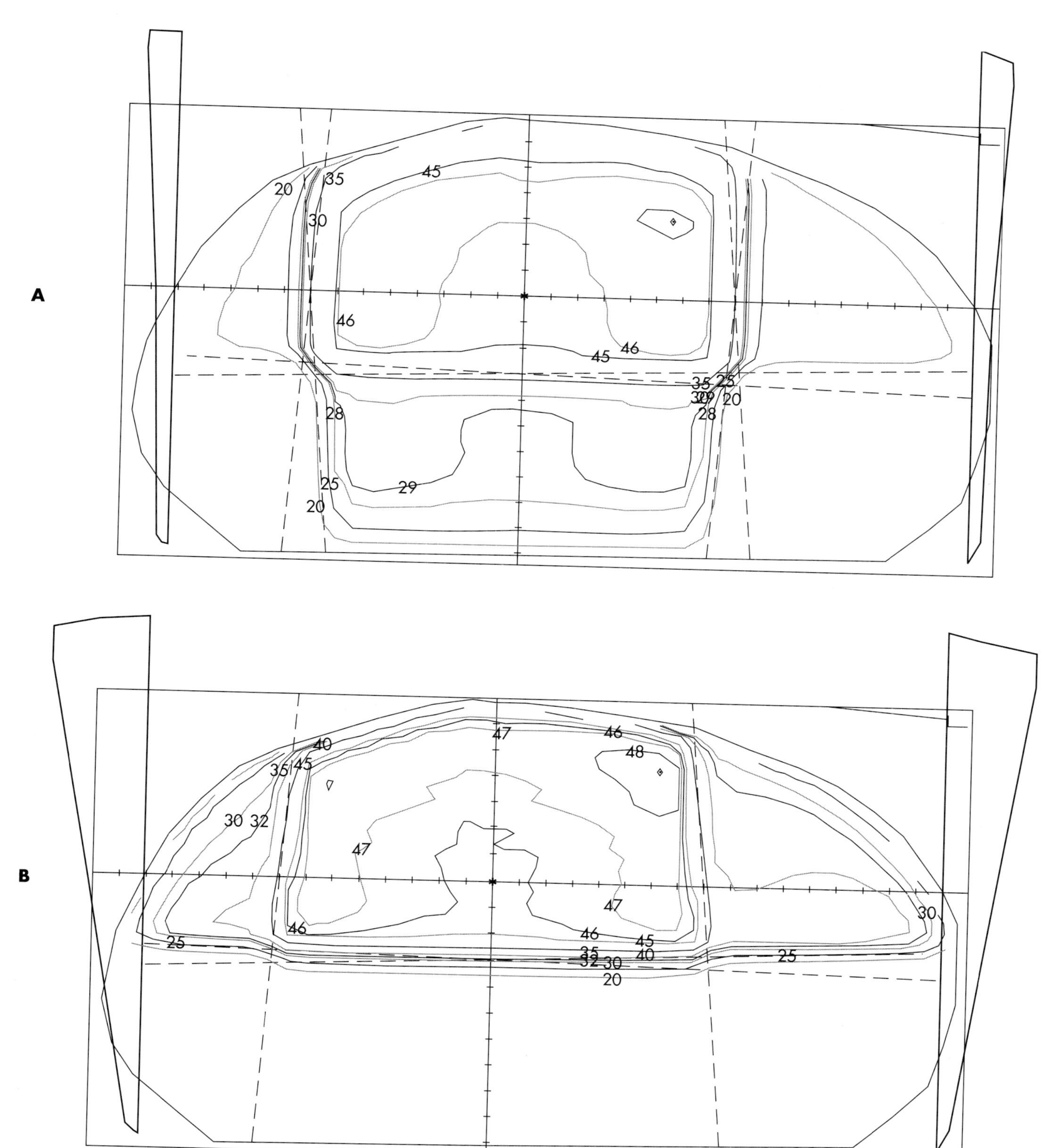

Fig 10-11 Isodose distribution of four-field pelvis technique **(A)** versus three-field technique **(B)**. Note the sparing of the anteriorly located small bowel with the three-field technique.

surface is treated with bolus. Skin reactions range from brisk erythema (treated with topical steroid creams) to moist desquamation (requiring sitz baths, Domeboro's solution, and possibly a treatment break). Therapists play an important role in monitoring the perineal area, which the patient cannot easily see. The therapist meets with the patient daily and can assess whether the reaction has intensified. The therapist can question patients to determine the way they are caring for their skin. If the patient has a moist desquamation, recommendations include taking sitz baths in tepid water, wearing loose undergarments or none at all, and allowing the area to be exposed to air and kept dry after the bath. These suggestions keep the area clean and dry.

Skin reactions in the perineal area of patients who have had a low anterior resection may be minimized by taping the patient's buttocks apart for the PA treatment field.[36] The buttocks create a natural bolus effect in the gluteal cleft. Taping them apart before treatment of the PA field reduces this skin fold. Two persons should tape simultaneously so that the patient is not rotated to one side or the other for treatment.

The physical side effects of treatment are often the most visible and easiest to address; however, the therapist must be alert to the emotional needs of the patient and family. The psychosocial aspect of a cancer diagnosis and treatment can be just as painful as the treatment or cancer itself. Therapists are not expected to diagnose but should *listen* to what the patient is saying and be available to offer suggestions and support. Sometimes, all the patient needs is for someone to listen and know someone cares. The therapist should provide the patient with information about community or hospital services, such as the American Cancer Society (ACS) "I Can Cope" series, the hospital oncology social worker or chaplain, and other support groups in the area. Patients with a colostomy may be having difficulty adjusting to their appliance, so the therapist can refer them to an endostomal therapist for assistance. The therapist should listen to patients and determine the way their diagnosis and treatment has affected their self-image and self-esteem. The ACS has a program called "Look Good, Feel Better" to assist patients in dealing with cosmetic side effects of cancer (primarily hair loss), but the program can also place a more positive outlook on a person's everyday life by stressing the message,"looking good and feeling better."

The ACS's written materials about specific types of cancer or other publications for cancer patients should be handed out or made available to the patient. These are documents patients can use as references and share with families and friends because the physician gives much of this information verbally to the patient, who may have trouble remembering it. After the patient has completed treatment, these written materials can still be referenced if the patient encounters a question. Being informed and knowledgable can lessen the anxiety associated with cancer and its treatment.

Case Study

A 60-year-old male with a 2- to 3-month history of rectal bleeding was examined by his local physician. The patient had noticed streaks of blood on his stool, which had changed in caliber to become progressively ribbonlike in diameter. The patient also complained of occasional rectal urgency and a full sensation in the lower abdomen and perineum. He also developed some urinary urgency. A rectal examination disclosed a mass. A flexible sigmoidoscopy was performed, which revealed a mass beginning 6 cm above the dentate line. The lesion was ulcerating and bleeding and occupied one third of the circumference of the bowel. A biopsy of the lesion revealed grade II adenocarcinoma. A further work-up included laboratory tests (complete blood count [CBC] and chemistry panel) and a CT scan with contrast of the abdomen and pelvis. The CT scan did not show any evidence of metastatic disease in the abdomen or pelvis, and all laboratory tests were normal.

The patient then underwent a low anterior resection in which 8 cm of the sigmoid colon and 12 cm of the rectum were removed. The pathology report indicated a grade II adenocarcinoma forming an ulcerating mass $3.5 \times 3.5 \times 1.0$ cm situated 2.5 cm from the distal resection margin. The tumor extended through the muscularis propria and just into the perirectal fat. The margins of resection were free of involvement, but the radial margins were close, with <1 cm of uninvolved fat. Of 11 perirectal lymph nodes, 1 contained micrometastasis. The patient's mass was staged as a MAC stage C2.

Because of the close surgical radial margins caused by the penetration of the tumor through the bowel wall and positive node, this patient was felt to be at high risk for local recurrence of the tumor with surgery alone. Therefore adjuvant postoperative radiation therapy with chemotherapy was recommended.

The patient received 5400 cGy with a shrinking four-field technique. The initial volume, including regional nodes, was 4500 cGy, and then successive cone down boost fields were used to bring the tumor bed and target volume up to the total dose of 5400 cGy. To safely achieve this dose, the patient was treated in the prone position on the false tabletop with full bladder distention for the boost fields to shift the small bowel out of the high-dose regions. If the small-bowel shift was not accomplished, the total dose would have been limited to 5040 cGY.

ANAL CANCER

Epidemiology and etiology

Cancers of the anus occur more often in women than men and constitute approximately 1% to 2% of all large-bowel malignancies. [45] The median age at the time of diagnosis is 60. A general age distribution of 30 to 90 years is reported, with an increased incidence of cancers in men less than 45 years of age. This trend has been attributed to male homosexuality and anal intercourse. The etiological factors for the development of anal cancer are associated with genital warts, genital infections, human papillomaviruses (HPVs), and immunosuppression. Cigarette smoking has also been associated with the development of anal cancer.[11,45]

Anatomy and lymphatics

The anal canal is 3 to 4 cm long and extends from the anal verge to the anorectal ring at the junction of the anus and rectum. The anal canal is lined with a hairless, stratified squamous epithelium up to the dentate or pectinate line. At this line the mucosa becomes cuboidal in transition to the columnar epithelium found in the rectum.[11,45]

Lymphatic spread occurs initially to the perirectal and anorectal lymph nodes. If the tumor extends above the dentate line, the nodal groups at risk are the internal iliac and lateral sacral nodes; this is similar to rectal cancer. With involvement below the dentate line, inguinal lymph nodes may be involved. Inguinal lymph node involvement is found in approximately 30% of patients.[45]

Clinical presentation

The most common presenting symptoms include bleeding, pain, and the sensation of a mass. Pruritus or itching has been reported less often and is associated with a perianal lesion.[11,45]

Detection and diagnosis

A thorough physical examination should be performed. This includes a digital anorectal examination (noting anal sphincter tone and direct extension to other organs) and palpation of the inguinal lymph nodes. A proctoscopic examination and biopsy should be obtained. A further work-up includes a CT scan of the pelvis, a chest radiograph, a CBC, and liver function tests.

Pathology, staging, and routes of spread

Squamous cell carcinoma is the most common histology of anal cancer, comprising approximately 80% of the cases. The next most frequent type is basaloid, or cloacogenic, cancer. These tumors occur in the region of the dentate line where the epithelium is in transition. Also found in this region are adenocarcinoma (arising from the anal glands), mucoepidermoid tumors, and melanoma. Cancers occurring in the perianal region are typically squamous or basal cell carcinomas consistent with skin cancers.

The most commonly used staging system is the AJCC system. This is a clinical system in which tumors are staged according to their size and extent (see the box above).

Tumors of the anal canal spread most frequently by direct extension into the adjacent soft tissues. Lymphatic spread occurs relatively early, whereas hematogoneous spread to the liver or lungs is less common.

Treatment techniques

An abdominoperineal resection with a wide perineal dissection is the most common surgical procedure for anal cancer.

TNM Staging System for Anal Cancer

Tis	Carcinoma in situ
T_1	Tumor ≤ 2 cm in largest dimension
T_2	Tumor 2.1-5 cm in largest dimension
T_3	Tumor >5 cm in largest dimension
T_4	Tumor of any size invades adjacent organs (vagina, urethra, bladder)
N_0	Negative nodes
N_1	Perirectal lymph node(s) involved
N_2	Unilateral internal iliac and/or inguinal lymph node(s)
N_3	Perirectal and inguinal lymph nodes and/or bilateral internal iliac and/or inguinal nodes

Modified from Beahrs OH et al, editors: *AJCC manual for staging of cancer*, ed 4, Philadelphia, 1992, JB Lippincott.

This procedure results in an overall survival rate of 50%. Radiation alone or in combination with chemotherapy (5-fluorouracil [5-FU] and mitomycin C) is now advocated as the preferred method of treatment. Studies have shown that the multimodality (radiation and chemotherapy) approach provides good local control and colostomy-free survival.[37,45] Most series report survival rates from 50% to 80% at 5 years, with a local control rate of 60% to 80%.[45]

A variety of radiation techniques exist for the treatment of anal cancer. Most use a four-field or AP/PA pelvic-field approach including a boost to the tumor bed with a perineal electron field or another multifield technique. The pelvic field extends from the lumbosacral-sacroiliac region to 3 cm distal to the lowest extent of the tumor (noted by a radiopaque marker at the time of simulation). The inferior border typically flashes the perineum, resulting in brisk erythema and moist desquamation of the perineal tissues. The lateral border may extend to include treatment of the inguinal lymph nodes on the AP field only, placing that field edge at the midlateral aspect of the femoral heads. The PA field is kept narrower because the anteriorly located inguinal nodes do not receive much contribution from the posterior field. This also avoids an excessive dose to the femoral heads, yet encompasses the tumor bed and deep pelvic nodes. Anterior electron fields centered over each inguinal region and abutting the PA lateral border are used to further supplement the dose to the inguinal lymph nodes.

The dose regimen used with radiation alone is 6000 to 6500 cGy delivered to the region of the primary tumor. This dose is reduced to approximately 4500 to 5040 cGy if concomitant chemotherapy is used. With either technique, field reductions are implemented after a dose of 4500 cGy to reduce small-bowel toxicity.

In conclusion, radiation therapy alone or in combination with chemotherapy is a viable treatment option, providing sphincter preservation and satisfactory cure rates in patients with anal cancer.

ESOPHAGEAL CANCER

Epidemiology and etiology

Cancer of the esophagus comprises 1% of all cancers in the United States, with approximately 11,000 cases estimated in 1994. Men are more commonly affected than women (8000 versus 3000, respectively), and a higher incidence is reported in blacks than in whites (13.1 versus 3.5 per 100,000).[5,15] Most of these cancers are diagnosed in patients between 55 and 65 years of age. Esophageal cancer is a nearly uniformly fatal disease, with the estimated deaths in the United States numbering 10,400 in 1994.[5]

Cancer of the esophagus occurs with the greatest frequency in northern China, northern Iran, and South Africa. In China one northern county (Hebi) has an incidence rate of 139.8 persons per 100,000 occurring in persons 30 years of age or older, whereas another county in China has a rate of only 1.4 persons per 100,000. This has been attributed to environmental and nutritional factors.[15,18,44]

The most common and important etiological factors in the development of squamous cell cancer of the esophagus in western countries are excessive alcohol and tobacco use. Alcohol and tobacco abuse are associated with 80% to 90% of all cases diagnosed in North America and western Europe. The combination of these two factors has a synergistic effect on the mucosal surfaces, increasing the risk of esophageal cancer and other aerodigestive malignancies. Esophageal cancer is commonly found as a second primary after a previous diagnosis of head and neck cancer.[15,18,44]

Dietary factors have also been implicated in the development of cancer of the esophagus. Diets low in fresh fruits and vegetables and high in nitrates (i.e., cured meats, fish, pickled vegetables) have been cited as risk factors for persons from Iran, China, and South Africa, respectively.

Other conditions predispose individuals to the development of esophageal cancer. They include achalasia, Plummer-Vinson syndrome, caustic injury, and Barrett's esophagus.

Achalasia is a disorder in which the lower two thirds of the esophagus has lost its normal peristaltic activity. The esophagus becomes dilated (termed *megaesophagus*), and the esophogastric junction sphincter also fails to relax, prohibiting the passage of food into the stomach. Clinical symptoms include progressive dysphagia and regurgitation of ingested food. Patients with achalasia have a 5% to 20% risk of developing cancer of the esophagus.[43,44]

Plummer-Vinson syndrome (also known as Paterson-Kelly syndrome) is an iron-deficient anemia characterized by esophageal webs, atrophic glossitis, and spoon-shaped, brittle fingernails. This syndrome occurs mostly in women.

Caustic injuries and burns caused by the ingestion of lye are responsible for 1% to 4% of esophageal squamous cell cancers. Malignancies develop in the scarred, or stricture, area years after an injury.[43,44]

Barrett's esophagus is a condition in which the distal esophagus is lined with a columnar epithelium rather than a stratified squamous epithelium. This mucosal change usually occurs with gastroesophageal reflux. One theory to explain this phenomenon is that chronic chemical trauma resulting from reflux causes the mucosa to undergo metaplasia.[43,44] Adenocarcinoma of the esophagus occurs in 2.4% to 8.3% of patients who have Barrett's mucosa.[18]

Prognostic indicators

Tumor size is an important prognostic tool. According to a series by Hussey et al., patients with tumors less than 5 cm in length had a better 2-year survival rate (19.2%) than patients with lesions larger than 9 cm (1.9%).[18] Tumors ≤ 5 cm in length were more often localized (40% to 60%), whereas tumors >5 cm had distant metastasis 75% of the time.[18,44] Other factors indicating a poor prognosis are weight loss of 10%, a poor performance status, and patients over age 65.

Anatomy and lymphatics

The esophagus is a thin-walled 25-cm-long tube lined with stratifed squamous epithelium. The esophagus begins at the level of C6 and traverses through the thoracic cage to terminate in the abdomen at the esophageal gastric (E-G) junction (T10-11).

For accurate classification, staging, and recording of tumors in the esophagus, the AJCC has divided the esophagus into four regions: cervical, upper thoracic, middle thoracic, and lower thoracic. Because lesions are localized by an endoscopy, reference is made to the distance of the lesion from the upper incisors (front teeth). This distance is also used in defining each region (Fig. 10-12).[2,44]

The cervical esophagus extends from the cricoid cartilage to the thoracic inlet (suprasternal notch [SSN]), corresponding to vertebral levels C6 to T3 and measuring about 18 cm from the upper incisors. The thoracic inlet (SSN) to the level of the tracheal bifurcation (carina)—24 cm from the incisors—defines the upper thoracic portion. The middle thoracic esophagus begins at the carina and extends proximally to the E-G junction, or 32 cm from the incisors. The lower thoracic portion includes the abdominal esophagus and is approximately 8 cm long at a level of 40 cm from the incisors.[2,13,44]

The esophagus lies directly posterior to the trachea and is anterior to the vertebral column. Located laterally and to the left of the esophagus is the aortic arch. The descending aorta is situated lateral and posterior to the esophagus (see Fig. 10-12). During an endoscopy an indentation is visible where the aorta and left main-stem bronchus are in contact with the esophagus. Because of the esophagus' intimate relationship with these structures, tumors are often locally advanced, fistulas may occur, and surgery is often not feasible.[13,39,44]

Histologically, the esophagus consists of the usual layers of the bowel common to the gastrointestinal tract (i.e., the mucosa, submucosa, and muscular layers). However, the esophagus lacks a serosal layer. The outermost layer, the adventitia, consists of a thin, loose connective tissue. This is another factor contributing to the early spread of these tumors to adjacent structures.[18,39]

The esophagus has numerous small lymphatic vessels in the mucosa and submucosal layers. These vessels drain outward into larger vessels located in the muscular layers (Fig. 10-13). Lymph fluid can travel the entire length of the esophagus and drain into any adjacent draining nodal bed, placing the entire esophagus at risk for skip metastasis and nodal involvement.[17,18,39,44]

Although the entire length of the esophagus is at risk for lymphatic metastasis, each region still has primary or regional nodes that specifically drain the area. For example, the upper

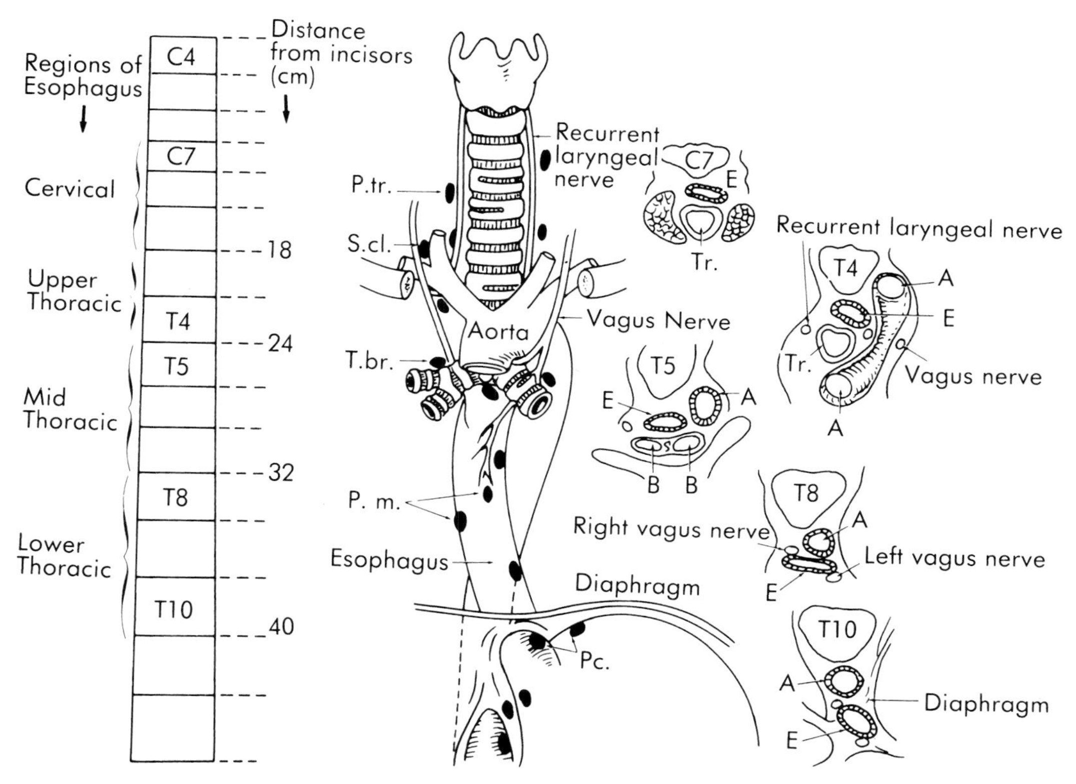

Fig. 10-12 The relationship of the esophagus with surrounding anatomical structures, including divisions of the esophagus and their location from the upper central incisors. (From Cox JD: *Moss' radiation oncology: rationale, techniques, results,* ed 7, St Louis, 1994, Mosby.)

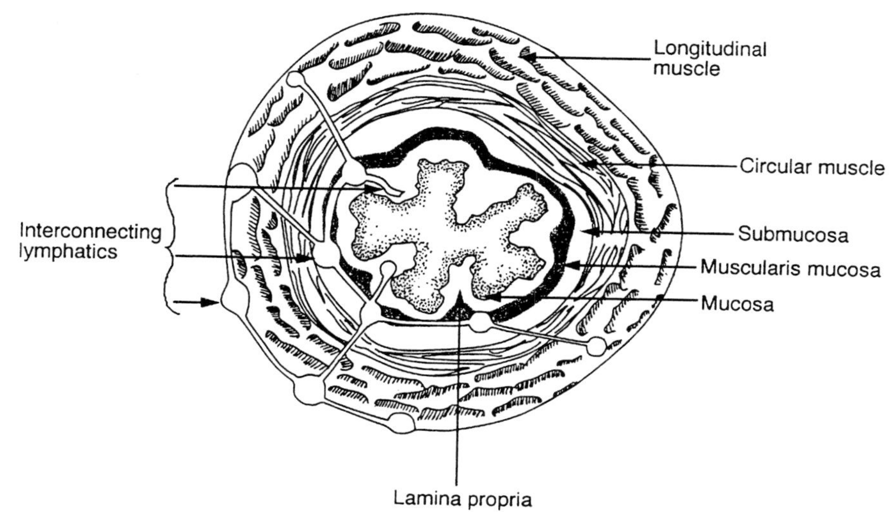

Fig. 10-13 Lymphatic vessels located in the wall of the esophagus. (From Cox JD: *Moss' radiation oncology: rationale, techniques, results,* ed 7, St Louis, 1994, Mosby.)

third (cervical area) of the esophagus drains into the internal jugular, cervical, paraesophageal, and supraclavicular lymph nodes. The upper and middle thoracic portion has drainage to the paratracheal, hilar, subcarinal, paraesophageal, and paracardial lymph nodes. Finally, the principal draining lymphatics for the distal or lower third of the esophagus include the celiac axis, left gastric nodes, and nodes of the lesser curvature of the stomach (Fig. 10-14). Lymphatic spread is unpredictable and may occur at a significant distance from the tumor. Positive nodes outside a defined region represent distant metastasis rather than regional spread. For example, supraclavicular nodal involvement in a primary tumor located in the cervical esophagus is considered regional lymph node involvement, but this would be a distant metastasis for tumors arising in the thoracic esophagus.[2,13]

Clinical presentation

The most common presenting symptoms are dysphagia and weight loss, which occur in 90% of patients. Patients complain of food sticking in their throat and may point to the location of this sensation. Initially, patients have difficulty with bulky foods, then with soft foods, and finally even with liquids. Patients may recall having this difficulty in swallowing for 3 to 6 months before the diagnosis. Regurgitation of undigested food and aspiration pneumonia may also occur. **Odynophagia** (painful swallowing) is reported in approximately 50% of patients. Symptoms of a locally advanced tumor include the following: hematemesis (vomiting blood), coughing (caused by a tracheoesophageal fistula), hemoptysis, Horner's syndrome, or hoarseness as a result of nerve involvement.[15,18,44]

Detection and diagnosis

A thorough history and physical examination should be performed. Information should be obtained regarding weight loss and the use of alcohol and tobacco. The physical examination should include palpation of the cervical and supraclavicular lymph nodes and abdomen to assess potential spread to the nodes or liver. A chest radiograph and esophagogram are necessary for localizing the lesions causing the dysphagia. Esophagograms depict characteristic features of esophageal cancers, such as those in Fig. 10-15. The reported incidence of tumors located in each third of the esophagus varies in the literature. Lesions in the upper third of the esophagus occur with the least frequency, comprising 10% to 25% of tumors. Approximately 40% to 50% of tumors are located in the middle third of the esophagus, and 25% to 50% are located in the lower third.[15,18,44]

A CT scan of the chest and upper abdomen should be obtained. This scan may demonstrate extra mucosal spread and invasion of adjacent structures such as the trachea or aorta. Spread to lymph nodes in the thorax and abdomen can be also assessed. Blood-borne spread to the liver and adrenals may be imaged via CT, although small lesions may not be detectable.

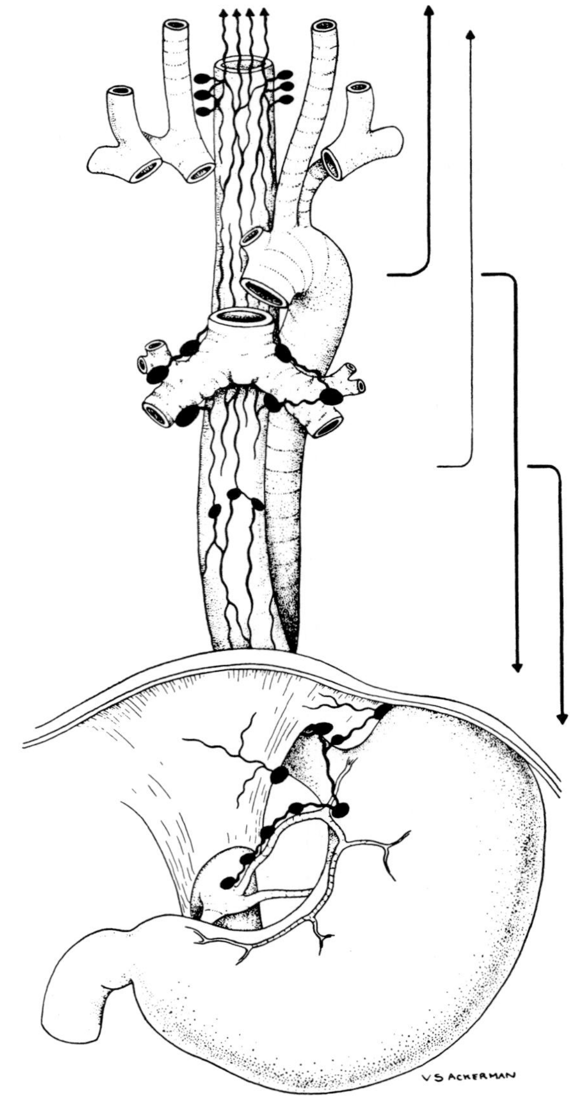

Fig. 10-14 Lymphatic drainage of the esophagus. The *arrows* represent potential spread to cervical, mediastinal, and subdiaphragmatic lymph nodes, based on the location of the esophageal lesion. Subdiaphragmatic involvement is unusual in the upper-third tumors. (From del Regato JA, Spjut HJ, Cox JD: *Ackerman and del Regato's cancer: diagnosis, treatment, and prognosis,* ed 6, St Louis, 1985 Mosby.)

An ultrasound of suspicious liver nodules is performed to differentiate metastasis from a cystic mass.[15,18,44] Laboratory studies include a CBC and blood chemistry group to assess the liver and kidney function.

A histological confirmation is obtained during an esophagoscopy. A rigid or flexible scope can be used to examine the entire esophagus, obtaining brushings and biopsies of all suspicious lesions. A bronchoscopy should also be performed for all upper- or middle-third lesions to detect any possible communication of the tumor with the tracheobronchial tree.[15,18,44]

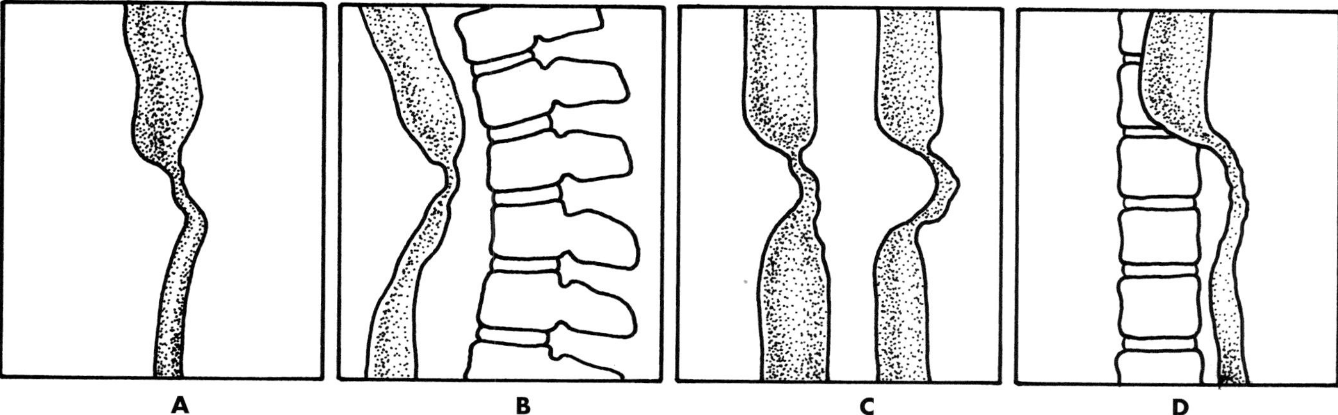

Fig. 10-15 Esophagograms demonstrating four characteristic features of unresectable tumors. **A,** Tortuosity of the esophageal axis proximal to the tumor. **B**, Esophageal axis angulation. **C,** Deviation of the axis above and below the tumor; deviation of the tumor axis. **D,** Displacement of the esophageal axis from the spine. (Redrawn from Akiyama H: Surgery for carcinoma of the esophagus, *Curr Probl Surg* 17:56, 1980.)

Pathology and staging

The most common pathological type of esophageal cancer is squamous cell carcinoma, accounting for 90% of all cases.[18] Adenocarcinoma is the next most frequent malignancy of the esophagus and typically occurs in the distal esophagus. Adenocarcinoma is often found with Barrett's esophagus or is believed to be an extension of a gastric cancer into the esophagus. In the United States, adenocarcinoma has been increasing in frequency. A variety of other epithelial tumors arise in the esophagus but are rare. These include adenoid cystic carcinoma, mucoepidermoid carcinoma, adenosquamous carcinoma, and undifferentiated carcinoma.[18,44]

Nonepithelial tumors also arise in the esophagus, although this is rare. Leiomyosarcoma (a tumor of the smooth muscle) is the most common nonepithelial tumor. Leiomyosarcomas yield a more favorable prognosis than squamous cell carcinomas. Malignant melanoma, lymphoma, and rhabdomyosarcoma are other nonepithelial tumors that can occur in the esophagus.[18,44]

The AJCC staging system for esophageal cancer is shown in the box to the right.

Routes of spread

Because the esophagus is distensible, lesions are quite large before causing obstructive symptoms. Spread is usually longitudinal. Occasionally, skip lesions may be present at a significant distance from the primary lesion. This is principally due to submucosal spread of the tumor through interconnecting lymph channels. Locally advanced disease, invasion into adjacent structures, and early spread to draining lymphatics are quite common in esophageal cancer. Distant metastasis can occur in many different organs, with the liver and lung being the most common.

TNM Staging of Esophageal Cancer

Tis	Carcinoma in situ
T_1	Tumor invades submucosa
T_2	Tumor invades muscularis propria
T_3	Tumor invades adventitia
T_4	Tumor invades adjacent structures
N_0	Negative regional nodes
N_1	Positive regional nodes
M_0	No distant metastasis
M_1	Distant metastasis (liver, lung, or nodes beyond region of primary; positive cervical nodes with a thoracic esophagus primary)

Modified from Beahrs OH et al, editors: *AJCC manual for staging of cancer,* ed 4, Philadelphia, 1992, JB Lippincott.

Treatment techniques

The treatment of esophageal cancer is highly complex and technically difficult. Most patients have locally advanced or metastatic disease at the time of diagnosis and require multimodality treatment. Treatment is usually categorized as curative or palliative and may be given with surgery or radiation for the local-regional problem. Patients who receive either modality (surgery or radiation) alone have a significant risk of local recurrence and distant metastasis. The primary goal of either treatment is to provide relief of the dysphagia and a chance for cure. The current nonsurgical standard for the treatment of esophageal cancer is combined chemotherapy and radiation therapy.[23,31]

A variety of surgical techniques exist for the resection of esophageal cancer. In many centers, surgical resection is limited to the middle and lower thirds of the esophagus. The cervical esophagus is not considered a surgically accessible site in many institutions and is often managed with radiation therapy and chemotherapy. Curative surgery usually involves a subtotal or total esophagectomy. The type of procedure chosen depends on the location of the lesion and extent of involvement. Typically, the entire esophagus is removed. The continuity of the gastrointestinal system is maintained by placing either the stomach or left colon in the thoracic cavity. The Ivor Lewis procedure consists of a laparotomy and right thoracotomy to remove the esophagus and mobilize the stomach into the thoracic cavity (Fig. 10-16). A total thoracic esophagectomy also requires multiple surgical incisions. A laparotomy is performed to mobilize the stomach, and a thoracotomy is performed to remove the esophagus. However, a third incision is made at the neck to assist in the anastomosis of the stomach to the remaining cervical esophagus (Fig. 10-17).[15,44]

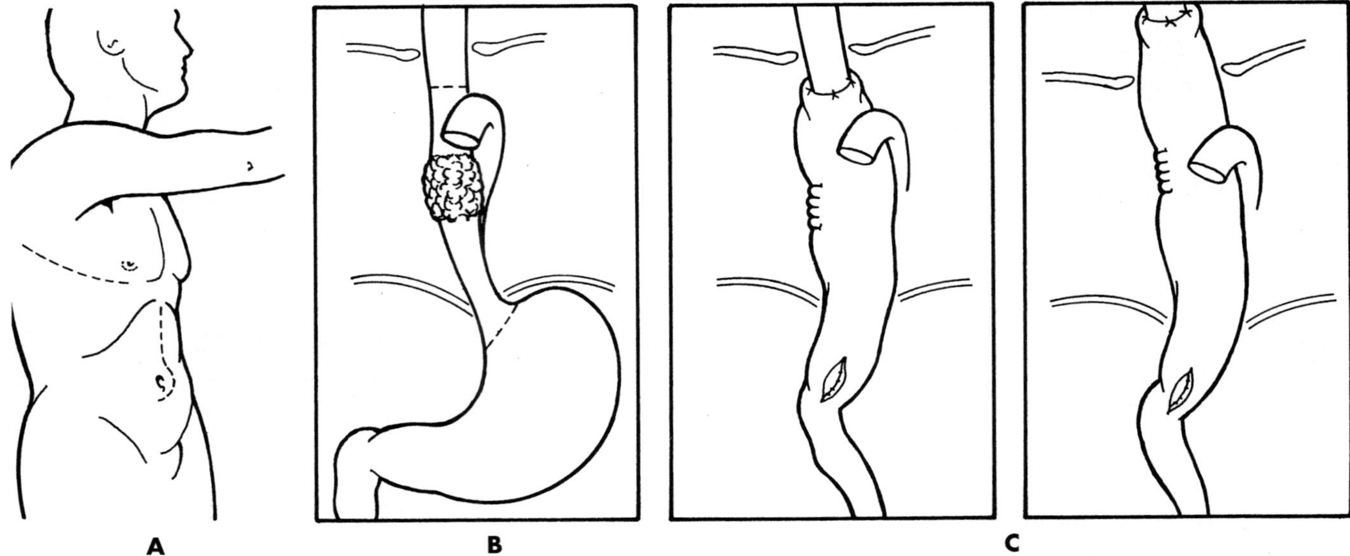

Fig. 10-16 The Ivor Lewis procedure. **A,** Laparotomy and right thoracotomy. **B,** Tumor and margin of resection. **C,** Mobilization of the stomach into the chest cavity with anastomosis to the remaining esophagus (esophagogastrostomy). (Redrawn from Ellis FH Jr: Esophagogastrectomy for carcinoma: technical considerations based on anatomic location of lesion, *Surg Clin North Am* 60:273, 1980.)

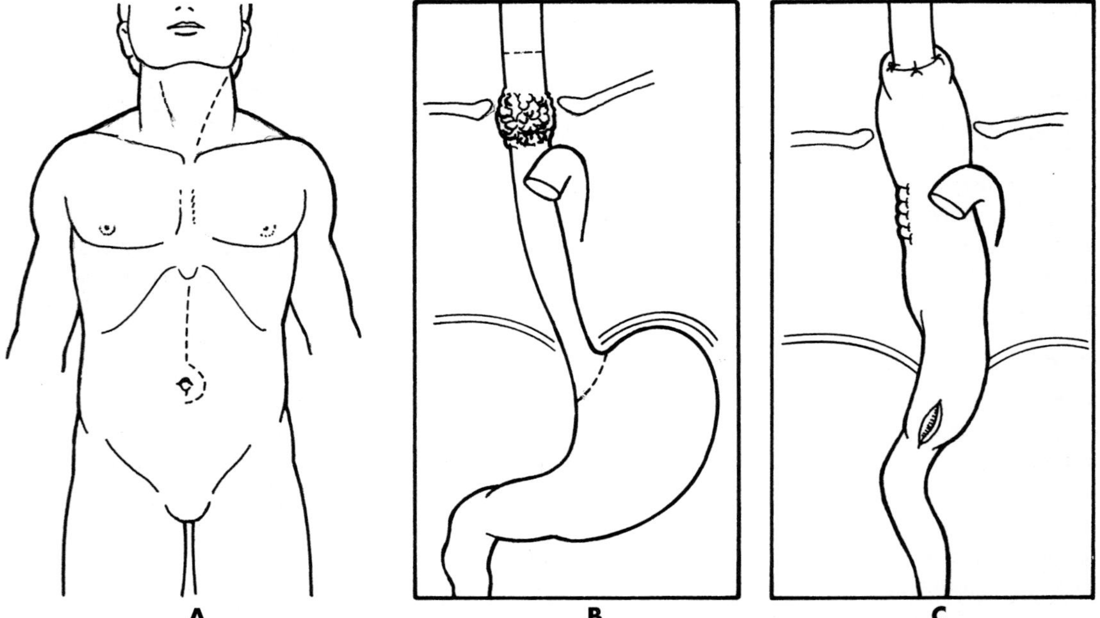

Fig. 10-17 **A,** Laparotomy and left cervical incision. **B,** Tumor and margin of the resection. **C,** Mobilization of the stomach into the chest cavity with anastomosis to the cervical esophagus via a neck incision. (Redrawn from Ellis FH Jr: Esophagogastrectomy for carcinoma: technical considerations based on anatomic location of lesion, *Surg Clin North Am* 60:275, 1980.)

Both of these procedures are technically difficult and associated with a high morbidity and mortality rate. Operative mortality rates from either procedure have ranged from 8% to 31%, although recent studies have demonstrated a decrease in these rates. Complications from surgery include anastomotic leaks (which can be life threatening), respiratory failure, pulmonary embolus, and myocardial infarctions. Strictures, difficulty in gastric emptying, and gastoresophageal reflux are mechanical side effects resulting from surgery.

Even after a curative resection the majority of patients fail distantly with blood-borne spread to the lungs, liver, or bone.

Radiation therapy. Radiation therapy alone or with chemotherapy has been routinely used for the treatment of esophageal cancer. Radiation therapy with chemotherapy is considered the current nonsurgical treatment of choice for esophageal cancer.[23,31,44] A recent study demonstrated a clear advantage for radiation therapy and chemotherapy compared with radiation therapy alone.[31]

Chemotherapy. The poor survival rates resulting from esophageal cancer are associated with the high percentage of patients who fail locally and with distant metastasis after curative treatment. The addition of combination chemotherapy has resulted in a decrease in local and distant failures and an increase in the overall survival rate compared with radiation alone (Figs. 10-18 and 10-19).[31] 5-FU and cisplatin are administered during weeks 1, 5, 8, and 11 of the radiation therapy treatments. Combined modality therapy has definite local control and survival benefits. However, the side effects from this regimen are worse.

Field design and critical structures. Esophageal cancer spreads longitudinally with skip lesions up to 5 cm from the primary. Regional spread to draining lymphatics is a common early presentation and must be taken into consideration in the design of the radiation field. The cervical, supraclavicular, mediastinal, and subdiaphragmatic (celiac axis) lymph node regions are at risk. The degree at which these nodal groups are at risk depends on the location of the primary tumor. Supraclavicular nodes are involved more often with a proximal lesion than a distal lesion. However, neck or abdominal nodal-disease involvement can occur with any esophageal primary site.[23]

Because of the potential for longitudinal spread of these cancers, radiation portals encompassing the areas at risk are typically quite large. For tumors of the thoracic esophagus the anatomical borders included in the treatment field extend from above the supraclavicular fossa to the esophagogastric junction. This volume is necessary for including the regional lymphatics and encompassing the primary tumor with a 5-cm margin above and below the gross disease.

Lesions of the upper third of the esophagus are treated with a field that begins at the level of the thyroid cartilage and ends at the level of the carina. In patients with tumors of the distal third of the esophagus the inferior margin must include the celiac-axis lymph nodes, which are located at the T12-L1 vertebral level. The superior extent of the treatment field should include the mediastinal nodes and may include the supraclavicular nodes because they are at a low risk of being involved.[18,23,44]

The standard technique for treating the initial large fields is an AP/PA field, followed by shrinking fields of various arrangements. For treatment with radiation alone the prescribed dose is 65 Gy. With combined radiation and chemotherapy the total dose is 50 Gy to minimize normal tissue toxicity. Both of these doses exceed the radiation-tolerance dose of the spinal cord, which is 45 to 50 Gy. Careful dosimetry planning is necessary to avoid overdosing the spinal cord. AP/PA fields are used initially; as cord tolerance is approached, an off-cord technique is implemented. A vari-

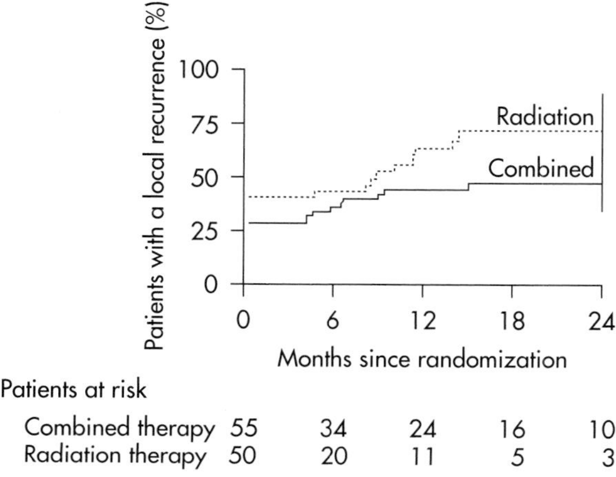

Fig. 10-18 A comparison of radiation alone with combined radiation and chemotherapy regarding the time to a local recurrence in patients with esophageal cancer. (From Herskovic A et al: Combined chemotherapy and radiotherapy compared with radiotherapy alone in patients with cancer of the esophagus, *N Engl J Med* 326:1596, 1992.)

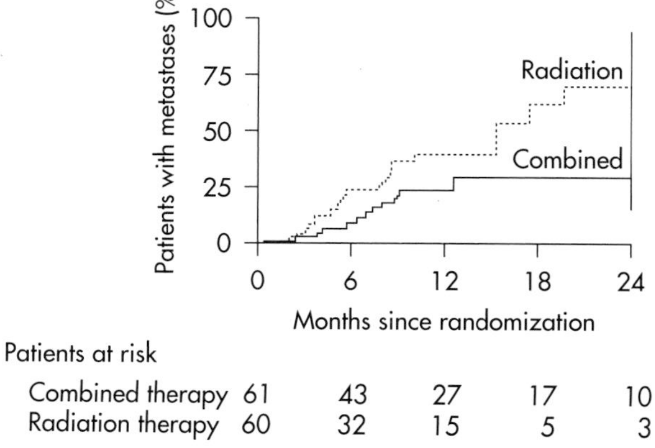

Fig. 10-19 A comparison of radiation alone with combined radiation and chemotherapy regarding the time to a distant metastasis in patients with esophageal cancer. (Modified from Herskovic A et al: Combined chemotherapy and radiotherapy compared with radiotherapy alone in patients with cancer of the esophagus, *N End J Med* 326:1595, 1992)

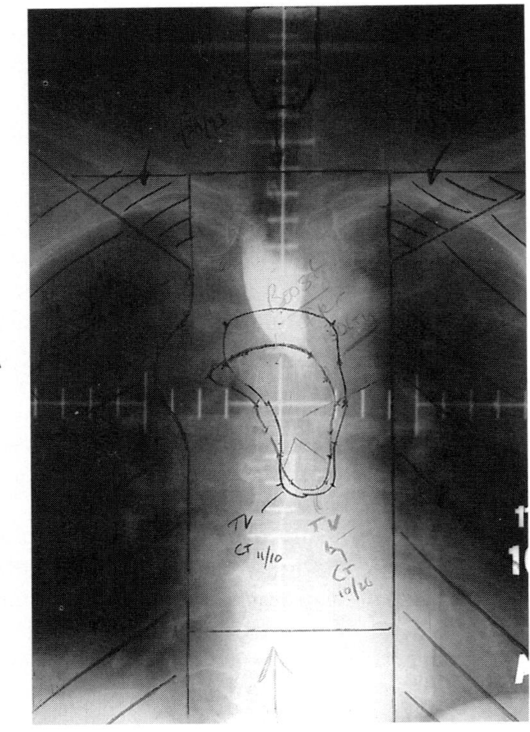

ety of off-cord field arrangements can be used, depending on the location of the tumor. The most common field arrangements are oblique radiation portals. Many institutions use a three-field approach: an anterior field and two posterior-wedged obliques, especially for lesions of the thoracic esophagus. Two anterior-wedged obliques or parallel-opposed oblique fields have also been used for lesions of the upper third of the esophagus (Fig. 10-20).[18,23,44] Another common off-cord technique in distal esophageal lesions is opposed laterals with AP/PA fields.

For the simulation of a patient with esophageal cancer a variety of patient positions have been advocated. Some authors advise placing the patient in the prone position, using gravity to help place the esophagus at a greater distance from the spinal cord. This facilitates lower cord doses without compromising the tumor dose.[9,18] More universal is the standard supine position for patient simulation and treatment. Older patients and those who are more ill can tolerate this position easier and for a longer time than the prone position.

Other patient-positioning issues deal with the placement of the patient's arms. Because lateral treatment-field arrangements may be used, the patient's arms are often positioned

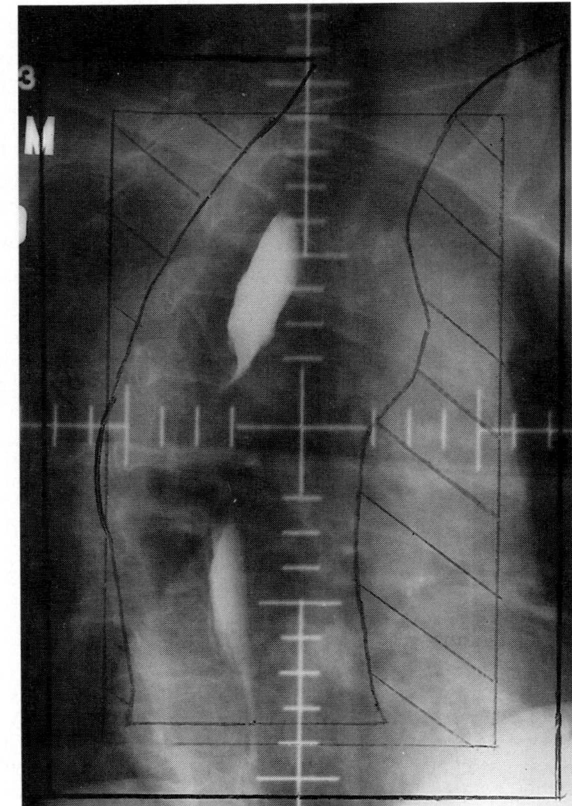

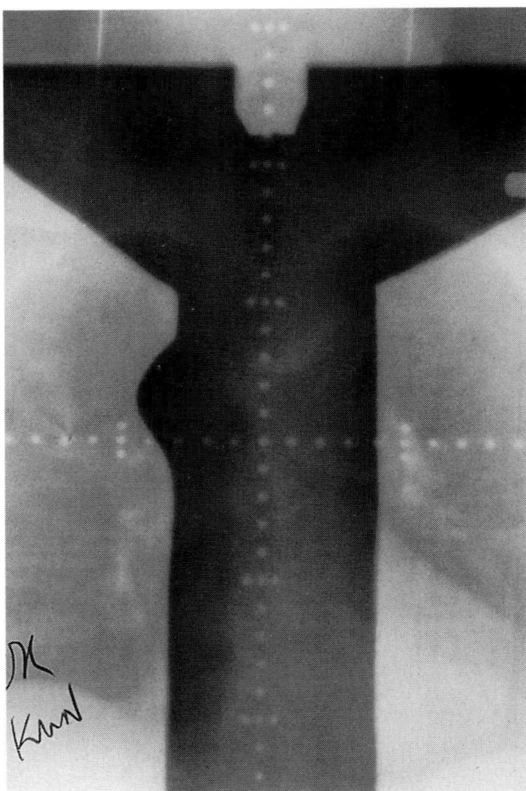

Fig. 10-20 Radiation treatment fields for cancer of the esophagus. **A,** An AP/PA field with barium to localize the esophageal lesion. **B,** Off-cord oblique fields. **C,** Port film of the initial AP field.

above the head, with the patient clasping the elbows or wrists. This position can be difficult for the patient to hold and maintain, causing reproducibility problems later during treatment. Custom-made immobilization devices such as body casts, foaming cradles, and vacuum-bag devices greatly assist the daily reproducibility of the setup. Without a custom-made device, measurements of the elbow-to-elbow separation will assist in the consistency of the daily setup.

For the simulation of patients with their arms along their sides for isocentric fields, the elbows should be bent slightly out from the body so that a set of marks can be placed on the thoracic cage for a **three-point setup**. This is extremely important if the lateral positioning marks are on the arms and shoulders, as they are in an upper-third esophageal lesion. The arms are quite mobile and are not reliable for positioning and maintaining the established isocenter daily. Therefore a second set of three reference points are placed lower on the thoracic cage and are used to establish the isocenter. The upper three points are used to maintain the shoulder position. The AP SSD, or setup distance, is double-checked and maintained, especially with oblique treatment fields.

Orthogonal radiographs are taken 90 degrees apart at the time of the initial simulation. This includes an anterior film (defining the actual treatment volume) and a lateral film (establishing the isocenter or depth). Both films should be taken with barium contrast in the esophagus to delineate the esophagus and its relationship to normal structures. These radiographs, along with multiple-level contours or a CT scan with the patient in treatment position, assist the dosimetrist in planning the necessary off-cord field arrangements (Fig 10-21). After the treatment plan is complete a second simulation is often needed to film the oblique treatment fields.

Side effects. After 2 weeks of radiation treatment, patients begin to experience **esophagitis.** They complain of substernal pain during swallowing and the sensation of food sticking in their esophagus. Patients may be unable to eat solid foods and require a diet of bland, soft, or pureed foods. In addition, patients should eat small, frequent meals that are high in calories and protein (Table 10-3). High-calorie liquid supplements such as Carnation Instant Breakfast and Ensure

Table 10-3 Dietary guidelines for patients receiving thoracic irradiation

Recommended foods	Foods to avoid
Cottage cheese, yogurt, and milk shakes	Hot and spicy foods
Puddings	Dry to coarse foods
Casseroles	Crackers, nuts, and potato chips
Scrambled eggs	Raw vegetables, citrus fruits, and juices
Meats and vegetables in sauces or gravies.	Alcoholic beverages

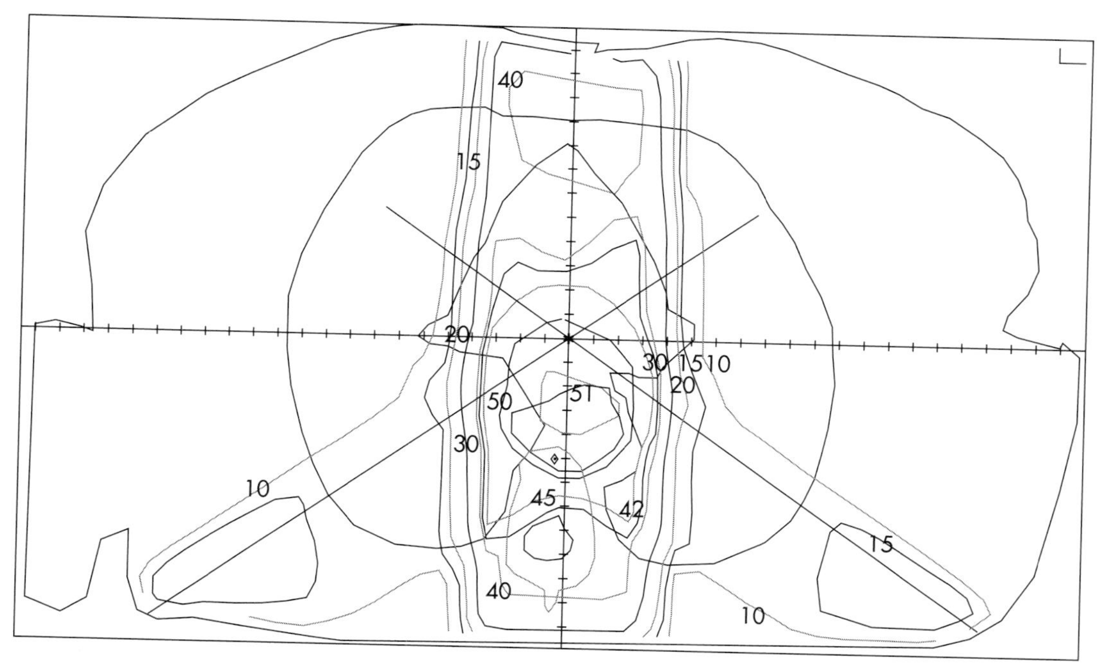

Fig.10-21 Isodose distribution resulting from AP/PA and parallel-opposed obliques. AP/PA fields are discontinued as cord tolerance is reached. Note the sparing of the spinal cord with oblique fields.

are good alternatives for a high-calorie snack during the day or at bedtime.[14,31,49]

To ease the pain of swallowing, the physician may suggest the patient take liquid analgesics or viscous lidocaine before meals. These drugs provide local and systemic pain relief. Esophagitis can become quite severe by the end of the treatment and may even require the placement of a nasogastric tube.

Concomitant chemotherapy increases the sensitivity of the esophageal mucosa to radiation. Therefore more severe esophagitis and possibly ulceration may occur. The radiation tolerance of the esophagus is 65 Gy delivered with 1.8- to 2.0-Gy fractions. When concurrent chemotherapy is administered the total radiation dose safely delivered is 50 Gy, based on the increased treatment-related toxicities associated with combined-modality treatment. Decreased blood counts, nausea, and vomiting also occur with chemotherapy. A break in a patient's treatment may be necessary if the leukocyte or platelet count becomes too low.

Radiation pneumonitis or pericarditis may occur if a large volume of lung or heart is in the radiation field. Proper field shaping with custom blocks, multiple fields per day, and careful dosimetry greatly reduce the likelihood of these complications being severe. Perforation and fistula formation can result from rapid shrinkage of a tumor that was adherent to the esophageal-tracheal wall.

Long-term side effects from irradiating the esophagus include stenosis or stricture as a result of scar formation. Dilatations of the esophagus can be performed, relieving the obstructive symptoms and restoring the patient's ability to swallow.[18,31,44] Transverse myelitis is a late complication that should not occur if the radiation treatments are delivered and planned precisely and accurately.

Role of radiation therapist

Patients receiving radiation therapy for esophageal cancer require a lot of supportive care. They usually experience substantial weight loss as a result of the tumor's obstructive process and are nutritionally compromised. Esophagitis, as a result of the treatment, can cause more weight loss and further debilitate the health of the patient. The therapist should question patients about the way they are feeling, their appetite, and their food intake. Dietary suggestions regarding recommended foods or those to avoid should be made available to the patient. Some radiation therapy centers have printed sheets for the therapist or nurse to give to the patient. Many centers also have a dietitian to whom the patient may be referred for meal planning and dietary supplements.

Esophagitis can be emotionally and physically draining for these patients. The therapist should try to monitor the patient's emotional well-being as much as the physical aspects. The therapist should inform the patient about local cancer support groups that assist in coping with side effects of radiation treatments and disease.

Case Study

A 73-year-old woman had a 1-month history of dysphagia to solid foods and eventually to liquids. A barium swallow of the upper gastrointestinal area was obtained, revealing a 4-cm narrowing in the distal third of the esophagus. An endoscopy indicated an ulcerative lesion 32 to 35 cm from the incisors, or 5 cm above the esophagogastric junction. A biopsy was performed on this lesion, revealing a grade III squamous cell carcinoma. A physical examination was negative for any masses or hepatosplenomegaly. A CT scan of the chest demonstrated a 4-cm-long circumferential lesion located in the distal third of the esophagus. A CT scan of the abdomen was negative for any metastasis to the liver.

The patient was informed of the treatment options and side effects and elected combined modality radiation and chemotherapy treatment. A dose of 50 Gy was delivered to the tumor and regional nodes. Anterior and posterior opposed fields were treated with a dose of 30 Gy, and then off-cord parallel-opposed obliques and opposed laterals were treated with an additional 20 Gy. Fluorouracil and cisplatin chemotherapy were administered concurrently with the radiation.

PANCREATIC CANCER

Epidemiology and etiology

Cancers of the pancreas account for approximately 2% (28,000) of all cancers diagnosed in 1994. Pancreatic cancer is the fourth-leading cause of cancer-related deaths in the United States, with 25,000 deaths occurring annually. It occurs with equal frequency in men and women, with the majority of patients in the 50- to 80-year-old age group.[5,46]

No known cause exists for the development of pancreatic cancer, although a higher incidence seems to occur in smokers. Exposure to industrial chemicals such as benzidene and beta napthylamine over an extended period is related to an increased incidence of pancreatic cancer. However, definitive evidence establishing a causal relationship is lacking.[6,30,46]

Anatomy and lymphatics

The pancreas is located retroperitoneally at the L1-L2 level and lies transversely in the upper abdomen. The pancreas is divided into three anatomical regions: the head, body, and tail. The head of the pancreas is located in the C-loop of the duodenum. The body lies just posterior to the stomach near the midline and is anterior to the inferior vena cava (IVC). Extending laterally to the left, the tail terminates in the splenic hilum. The pancreas is in direct contact with the duodenum, jejunum, stomach, major vessels (IVC), spleen, and kidney. Tumors of the pancreas commonly invade these structures and are therefore usually unresectable at the time of diagnosis.[6,13,30]

Numerous lymph node channels drain the pancreas and its surrounding structures. The main lymph node groups include the superior and inferior pancreaticoduodenal nodes, porta hepatis, suprapancreatic nodes, and paraaortic nodes. Tumors arising in the tail of the pancreas drain to the splenic hilar nodes (Fig. 10-22). Most patients have advanced local and/or metastatic disease at the time of diagnosis.[2,6,13,30]

Clinical presentation

The four most common presenting symptoms of pancreatic cancer are abdominal pain, anorexia, weight loss, and jaundice. Tumors arising in the head of the pancreas may obstruct the biliary system, resulting in jaundice. Tumors that occur in the body or tail of the pancreas are not associated with obstruction of the biliary system and commonly involve severe pain and weight loss. Pancreatic cancers occur most frequently in the head of the pancreas.[6,30]

Detection and diagnosis

A thorough history and physical examination are extremely important. The abdomen should be assessed for palpable masses. The tumor's obstruction of the biliary system can result in an enlarged pancreas, gallbladder, or liver. Palpable supraclavicular nodes or rectal masses discovered during a digital rectal examination indicate peritoneal spread. All these signs suggest an advanced-stage disease. The presence or absence of jaundice is assessed by paying particular attention to the sclera, skin, and oral-cavity mucosa.[6,30]

The most valuable and important diagnostic test is a CT scan of the abdomen. This scan provides a complete view of the abdominal structures most likely involved with the tumor. This image localizes the mass in the pancreas and depicts whether it is a head, body, or tail primary. The scan also demonstrates whether the tumor has invaded surrounding structures such as the duodenum, superior mesenteric vessels, or celiac-axis vessels. Spread to the regional lymph nodes and distant metastasis to the liver can also be assessed.

The resectability of the tumor can be determined by the information found on the CT scan. Liver metastasis and the involvement of the superior mesenteric artery or other major vessels are two contraindications to surgery. A CT-guided fine-needle biopsy of the primary tumor or metastatic lesions may be performed to establish the diagnosis.[6,30]

Endoscopic retrograde cholangiopancreatography (ERCP) is used in evaluating the obstruction and potential involvement of the biliary system. This procedure is more beneficial for the diagnosis of a primary tumor of the biliary system. Ultrasonography has also been used to assess ductal obstruction, blood-vessel invasion, and liver metastasis.

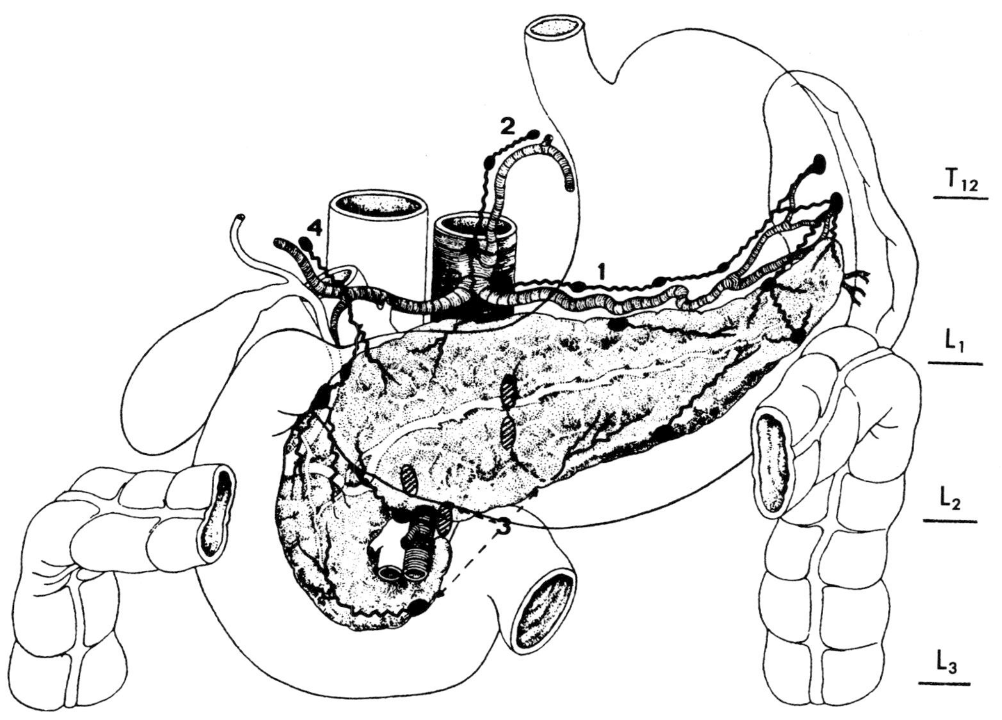

Fig. 10-22 Anatomy and lymphatic drainage of the pancreas. Note the intimate relationship of the pancreas with the duodenum, stomach, transverse colon, spleen, and common bile duct. The four main trunks of lymphatic drainage: The left side drains along the tail into splenic hilar nodes *(1)*; superior pancreatic lymph nodes and the celiac axis *(2)*; inferior pancreatic, mesenteric, and left paraaortic nodes *(3)*; right-side drainage to anterior and posterior pancreaticoduodenal nodes and right paraaortic nodes *(4)*. (From del Regato JA, Spjut HJ, Cox JD: *Ackerman and del Regato's cancer: diagnosis, treatment, and prognosis,* ed 6 St Louis, 1985, Mosby.)

A laparoscopy performed before any surgical intervention may rule out small liver metastases (1 to 2 mm) that were undetectable on a CT scan.[30] According to a study done by Warshaw et al.,[48] laparotomies indicated that 40% of patients had small metastases in the liver or on parietal peritoneal surfaces. These patients were spared the morbidity of unnecessary abdominal surgery. If the patient's tumor appears to be resectable, based on the diagnostic work-up, exploratory surgery and a biopsy are performed to determine the histology of the pancreatic mass.

Pathology and staging

Adenocarcinomas comprise 80% of pancreatic cancers. Other histological types include islet cell tumors, acinar cell carcinomas, and cystadenocarcinomas.[6,30]

A formal TNM staging system for pancreatic cancer is available. Most institutions, however, simply classify tumors as resectable or unresectable.

Routes of spread

Cancers of the pancreas are locally invasive. Lymph node involvement or direct extension into the duodenum, stomach, and colon is not uncommon at the time of diagnosis. The tumor often encases or invades the superior mesenteric artery, portal vein, and celiac axis artery, rendering the tumor unresectable. Hematogenous spread to the liver via the portal vein is another common pathway of spread. Because of the propensity of these tumors to invade other abdominal structures, peritoneal seeding of tumor cells can also occur.[6,19,30]

Treatment techniques

Surgery is the treatment of choice. Most tumors, however, are unresectable. Contraindications for undergoing a curative surgical procedure are liver metastasis, extra pancreatic serosal implantation, and invasion or adherence to major vessels.[6]

The most common potentially curative surgical procedure is a pancreaticoduodenectomy (Whipple procedure), which involves a resection of the head of the pancreas, entire duodenum, distal stomach, gallbladder, and common bile duct (Fig. 10-23). Reconstruction is done to maintain the continuity of the biliary-gastrointestinal system. The remaining pancreas, bile ducts, and stomach are anastomosed onto various sites of the jejunum (Fig. 10-24). The operative mortality rate from this procedure has greatly improved in recent years; it has been as high as 30%, but it is now less than 10%. The surgeon should place clips outlining the extent of the tumor to assist the radiation oncologist in planning adjuvant radiation therapy fields.[6,30]

Palliative biliary bypass procedures are often performed for unresectable tumors to redirect the flow of bile from obstructed ducts back into the gastrointestinal system. Typically, this is done by anastomosing the uninvolved bile ducts into the jejunum. Resolving the obstruction provides patients with relief of jaundice.

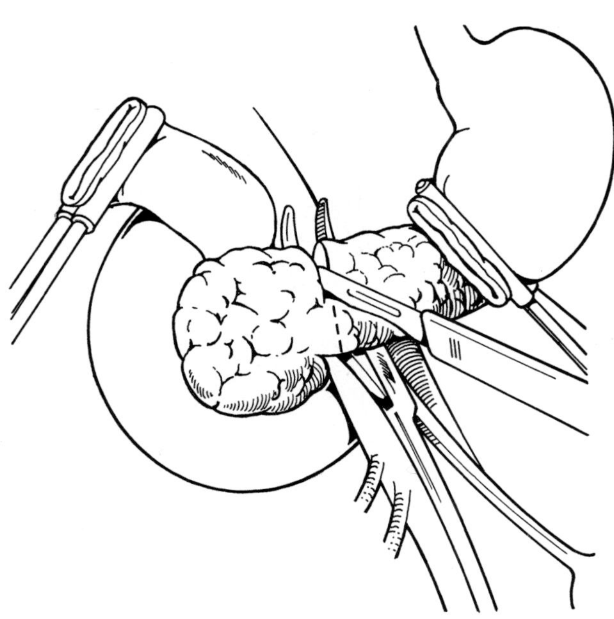

Fig. 10-23 Pancreaticoduodenectomy (Whipple Procedure); resection of the head of the pancreas, duodenum, distal stomach, gallbladder, and common bile duct. (From Beazley RM, Cohn I, Jr: Tumors of the pancreas, gallbladder, and extrahepatic ducts. In Holleb AI et al: *Textbook of clinical oncology,* Atlanta, 1991, American Cancer Society.)

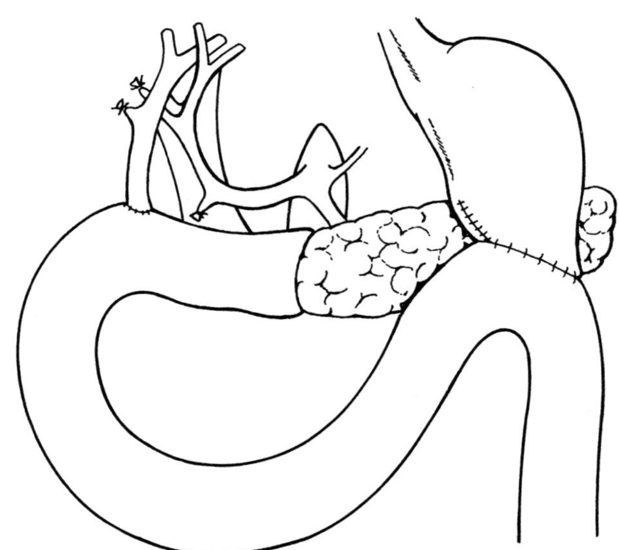

Fig. 10-24 Reconstruction of the biliary and gastrointestinal system. The remaining pancreas, stomach, and bile ducts are anastomosed to the jejunum. (From Beazley RM, Cohn I, Jr: Tumors of the pancreas, gallbladder, and extrahepatic ducts. In Holleb AI et al: *Textbook of clinical oncology,* Atlanta, 1991, American Cancer Society.)

Even with a potentially curative resection, the 5-year survival rate is usually less than 10%, with a median survival time of approximately 11 months.[32] This is due to a high local-regional recurrence rate and a high risk of distant metastases.[19,23,32]

Radiation therapy. Because of the high rate of distant metastasis and local-regional failure rate after surgery alone, combined-modality therapy versus observation was investigated in a randomized trial of patients with resected tumors. Adjuvant combined-modality treatment after surgery resulted in a significant improvement in the overall survival rate compared with no further treatment.[32]

Radiation therapy and chemotherapy are considered the preferred treatments for locally advanced, unresectable pancreatic cancers. Studies comparing radiation alone with radiation and chemotherapy alone have demonstrated that the combined-modality treatment provides modestly improved survival rates.[38]

Specialized radiation therapy techniques have been investigated to determine whether higher doses to the tumor bed would translate into an increase in local control and better survival rates. One method of delivering a higher dose to the primary tumor is intraoperative radiation therapy (IORT). A single dose of 20- to 25-Gy intraoperative electrons is delivered as a boost dose, following 50.4 Gy delivered by external beam radiation therapy. The main theoretical advantage of IORT is that it allows a higher dose to be delivered to the primary site than conventional external beam therapy because of the many dose-limiting structures located in the upper abdomen. Critical structures such as the kidney, liver, stomach, and small bowel can be moved out of the way or shielded during IORT. Studies evaluating the efficacy of this specialized boost technique have demonstrated an increase in local control when this method is added to the standard external beam therapy and chemotherapy treatment regimen. However, overall survival rates were not improved because of systemic failures in the liver or peritoneal seeding. Accordingly, IORT should not be used for pancreatic cancer in routine clinical practice. Different chemotherapy regimens are being investigated that may improve the systemic failures and increase survival rates.[20]

Chemotherapy. As mentioned, chemotherapy is standardly used with radiation therapy as an adjuvant treatment in resected pancreatic tumors and as the primary treatment with radiation for unresectable disease. 5-FU is the drug of choice and is delivered concomitantly with the radiation. Even with combined-modality treatment, the overall survival rate of patients with pancreatic cancer is extremely poor. Different drug combinations and sequences are being investigated for improving survival rates. Future trials of continuous-infusion 5-FU combined with leucovorin are currently being investigated at the Mayo Clinic and NCCTG.[20]

Field design and critical structures A four-field technique (AP/PA/LATS) is used for encompassing the primary tumor bed and draining lymphatics as defined by surgical clips or CT. A dose of 45 to 50 Gy is delivered in 1.8-Gy fractions with high-energy photons and a reduction in the field volume after 45 Gy. The upper abdomen contains many dose-limiting structures that must be considered for the designing and planning of radiation treatments. These structures include the kidneys, liver, stomach, small bowel, and spinal cord. The dose through the lateral fields is limited to 18 to 20 Gy because of the large volume of liver and kidneys in these fields.

Typical AP/PA field volumes for the head of a pancreatic lesion extend approximately from T10-11 for inclusion of the tumor bed, draining lymphatics, and celiac axis (T12-L1). The width of the field should encompass the entire duodenal loop and the margin extending across the midline on the left. The lateral fields are designed to provide a 1.5 to 2-cm margin anteriorly beyond the known disease. Posteriorly, the field extends 1.5 cm behind the anterior vertebral body for adequate coverage of the paraaortic nodes (Fig. 10-25). For body or tail lesions the volume treated does not need to include the duodenal loop but must extend farther to the left to provide an adequate margin on the primary tumor and to include the splenic hilar nodes.[30]

For simulation the patient is placed in the supine position with the arms along the side of the body and the elbows bent off the table or with the arms above the head for easier placement of the lateral isocenter marks. Preliminary borders and an isocenter are established and marked on the patient's skin. At many centers, renal contrast is injected, and a reference AP and/or lateral film is taken to determine the kidney location relative to other structures. This film assists in the design of custom shielding blocks to avoid unnecessary irradiation to the kidneys. The location of the kidneys may also be transferred from measurements of a CT scan onto the simulation film. For treating a head of pancreas lesion, approximately 50% of the right kidney is in the treated volume; therefore at least two thirds of the left kidney should be shielded to preserve normal kidney function.

After the films for kidney localization are completed, the patient is instructed to drink barium for localization of the duodenum and stomach. This is done to ensure adequate margins on the duodenum, especially for unresectable head of pancreas lesions. Another set of AP and lateral radiographs are then taken. This final set of films is representative of the actual volume to be treated. Custom-made blocks are fabricated from these films. Shielding blocks are designed to block as much as possible of the kidneys, liver, and stomach on the AP/PA fields, while the lateral film is used to block the spinal cord and small bowel.[30]

Side effects. The most common complaints of patients receiving radiation for pancreatic cancer are nausea and vomiting. Antiemetics may be given to mitigate these adverse effects. Other potential acute side effects include leukopenia, thrombocytopenia, diarrhea, and stomatitis. Long-term side effects, such as renal failure, are rare and suggest the possibility of improper shielding of the kidney.[4,38]

A 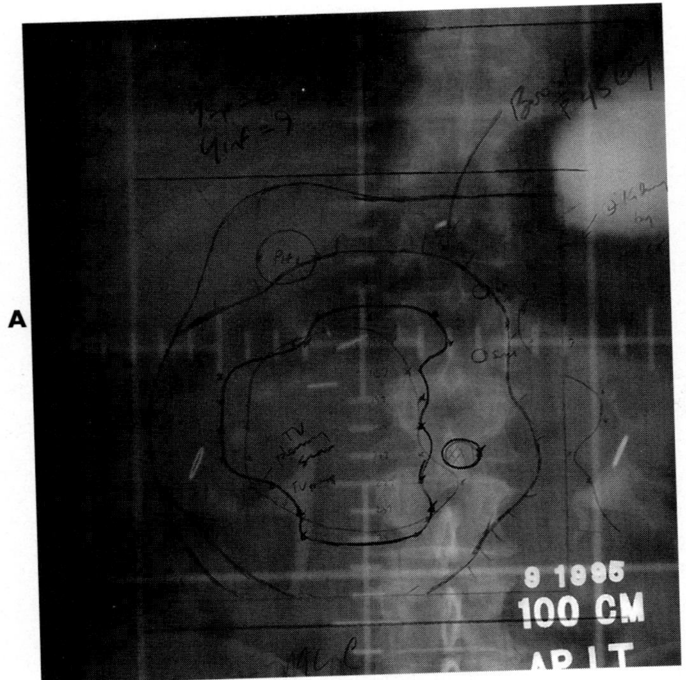

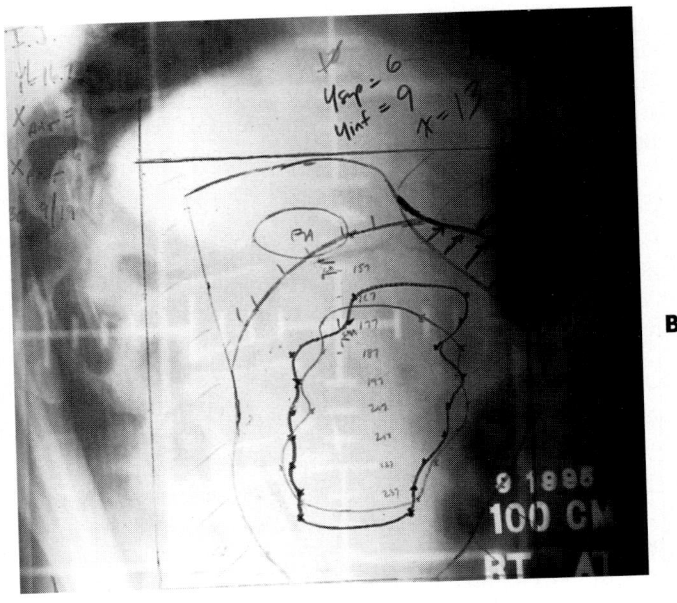 **B**

Fig. 10-25 Radiation therapy treatment fields for pancreatic cancer. **A,** AP/PA. **B,** Opposed laterals.

Case study

A 60-year-old female experienced a 26-pound weight loss, epigastric pain, and nausea and vomiting after eating. A CT scan revealed a 4-cm mass in the head of the pancreas, atrophy of the body and tail of the pancreas, and dilatation of the pancreatic duct, with a soft density mass that may have represented adenopathy. No evidence of liver metastasis was present. The mass appeared immediately adjacent to the superior mesenteric vein and was considered surgically unresectable. A CT-guided needle biopsy was performed and revealed a grade III adenocarcinoma of the head of the pancreas.

A physical examination was performed. Palpable masses in the abdomen; hepatosplenomegaly; and palpable lymphadenopathy in the cervical, supraclavicular, axillary, and inguinal regions were absent.

The tumor was surgically unresectable, and the patient was referred for primary radiation therapy combined with 5-FU chemotherapy. The goal of the treatment was to relieve her pain and increase the duration of her survival. A dose of 45 Gy was delivered to the initial large tumor-nodal fields via a four-field technique with a cone down boost for the final three treatments, arriving at a total dose of 50.4 Gy.

Review Questions

Essay

1. Describe the three mechanisms by which cancer of the colon or rectum spreads.
2. List and describe the dietary and medical-management recommendations of radiation-induced diarrhea.

Multiple Choice

3. What is the principal lymph node group involved in patients with rectal cancer?
   a. Common iliac nodes
   b. Inguinal nodes
   c. Paraaortic nodes
   d. Internal iliac nodes
4. What are the principal etiological factors in the development of esophageal cancer in North America?
   a. A diet high in fat and high in nitrate content
   b. A diet low in fat and high in vegetables and fruits
   c. Excessive alcohol and tobacco use
   d. Achalasia and Plummer-Vinson syndrome

5. What is a common site of blood-borne metastasis from rectal, pancreatic, or esophageal malignancies?
   a. Brain
   b. Bone
   c. Adrenal gland
   d. Liver
6. For radiation treatment to the thorax for esophageal cancer, what is the dose-limiting structure attracting the most concern?
   a. Spinal cord
   b. Heart
   c. Esophagus
   d. Trachea
7. What radiation-field design is most commonly used to avoid the critical structure in question # 6?
   a. Lateral-opposed fields
   b. AP/PA fields
   c. Oblique fields
8. Which of the following are common presenting symptoms of pancreatic cancer?
   I. Jaundice
   II. Nausea and vomiting
   III. A 10% weight loss
   IV. Anorexia
   a. I and II
   b. II and III
   c. I, II, and IV
   d. I, III, and IV
   e. I, II, III, and IV
9. Which of the following statements regarding pancreatic cancer is *not* correct?
   a. It is locally invasive into surrounding structures.
   b. Hematogenous spread to the liver at the time of diagnosis is common.
   c. The 5-year survival is rate 80%.
   d. Most tumors are unresectable.
10. For irradiation of the upper abdomen for pancreatic cancer, what is the most radiosensitive dose-limiting structure?
    a. Kidneys
    b. Liver
    c. Small bowel
    d. Spinal cord

Questions to Ponder

1. Describe the rationale for the addition of adjuvant postoperative radiation therapy after a curative surgical resection for rectal cancer.
2. Compare and contrast the postoperative radiation treatment field design used for a rectal cancer patient who has undergone an anterior resection versus an abdominoperineal resection.
3. What are the theoretical advantages of using IORT as a boost technique for the treatment of colorectal or pancreatic cancer?
4. What techniques are used to decrease or limit the radiation dose to the small bowel? Why are these important?
5. In treating the thorax for esophageal cancer, the arms and shoulders can create problems with the reproducibility of the setup. What can be done to ensure consistency in the daily setup of the treatment fields?

REFERENCES

1. Beahrs OH et al, editors: *AJCC manual for staging of cancer,* ed 3, Philadelphia, 1988, JB Lippincott.
2. Beahrs OH et al, editors: *AJCC manual for staging of cancer,* ed 4, Philadelphia, 1992, JB Lippincott.
3. Beart RW: Colorectal cancer. In Holleb AI, Fink DJ, Murphy GP, editors: *ACS clinical oncology,* Atlanta, 1991, American Cancer Society.
4. Bentel GC: *Radiation therapy planning,* New York, 1992, Macmillan.
5. Boring CC et al: Cancer statistics, 1994, *CA Cancer J Clin* 44:7-26, 1994.
6. Brennan MF, Kinsella TJ, Casper ES: Cancer of the pancreas. In Devita VT, Hellman S, Rosenburg SA, editors: *Cancer principles and practice of oncology,* Philadelphia, 1993, JB Lippincott.
7. Cohen AM, Minsky BD, Friedman MA: Rectal cancer. In Devita VT, Hellman S, Rosenburg SA, editors: *Cancer principles and practice of oncology,* Philadelphia, 1993, JB Lippincott.
8. Cohen AM, Minsky BD, Schilsky RL: Colon cancer. In Devita VT, Hellman S, Rosenburg SA, editors: *Cancer principles and practice of oncology,* Philadelphia, 1993, JB Lippincott.
9. Corn BW et al: Significance of prone positioning in planning treatment for esophageal cancer, *Int J Radiat Oncol Biol Phys,* 21:1303-1309, 1991.
10. Cummings BJ: Adjuvant radiation therapy for colorectal cancer, *Cancer Suppl* 70(5):1372-1381, 1992.
11. Cummings BJ: Anal canal. In Perez CA, Brady LW, editors: *Principles and practices of radiation oncology,* Philadelphia, 1987, Lippincott.
12. DeCosse JJ, Tsioulias GJ, Jacobson JS: Colorectal cancer: detection, treatment, and rehabilitation, *CA Cancer J Clin* 44:27-42, 1994.
13. Del Regato JA, Spjut HJ, Cox JD: Cancer of the digestive tract. In Ackerman LV, Del Regato JA, editors: *Cancer: diagnosis, treatment and prognosis,* ed 6, St Louis, 1985, Mosby.

14. *Eating hints,* U.S. Department of Health and Human Services, NIH, pp. 10-11, 1983.
15. Ellis FH Jr, Levitan N, Lo TCM: Cancer of the esophagus. In Holleb AI, Fink DJ, Murphy GP, editors: *ACS clinical oncology,* Atlanta, 1991, American Cancer Society.
16. Enker WE: Adenocarcinomas of the appendix and colon: surgical management. In Copeland EM, editor: *Surgical oncology,* New York, 1983, John Wiley & Sons.
17. Fisher SA, Brady LW: Esophagus. In Perez CA and Brady LW, editors: *Principles and practices of radiation oncology,* Philadelphia, 1987, JB Lippincott.
18. Fisher SA, Brady LW: Esophagus. In Perez CA, Brady LW, editors: *Principles and practices of radiation oncology,* Philadelphia, 1992, JB Lippincott.
19. Foo ML et al: Patterns of failure in grossly resected pancreatic ductal adenocarcinoma treated with adjuvant irradiation ±5 fluorouracil, *Int J Radiat Oncol Biol Phys* 26:483-489, 1993.
20. Garton GR et al: High-dose preoperative external beam and intraoperative irradiation for locally advanced pancreatic cancer, *Int J Radiat Oncol Biol Phys* 27:1153-1157, 1993.
21. Gunderson LL: Colorectal cancer. In Perez CA, Brady LW, editors: *Principles and practice of radiation oncology,* Philadelphia, 1987, Lippincott.
22. Gunderson LL et al: Indications for and results of intraoperative irradiation for locally advanced colorectal cancer, *Front Radiat Ther Oncol* 25:284-306, 1991.
23. Gunderson LL et al: Upper gastrointestinal cancers: rationale, results, and techniques of treatment, *Front Radiat Ther Oncol* 28:121-139, 1994.
24. Gunderson LL, Dozois RR: Intraoperative irradiation for locally advanced colorectal carcinomas, *Perspect Colon Rectal Surg* 5:1-23, 1992.
25. Gunderson LL, Martenson JA: Cancers of the colon and rectum. In Levitt S, Khan F, Potish R, editors: *Technological basis of radiation therapy,* ed 2, Philadelphia, 1991, Lea & Febiger.
26. Gunderson LL, Martenson JA: Colorectal cancer: radiation therapy. In *Current therapy in hematology-oncology,* ed 4, Philadelphia, 1992, BC Decker.
27. Gunderson LL, Martenson JA: Gastrointestinal tract radiation tolerance, *Front Radiat Ther Oncol* 23:277-298, 1989.
28. Gunderson LL, Martenson JA: Postoperative adjuvant irradiation with or without chemotherapy for rectal carcinoma, *Semin Radiat Oncol,* 4(1):55-63, 1993.
29. Gunderson LL, Martenson JA, Smalley SR: Gastrointestinal toxicity. In John MJ et al, editors: *Chemoradiation: an integrated approach to cancer treatment,* Philadelphia, 1993, Lea & Febiger.
30. Gunderson LL, Willett CG: Pancreas and hepatobiliary tract. In Perez CA, Brady LW, editors: *Principles and practices of radiation oncology,* Philadelphia, 1992, JB Lippincott.
31. Herskovic A et al: Combined chemotherapy and radiotherapy compared with radiotherapy alone in patients with cancer of the esophagus, *N Engl J Med* 326:1593-1631, 1992.
32. Kalser MH, Ellenberg SS: Pancreatic cancer: adjuvant combined radiation and chemotherapy following curative resection, *Arch Surg* 120:899-903, 1985.
33. Krook JE et al: Effective surgical adjuvant therapy for high-risk rectal carcinoma, *N Engl J Med* 324:709-715, 1991.
34. Lynch HT et al: Familial colon cancer : delineation of clinical subsets with etiologic and treatment considerations. In Levin B, editor: *Gastrointestinal cancer: current aproaches to diagnosis and treatment,* Austin, Texas, 1988, University of Texas Press.
35. Martenson JA et al: Prospective phase I evaluation of radiation therapy, 5-fluorouracil, and levamisole in locally advanced gastrointestinal cancer, *Int J Radiat Oncol Biol Phys,* 28:439-443, 1994.
36. Martenson JA, Gunderson LL: Colon and rectum. In Perez CA, Brady LW, editors: *Principles and practices of radiation oncology,* Philadelphia, 1992, JB Lippincott
37. Martenson JA, Gunderson LL: External radiation therapy without chemotherapy in the management of anal cancer, *Cancer* 71:1736-1740, 1993.
38. Moertel CG et al: Therapy of locally unresectable pancreatic carcinoma: a randomized comparison of high dose (6000 rads) radiation alone, moderate dose radiation (4000 rads + 5-fluorouracil), and high dose radiation + 5-fluorouracil, *Cancer* 48:1705-1710, 1981.
39. Netter FH: Digestive system, vol 3 part I & II. In Oppenheimer E, editor: *CIBA collection of medical illustrations,* West Caldwell, New Jersey, 1987, Donelly & Sons.
40. O'Brien MJ et al: Precursors of colorectal carcinoma, *Cancer Suppl* 70(5):1317-1325, September 1992.
41. Papillon J: *Rectal and anal cancers: conservative treatment by irradiation-an alternative approach to radical surgery,* New York, 1982, Springer-Verlag.
42. Peacock JL, Keller JW, Asbury RF: Alimentary tract cancers. In Rubin P, editor: *Clinical oncology: a multidisciplinary approach for physicians and students,* ed 7, Philadelphia, 1993, WB Saunders.
43. Robbin SL, Cottran RS: *Pathologic basis of disease,* ed 2, Philadelphia, 1979, WB Saunders.
44. Roth JA et al: Cancer of the esophagus. In Devita VT, Hellman S, Rosenburg SA, editors: *Cancer principles and practice of oncology,* Philadelphia, 1993, JB Lippincott.
45. Shank B, Cohen AM, Kelsen D: Cancer of the anal region. In Devita VT, Hellman S, Rosenburg SA, editors: *Cancer principles and practice of oncology,* Philadelphia, 1993, JB Lippincott.
46. Steele GD Jr et al: Clinical highlights from the National Cancer Data Base: 1994, *CA Cancer J Clin* 44:71-80, 1994.
47. Vargas PA, Alberts DS: Primary prevention of colorectal cancer through dietary modification, *Cancer Suppl* 70(5):1229-1233, 1992.
48. Warshaw AL, Swanson RS: What's new in general surgery: pancreatic cancer in 1988, possibilities and probabilities, *Ann Surg* 208:541, 1988.
49. Yasko JM: *Care of the client receiving external radiation therapy,* Reston, Virginia, 1982, Reston Publishing.

BIBLIOGRAPHY

O'Connell JM et al: Improving adjuvant therapy for rectal cancer by combining protracted-infusion fluorouracil with radiation therapy after curative surgery, *N Engl J Med* 331:502-507, 1994.

O'Connell MJ, Gunderson LL: Adjuvant therapy for adenocarcinoma of the rectum, *World J Surg* 16:510-515, 1992.

Urba SG et al: Concurrent preoperative chemotherapy and radiation therapy in localized esophageal adenocarcinoma, *Cancer* 69:285-291, 1992.

CHAPTER

11

Gynecological Tumors

Timothy Dziuk
J. Michael Kerley

Outline

Key terms

Cervical cancer
Endometrial cancer
Interstitial implant
Intrauterine tandem
Midline block
Ovarian cancer
Parametrium
Pelvic inlet
Perineum
Sensitive test
Specific test
Vaginal cancer
Vaginal colpostats
Vaginal cuff
Vaginal cylinder implant
Vulvar cancer

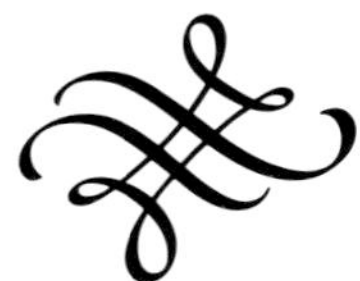

This chapter provides radiation therapists with basic knowledge of gynecological malignancies. An initial section on epidemiology and etiology discusses the relative number of cancers and deaths resulting from the various sites. This section is followed by a site-specific discussion regarding the populations at risk and various risk factors. The anatomy of the pelvic gynecological structures is then reviewed. Knowledge of radiation tolerances and lymphatic drainage is of critical importance in radiation therapy treatment planning. These issues are discussed in depth.

Following this general review, the organ areas (vulva, vagina, cervix, endometrium, and ovaries) are discussed in individual sections. Each section begins with a clinical presentation that includes symptoms, as well as data regarding lymphatic spread and prognostic features. This is followed by a brief description of the clinical work-up, expected pathology, and staging. To minimize confusion, the staging is limited to the system provided by the International Federation of Gynecology and Obstetrics (FIGO).[15] Treatment considerations specific to each organ are then presented. This is done to orient the radiation therapist to required modifications in the treatment design beyond the basic pelvic treatment plan and to provide the rationale for these modifications. Each section closes with a case study that synthesizes the principles presented.

After the sections concerning specific organs, general principles of external beam radiation therapy and brachytherapy are discussed in detail. The goal is to promote a clear knowledge of the basic design of treatment fields and enable the radiation therapist to understand the rationale underlying the various simulations. Dose schedules are presented generally and with the specific sites. In general, the radiation therapist should be able to use data in this section to understand and critique most gynecological treatment plans.

The chapter closes with a discussion of expected side effects from radiation therapy and the radiation therapist's role in evaluating and managing these sequelae. The radiation therapist has three main functions during the course of therapy: treatment delivery, ongoing patient assessment, and patient reassurance.

EPIDEMIOLOGY AND ETIOLOGY

In 1995 approximately 80,000 patients developed gynecological cancer in the United States. This type of malignancy is divided into endometrial (40%), ovarian (33%), cervical (20%), and other gynecological cancers (7%). An estimated 26,400 deaths occurred, with ovarian being the most prevalent (55%), followed by endometrial (22%), cervical (18%), and other gynecological cancers (5%).[3]

Alternatively, considering the ratio of deaths to new cases, ovarian cancer has the highest death rate at 55%, followed by cervical cancer (excluding carcinoma in situ) at 30%, and endometrial cancer at 18%. Although there are 25% more endometrial than ovarian cancers, ovarian cancer deaths are 250% the incidence of endometrial-related deaths. The high death rate for ovarian cancer is primarily due to the relatively nonspecific early symptoms with a consequent diagnosis of later-stage disease. A secondary reason is less effective treatment. Endometrial cancer has a relatively higher cure rate because the early symptom of postmenopausal bleeding usually results in a physical evaluation at an earlier stage, during which effective local therapy can be initiated.

Cervical carcinoma is more prevalent than other gynecological cancers among younger women and those of lower socioeconomic status. The incidence of invasive cervical cancer rises rapidly to a plateau between ages 45 and 55, with an average age of 48.[10] Early sexual activity, multiple partners, and multiple pelvic infections (especially with genital warts and human papillomaviruses [HPV] and herpes simplex type 2 [HSII]) have been associated with an increase in the risk of this disease and an earlier onset. Incidence is also higher among wives of men with penile cancer. As with vaginal cancers, there is an increased risk of clear cell adenocarcinoma in women whose mothers used diethylstilbestrol (DES) during the early months of pregnancy. However, all women are at some risk and need effective and safe screenings. The widespread use of pap smears has resulted in early detection; two thirds of cervical cancers are now detected in the noninvasive stage and are therefore highly curable with local therapy.

The prevalence of endometrial cancer has increased as a result of the aging population, high-calorie and high-fat diets, and the use of unopposed estrogen in the 1960s and 1970s. The incidence peaks at about 58 years, and over 75% of patients are women over the age of 50. Diabetes and hypertension are linked with an increase in the prevalence. Women who are 50 pounds overweight have a ninefold increase in risk. A higher risk also results from an increase in estrogen or the estrogen-to-progesterone ratio, as occurs with nulliparity, infertility secondary to anovulation (with a deficit in progesterone), dysfunctional bleeding during menopause (secondary to estrogen overstimulation), or prolonged oral estrogen administration without progesterone.

Vaginal and vulvar cancers are rare and usually occur in older women. Vulvar carcinoma, which is three times as common as vaginal cancer, has been associated with medical illnesses, such as hypertension, obesity, and diabetes, and with sexually transmitted diseases.[7,8] Atrophic-dysplastic changes in the normal vaginal lining, a loss of hormone stimulation, and poor hygiene may also be associated with vulvar cancers. An unusual clear-cell variant of vaginal cancer seen in young women (median age of 19) has been associated with DES use by their pregnant mothers while they were in utero. If the cervix is involved with a vaginally located cancer, the tumor is instead classified as a cervical cancer with vulvovaginal spread and is treated in the same way as other advanced cervical cancers.

Ovarian carcinoma occurs primarily in women between the ages of 50 and 70. At 14,500 estimated deaths in 1995, it is the fourth-leading cause of cancer deaths in women, following lung (62,000), breast (46,000), and colon (24,500) cancer. Risk factors include an older age, late or few pregnancies, late menopause, a lack of oral contraceptive use, a family history of ovarian cancer, and a personal history of breast, colon, or endometrial cancer.[26] Diets high in meat and/or animal fat and living in industrialized nations (except Japan) are risk factors. Screening is poor because the disease is detectable during physical examinations, radiographic studies, and seriological tests only intermittently and usually at an advanced stage. With the low prevalence of this disease, even a 100% **sensitive test** (0% false-negative) for detecting tumors and a 99% **specific test** (1% false-positive) for patients with disease result in over 100 laparotomies for every early ovarian cancer detected with an iatrogenic death rate equal or higher than the disease. For patients with hereditary ovarian cancer syndrome the lifetime risk increases from 1% to 40%, and a screening with an annual rectovaginal pelvic examination, CA 125 serum determinations, and transvaginal ultrasound* is recommended to reduce this significant risk.

ANATOMY AND LYMPHATICS

The vulva is the outermost portion of the gynecological tract. The major parts include the labias majora and minora, the clitoris, and the area bound by these three, called the *vestibule.* The vestibule is triangular, is located anterior to the

*Until childbearing is completed, at which time a prophylactic bilateral oophorectomy can be done.

vaginal opening, and usually contains the urethral meatus, unless the meatus exits the outer third of the vaginal canal. The **perineum** refers to the area between the vulvovaginal complex and anal verge. The vagina is a muscular tube that extends 6 to 8 inches superiorly from the vulva and is located anterior to the rectum and posterior to the bladder. The cervix (the part of the womb that extends into the apex of the vagina) is a firm, rounded structure from 1.5 to 3 cm in diameter. The cervix often protrudes into the vagina, producing lateral spaces in the vaginal apex called the *fornices.* A canal called the *cervical os* extends from the vagina, through the central cervix, and into the uterine cavity, or pelvic portion of the womb. The uterus is a hollow, muscular structure that extends at a right angle from the vagina to overlie the bladder. Extending laterally from the superior uterus are the twin fallopian tubes. These are hollow structures designed to transmit the ova from the ovaries located adjacent to them. The **parametrium** refers to the area immediately lateral to the uterine (womb) body (Fig. 11-1).

Radiation therapy treatment requires an understanding of the radiosensitivity of the various gynecological structures and their lymphatic drainage. The vulva and perineum usually show the most acute short-term side effects, partly because of their radiation sensitivity and the often parallel and tangential nature of the treatment beams applied to them. Doses above 40 Gy at standard fractions (1.8 to 2 Gy) often cause significant acute erythema and desquamation, and doses above 50 Gy cause late telangiectasis. Significant fibrosis can result from doses approaching 70 Gy. The vagina is more tolerant, with the upper vaginal mucosa tolerating up to 140 Gy and the lower up to 100 Gy before extensive fibrosis.[14] Early mucositis and later telangiectasis occur with much lower treatment-range doses (60 to 85 Gy). The uterus and cervix tolerate extremely high doses of radiation and allow the effectiveness of high-dose brachytherapy to the womb. Up to 200 Gy can be delivered locally to the canal without necrosis. The ovary is the most radiosentive gynecological structure. The dose response is age dependent. For example, a dose of 4 to 5 Gy produces the permanent cessation of menses in about 65% of women under age 40, 90% of those aged 40 to 44, and 100% of those 50 years or older.[20]

Many other organs surrounding the gynecological structures have dose tolerances that must be respected. The bladder, which is located anterior to the vagina and cervix and somewhat under the uterus, expands forward and away from these structures when it is filled. The point tolerance is about 70 Gy, but whole-bladder treatment results in acute cystitis at doses as low as 30 Gy. This results in acute bladder irritation

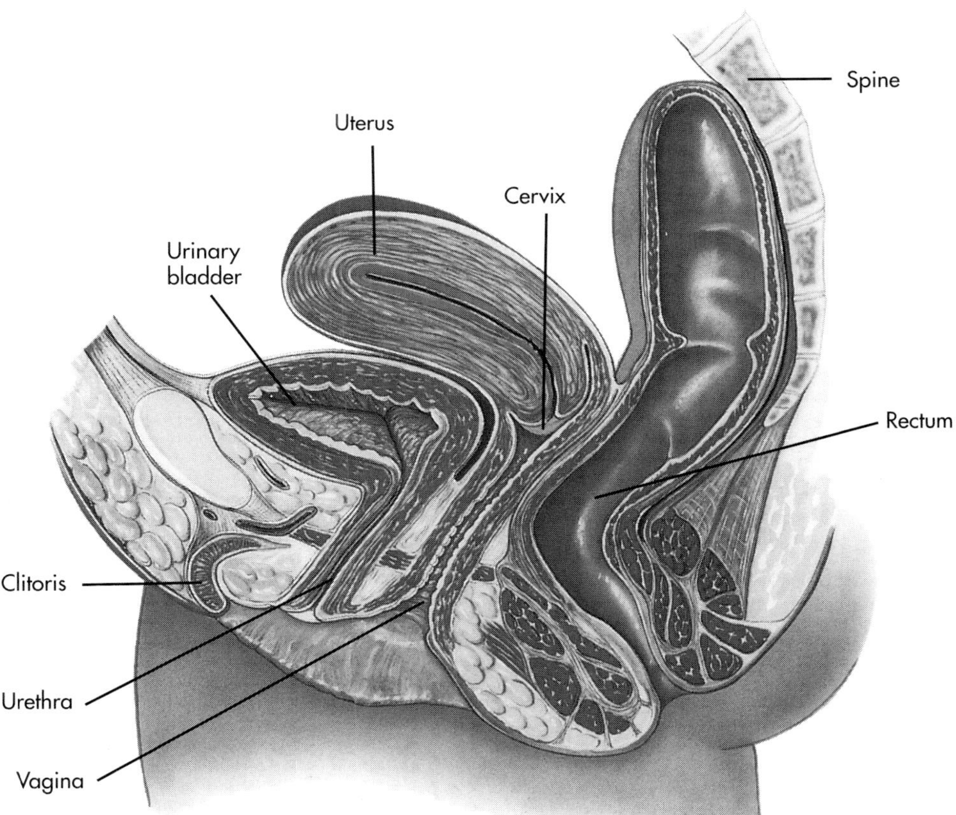

Fig. 11-1 A sagittal view of the female pelvis. (From Seely R: *Essentials of anatomy and physiology,* St Louis, 1991, Mosby.)

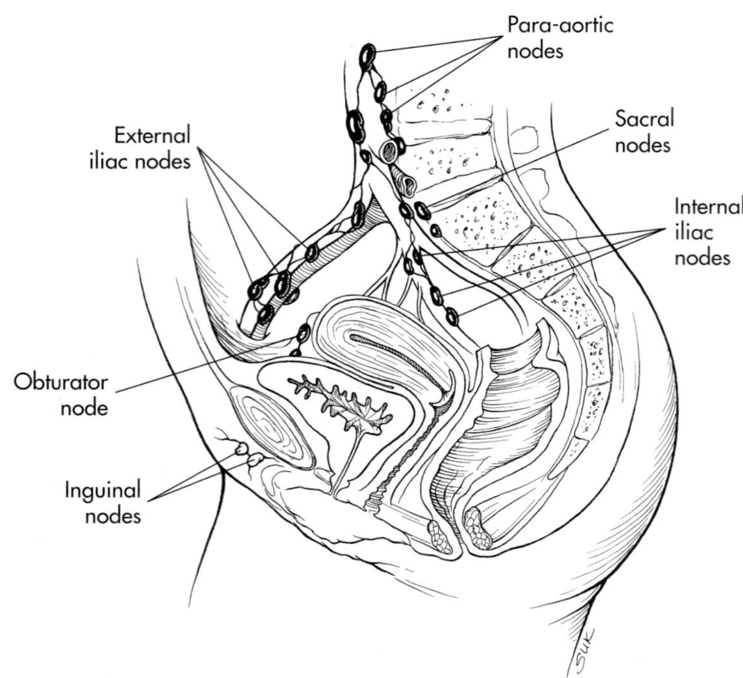

Fig. 11-2 Lymph node drainage of the pelvis.

with dysuria, frequency, and urgency but usually resolves in a couple of weeks. Chronic cystitis occasionally occurs 6 months after radiation with doses above 50 to 60 Gy, and contracture and/or hemorrhagic cystitis occurs with doses above 65 Gy. The rectum, which is immediately posterior to the vagina and cervix, also has a point tolerance of about 70 Gy. The rectum continues superiorly with the sigmoid colon, with a whole-organ tolerance of about 50 Gy. Diarrhea, bleeding, urgency, and pain can occur acutely at 30 to 40 Gy. Stricture, bleeding, and perforation are late complications that occur with doses above the tolerance level. The small bowel is variably looped down in the pelvis and may overlie the uterus and bladder. This bowel has a lower tolerance at 45 Gy, can yield the same acute toxicity as the large bowel (but at lower doses), and is more likely to obstruct as a chronic complication.

The treatment design must consider the extent of the primary lesion and the probability of metastases to the draining lymph nodes. Lymphatic drainage includes the inguinal lymph nodes (external and internal), pelvic nodes (the internal iliac chain, which originates approximately with the obturator node, and external iliac chain), and periaortic nodes (Fig. 11-2). The deep inguinals drain into the external iliac chain, and the internal and external iliac chains join and then drain into the periaortics. Drainage is approximately contiguous. Therefore if involvement of the nodes occurs at one level, including the next higher nodal group in the treatment field may be appropriate.

Ovarian and upper endometrial lymphatics follow the ovarian blood supply to terminate in periaortic lymph nodes at the level of the kidneys and follow the round ligament to involve the inguinal lymphatics. The primary drainage pattern of the cervix and additional drainage patterns of the ovary and uterus are to the external iliac, obturator, and hypogastric chains. Upper vaginal drainage follows the cervical pathways. Lower vaginal drainage may follow the vulvar drainage into the inguinal nodes.

VULVA

Clinical presentation

Vulvar cancer patients usually have a subcutaneous lump or mass. Patients with more advanced disease have an ulcerative exophytic mass. The disease is usually unifocal, with the labia majora as the most common location. Often, the patient has a long history of irritation. Lymphatic spread is predictable, involving the superficial inguinal nodes first, then the deep femoral nodes, and eventually the pelvic nodes. However, lymph nodes are falsely enlarged in about 40% of patients. The incidence of lymph node involvement is related to the depth of invasion (less than 10% at 1 to 3 mm and about 25% at 3 to 4 mm) and tumor size (38% for tumors greater than 5 mm and 46% for those greater than 20 mm).[22] Occult disease is common, as is inflammation, so a high level of false-negatives and -positives are based on the examination and clinical suspicion alone. Prognostic factors include the size of the lesion, depth of invasion, and histological subtype. The presence and extent of lymph node involvement is the strongest predictor of overall survival rates.

Detection and diagnosis

A work-up should include a biopsy, a cytological examination, a history, a physical examination, blood counts and chemistries, a urinalysis, chest radiographs, an intravenous pyelogram (IVP) and/or a computed tomography (CT) scan, and a cystoscopy. Liver scans, a bone scan, a sigmoidoscopy, and a pelvic CT scan are usually performed if the tumor is advanced clinically or found on the other staging studies.

Pathology and staging

Squamous cell carcinomas comprise about 95% of vulvar cancers, and adenocarcinomas represent the remaining 5%. Staging is as follows:

- I All lesions confined to the vulva with a maximum diameter of 2 cm or less and no suspicious groin lymph nodes
- II All lesions confined to the vulva with a maximum diameter greater than 2 cm and no suspicious groin nodes
- III Lesions extending to the lower urethra, vagina, anus, or perineum without grossly positive groin lymph nodes; any lesion with grossly positive unilateral inguinal or femoral lymph nodes
- IV Lesions that extend to the upper urethra, bladder, rectal mucosa, or bone; or with positive bilateral inguinal or femoral nodes (IVa), lesions with pelvic node involvement or distant metastases (IVb)

Treatment techniques

Historically, treatment has involved a radical vulvectomy with a groin node dissection. For Stage III disease with positive inguinal nodes, deep pelvic nodes must be addressed, either with a pelvic node dissection or pelvic irradiation. Recently, a more conservative approach using lesser surgery (such as a wide local excision or a simple vulvectomy) with external irradiation of the primary and inguinal nodes has been encouraged.[11,12]

Radiation therapy may be administered preoperatively but is seldom used as the sole treatment. (Simulation techniques are discussed at the end of the chapter.) For Stages I and II disease, radiation therapy is usually given after a simple vulvectomy (50 Gy) and a wide local excision (60 Gy plus a 5- to 10-Gy boost if margins are positive). With radiation therapy alone, doses of 65 to 70 Gy are delivered.[21] For Stage III disease, radiation therapy is given postoperatively if the primary is >4 cm, margins are positive, or three or more lymph nodes are positive. A dose of 50 Gy is delivered to control microscopic disease, with a 15-Gy boost if margins are microscopically positive and 20 Gy for grossly involved margins. Boosts may be delivered using photons, en face perineal electrons, and via brachytherapy. The inguinal region (nodes) is treated to 45 to 50 Gy for control of microscopic disease and to 65 to 70 Gy for palpable disease. If the pelvic nodes are included, 45 to 50 Gy is delivered for microscopic disease and 60 Gy for macroscopic disease. Treatment interruptions are usually needed at 40 Gy or less if chemotherapy is given concomitantly. The vulva and perineum usually develop significant moist desquamation as a result of the decreased thickness of the region, the parallel delivery of the external beam, and the need for bolus.

The overall 5-year survival rate is about 50%, and the disease-free survival rates in surgically treated patients with Stages I through IV disease are 90%, 81%, 68%, and 20%, respectively.[25] Hacker[11,12] has shown the influence of regional lymph node involvement, with actuarial 5-year survival rates of 96% for node negative, 94% with one node positive, 80% with two nodes positive, and 12% with three or more nodes positive.

Case Study

M.M. is an 83-year-old white female with underlying vascular disease from her hypertension, diabetes, and hypercholesterolemia. She consulted her gynecologist and exhibited a 5-cm right labial mass. A wide local excision and bilateral lymph node dissections revealed no positive nodes. The mass recurred 6 months later on the right side, and the patient underwent a simple vulvectomy and rhomboid skin flap grafts. Because of the recurrence, deep invasion, and close margins, she was referred for postoperative radiation therapy. Her disease was considered Stage II initially before the recurrence.

The treatment design included AP/PA lower pelvic fields and anteriorly treated inguinal fields. Initially, 6-MV photons were used with anterior bolus. The initial dose was 50.4 Gy at 1.8 Gy per fraction. The perineum and operative sites received a boost of 10 Gy with en face 9-MeV electrons at 2 Gy per fraction. The patient required several treatment breaks for wet desquamation and urethral irritation. Diarrhea was not a major problem.

M.M. remained free of disease for 18 months, until a recurrence in the periurethral area. An iridium **interstitial implant** was performed to a small volume surrounding the area of recurrence at a dose of 40 Gy over 4 days. This treatment controlled the local disease, but she experienced recurrence again in the peroneal body and anal canal. M.M. is considering some type of exenterative procedure.

VAGINA

Clinical presentation

Vaginal cancer is a malignancy that arises in the vagina and does not extend to the vulva or cervix. This definition helps make vaginal cancer a rare disease that accounts for approximately 2% of all gynecological cancers. No etiological associations are definite, except for the rarer clear cell variant seen in 1 per 1000 women exposed to DES while they were in utero. The usual squamous cell carcinomas occur in older women (median age of 65), whereas clear cell carcinomas occur in young women (median age of 19).[13] Abnormal vaginal bleeding and/or painful intercourse are the usual presenting symptoms. The most common location is the posterior upper third of the vagina. The risk of lymphatic involvement increases with the depth of invasion. Pelvic lymphatic involvement is similar to cervical cancer, with lesions of the lower third of the vagina also involving the inguinal nodes.

Detection and diagnosis

The work-up should include a biopsy, a cytological examination, a careful history, a physical examination, blood counts and chemistries, a urinalysis, chest radiographs, an IVP or abdomenopelvic CT scan, and a cystoscopy. If the disease is advanced, liver and bone scans, a sigmoidoscopy, and a pelvic CT scan are recommended.

Pathology and staging

Squamous cell carcinomas total 80% to 90% of vaginal cancers. Malignant melanomas comprise about 5% of vaginal cancers. Other vaginal cancers include sarcomas, malignant lymphomas, and clear cell adenocarcinomas. Staging is as follows:

- I Carcinoma confined to the vaginal wall
- II Carcinoma extends to the subvaginal tissue but not to the pelvic wall
- III Carcinoma extends to the pelvic wall
- IV A—Carcinoma involves the mucosa of the bladder or rectum or extends outside the pelvis
  B—Distant metastases.

Treatment techniques

Radiation therapy is the treatment of choice for most vaginal cancers. Surgery is used for recurrent or persistent squamous cell cancers and in young women who have early clear cell adenocarcinoma. For small, superficial lesions, only the vaginal tissues are treated (via local excision or brachytherapy), but for invasive lesions the entire pelvis must be treated. Doses of 45 to 50 Gy are given to the pelvis, and the entire vagina is included in the external beam field. If the tumor involves the middle or lower third of the vagina, the inguinal nodes are also treated as in vulvar cancer. Microscopic disease is treated to 50 Gy and macroscopic to 65 to 80 Gy. Brachytherapy implants are used to bring the primary and adjacent macroscopic disease to curative doses. Problems with early acute dermatitis are quite similar to those seen in vulvar cancer patients. (Details concerning teletherapy simulation, brachytherapy, and overall side effects are given in the final sections of this chapter.)

Case Study

O.A. is a 61-year-old white female with underlying chronic obstructive pulmonary disease (COPD) and hypertension. She complained to the gynecologist of 2 months of vaginal bleeding, especially after intercourse. A pelvic examination revealed a mass at the lateral aspect of the vagina and discontinuous from the cervix. A biopsy confirmed poorly differentiated, invasive squamous cell carcinoma. The results of other staging studies were negative. Her disease was classified as Stage II (T_2, N_0).

Radiation therapy consisted of AP/PA pelvic and vaginal treatment, with 18-MV photons at 2 Gy per fraction to 20 Gy. A midline block was then added, and she was treated to an additional 20 Gy. A reduced parametrial boost with midline blocking and off the small bowel was given an additional 10 Gy.

Brachytherapy consisted of a **vaginal cylinder implant,** giving the mucosa 20 Gy over 2 days at the beginning of the midline-blocked pelvic treatment, and a second complex implant with a vaginal cylinder and right-sided interstitial needles given at the end of the initial pelvic treatment. The second implant yielded an additional 40 Gy to the vaginal mucosa and 25 Gy to the right-sided vaginal extension of the tumor.

The patient experienced some diarrhea, cystitis, and vaginal dryness but is still sexually active and free of disease 2 years later.

CERVIX

Clinical presentation

Cervical cancer is a slowly progressive disease, with the earliest phase (noninvasive carcinoma in situ) occurring approximately 10 years earlier than invasive cancer. The earlier cervical cancer is detected, the better the local and overall control. Routine Papanicolaou smears have played a crucial role in the early detection of cervical cancer and in the improved overall survival rate. Screening should begin at age 18 or earlier in sexually active women.

Common presenting signs of invasive cancer are postcoital bleeding, increased menstrual bleeding, and discomfort with intercourse. A foul-smelling discharge, pelvic pain, and urinary or even rectal symptoms may accompany more advanced disease. Invasive cancer appears as a friable, ulcerative, or exophytic mass originating from or involving the cervix. The mass may extend into the vaginal canal and onto the vaginal sidewalls, or it may invade adjacent tissues such as the parametrium, bladder, or rectum. Lymphatic involvement is usually orderly, involving parametrial nodes, followed by pelvic, common iliac, pariaortic, and even supraclavicular nodes. The incidence of pelvic and periaortic nodal involvement is local-stage dependent, with <5% and <1% for Stage I, 15% and 5% for Stage IB, 30% and 15% for Stage II, and 50% and 30% for Stage III.[17] With periaortic nodal involvement a 35% risk exists for supraclavicular spread.[1]

Survival rates and local control decrease as the stage and bulk of the disease increase. Uteral invasion has been associated with a reduction in 5-year survival rates from 92% to 54%.[18] Bulky or barrel-shaped cervical cancer is associated with a 15% to 20% increase in distant metastases and a decrease in local control.[23,24] For Stages IB and IIA the involvement of lymph nodes results in approximately a 50% reduction in survival rates.[4-6] Host factors associated with decreased local control or survival rates include anemia (hemoglobin of less than 10 or 11 grams), hypertension (diastolic pressure above 110 mm Hg), and a temperature over 100° F.[2,16,27]

Detection and diagnosis

The work-up should initially include a pelvic examination, pap smear, and biopsy of any suspicious lesions. Further staging studies include a complete history, a physical examination under anesthesia, dilatation and curettage to assess uterine involvement, complete blood counts, chemistries, and a urinalysis. Chest radiographs, barium enema, and an IVP are used for International Federation of Gynecology and Obstetrics (FIGO) staging. For more advanced disease, abdominopelvic CT or magnetic resonance imaging (MRI) scans, a cystoscopy, and a proctoscopy are recommended. A lymphangiogram and laparotomy may also be used to help with the treatment design but are not used for the initial staging. Surgical evaluation with lymph node dissection is associated with a significant increase in pelvic side effects, but a laparoscopic or CT-directed biopsy may be useful in designing treatment portals.

Pathology and staging

Pathologically, most cervical, vaginal, and vulvar cancers are squamous cell types. Adenocarcinomas of the cervix arise from the mucous-secreting endocervical glands and comprise about 8% of these tumors. Small cell and clear cell types comprise about 2% of the remaining tumors and have a higher metastatic potential. Staging is as follows:

- 0 Carcinoma in situ
- I Cervical cancer confined to the cervix
  - Ia1—minimal (<3 mm) microscopic invasion
  - Ia2—lesions that do not invade deeper than 5 mm or have horizontal spread greater than 7 mm
  - Ib—lesions larger than Ia2 but confined to the cervix and corpus
  - Ib B—barrel-shaped lesions confined to the cervix but variously defined according to size and usually greater than 4 cm
- II Cervical cancer extending beyond the cervix and corpus but not to the pelvic sidewalls or lower third of the vagina
  - IIa—tumor that extends to the upper two-thirds of the vagina
  - IIb—tumor that extends to the parametria but not to the pelvic sidewall
- III Cervical cancer extending to the pelvic sidewall or to the lower third of the vagina
  - IIIa—no tumor to the pelvic sidewall (i.e., to the lower third of the vagina)
  - IIIb—extension to the pelvic sidewall, hydronephrosis, or a nonfunctioning kidney
- IV Extension outside the pelvis and invasion of the bladder or rectum
  - IVa—bladder or rectal invasion
  - IVb—distant metastases

Staging is based on a clinical examination before the initiation of therapy and may be supplemented by a blood analysis, chest radiographs, an IVP, a cystoscopy, a barium enema, and bone scans. A CT scan, laparatomy findings, an MRI scan, and lymphangiograms may modify treatment but do not change the FIGO staging. For statistical purposes the cancer is staged at the earlier level if disagreement or doubt exists.

Treatment techniques

For early Stage 0 (carcinoma in situ) and for Stage Ia1 invasive cancer, the usual treatment is a total abdominal hysterectomy (TAH) with a small amount of vaginal tissue, known as the **vaginal cuff.** Alternately, a conization limited to the cervix itself may be performed in women who desire additional children. A tandem and ovoid implant, delivering 45 to 55 Gy to point A, is occasionally used for medically inoperable patients. For Stage Ia2, TAH or a more aggressive modified radical hysterectomy is usually performed. In the medically inoperable patient, 60 to 70 Gy may be delivered with the use of a tandem and ovoid implant. Stages Ib and IIa are somewhat controversial because surgery and radiation therapy yield similar control and survival data. Because of the preservation of vaginal pliability and ovarian function, surgery is often used for younger women, whereas radiation is used for women who have a higher risk for surgical complications. Radiation is used with a combination of external beam therapy and implants. For bulky cervical disease, radiation therapy is the initial treatment of choice and may be delivered at doses slightly higher than usual or followed by a simple hysterectomy for barrel-type lesions. Postoperative irradiation is usually given for positive pelvic nodes, disease more advanced than originally staged, positive margins, and if disease is an incidental finding in a less-than-definitive surgical procedure. Patients with Stages IIb, III, and IVa are usually treated with irradiation, with or without chemotherapy. Total tumor doses are increased from 70 Gy for low-volume disease to 85 Gy for advanced or bulky disease. The external beam dose increases with more advanced disease, whereas the implant dose may stay the same or actually decrease, depending on critical organ doses. (External beam treatment, implant doses and techniques, and side effects are further discussed later in this chapter.)

Approximate 5-year survival rates are 95% for Stage Ia cervical cancer, 85% for Stage Ib, 70% for Stage II, 50% for Stage III, and <10% for Stage IV. Local control rates are 92% for Stage Ib, 85% for Stage IIa, 75% for Stage IIb, and 60% for Stage IIIb.

Case Study

C.W. is a 42-year-old female who had a 6-month history of slowly progressive bleeding after intercourse. Her periods were otherwise normal, and she did not have any pelvic or vaginal pain. She had pap smears performed in her twenties and early thirties, but none recently.

During an examination, the cervix was enlarged to about 5 cm, and an ulcerative lesion was seen extending from the inferior cervix into the posterior fornix. The pap smear was positive for squamous cell carcinoma, and biopsies from the lesion, endocervix, and endometrium demonstrated invasive, poorly differentiated squamous cell carcinoma. A pelvic examination confirmed the bulky lesion, and the extension onto the vaginal wall was palpable; no appreciable parametrial extension was present (Stage IIa). A chest radiograph and IVP were negative for metastatic disease. A pelvic CT scan confirmed the presence of an enlarged cervical mass, but no discernible pelvic adenopathy or masses were present.

Because of the lesion's bulk, the patient was not considered a surgical candidate and definitive radiation therapy was initiated. She received 4500 cGy via a four-field technique, with the treatment of customized 16 × 18.5 cm AP/PA and 14 × 18.5 cm right/left parallel-opposed fields. Photons of 15 Mv were used to deliver 180-cGy daily fractions. She was evaluated during the fifth week, and marked shrinkage was noted in the tumor. The first tandem and ovoid implant procedure was performed 3 days after the completion of the 4500-cGy dose. The tandem was loaded with 15-, 10-, and 10-mg radium-equivalent Cs 137 sources, and the small ovoids were each loaded with 15-mg sources. The point-A dose rate was 50 cGy per hour, and the implant was left in place for 48 hours. The dose rate at the pelvic sidewall was 12 cGy per hour, whereas the bladder and rectum maximum dose rates were 30 cGy per hour. The week after the first implant, 540 cGy was delivered in three fractions as a pelvic-sidewall boost via 16 × 16 cm AP/PA fields, with a midline (rectal and bladder sparing) block designed from the isodose distribution of the implant. A second, nearly identical implant was performed the week after the boost field, with a total implant time of 30 hours. The cumulative dose to point A was 8400 cGy, whereas the pelvic sidewall received 5980 cGy. The doses for the bladder and rectal points were each 6000 cGy.

Beginning the fourth week of treatment, the patient experienced diarrhea which was initially managed with a low-fiber diet and eventually required antidiarrheal agents. The diarrhea gradually improved through the implants, and the patient was without a complaint for 4 days after the second implant. She otherwise tolerated the treatment quite well.

At a follow-up 1 week after the second implant, the cervix's size was normal. Considerable necrotic debris was present at the vaginal apex, but bleeding did not occur during the examination. The following month she described a brown vaginal discharge with sparse matter that resembled coffee grounds. At her next examination, there were patchy, hypopigmented areas alternating with telangiectasis (fine, superficial blood vessels) of the vagina, and the cervix was nearly healed.

She continued to have control of the local disease and no pelvic side effects. About 1 to 1½ years after therapy, she exhibited multiple lung nodules. A chemotherapeutic regimen was begun, but the patient expired 5 months later.

ENDOMETRIUM

Clinical presentation

About 75% of women with **endometrial cancer** experience vaginal bleeding, and about 30% have a foul-smelling vaginal discharge. Approximately one third of postmenopausal bleeding is cancer related, usually cervical or endometrial. Screening is most reliably and comfortably performed by aspiration curettage because the pap smear has only a 50% or less diagnostic accuracy in endometrial cancer. Most endometrial cancers are early stage, with about 70% in Stage I and 10% each in Stages II, III, and IV. Poor prognostic factors include higher grade, increased depth of invasion into the myometrial muscle, lymph node involvement, and cancer cells in the peritoneal fluid (positive peritoneal cytology) or on serosal surfaces.

Lymphatic spread occurs initially to the internal and external iliac pelvic nodes. For Stage I disease, about 10% of patients are node positive. This increases to between 25% and 35% for Stage II disease, a poorly differentiated histology, or a deep myometrial invasion. If pelvic nodes are involved, about a 60% chance exists for periaortic node involvement.

Detection and diagnosis

The work-up should include suction curettage of the endometrial cavity for the initial diagnosis. A dilatation and curettage with cervical biopsies are necessary for full staging. A thorough history is taken, and a physical examination is performed. Additional studies include chest radiographs, blood counts and chemistries, and a urinalysis. Surgery is most often the initial definitive management. Before proceeding, an ultrasound, a pelvic CT, or an MRI scan is often attempted to assess uterine invasion and lymph node involvement. Standard surgery includes an exploratory laparotomy with staging biopsies, washings, and a radical hysterectomy.

Pathology and staging

Adenocarcinoma of the endometrial lining is the most common type of endometrial cancer. Adenosquamous cancer is a variant seen about 20% of the time and is usually more advanced in stage. Papillary serous adenocarcinoma is an extremely malignant form of endometrial carcinoma that tends to spread quite rapidly and widely throughout the abdominal cavity and usually has a poor outcome. Sarcomas rarely have a good outcome and deserve aggressive combined-modality therapy (usually surgery and radiation therapy). Staging is as follows:

- IA* Tumor limited to the endometrium
- IB Tumor invading the inner half of the myometrium
- IC Tumor invading the outer half of the myometrium
- IIA Involvement of the endocervical glands
- IIB Invasion of the cervix tissues
- IIIA Tumor that invades through the myometrium or cancer cell in the peritoneal fluid
- IIIB Vaginal involvement
- IIIC Involvement of pelvic or periaortic lymph nodes or metastases to distant organs

Treatment techniques

Treatment can involve surgery and/or radiation therapy, depending on the stage, grade, medical condition of the patient, and experience of the institution administering the therapy. Preoperative therapy is given in some institutions for high grade and high clinical stages to downstage the patient before surgery. Usually, patients who have already undergone operations are referred for postoperative therapy, and nonoperative candidates are referred for definitive therapy. After a total abdominal hysterectomy, patients with Stage Ia, Grade 1 disease are not treated further. At many institutions, patients with Stage Ib, Grades 1 and 2 and sometimes Stage Ia, Grade 2 disease are treated postoperatively with brachytherapy alone. Low surface doses of 60 to 70 Gy are typically used in one application, or high doses of 5 to 7 Gy to a 0.5-cm depth are used for three applications. Patients with Stage Ic (or higher) or Grade 3 disease have an increased risk of pelvic node involvement, so external beam radiation therapy is a component of postoperative treatment. Minimal nodal doses of 45 to 50 Gy are supplemented with implants to bring the vaginal mucosa dose up to 80 Gy or more. Residual pelvic nodes or masses can be boosted up to 60 to 65 Gy with shaped, small-volume external fields.

Irradiation alone may be used for medically inoperable patients and for Stages III and IV. Usually, at least a 50-Gy external beam pelvic dose is recommended with an implant sufficient to bring the tumor dose above 75 Gy. Bulky disease can be brought to 100 Gy with careful implant techniques and midline shielding. (See the section on simulation techniques at the end of the chapter.)

For Stage I disease the local recurrence rate can be reduced from 12% with surgery alone to 3% with preoperative radiation therapy and to 0% with postoperative therapy.[9] The 5-year survival rates are 64%, 76%, and 81%, respectively. Overall, there is a 90% 5-year survival rate for all Stage I patients, including the most common and nonradiated Stage I, Grade 1 patients. For Stage II, 5-year disease-free survival rates are about 80% with surgery and radiation therapy versus 50% for radiation therapy alone. The 5-year survival rate for Stage III disease treated with radiation therapy alone is only 25%.

*Before 1989, Stage I was differentiated by the uterine cavity length, with Ia less than 8 cm, and Ib greater than 8 cm.

Case Study

C.G. is a 62-year-old postmenopausal female who had been having routine (biannual) pap smears, which were normal. She developed intermittent vaginal bleeding and consulted her gynecologist the same week. Another pap smear was normal, but an endometrial biopsy showed a moderately differentiated endometrial carcinoma. A chest radiograph, blood work, and a pelvic CT scan were normal. She underwent an abdominal hysterectomy and the removal of both ovaries. No lymph nodes were palpable during the surgery. A pathology report confirmed a moderately differentiated adenocarcinoma that invaded nearly the entire myometrium. The cervix and parametrial tissues were not involved, and her disease was classified as Stage IC.

Her postoperative course was unremarkable, and she was referred for adjuvant radiation therapy. She was treated with 18-MV photons to 4500 cGy in 180-cGy daily fractions via a four-field technique with customized 16 × 16 cm AP/PA and 16 × 14 cm right/left parallel-opposed fields. After the external beam radiation therapy, she underwent a 60-hour vaginal cylinder implant. A 3-cm domed cylinder was placed and loaded with two 15-mg radium-equivalent Cs 137 sources, which delivered 60 cGy per hour at the vaginal surface. The patient tolerated the treatment quite well, experiencing mild diarrhea and fatigue at the completion of the external irradiation. The implant was well tolerated. About 6 years after treatment, she was without evidence of disease. She complained of having to urinate more frequently, but this was not problematic, and she was without dysuria. She had periodic rectal irritation, which responded after several days to steroid suppositories.

OVARIES

Clinical presentation

Ovarian cancer is the most deadly of the gynecological cancers because it has few symptoms until it is widely disseminated. The most common presenting symptoms are abdominal and/or pelvic pain, abdominal distension, or nonspecific gastrointestinal symptoms (e.g., nausea, constipation, and heartburn). These are due to the presence of the tumor or fluid in the abdominal cavity. Occasionally, ovarian cancer may be diagnosed in early stages as a palpable mass adjacent to the uterus.

The disease is most common in women 50 to 70 years old. It is considered early if confined to the ovaries. Progression occurs to the pelvis, abdominal cavity, and nodes. CA 125 is often elevated in the serum but is a poor screening test and is best used to follow disease during and after therapy. In apparently early ovarian cancer, subclinical metastases are noted during surgery to the peritoneal fluid, aortic nodes, and diaphragm in 33%, 10%, and 10% of the tumors, respectively.[23,24] About 80% of ovarian cancer patients have abdominal cavity involvement at the time of presentation. Spread occurs through the lymphatics and peritoneal fluid distributions. Survival rates are 90% at 5 years for Stage I, 20% for Stage III, and 5% for Stage IV disease. About 22 months of increased survival time occurs with optimal versus suboptimal surgical reduction of intraabdominal disease.[19]

Detection and diagnosis

Diagnosis and staging are surgical. The preoperative work-up usually includes a history, a physical examination, liver and renal function blood work, chest radiographs, pelvic ultrasound (including transvaginal views), abdomenopelvic CT or MRI scans, and serum CA 125. Some work-ups include a barium enema (BE), an endoscopy, and upper gastrointestinal (UGI) series. The surgical evaluation includes a cytological evaluation of the peritoneal fluid, an intraoperative evaluation of adnexal masses, and an examination and biopsy of the peritoneal fluid drainage pathways. Removal of as much of the tumor as possible produces the best outcomes.

Pathology and staging

About 90% of ovarian cancers are epithelial (from ovary surfaces), 7% are stromal, and 3% are from the ovarian germ cell itself. These include dysgerminomas, which are treated like seminomas. Staging is as follows:

- I Tumor limited to the ovaries
  - Ia Tumor limited to the ovary, surface intact and uninvolved, and no malignant ascites
  - Ib Tumor limited to both ovaries, surface intact and uninvolved, and no malignant ascites
  - Ic Tumor on the ovarian surface, capsule ruptured, or malignant ascites or washings
- II Tumor with pelvic extension
  - IIa Extension or implants on the fallopian tubes or uterus
  - IIb Extension to other pelvic organs
  - IIc Extension to other pelvic organs, with the tumor on the ovarian surface, the capsule ruptured, or malignant ascites or washings
- III Tumor involves the peritoneal surfaces or extends outside the pelvis and/or regional node metastases
  - IIIa Microscopic abdominal peritoneal metastases
  - IIIb Macroscopic peritoneal metastases less than 2 cm in diameter
  - IIIc Abdominal implants greater than 2 cm or positive retroperitoneal or inguinal nodes
- IV Distant metastases

Treatment techniques

For epithelial tumors the initial treatment involves surgical evaluation and debulking. Postoperative therapy may include single-agent or combination chemotherapy and/or whole abdominal and pelvic radiation therapy. Radiation therapy is controversial and may include radioisotopes placed into the peritoneal cavity or all external beam treatment. For most epithelial tumors, postoperative therapy includes platinum-based chemotherapy, although abdomenopelvic radiation therapy yields similar results.[4-6,19]

The two approaches are not additive, but toxicities are. Peritoneal radioisotope treatment is best not used in addition to external beam therapy for similar reasons.

For well-differentiated Stages Ia and Ib, the 5-year survival rates are between 90% and 100%. The 5-year survival rate for radiation-therapy-treated Stage II is 74% for microscopic residual disease, 58% for residual disease less than 2 cm, and 39% for residual disease greater than 2 cm. Comparable results for Stage III are 48%, 43%, and 18%.[4-6]

SIMULATION AND TREATMENT

Vulvar fields include the primary site and inguinal region. A pelvic field is added to the top or bottom of L5 if the primary is greater than 2 cm or if deep femoral nodes are positive. Pelvic fields should include the **pelvic inlet,** which is the opening in the pelvis into which a baby's head enters. The pelvic inlet includes the sacral promontory, the pelvic inner side walls, and the pubic bones, with a 2-cm lateral margin to cover pelvic lymph nodes. The patient is usually simulated in the "frog-leg" position, with wires over surgical scars and palpable nodes. Bolus is placed over the vulva and perineum. The fraction size is limited to 1.8 Gy, and frequent splits are often necessary by 40 Gy because of severe perineal reactions (Fig. 11-3). Inguinal nodes are best treated from the anterior to minimize doses to the femoral head and neck. Techniques to accomplish this include partial transmission blocks, weighting of the anterior field more heavily, anterior bolus, use of lower energies anteriorly and higher energies posteriorly, and anterior electron fields for boosts.

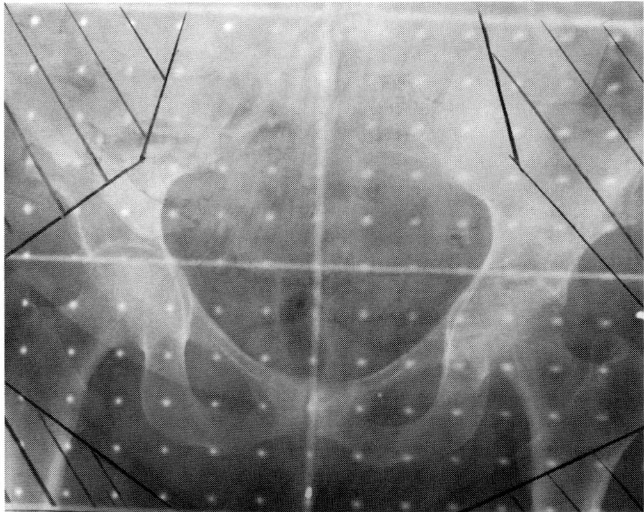

Fig. 11-3 A simulation radiograph demonstrating a treatment field used to treat the vulva, pelvic, and inguinofemoral lymph nodes.

Vaginal cancers are usually treated with radiation therapy. Surgery is most often reserved for recurrences, clear cell adenocarcinoma at an early stage, and persistent masses. Brachytherapy alone or as a boost depends on the size of the primary and nodal status. For carcinoma in situ and Stage I well-differentiated cancer the entire vagina can be treated via brachytherapy alone with a dose to 60 Gy through a device called a *vaginal cylinder,* which is a canal-filling cylinder into which an isotope can be placed to ensure an even dose to the vaginal mucosa. Further brachytherapy can be done as a boost of 20 Gy to minimal disease, with the cylinder and/or another brachytherapy device consisting of needles placed directly into the at-risk tissues (an interstitial implant) for more deeply invasive tumors. For more aggressive lesions other than early Stage I, doses of 45 to 50 Gy are given to a pelvic field and the entire vagina. AP/PA fields with anterior weighting are customarily used to cover the at-risk tissues, to make blocking easier, and to deliver a lower dose to the femoral head and neck. The inguinal nodes are included for tumors involving the lower two thirds of the vagina. Brachytherapy implants are used to bring the primary and adjacent macroscopic disease to doses up to 65 to 85 Gy (Fig. 11-4, *A* and *B*). Perez recommends a **midline block** after 20 Gy for earlier invasive disease and after 40 Gy for Stages IIb or greater so that a greater tumor-to-critical structure (bladder-rectum) dose can be given.[21,22] A midline block consists of a block placed in an AP/PA field to shield tissues that will be or already are treated by a brachytherapy device. Often the edges of the block have different value layers of blocking material to feather the junction of tissues treated with teletherapy and brachytherapy. Deeply invasive disease requires boosting with combination implants that include an interstitial component (Fig. 11-5, *A-C*).

Radiation therapy is the best treatment for cervical cancer. Surgery is reserved for medically operable patients in earlier stages (I to IIa) for whom cure rates are similar and morbidity may be less. For bulky cervical disease, radiation may be followed by an extrafacial hysterectomy. Conversely, surgery may be followed by radiation therapy for positive pelvic nodes, positive margins, and disease more advanced than originally suspected. Patients with Stages IIb, III, and IVa are usually treated with irradiation alone or in combination with chemotherapy.

Cervical fields can be administered via a four-field or high-energy AP/PA technique. The lower border is at the bottom of the obturator foramen, unless the vagina is involved, in which case the lower extent of the border is at least 4 cm below the lowest extent of the disease (some include the entire vaginal length). The upper border is usually at the top or bottom of L5 or may be extended upward to L4 for a portion of the treatment if nodal involvement is suspected. The lateral borders are 1.5 to 2.0 cm lateral to the pelvic sidewall in the AP/PA plane. Laterally, the anterior border is at or anterior to the pubic symphysis, with a block designed to include the external iliac nodes; the posterior border includes S3. In patients with anterior or posterior extension, AP/PA fields alone or widening of the laterals to extend anterior to the pubis or posterior to include S4 and S5 is necessary. AP/PA fields allow midline blocking early so that a greater percentage of the dose is given with brachytherapy and less of the dose is given to the rectum and bladder. The four-field technique allows exclusion of the anterior bladder and posterior rectum in patients for whom brachytherapy plays a lesser role (e.g., bulkier disease) (Fig. 11-6, *A-E*). In patients with a high risk for pariaortic involvement, matching AP/PA fields can be con-

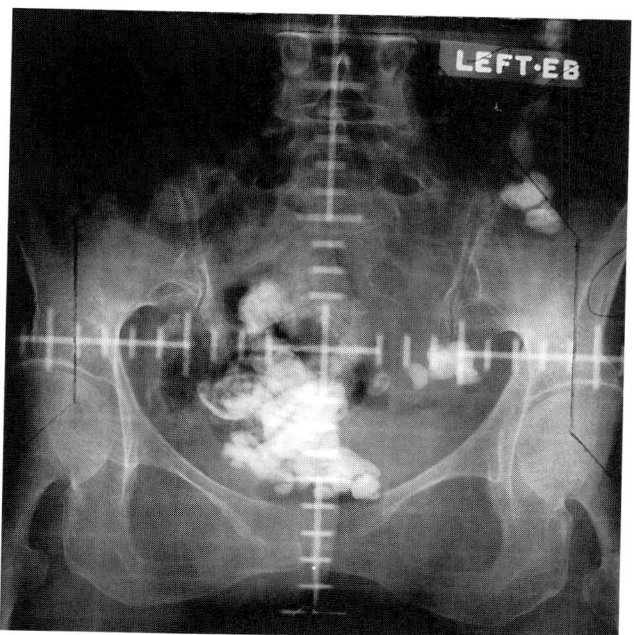

A

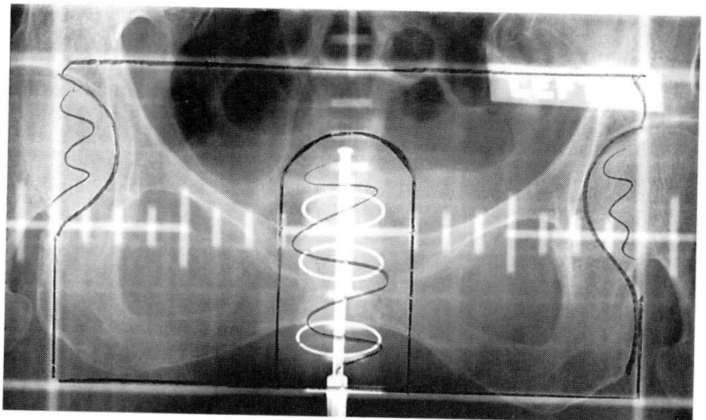

B

Fig. 11-4 Radiographs of vaginal simulation and brachytherapy implant procedures. **A,** A typical AP/PA simulation portal for a vaginal cancer treatment. **B,** A brachytherapy implant using a domed-cylinder technique. Note that the midline is blocked. The parametrial boost field with midline block is also shown.

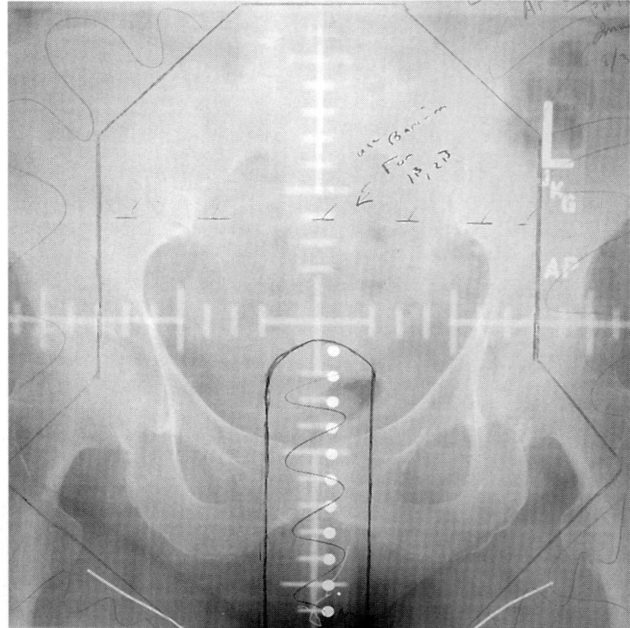

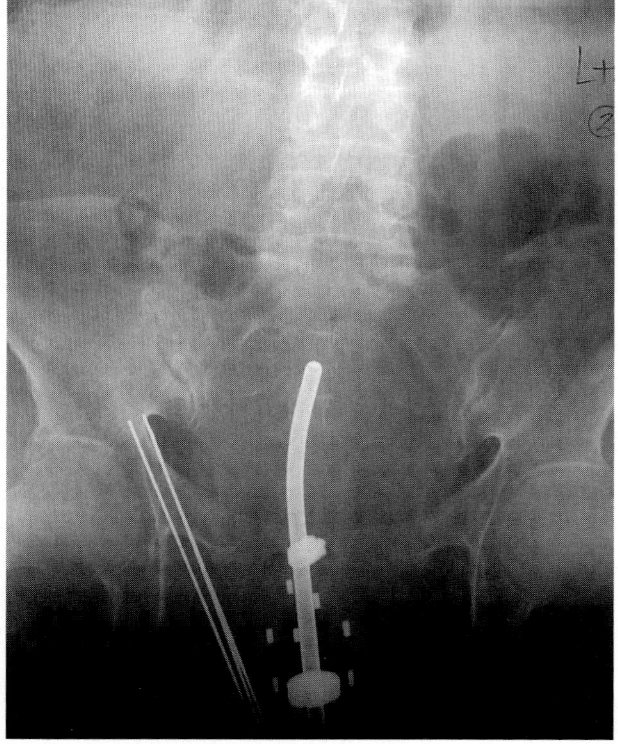

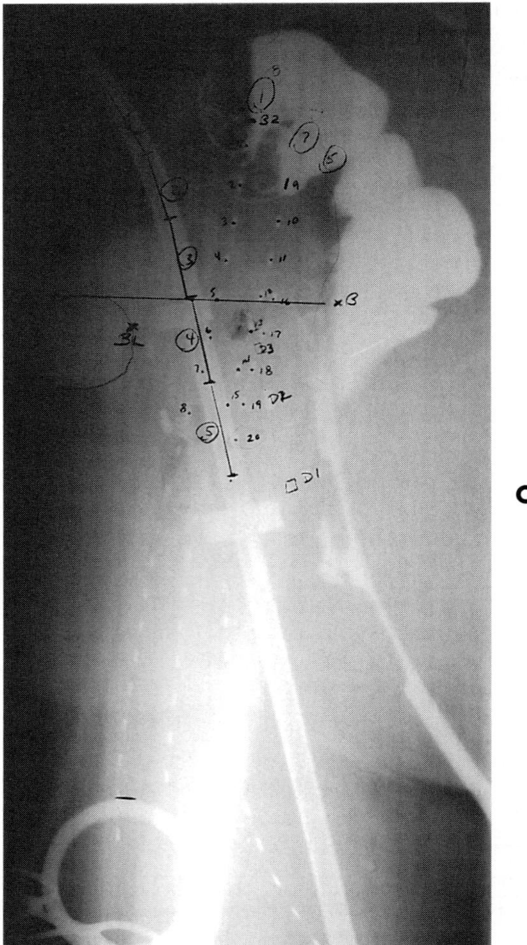

Fig. 11-5 Treatment of vaginal cancer. **A,** Pelvic AP/PA ports with a midline block. This particular arrangement used a 6-MV anterior field and an 18-MV posterior field. **B,** An AP view of an intrauterine tandem, vaginal cylinder, and interstitial needles used during a brachytherapy boost. **C,** A lateral view of an intrauterine tandem, vaginal cylinder, and interstitial needles used during a brachytherapy boost.

structed and even lateral boosts can be given for a small portion of the treatment (Fig. 11-7).

Anal markers, rectal barium, vaginal markers, and bladder contrast can be used to help delineate critical structures during the simulation process. Often, placing the patient prone with a belly board or full bladder allows the exclusion of the small bowel without jeopardizing the tumor coverage. Small-bowel contrast can allow minor field reductions that prevent complications while allowing higher tumor or nodal doses.

Doses are escalated, depending on the stage and volume of the disease. The higher the volume of the tumor, the later implants are done in the course of treatment. Also, the greater the bulk and stage, the smaller the percentage of the dose contribution from implants. These two factors allow better coverage of the tumor by the implant* and partially compensate for the poor geometry associated with increased volume disease. A standard **intrauterine tandem** (a small, hollow, curved cylinder that fits through the cervical os into the

*The tumor is shrunk first to fit the implant dose distribution.

A

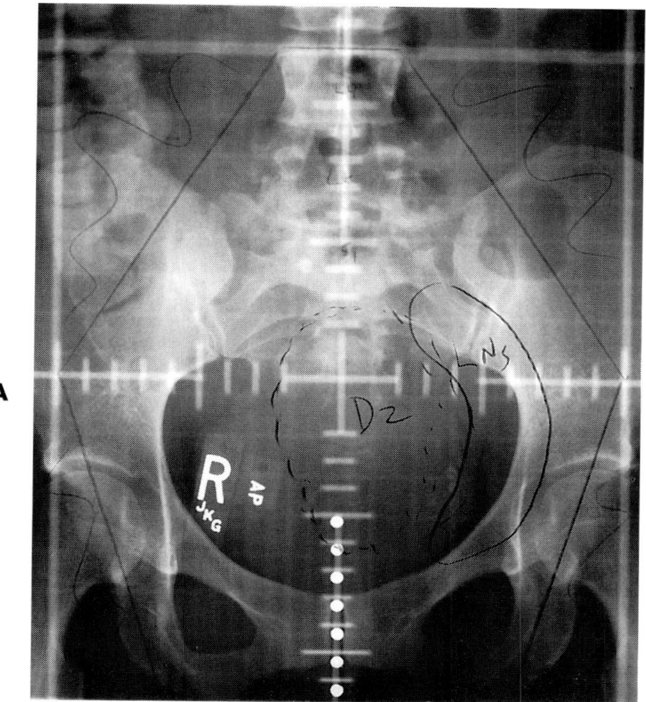

B

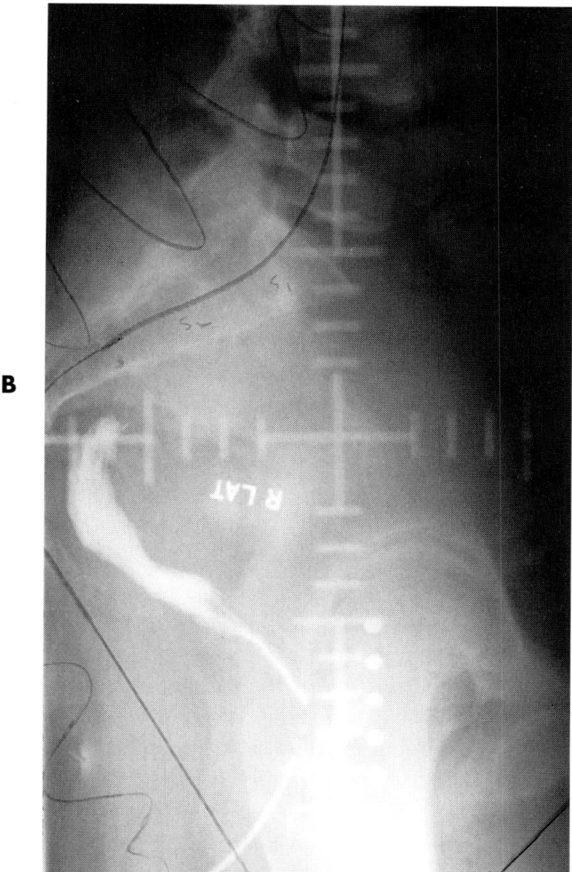

C

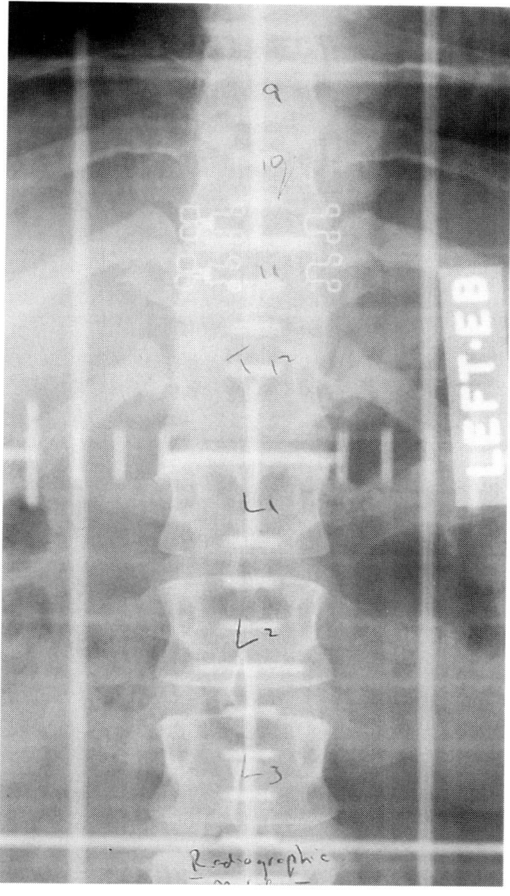

Fig. 11-6 Radiographs of cervical simulation and implant procedures. **A,** AP/PA radiographs of a four-field technique for a bulky cervical cancer. Note the vaginal marker in place. **B,** A lateral view of a four-field technique for a bulky cervical cancer with rectal contrast and a vaginal marker. **C,** Matched AP/PA paraaortic fields used in the treatment of lymphatic drainage involved in regionally advanced cervical cancer.

Continued.

uterus) and **vaginal colpostats** (two golf-club-shaped, hollow tubes placed laterally to the tandem into the vaginal fornices) implants can also be supplemented with interstitial or cylinder components. Numerous dose, field, and timing arrangements are possible for external beam radiation therapy and brachytherapy. The actual protocol used is based on the radiation oncologist's clinical experience. Examples of doses and configurations include the following: a 70-Gy tumor dose via an implant alone for Stage Ia disease, 75 Gy via 40-Gy pelvic radiation therapy plus 10 Gy with midline blocking plus a 35-Gy tumor dose from brachytherapy for Stages Ib and IIa disease, 80 Gy via 40-Gy pelvic radiation therapy plus 20 Gy with midline blocking plus 40 Gy from brachytherapy for Stages IIb and IIIa disease, and 85 Gy via 40-Gy pelvic radiation therapy plus 20 Gy with midline

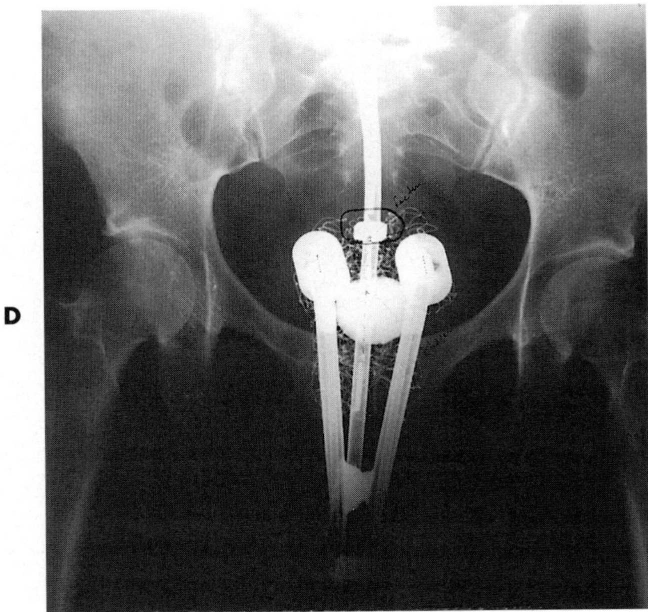

D

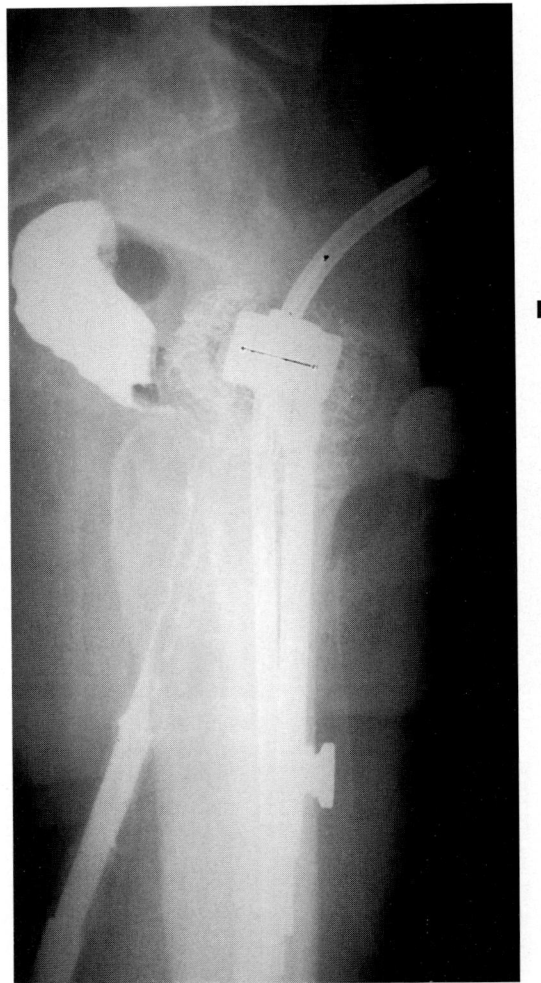

E

Fig. 11-6—cont'd **D,** An AP view of an intrauterine tandem and a vaginal colpostat cervical implant. **E,** A lateral view of an intrauterine tandem and a vaginal colpostat cervical implant.

blocking plus 45 Gy from brachytherapy for Stages IIIb and IVa disease. Some centers give a greater percentage of the dose with midline blocking to allow higher implant doses, and some give higher pelvic radiation therapy doses without midline blocking to cover the volume more evenly and sacrifice the amount of the brachytherapy dose. Low-dose-rate implants are usually paired (i.e., two are given approximately 2 weeks apart to achieve higher tolerated doses and allow further tumor regression). This also allows some correction in imperfections in the first implant dose distribution and in the patient's geometry. High-dose-rate implants are further fractionated for biological reasons. The goal is to deliver 50 to 60 Gy to microscopic disease, 60 to 70 Gy to small macroscopic disease, and 70 to 90 Gy to large macroscopic disease while limiting the volume and dose to the bladder, colorectal tissues, and small intestine. Central doses are prescribed to the point A prescription point, usually defined as 2 cm superior to the cervical os and 2 cm lateral to the endocervical canal. Point B is 3 cm lateral to point A.

Most endometrial cancers are seen postoperatively. For Stage Ib, Grades 1 and 2 and sometimes Stage Ia, Grade 2, a vaginal cylinder or colpostats alone are used to treat the vaginal cuff. Typical low-dose-rate doses, a 60- to 70-Gy surface dose, or high-dose-rate doses of 5 to 7 Gy × 3 to a 0.5-cm depth are prescribed. For Stage Ic or higher or for Grade 3 disease, an increased risk of pelvic nodal involvement exists and pelvic radiation therapy is given. Fields are similar to cervical fields, and midline blocking may be used if brachytherapy is included as part of the preoperative, postoperative, or definitive treatment. Heyman capsule techniques or an intrauterine tandem is used if a uterus is still available for implantation. Domed cylinders or vaginal colpostats are used if brachytherapy is necessary and a uterus is no longer available. Pelvic nodal doses of 50 to 60 Gy are recommended, with boosting up to 65 Gy for gross involvement. The endometrial cavity can be taken to 75 to 90 Gy with brachytherapy, but the bladder and rectum must be kept to about 60 to 65 Gy or less maximally, and the small bowel must be kept at or below 50 Gy maximally (Fig. 11-8).

Ovarian fields are also treated postoperatively after maximal debulking and staging by the gynecological oncologist. The entire peritoneal cavity must be covered, and an open-field technique is preferred. When no liver shielding is used, the upper abdominal dose is limited to 25 to 28 Gy in 1.0- to 1.2-Gy fractions. Partial renal blocking is used to limit the dose to a total of 18 to 20 Gy. The pelvis is then boosted up to a total dose of 50 Gy at 1.8 Gy per fraction. Higher-energy photons are recommended with AP/PA fields to limit the dosage variation to less than or equal to 5% (Fig. 11-9, *A* and *B*).

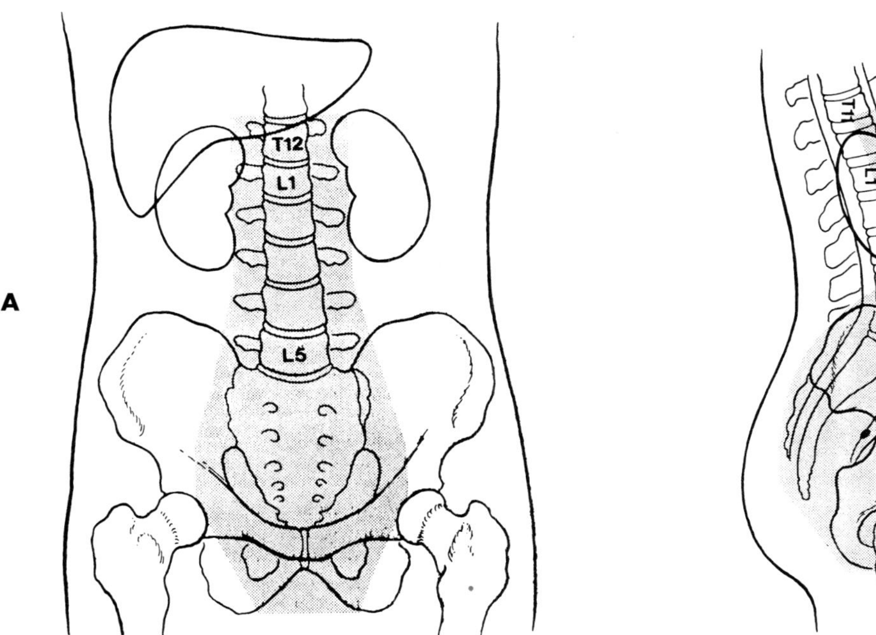

Fig. 11-7 Extended field irradiation. **A,** Anterior and posterior portals. **B,** Lateral portals. (From Russel A et al: High dose para-aortic lymph node irradiation for gynecological cancer: technique, toxicity and results, *Int J Radiat Oncol Biol Phys* 13:267-271, 1987.)

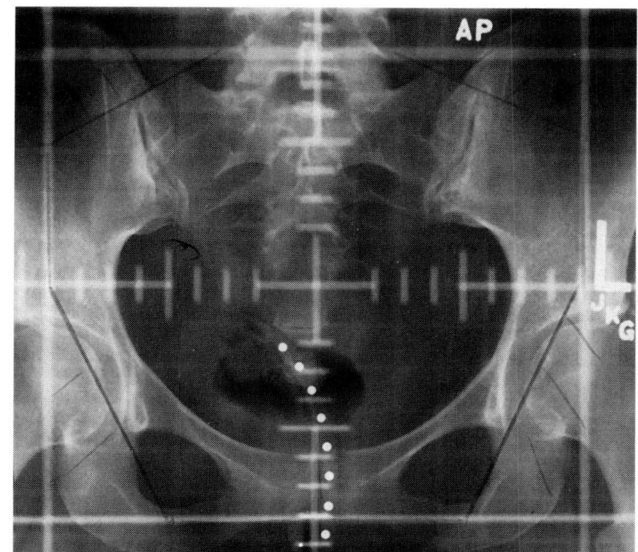

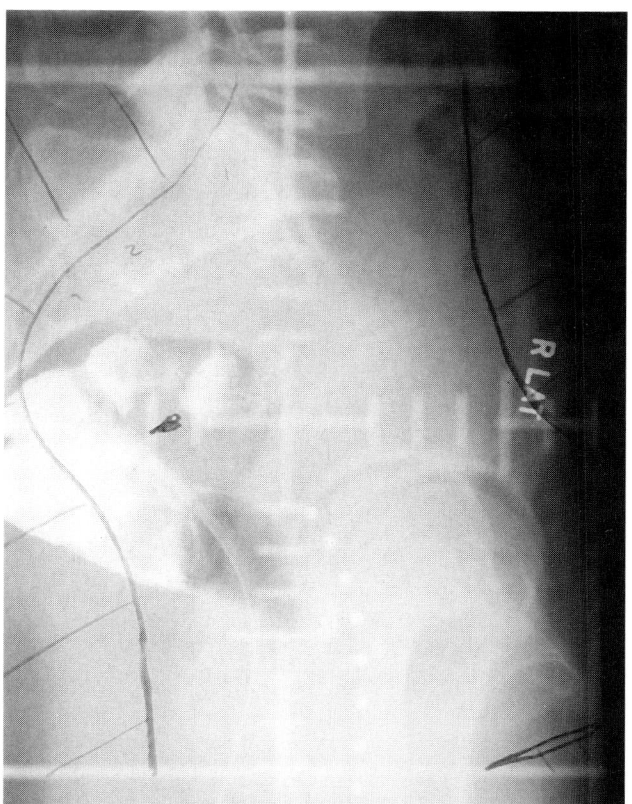

Fig. 11-8 Radiographs of endometrial simulation and implant procedures. **A,** AP/PA simulation radiographs of a four-field treatment for postoperative endometrial cancer. Note the placement of the vaginal marker. **B,** A right and left lateral radiograph of a four-field treatment for postoperative endometrial cancer. Note the placement of the vaginal marker along with rectal contrast.

Continued.

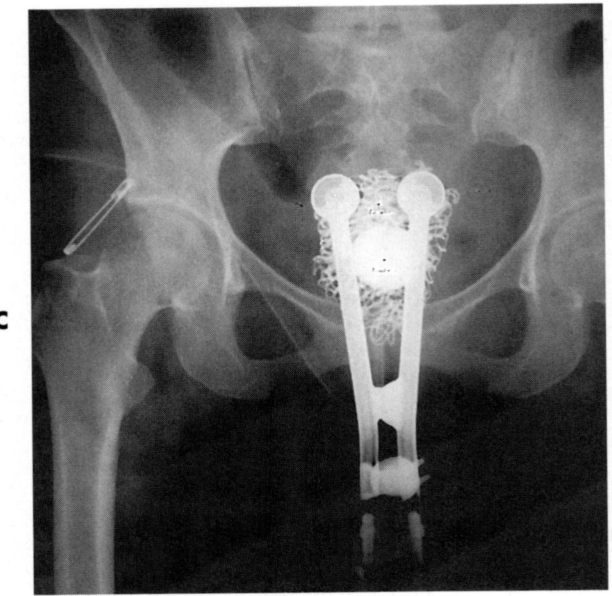

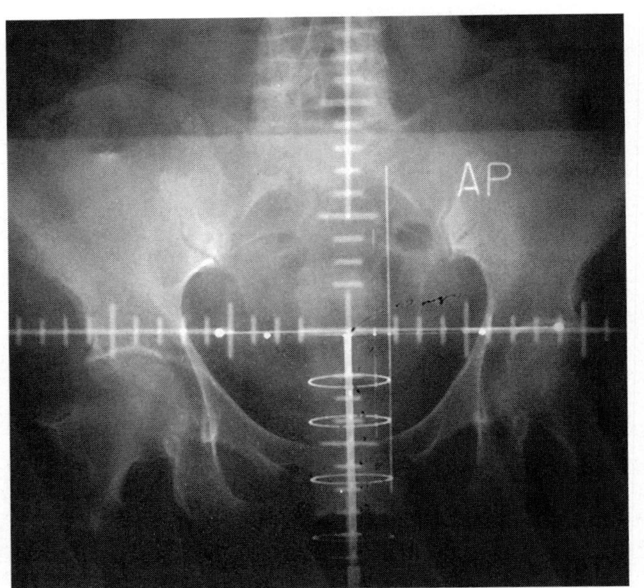

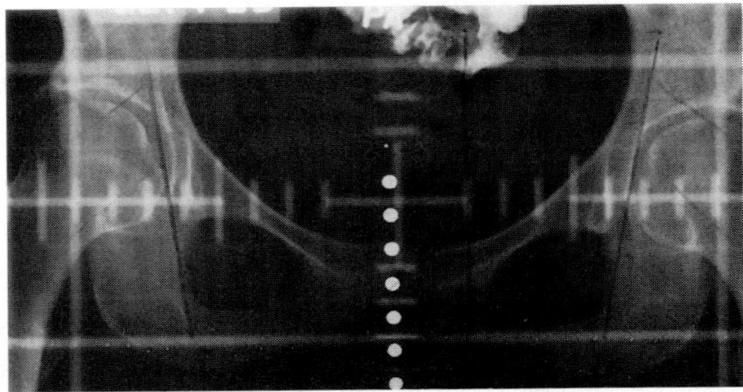

Fig. 11-8—cont'd C, A brachytherapy implant for postoperative endometrial cancer using colpostats. **D,** A brachytherapy implant using a high-dose-rate domed cylinder. **E,** A midline-blocked parametrial boost (small bowel excluded).

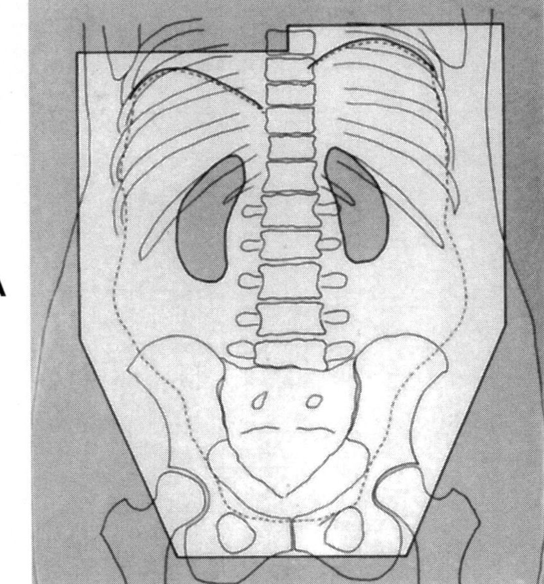

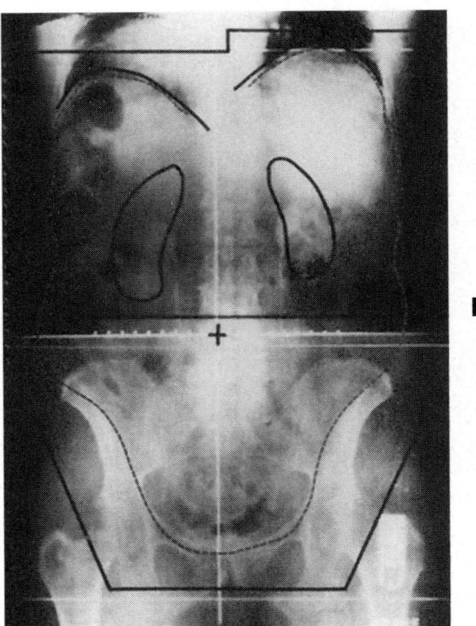

Fig. 11-9 A line drawing (**A**) and prone simulator radiograph (**B**) showing the field margin for abdominopelvic irradiation (*nonshaded area*), peritoneal outline (*dotted line*), and renal shields. The pelvic boost field is not shown. (From Cox JD: *Moss' radiation oncology: rationale, techniques, results,* ed 7, 1994, Mosby.)

SIDE EFFECTS OF TREATMENT

Acute side effects of pelvic radiation therapy include fatigue, diarrhea, dermatitis, and dysuria. Fatigue can occur the first week of treatment and can be exacerbated or complicated by anemia and depression as the patient comes to grips with the disease. Rest, reassurance, adequate nutrition, and antidepressants can make the course of treatment easier. Anemia, secondary to the disease or its treatment or as a separate problem, should be corrected to at least maintain a hemoglobin level above 10 and ideally above 11. Diarrhea usually occurs the second or third week of treatment and is related to large- and small-bowel treatment. Chemotherapy can significantly worsen this problem. Low-fiber diets, Carafate as a small-bowel coating agent, Lomotil, and loperamide are useful in alleviating this problem. Excluding as much bowel as possible from the radiation therapy fields also helps. This is done with the use of belly boards, the prone position with a full bladder on smaller fields, custom blocking, and serial field-size reduction. Dermatitis is more common with low-energy treatment, AP/PA fields, perineal flash or bolus when indicated, and concomitant chemotherapy treatment. Dome bond soaks Aquaphore ointment, and natural care gels can lessen the severity and speed healing. The prevention of local infection and correction of anemia and nutritional problems can also speed healing. Dysuria usually occurs the third or fourth week of treatment and can be lessened by treatment with a full bladder, partial bladder exclusion on lateral fields, and maintenance of a partially full bladder during brachytherapy.* Medications such as Pyridium and urised can be used to anesthetize the bladder, or Ditropan, levsin, and Hytrin can be used to relax the bladder. Infections should be treated aggressively. Bleeding can also complicate the treatment from anal irritation, bladder irritation, and a hemorrhagic tumor. Superficial en face radiation therapy can be applied directly to vaginal and cervical tumors with a large fraction size and not count against the total prescribed dose. (This can rapidly correct tumor bleeding.) Rectal irritation can be treated with hemorrhoidal preparations, steroids, topical anesthetic agents, and sitz baths.

Subacute side effects can include menopause, vaginal dryness and shrinkage, chronic cystitis, proctosigmoiditis, enteritis, and obstruction. Menopausal symptoms can be treated with cyclic hormonal therapy, vaginal dryness can be treated with moisturizing agents such as replens or hormonal creams, and shrinkage can be prevented with vaginal dialators or regular sexual activity. The inflammatory problems listed can be treated with local medications, Trental, nutritional support, antiinflammatory agents, and pain medications. Obstruction is a surgical problem.

*The foley should be clamped part of the time to fill the bladder and push it away from the implant.

Abdominal fields can also cause diarrhea, nausea, and upper gastrointestinal bleeding. Nausea can be treated prophylactically with agents such as Compazine or Kytril, and gastritis can be treated with H2 blockers (e.g., Tagamet, Zantac, Pepcid, and Axid), Carafate, or other acid inhibitors.

ROLE OF RADIATION THERAPIST

Treatment delivery

The primary role of the radiation therapist in the control of disease is simulation and treatment delivery. Patient positioning is an important component. Radiation therapists must often rely on their own experience regarding the way to position a particular patient for optimal comfort and stability. The pelvis can present considerable difficulty for simulation and reproducibility, especially when body habitus requires marking placement on loose skin overlying fat folds. The meticulous assessment of the patient's rotation is critical to prevent the shifting of the marks. Reminding the patient to maintain a full bladder when it is used to exclude the small bowel, encouraging the patient to remain on a low-residue diet when diarrhea is a problem, and remaining open and responsive to patient concerns helps to get the patient through treatment in the shortest possible time (optimal cure) and with minimal discomfort.

Patient assessment

The radiation therapist is a critical link in patient assessment. The radiation therapist is in daily contact with the patient, allowing monitoring of early changes in the patient's physical status. In addition, there is often better, closer communication between the patient and radiation therapist compared with the physician. Concerns and observations should be communicated to the medical staff members initially for more in-depth assessment. In some institutions, standing orders are written with specific expectations for suggestions to the patient and communications with medical staff members. Knowledge of institutional policy is important. The skin should be carefully assessed beginning the third week of radiation therapy. The gluteal and inguinal folds are the earliest to show a skin reaction. Pelvic irradiation can cause diarrhea, with consequent weight loss and electrolyte imbalance. A loose or soft stool is common, but the primary concern is watery diarrhea, which should be communicated immediately to medical staff members.

Reassurance

The radiation therapist has a responsibility to maintain a caring, professional atmosphere. Questions should be answered as much as knowledge permits, and medical staff members should be kept aware of patient concerns and questions. Chart rounds are an excellent format for this communication, but when in doubt, the radiation therapist should communicate with the nurse or physician.

SUMMARY

Gynecological malignancies are common and can comprise a significant proportion of the routine workload at a radiation oncology facility. For no other group of malignancies are the treatment options so diverse. The basic knowledge presented should enhance the radiation therapist's role in managing these patients while enabling a deeper understanding of the treatment rationale and potential outcome.

Review Questions

True or False

1. The vulva is more radiation tolerant than the endocervical and uterine canals.
   True _______ False _______
2. The vagina is the most radiosensitive gynecological structure.
   True _______ False _______
3. The dose response for radiation side effects in gynecological structures is age dependent.
   True _______ False _______
4. Lymphatic drainage is more important for gynecological radiation therapy planning than arterial blood supply or venous drainage.
   True _______ False _______
5. Bladder and rectal doses are more important to gynecological radiation therapy planning than kidney or ovarian doses.
   True _______ False _______

Matching (match the average age of onset)

6. Ovarian cancer
7. Cervical cancer
8. Uterine cancer
9. Clear cell vaginal cancer
10. Vulvar cancer
    a. 48 years
    b. 60 years
    c. 19 years
    d. 58 years
    e. 65+ years

Questions to Ponder

1. Why is the point A dose more important in the treatment design for cervical cancer than in that for uterine cancer?
2. What important structures in and around the pelvis may custom blocking help to reduce the dose while allowing full doses to at-risk tissues?
3. What are the tolerated (expected to have minimal long-term toxic effects) radiation therapy doses to the various pelvic structures?
4. Why is surgery less important for moderately advanced cervical cancer than for endometrial cancer?
5. In the United States, is preoperative or postoperative radiation therapy more commonly used for endometrial cancer? Explain the potential rationale for the most common approach.

REFERENCES

1. Buchsbaum HJ: Extrapelvic lymph node metastases in cervical carcinoma, *Am J Obstet Gynecol* 133:814-824, 1979.
2. Bush RD: The significance of anemia in clinical radiation therapy, *Int J Radiat Oncol Biol Phys* 12:2047-2050, 1986.
3. *Cancer facts and figures—1995,* Atlanta, 1995, American Cancer Society.
4. Dembo AJ: Abdominopelvic radiotherapy in ovarian cancer: a 10 year experience, *Cancer* 55:2285-2290, 1985.
5. Dembo AJ, Bush RD: Choice of postoperative therapy based on prognostic factors, *Int J Radiat Oncol Biol Phys* 8:893-897, 1982.
6. Dembo AJ, Thomas GM, Freidlander ML: Prognostic indices in gynecologic cancer, *Dev Oncol* 48:239-250, 1987.
7. Franklin EW, Rutledge FD: Epidemiology of epidermoid carcinoma of the vulva, *Obstet Gynecol* 39:165, 1972.
8. Friedrich EG Jr, Wilkinson EJ, Fu Ys: Carcinoma in situ of the vulva: a continuing challenge, *Am J Obstet Gynecol 136:880, 1980.*
9. Graham J: The value of preoperative or postoperative treatment by radium for carcinoma of the uterine body, *Surg Gynecol Obstet* 132:855, 1971.
10. Gusberg SB, McKay DG: Malignant lesion of the cervix and corpus uteri. In Danforth DN, editor: *Textbook of obstetrics and gynecology,* ed 2, New York, 1971, Harper & Row.
11. Hacker NV et al: Management of regional lymph nodes and their prognostic influence in vulvar cancer, *Obset Gynecol* 61:408-412, 1983.

12. Hacker NV et al: Vulva. In Hoskine WJ, Perez CA, Young RC, editors: *Principles and practices of gynecologic oncology,* Philadelphia, 1992, JB Lippincott.
13. Herbst AL, Ulfelder H, Poskanzer DC: Adenocarcinoma of the vagina. Association of maternal stilbestrol therapy with tumor appearance in young women, *N Engl J Med* 284:878-881, 1971.
14. Hintz GL et al: Radiation tolerance of the vaginal mucosa, *Int J Radiat Oncol Biol Phys* 6:711-716, 1980.
15. International Federation of Gynecology and Obstetrics (FIGO) classification, *FIGO* 18:190,1989.
16. Jenkin RD, Stryker JA: The influence of the blood pressure on survival in cancer of the cervix, *Bri J Radiol* 41:913-920, 1968.
17. Lanciano RM, Corn BW: Gynecologic cancer. In Coia LR, Moylan DJ, editors: *Introduction to clinical radiation oncology,* ed 2, Madison, Wisconsin, 1994, Medical Physics Publishing.
18. Noguchi H et al: Uterine body invasion of carcinoma of the uterine cervix as seen from surgical specimens, *Gynecol Oncol* 30:173-182, 1988.
19. Ozols RF et al: Epithelian ovarian cancer. In Hoskins WJ, Perez CA, Young RD, editors: *Principles and practice of gynecologic oncology,* Philadelphia, 1992, JB Lippincott.
20. Peck WS et al: Castration of the female by irradiation, *Radiology* 34:176-186, 1940.
21. Perez CA et al: Definitive irradiation in carcinoma of the vagina: long term evaluation of results, *Int J Radiat Oncol Biol Phys* 15:1283-1290, 1988.
22. Perez CA, Grigsby PW: Vagina & vulva. In Perez CA, Brady LW, editors: *Principles and practices of radiation oncology,* ed 2, Philadelphia, 1992, JB Lippincott.
23. Piver MS, Barlow JJ, Lele SB: Incidence of subclinical metastasis in stage I and II ovarian carcinoma, *Obstet Gyneco* 52:100, 1978.
24. Piver MS, Chung WS: Prognostic significance of cervical lesion size and pelvic node metastasis in cervical carcinoma, *Obstet Gynecol* 46:507-510, 1975.
25. Podratz KC et al: Carcinoma of the vulva: analysis of treatment and survival, *Obstet Gynecol* 61:63-74, 1983.
26. Reimer RR, Hoover R, Fraumeni JF Jr: Second primary neoplasms following ovarian cancer, *J Natl Cancer Inst* 61:1195, 1978.
27. Van Herik M: Fever as a complication of radiation therapy for carcinoma of the cervix, *Am J Roentgenol Radium Ther Nucl Med* 43:104-109, 1965.

BIBLIOGRAPHY

Anderson KN, Anderson E: *Mosby's pocket dictionary of medicine, nursing & allied health,* ed 2, St Louis, 1994, Mosby.

Brickner JT, editor: Carcinoma of the cervix. In *Patterns of care study newsletter,* Philadelphia, 1990-1991, American College of Radiology.

Cox JD: *Moss' radiation oncology: rationale, technique, results,* ed 7, St Louis, 1994, Mosby.

Glassburn JR, Brady LW, Grisby PW: Endometrium. In Perez CA, Brady LW, editors: *Principles and practice of radiation oncology,* ed 2, Philadelphia, 1992, JP Lippincott.

Grisby PW et al: Clinical Stage I endometrial cancer: results of an adjuvant irradiation and patterns of failure, *Int J Radiat Oncol Biol Phys* 21:379, 1991.

Grisby PW et al: Stage II carcinoma of the endometrium: results of therapy and prognostic factors, *Int J Radiat Oncol Biol Phys* 11:1915, 1985.

Hoskins WJ, Perez CA, Young RC: *Principles and practice of gynecologic oncology,* Philadelphia, 1992, JP Lippincott.

Josey WE, Nahamias AJ, Naib ZM: Viruses and cancer of the lower genital tract, *Cancer* 38:526, 1976.

Lanciano RM, Corn BW: Gynecologic cancer. In Coia LR, Moylan DJ, editors: *Introduction to clinical radiation oncology,* ed 2, Madison, Wisconsin, 1994, Medical Physics Publishing.

Mack T, Gasagrande JT: Epidemiology of gynecologic cancer. II Endometrium, ovary, vagina, vulva. In Munoz N, Bosch FX, Jenson OM, editors: Human papillomavirus and cervical cancer, New York, 1989, Oxford Press.

Perez CA, Bedwinek JM, Breaux SR: Patterns of failure of gynecologic tumors, *Cancer Treatment Sym* 2:226-227, 1984.

Perez CA, Brady LW, editors: *Principles and practices of radiation oncology,* ed 2, Philadelphia, 1992, JP Lippincott.

CHAPTER

12

Male Reproductive and Genitourinary Tumors

Carlos A. Perez
Russell L. Gerber
Janice M. Manolis

Outline

Key terms

Benign prostatic hypertrophy
Conformal radiation therapy
Cryptorchidism
Cystectomy
Hematuria
Impotence
Intravenous pyelogram
Prostate
Prostate-specific antigen (PSA)
Seminal vesicles
Seminomas
Smegma
Trigone
Transurethral resection

PROSTATE

Epidemiology

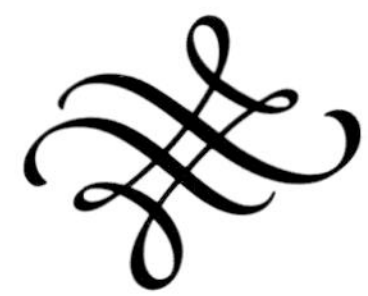

Carcinoma of the **prostate** (the walnut-shaped organ that surrounds the male urethra) is one of the most common malignancies in males in the United States. Approximately 1 in 11 men will develop prostate cancer. In 1996 317,000 new cases of prostate cancer were diagnosed in the United States, and approximately 41,000 men died of the disease.[2] The incidence increases with each decade of life; 80% of prostate carcinomas occur in men over 65 years of age. African-American men in the United States have the highest incidence of prostate cancer in the world, significantly higher than that of white men of comparable age.

Prognostic indicators

Tumor stage and histological differentiation. Strong prognostic indicators of prostate carcinoma are the clinical stage and pathological grade of tumor differentiation. Larger and less-differentiated tumors (those with a Gleason score ≥7) are more aggressive and have a greater incidence of lymphatic and distant metastases.

Age. Decreased survival rates have been reported for patients younger than 50 years. One study found a higher locoregional failure rate in patients younger than 60 years; however, survival was not significantly correlated with age.[75]

Race. Several authors have observed lower survival rates for African-American men with disease compared with white patients.[3,75] Although this observation was not confirmed in patients with Stages A2 and B disease, it was in patients with Stage C lesions.[3,70] This difference may be related to lower immune competence, biologically aggressive tumors, testosterone levels, environmental or socioeconomic conditions, and genetic or other unknown factors.[3,61]

Prostate-specific antigen level. Several reports strongly suggest a close correlation between pretreatment or post-treatment follow-up **prostate-specific antigen (PSA)** levels and the incidence of failure and survival.[54,100] Elevated PSA values after a radical prostatectomy or 6 months after definitive irradiation are sensitive indicators of persistent disease.

Lymph node status. The frequency and location of lymph node metastases have great prognostic significance.[44] Bagshaw, Ray, and Cox[5] reported disease-free survival rates of 86% in patients with negative lymph nodes, 71% with pelvic lymph node involvement, and only 30% with periaortic lymph node involvement. In contrast, Perez et al.[70] noted that Stage B patients treated with irradiation showed no significant difference in survival rates whether the lymph nodes were positive or negative at staging lymphadenectomy, but Stage C patients with negative nodes had a 7-year survival rate of over 80%, and patients with positive lymph nodes had a 20% survival rate. Similar results have been reported in Stage C patients treated with a radical prostatectomy and bilateral pelvic lymphadenectomy.

Transurethral resection. Lower survival rates have been described in patients undergoing a transurethral resection of the prostate (TURP) compared with those diagnosed by a needle biopsy, which is correlated with a higher incidence of distant metastases. A multivariate analysis of 702 patients revealed a statistically significant difference in survival rates between the needle biopsy and TURP groups in Stages B and C combined (65% and 59% at 5 years and 50% and 43% at 10 years, respectively).[60] However, in patients with Stages B1 and B2 tumors, no difference in disease-free survival was found between the needle biopsy and TURP groups. In the more advanced stages B2 and C patients, better disease-free survival was found in patients diagnosed via a needle biopsy.

A comparison was made between patients undergoing TURP and those diagnosed via a needle biopsy. Patients with T_3 and T_4, moderately or poorly differentiated tumors (a Gleason score of 8 to 10) who underwent TURP had a greater frequency of distant metastases and decreased survival rates.[74]

An analysis of the method of diagnosis (needle biopsy or TURP) and degree of histological tumor differentiation showed no statistically significant difference in the survival rates or failure patterns of patients with Stage B tumors.[70] With Stage C, moderately differentiated tumors, the 10-year disease-free survival rate was 48% for patients diagnosed by a needle biopsy and 15% for those diagnosed by TURP. McGowan[60] concluded that the adverse effect of TURP on the prognosis has not been definitely confirmed or refuted.

Anatomy

The prostate gland surrounds the male urethra between the base of the bladder and the urogenital diaphragm. The prostate is a walnut-shaped, solid organ that consists of fibrous, glandular, and muscular elements. It is attached anteriorly to the pubic symphysis by the puboprostatic ligament and separated posteriorly from the rectum by Denonvilliers' fascia (retrovesical septum), which attaches above to the peritoneum and below to the urogenital diaphragm. The seminal vesicles and vas deferens pierce the posterosuperior aspect of the gland and enter the urethra at the verumontanum (Fig. 12-1).

Natural history of disease

Local growth patterns. Most prostate carcinomas are multifocal and develop in the peripheral glands of the prostate, whereas benign prostatic hyperplasia arises from the central (periurethral) portion. As the tumor grows, it may extend into and through the capsule of the gland, invade periprostatic tissues and seminal vesicles, and if untreated, involve the bladder neck or rectum. The incidence of microscopic tumor extension beyond the capsule of the gland (at the time of a radical prostatectomy) in patients with clinical Stages A2 or B disease ranges from 15% to 50%. Seminal vesicle involvement has been observed in 10% of patients with Stage A2 tumors and in 30% of patients with Stage B2 lesions. The tumor may invade the perineural spaces, lymphatics, and blood vessels, producing lymphatic or distant metastases.

Regional lymph node involvement and distant metastases. The tumor size and degree of differentiation affect the tendency of prostatic carcinoma to metastasize to regional lymphatics. As smaller, nonpalpable tumors are diagnosed with the use of a PSA screening (a procedure that involves an evaluation of plasma levels), the incidence of metastatic pelvic lymph nodes decreases (Table 12-1). The involvement of multiple lymph nodes frequently occurs in well-differentiated and poorly differentiated lesions.

Periprostatic and obturator nodes are involved first, followed by external iliac, hypogastric, common iliac, and periaortic nodes (Fig.12-2). Approximately 7% of patients have involvement of the presacral lymph nodes (including the promontorial and middle hemorrhoidal group) without evidence of metastases in the external iliac or hypogastric lymph nodes. Metastases to the periaortic nodes occur in 5%

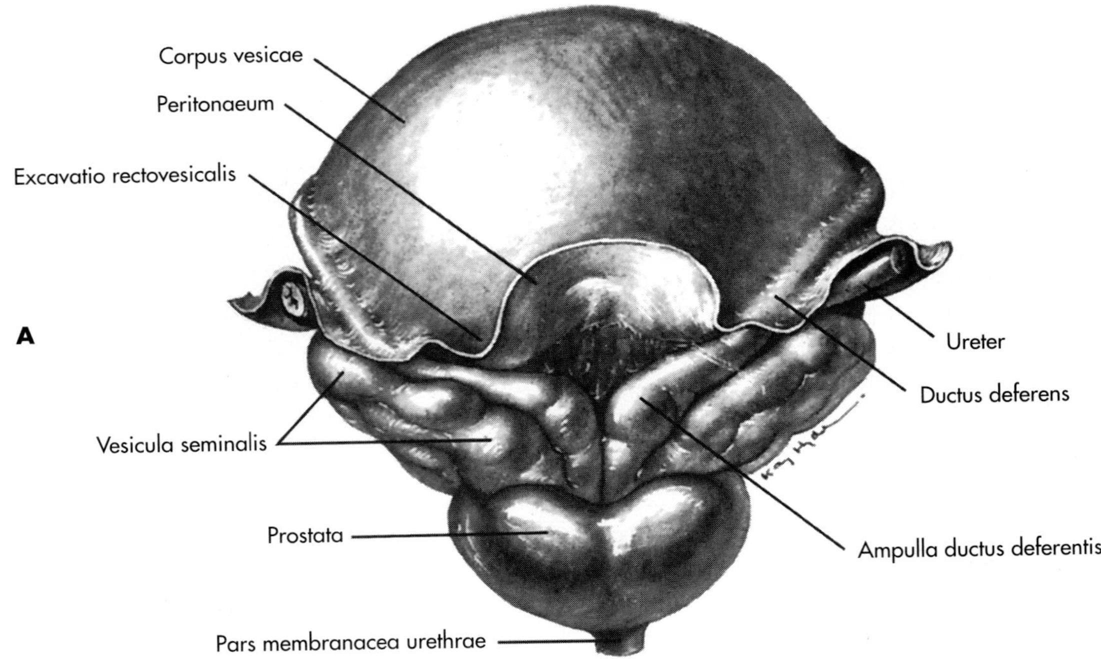

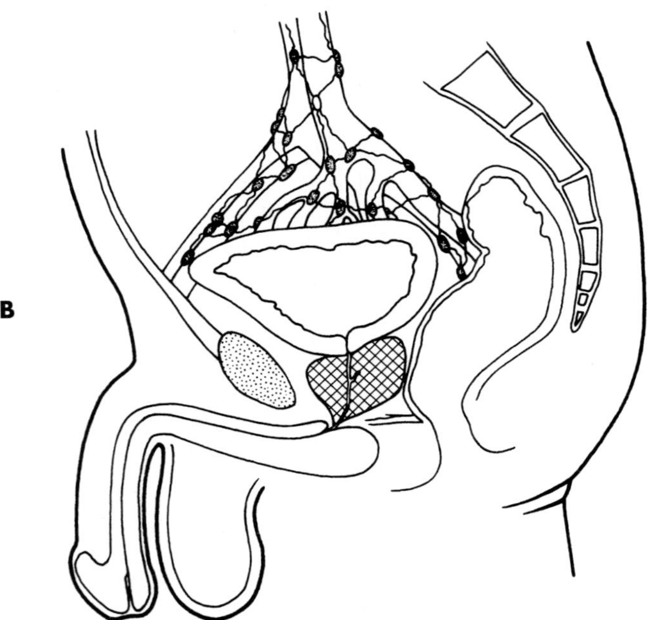

Fig. 12-1 **A,** A view of the posterior urinary bladder, illustrating the close relationship of the prostate and seminal vesicles. **B,** A sagittal view. (**A** from Anson BJ, McVay CB: *Surgical anatomy,* vol 2, ed 5, Philadelphia, 1971, WB Saunders.)

Table 12-1 Incidence of metastatic pelvic lymph nodes in carcinoma of the prostate

Clinical stage	Nerve-sparing radical prostatectomy*	Radiation therapy series: lymph node dissection†
A2 (T_{1b})	2/61 (3.3%)	1/21 (5%)
B (T_2)	33/425 (7.8%)	38/135 (28%)
C (T_3, T_4)	—	48/95 (51%)

Perez CA et al: Localized carcinoma of the prostate (stages T1B, T1C, T2, and T3): review of management with external beam radiation therapy, *Cancer* 72:3156-3173, 1993.
* Data from Petros J, Catalona WJ: Lower incidence of unsuspected lymph node metastases in 521 consecutive patients with clinically localized prostate cancer, *J Urol* 147:1574, 1992.
† Data from Hanks G et al: Comparison of pathologic and clinical evaluation of lymph nodes in prostate cancer: implications of RTOG data for patient management and trial design and stratification, *Int J Radiat Oncol Biol Phys* 23:293, 1992.
T, Tumor.

to 25% of patients. Patients with positive pelvic lymph node metastases are more likely to develop distant metastases than those with negative nodes. The incidence of distant metastases ranges from 20% in Stage A2 to 65% in Stage D1.

Clinical presentation

Patients with prostate carcinoma may complain of decreased urinary stream flow, frequency, difficulty in starting urination, dysuria, and infrequently even hematuria. These symptoms may also be caused by conditions other than cancer, such as **benign prostatic hypertrophy** (enlargement of the prostate gland, leading to narrowing of the urethra) and infection. Some tumors are diagnosed at the time of a **transurethral resection** (a surgical procedure of the prostate performed for lower urinary tract obstructive symptoms), although this procedure is being performed less often. Bone pain or other symptoms associated with distant metastasis are seen less frequently at the time of the initial diagnosis.

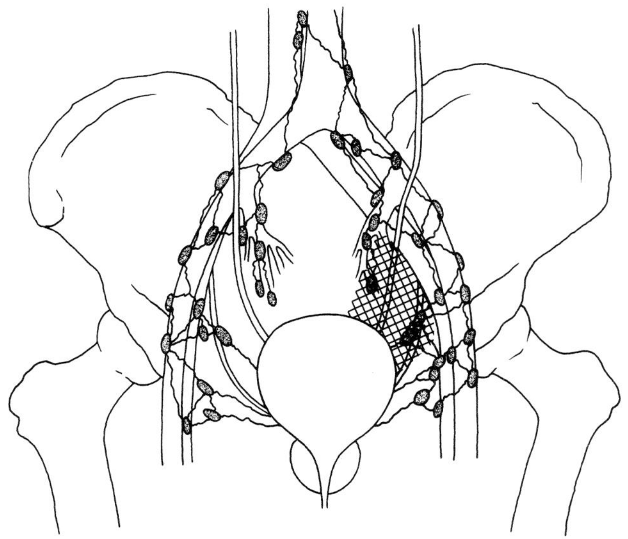

Fig. 12-2 The location of lymph nodes most frequently involved in carcinoma of the prostate. The hatched area outlines the zone usually dissected in a limited staging lymphadenectomy. (From Perez CA: Prostate. In Perez CA, Brady LW, editors: *Principles and practice of radiation oncology,* ed 2, Philadelphia, 1992, JB Lippincott.)

Diagnostic Work-up for Carcinoma of the Prostate

Routine
- Clinical history and clinical examination
- Rectal examination

Laboratory
- CBC and blood chemistry
- Serum PSA
- Plasma acid phosphatases (prostatic/total)

Radiographic imaging
- Computed tomography or magnetic resonance imaging scan of the pelvis and abdomen
- Chest x-ray examination
- Radioisotope bone scan
- Transrectal ultrasonography

Cystourethroscopy
- Needle biopsy of prostate (transrectal, transperineal)

From Perez CA: Prostate. In Perez CA, Brady LW, editors: *Principles and practice of radiation oncology,* ed 2, Philadelphia, 1992, JB Lippincott. *CBC,* Complete blood count; *PSA* prostate-specific antigen

Almost 40% of patients diagnosed with carcinoma of the prostate 20 years ago had Stage D disease (distant metastasis). Increasing awareness by the public and physicians and the growing use of PSA have reduced this percentage to about 20%.

Detection and diagnosis

Complete physical and rectal examinations are mandatory. In most patients the seminal vesicles cannot be palpated, but a firm area extending above the prostate suggests that the seminal vesicles are involved by malignancy. Approximately 50% of prostatic nodules found during the rectal examination are confirmed to be malignant at the time of a biopsy.

The diagnosis of prostatic carcinoma can be obtained only through a histological confirmation. A perineal or transrectal needle biopsy is still the standard method of diagnosis in the United States. In Europe, especially Scandinavia, an aspiration biopsy has been used for many years with impressive results.[8] False-negative diagnoses range from less than 5% to 30%.

The standard tests required in the evaluation of patients with prostatic carcinoma are listed in the box above.

Some authors have concluded that in many cases there are no specific characteristics on transrectal sonograms that differentiate benign prostatic disease from malignancy. Therefore a biopsy is always required.[84] A sensitivity rate of 86% and a specificity rate of only 41% have been reported. Tumors less than 1 cm are the most difficult to detect.[13] Transrectal magnetic resonance is increasingly used in the evaluation of these patients with promising preliminary results.[91]

Screening. Carcinoma of the prostate can be asymptomatic until attaining a significant size. An annual digital rectal examination of the prostate should be performed in all men over 40 years of age. A digital rectal examination has about a 70% sensitivity rate and a 50% specificity rate in detecting prostate cancer. Radioimmunoassays for prostatic acid phosphatase (PAP) have a sensitivity rate of only 10% and a specificity rate of 90% for malignant tumors and have been largely replaced by PSA testing.

PSA plasma levels are routinely obtained in men over 50 years of age. Prostatic antigen is detected in the normal prostatic tissue benign hyperplasia, malignant tumors, seminal fluid, and sera of patients with prostatic hyperplasia or cancer. The normal PSA value is 0.4 to 4 ng/ml. Recently, the recommendation was made that the upper normal PSA level be adjusted according to age (up to 6 ng/ml in men older than 70 years). Elevated PSA titers at the time of the diagnosis of carcinoma are associated with a greater probability of lymph node metastases or distant dissemination (Fig. 12-3).

Some authors have concluded that PSA is more sensitive than PAP and a rectal examination in the detection of prostate carcinoma and that PSA will be more useful in monitoring the response and recurrence after therapy. However, PSA and PAP may be elevated in benign prostatic hyperplasia.[43] In a study of 1653 healthy men 50 years or older who participated in a PSA screening project, PSA determinations increased to

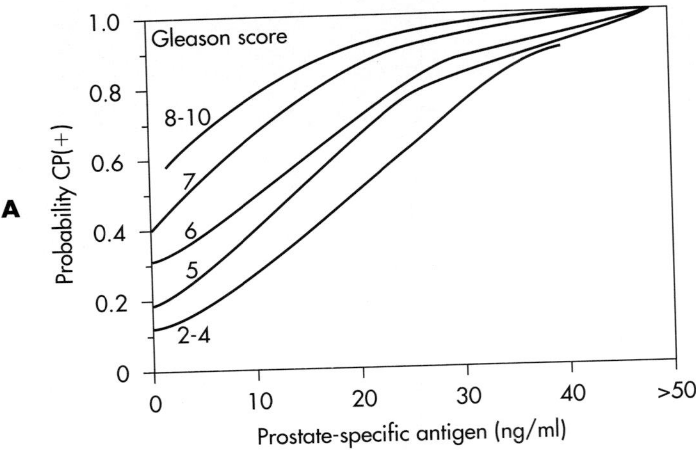

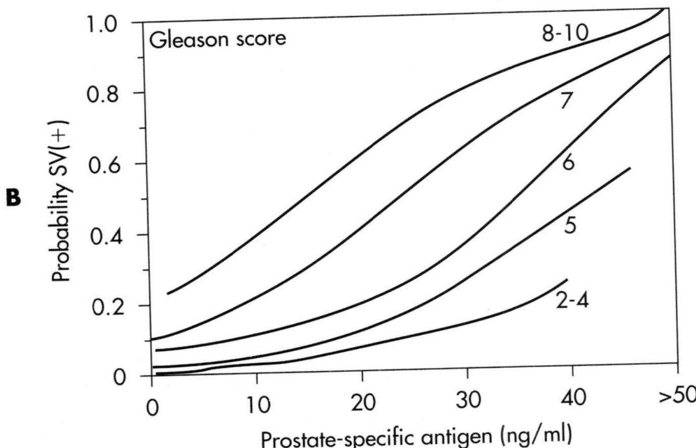

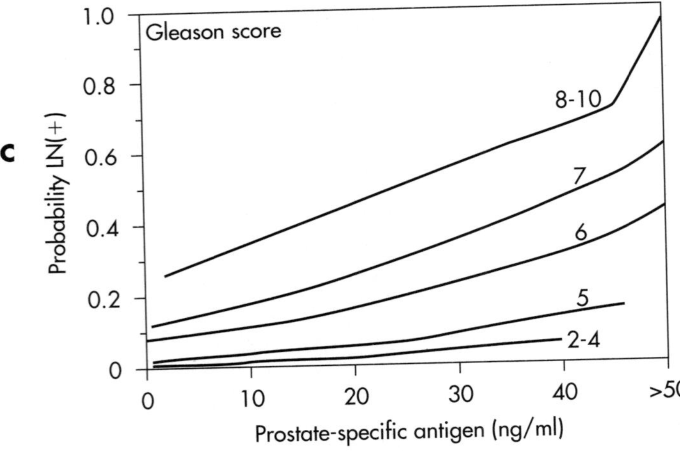

Fig. 12-3 **A,** The probability of capsular penetration *(CP+)* as a function of the serum PSA and preoperative Gleason score. **B,** The probability of seminal vesicle involvement *(SV+)* as a function of the serum PSA and preoperative Gleason score. **C,** The probability of lymph node involvement *(LN+)* as a function of the serum PSA and preoperative Gleason score. (From Partin AW et al: *J Urol* 150:110-114, 1993.)

70% the proportion of prostatic carcinomas localized to the gland at the time of diagnosis, in contrast to only 30% of carcinomas diagnosed by a routine rectal examination.[12] This should eventually result in decreased cancer mortality.

Transrectal ultrasound has been used to detect smaller lesions, even before they are clinically palpable. However, many detected lesions are not malignant; therefore the specificity rate of the test is only 40% to 50%. Ultrasound is used to guide needle biopsies of small, nonpalpable lesions, although multiple biopsies of both prostate lobes detect more cancers.

PSA in the selection of patients for therapy and post-treatment evaluation. Several authors have shown a close correlation between PSA levels and clinical and pathological tumor stage, and in conjunction with Gleason score, a predictable correlation with incidence of lymph node metastasis. The Gleason score indicates the histological grade of the tumor (<4, well differentiated; 5 to 7, moderately differentiated; 8 to 10, poorly differentiated). A group of patients with a PSA level below 2.8 ng/ml and a Gleason score below 4 had about a 1% incidence of nodal disease or seminal vesicle involvement at the time of a prostatectomy, but 60% of patients with a PSA level above 40 ng/ml and a Gleason score above 8 had these findings.[67] PSA may be of great value in the follow-up of patients treated with radical prostatectomy or radiation therapy for localized prostatic cancer or after hormonal therapy.

Pathology and staging

Most malignant tumors of the prostate are adenocarcinomas. Gleason[33] devised a quantitative histological grading system initially based on the clinical stage and morphological tumor characteristics. The pathologist evaluates the predominant degree of differentiation of the tumor (primary pattern) and the less-apparent component (secondary pattern) based on the morphology of the lesion (e.g., glandular pattern, distribution of glands, stromal invasion) (Fig.12-4, *A*). The primary and secondary scores are individually expressed from 1 to 5. Pathological features are scored from 2 to 10 (<4, well differentiated; 5 to 7, moderately differentiated; 8 to 10, poorly differentiated tumor). The Gleason score also correlates closely with prognosis (Fig. 12-4, *B*). At Washington University the histological differentiation of the tumor was strongly correlated with the incidence of distant metastases and survival but not as closely as with locoregional failure.[70]

Findings from the digital examination of the prostate and from other studies determine the stage of the disease, which is classified according to the American Joint Committee on Cancer (AJCC) or the Jewett-Whitmore system (Table 12-2). A substantial correlation exists between the PSA levels, tumor stage, and incidence of metastatic pelvic lymph nodes or distant metastasis.

Stage A1 (T_{1a}) lesions are well-differentiated adenocarcinomas that are not clinically apparent (5% or less of tissue

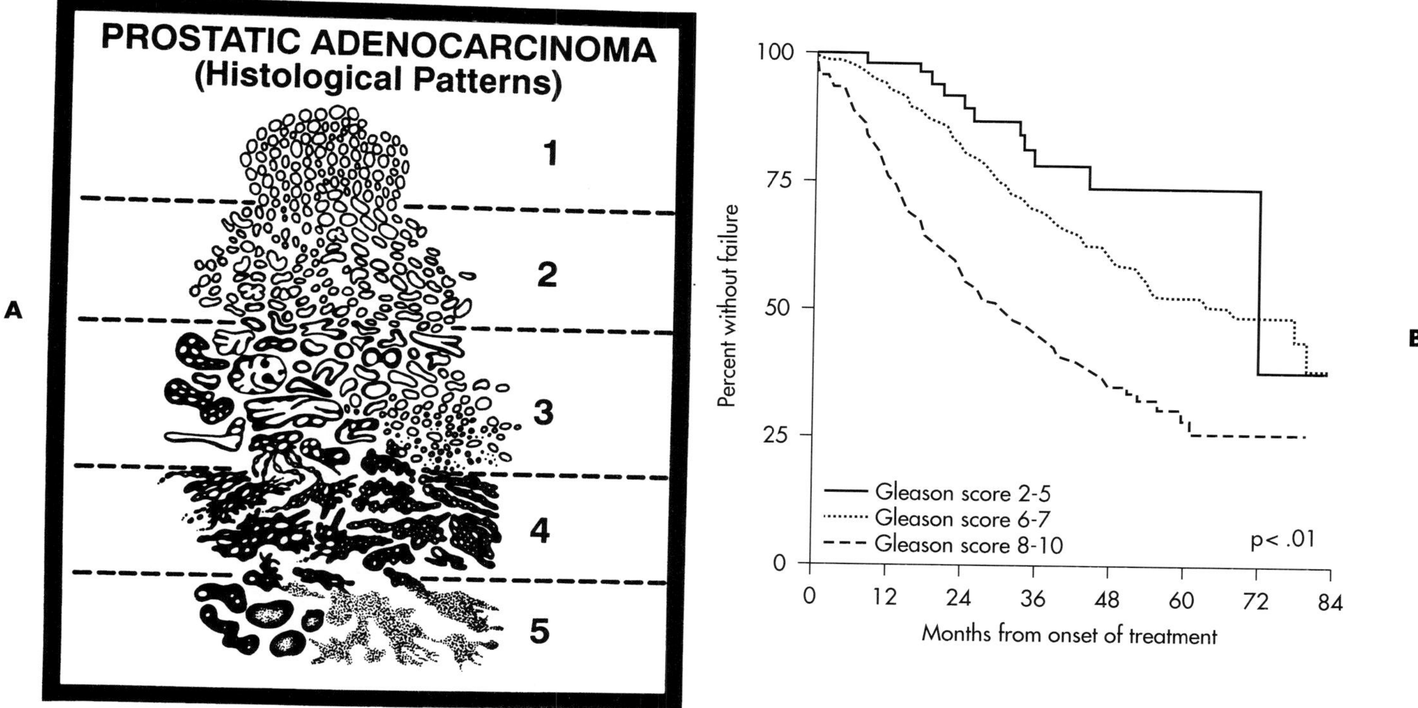

Fig. 12-4 **A,** A simplified drawing of histological patterns, emphasizing the degree of glandular differentiation and relation to stroma. The all-black area in the drawing represents the tumor tissue and glands with all cytological detail obscured, except in the right side of pattern 4, where tiny open structures are intended to suggest the hypernephroid pattern. **B,** Survival correlated with the Gleason score (N = 566). (**A** from Gleason DF et al: Histologic grading and clinical staging of prostatic carcinoma. In Tannenbaum M, editor: *Urologic pathology: the prostate,* Philadelphia, 1977, Lea & Febiger; **B** from Pilepich MV et al: Prognostic factors in carcinoma of the prostate: analysis of RTOG Study 75-06, *Int J Radiat Oncol Biol Phys* 13:339-349, 1987.)

Table 12-2 Staging of prostate cancer

Jewett-Whitmore system	Staging classification	TNM system
A1	No clinical disease; fewer than three fragments contain tumor	T_0, N_0, M_0
A2	No clinical disease; more than three fragments contain tumor	
B1	Palpable nodule confined to one lobe	
	Less than 1 cm	T_{1a}, N_0, M_0
	Greater than 1 cm	T_{1b}, N_0, M_0
B2	Tumor involvement of both lobes	T_{1c}, N_0, M_0
	Invasion of but not through the capsule	T_2, N_0, M_0
C1	Penetration of capsule; minimal extension	T_3, N_0, M_0
C2	Extensive local disease; ureteral-bladder obstruction	T_4, N_0, M_0
D1	Nodal metastases not clinically appreciated	T_2, N–, M_0
	Widespread metastases not clinically appreciated	T_2, N_2, M–
D2	Nodal metastases clinically manifest	T_2, N–, M_0
	Widespread metastases clinically manifest	T_2, N_2, M_2

T, Tumor; *N,* node; *M,* metastasis.

resected). They are incidentally found during a transurethral resection or needle biopsy of the prostate. Stage A2 (T_{1b}) tumors are also subclinical, but they are more diffuse or have a larger volume, frequently with multifocal involvement of the prostate. T_{1c} tumors are identified by a needle biopsy (e.g., because of elevated PSA levels).

Stage B (T_2) tumors are palpable and confined in the capsule of the prostate gland. Stage B1 (T_{2a}) tumors involve less than half a lobe; Stage B2 (T_{2b}) represents a more extensive intraglandular palpable tumor.

Stage C ($T_{3a,b}$) lesions have extracapsular extension and are subclassified as Stage C1 (T_{3a}) if they involve the periprostatic tissues or one seminal vesicle. Tumors that involve both seminal vesicles or are larger than 6 cm are subclassified as Stage C2 (T_{3b}).

Stage D (T_4) tumors are subclassified as D1 if there is metastatic disease to the regional lymph nodes or if, according to Perez, Pilepich, and Zivnuska,[73] there is extensive involvement of the bladder, rectum, or pelvic tissues extending to the pelvic wall (detected through a clinical examination). D2 represents distant dissemination.

Treatment techniques

Several areas of controversy surround the management of patients with prostatic carcinoma. The natural history of this tumor is variable and influenced by multiple prognostic factors. The different forms of therapy can affect the quality of life and sexual function in varying degrees.

Localized carcinoma of the prostate has a fairly slow clinical course. The National Cancer Institute Consensus Development Conference on Management of Localized Prostate Cancer concluded that radical prostatectomy and radiation therapy are clearly effective treatments in appropriately selected patients for tumors limited to the prostate.

Several authors have reported on patients aged 60 to over 80 who, after a histological diagnosis of prostatic carcinoma, were managed conservatively and monitored without specific anticancer treatment until symptoms developed.[1,48] The literature indicates that these tumors have a protracted course associated with a significant competing mortality and marginal benefit from radical prostatectomy at 10 years.[1] Calculated 10-year disease-specific survival rates of 93% for radical prostatectomy, 83% for deferred treatment, and 62% for external radiation therapy have been observed. Observation is reported to be reasonable management for patients over 75 years of age. Radical prostatectomy or radiation therapy offers the same therapeutic benefits to patients 60 to 65 years old with moderately or poorly differentiated tumors.[27] In today's health environment in the United States, delaying definitive therapy in most patients with localized carcinoma of the prostate is almost impossible, except in certain older patients or those with less-than-ideal general health and well-differentiated Stage A or B1 tumors.

According to many urologists, Stage A1 (T_{1a}) disease found incidentally requires no treatment; many years of natural evolution may pass before the disease becomes a clinical problem. According to one study, only 6.8% of 148 patients with Stage A focal carcinoma (treated conservatively or not) had progression of disease. A literature review showed a death rate of only 1.9% in 262 patients with Stage A1 carcinoma.[10]

Some authors have noted decreased survival rates with poorly differentiated (G3) tumors but not with well-differentiated lesions in Stage A1 adenocarcinoma of the prostate.[42,48] In 313 patients who had T_1, N_0 tumors treated with external irradiation, the 5-year survival rate was comparable to that of a matched-age normal male group (77% and 81%, respectively), but the 10-year survival rate was below the normal life expectancy (51% and 62%, respectively).[41]

Traditionally, the treatment of choice for patients with resectable Stage A2 or B (T_1 or T_2) prostate carcinoma has been radical prostatectomy. Impetus has been given to the use of nerve-sparing surgery because an increasing number of tumors are being diagnosed at earlier stages, and a lower incidence of sexual **impotence** (the inability to obtain an erection or ejaculate after an erection) has been reported with this surgery (40% to 60%, depending on the patient's age and tumor extent) compared with classical radical prostatectomy (close to 100%). Radiation therapy has been nearly as effective in the treatment of these patients, some of whom prefer this modality instead of surgery. In an analysis of 104 patients with Stage $T_{1b2,}N_0$ disease treated with definitive irradiation, the tumor-free survival rate was 96% at 5 years and 86% at 10 years.[40] Locoregional tumor control was 93% at 5 years and 84% at 10 years. These results are comparable to those reported for radical prostatectomy.

For stage C (T_3) disease most urologists and radiation oncologists agree that external beam irradiation is the treatment of choice, although hormonal therapy is an alternative.

Cryosurgery, in which tissues are coagulated through their exposure to extremely low temperatures, has been introduced for the treatment of prostate cancer. Although therapy results are not available at this time, preliminary reports indicate that this procedure is associated with low morbidity.[65]

Hormonal therapy. In 1941, Huggins, Stevens, and Hodges[46] demonstrated prostate tumor regression and diminished serum acid phosphatase levels after orchiectomy or estrogen administration. Many types of hormonal therapy, all seeking to reduce the androgenic stimulation of prostatic carcinoma, have been used since then. Orchiectomy removes 95% of circulating testosterone and is followed by a prompt, long-lasting decline in serum testosterone levels. Estrogen appears to suppress pituitary gonadotropin, causing reduced stimulus for testicular testosterone synthesis, direct interference with hormonal synthesis, or a direct effect on the prostatic cell competing with hormonal receptors. Gonadotropin-releasing hormone agonists such as goserelin (Zoladex) and Buserelin cause an initial rise in gonadotropin levels, followed by a sharp decline within 2 to 3 weeks. Parallel changes occur in levels of circulating testosterone, interfering with androgen production in the adrenal gland. Results with these compounds are similar to those obtained with bilateral orchiectomy.

Aminoglutethimide, which is administered with a glucocorticoid, inhibits the synthesis of all adrenal steroids and can further reduce serum testosterone levels in castrated patients.[109]

Flutamide (Eulexin) is a nonsteroidal antiandrogen that blocks the effect of 5α-reductase, inhibiting the formation of dihydrotestosterone and the androgen uptake and nuclear binding in the prostate cell.

Hormonal therapy has definite palliative value in prostatic cancer, and survival beyond 10 years occurs in 10% of patients with bony metastases responding to such treatment. However, adjuvant therapy with diethylstilbestrol in patients treated with prostatic or pelvic irradiation confers no overall survival advantage.

Chemotherapy. Several drugs have been evaluated in patients for whom hormonal therapy failed. Response rates with single-agent doxorubicin (Adriamycin) are 25% to 35%. With cyclophosphamide the rate of partial response plus stable disease ranges from 26% to 41%, but only 5% of patients have complete or partial responses. In about 10% of patients 5-fluorouracil has induced partial responses. A partial response rate of only 8% was observed with hydroxyurea. Prospective randomized trials have not supported the superiority of combination chemotherapy over single drugs in metastatic prostate cancer. In five randomized studies of single-agent versus combination chemotherapy, there was no or minimal difference in the percentage of patients with partial response plus stable disease; the response duration and survival rates were essentially the same. Less than 10% complete or partial response occurred in over 3000 patients with advanced or recurrent metastatic carcinoma of the prostate treated with various chemotherapeutic agents.[23]

Radiation therapy.

External irradiation. When the pelvic lymph nodes are treated, as is selectively done at Washington University, the field size for Stage A2, B, or C lesions is 15 × 15 cm at the patient surface (16.5 cm at the isocenter) (Fig. 12-5, *A*). The reduced field for treatment of the prostatic volume can be about 8 × 10 cm for Stages A2 and B to 10 × 12 cm or larger for Stages C and D1. In most institutions computed tomography (CT) or magnetic resonance imaging (MRI) is used to determine the exact size and location of the prostate and to establish the tumor extent. The inferior margin of the field should be at the junction of the prostatic and membranous urethra (usually at the bottom of the ischial tuberosities). The lateral margins should be about 2 cm from the lateral bony pelvis.

When lateral portals are used, either for the box technique (including the lymph nodes) or for irradiation of the prostate with rotational techniques, it is important to delineate with the aid of CT or MRI the anatomical structures of the pelvis and location of the prostate in relation to the bladder, rectum, and bony structures.

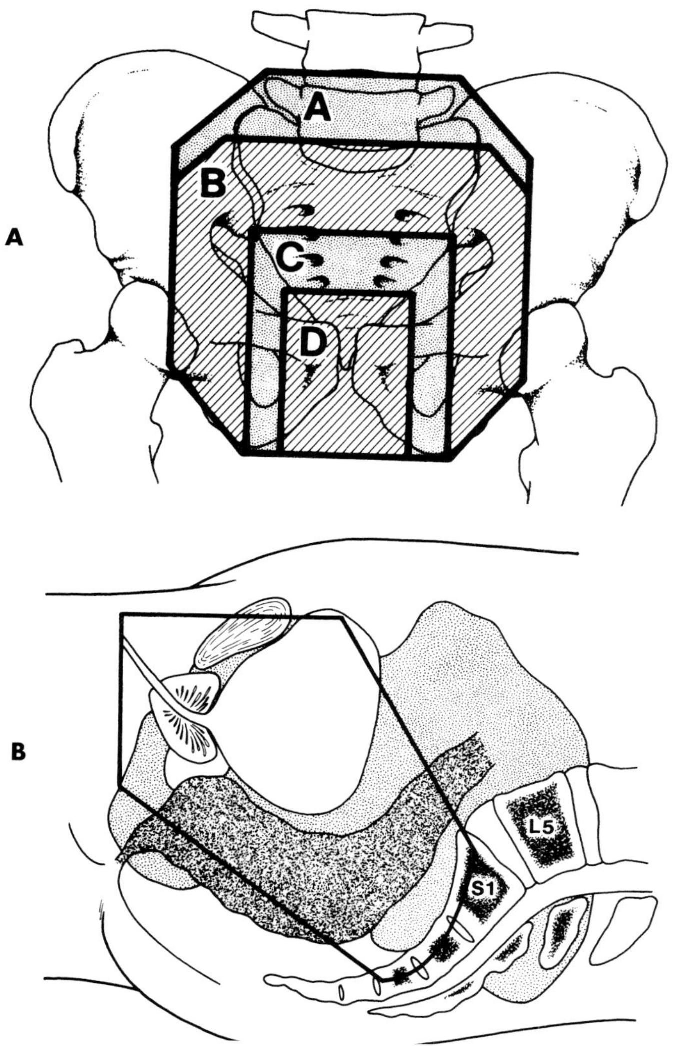

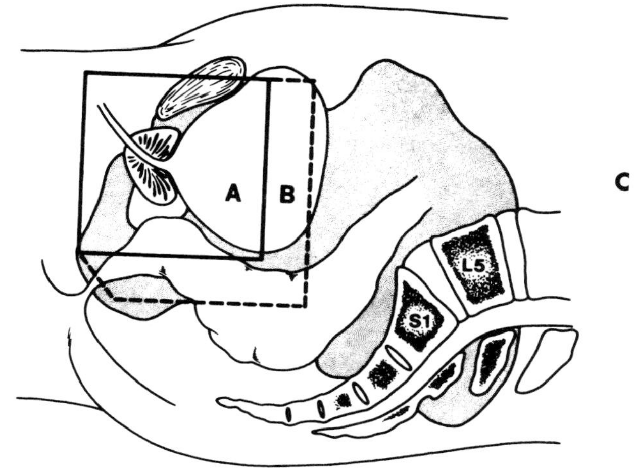

Fig. 12-5 **A,** A diagram of the pelvis showing volumes used to irradiate the prostate and pelvic lymph nodes. The lower margin is at or even 1 cm below ischial tuberosities. *A* and *B* indicate pelvic portals used for patients with Stages C or D1 and A2 or B disease, respectively. *C* illustrates the prostate boost for Stage C or D1 disease, and *D* shows the boost for Stage A2 or B disease. **B,** The lateral portal used in the box technique to irradiate pelvic tissues and the prostate. The anterior margin is 0.5 to 1 cm posterior to projected cortex of pubic symphysis. Presacral lymph nodes are included down to S3; inferiorly, the posterior wall of the rectum is spared. **C,** A lateral diagram of reduced fields used to irradiate the prostate and immediately adjacent tissues. (From Perez CA: Prostate. In Perez CA, Brady LW, editors: *Principles and practice of radiation oncology,* ed 2, Philadelphia, 1992, JB Lippincott.)

The initial lateral field encompasses a volume similar to that treated with AP/PA pelvic portals, including the pelvic and presacral lymph nodes above the S3 segment, allowing for sparing of the posterior rectal wall distal to this level. The anterior margins should be 1 cm posterior to the projection of the anterior cortex of the pubic symphysis (Fig. 12-5, *B*). Some of the small bowel may be spared anteriorly, following the anatomical location of the external iliac lymph nodes.

For simulation of these portals the patient is placed in the supine position. A small plastic rod with radiopaque markers 1 cm apart is inserted in the rectum. After thorough cleansing of the penis and surrounding areas with Betadine (via a sterile technique), 40% iodinated contrast material is injected in the urethra until the patient complains of mild discomfort. This procedure documents the junction of the prostatic and bulbous urethra, thus accurately localizing the apex of the prostate, which is more difficult to identify on a CT or MRI scan. AP and lateral radiographs are taken after the position of the small portals is determined from a fluoroscopic examination. Fig. 12-6 shows an example of simulation films outlining the AP and lateral portals used for the pelvic box technique.

For the boost the upper margin is 3 to 5 cm above the superior pubic ramus, depending on the extent of disease and volume to be covered (i.e., prostate or seminal vesicles). The anterior margin is 1 cm posterior to the anterior cortex of the pubic bone, the inferior margin is 2 cm caudal (distal) to the junction of the prostatic and membranous urethra, and the posterior margin is 2 cm behind the radiopaque marker in the rectum (Fig. 12-5, *C*).

The different boost portal sizes should be individually determined for each patient, depending on the clinical and radiographic assessment of the tumor extent. Policies of treatment and average field sizes are recommended in Table 12-3.

After the appropriate portals have been determined, the corners of the reduced portals and the isocenters for both portals are tattooed with india ink.

When indicated, the periaortic lymph nodes can be treated through a single extended portal that includes the pelvic and periaortic lymph nodes (Fig. 12-7, *A*) if large-field linear accelerator beams are available. Otherwise, a separate periaortic portal is placed above the pelvic fields, and calculations for an appropriate gap (about 3 cm) should be made (Fig. 12-7, *B*). The portal's superior margin should be at the T12-L1 vertebral interspace to cover all the periaortic lymph nodes. The width, which usually is about 10 cm, can be determined with the aid of a lymphangiogram or CT. If these studies are not available, the **intravenous pyelogram** (a radiographic procedure using contrast media) indicates the trajectory of the ureters, which although not 100% accurate, may be used as landmarks. The dose to the distal spinal cord should be limited to 4500 cGy, with a small posterior 5 half-value layer block above the L2-3 interspace.

Ideally, high-energy photon beams (above 15 MV) should be used to treat these patients, thus simplifying techniques and decreasing morbidity. With 18-MV photons, up to a 4500-cGy total dose can be delivered with AP/PA portals in patients less than 20 cm in AP diameter. The additional dose is administered with lateral portals. With photon beam energies below 18 MV, lateral portals are always necessary to deliver part of the dose, in addition to the AP/PA portals (box technique). An additional dose is administered with bilateral 120-degree arc rotations, skipping the midline anteriorly and posteriorly (60-degree vectors) to provide adequate dose distributions (Fig. 12-8). Small fields alone are used for the irradiation of selected patients with Stage A2 or B disease, after

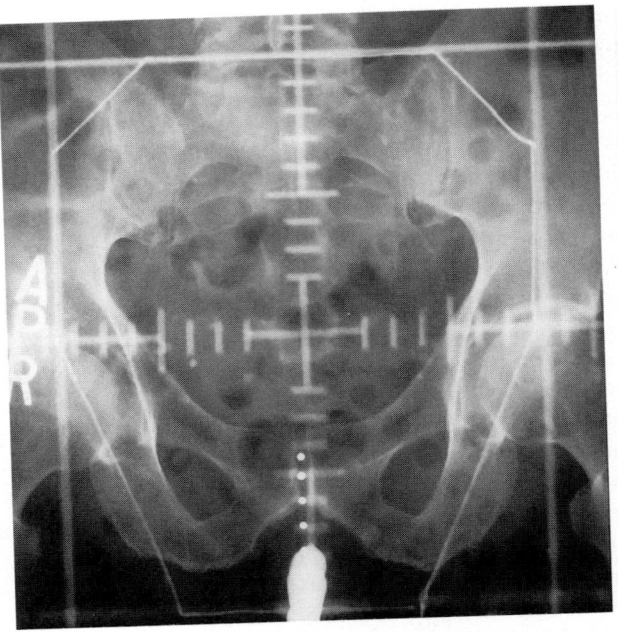

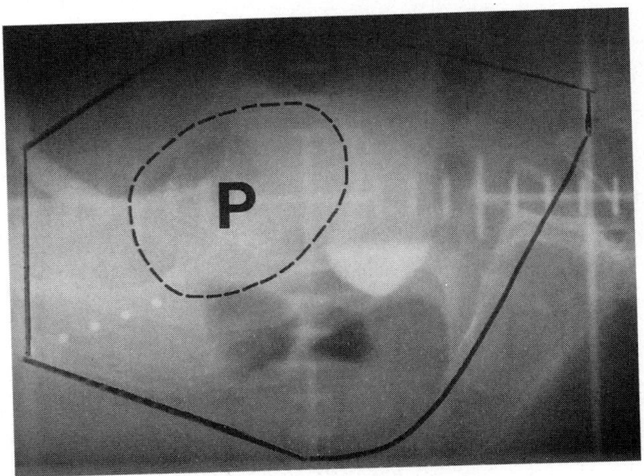

Fig. 12-6 AP (**A**) and lateral (**B**) portals for carcinoma of the prostate as shown on simulation films. The junction of the prostatic and bulbous urethra (distal margin of the prostate) is identified by a urethrogram. Note the relationship of the portals to the roof of the acetabulum, the pubic symphysis anteriorly, and the ischial tuberosities posteriorly. (From Perez CA: Prostate. In Perez CA, Brady LW, editors: *Principles and practice of radiation oncology,* ed 2, Philadelphia, 1992, JB Lippincott.)

Table 12-3 Summary of treatment guidelines for prostatic adenocarcinoma through the use of high-energy photons at Mallinckrodt Institute of Radiology with conventional techniques

Stage	Portal size (cm at isocenter)		Technique		Tumor doses* (cGy)	
	Pelvic	Prostatic	Pelvic	Prostatic	Pelvic lymph Nodes	Boost
A1 (less than well differentiated)		8 × 10	None	120-degree bilateral arcs		6400/6.5 wk
A2, B—Staging lymphadenectomy, negative pelvic lymph nodes		8 × 10 or 10 × 12		120-degree bilateral arcs	0	6800/7 wk
A2-B1 (well differentiated)—No staging		10 × 12	AP/PA	120-degree bilateral arcs	0	6800/7 wk
A2, B—No lymphadenectomy	16.5 × 16.5	8 × 10	AP/PA	120-degree bilateral arcs	4500/5 wk	2200/2 wk
A2, B—Any histology, patients older than 70 years		8 × 10 or 10 × 12		120-degree bilateral arcs	0	6800/7 wk
A2, B—Positive common iliac nodes* (plus 4500 cGy to periaortic nodes†)	16.5 × 21	8 × 10	AP/PA	120-degree bilateral arcs	4500/5 wk	2200/2 wk
C—Negative lymphadenectomy	16.5 × 16.5	12 × 12 or 12 × 14	AP/PA	120-degree bilateral arcs	4500/5 wk	2600/2.5 wk
C—Positive external iliac of hypogastric nodes by any evaluation	16.5 × 21	10 × 12 or 12 × 14	AP/PA	120-degree bilateral arcs	4500/5 wk	2600/2.5 wk
C—Positive common iliac or periaortic nodes (plus 4500 cGy to periaortic nodes†)	16.5 × 21	8 × 10 or 10 × 12	AP/PA	120-degree bilateral arcs	4500/5 wk	2600/2.5 wk
D1	16.5 × 21	10 × 12 or 12 × 14	AP/PA	120-degree bilateral arcs	4500/5 wk	2000/2 wk

Modified from Perez CA: Prostate. In Perez CA, Brady LW, editors: *Principles and practice of radiation oncology*, ed 2, Philadelphia, 1992, JB Lippincott.
*Daily dose: large pelvic fields, 180 cGy; boost prostatic portals, 200 cGy.
†For grossly positive periaortic nodes, add 500 to 1000 cGy with reduced portals. In Stage C, if seminal vesicles are involved (C2), the boost portal may be 12 × 14 cm.
AP/PA, Anteroposterior/posteroanterior.

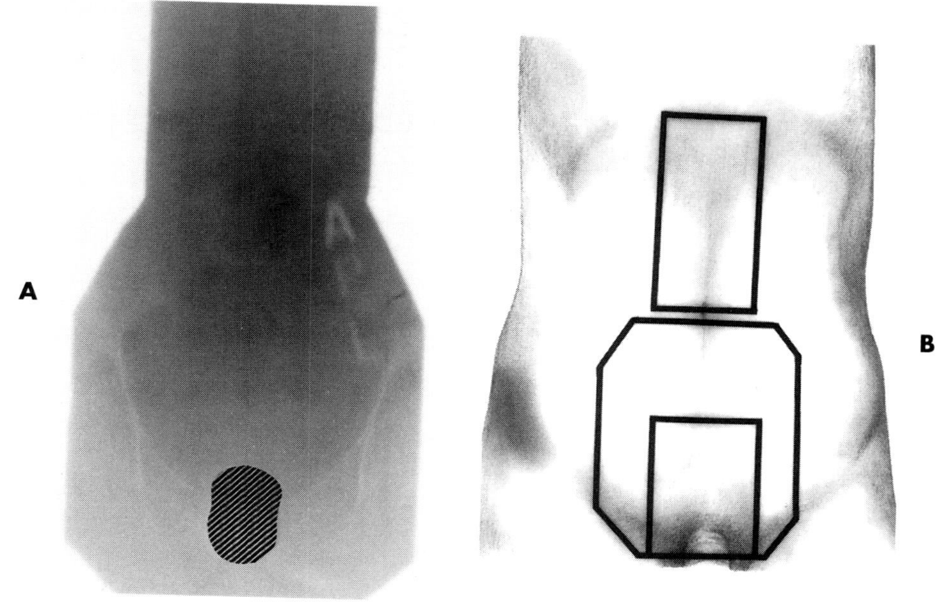

Fig. 12-7 **A,** A localization film showing an extended portal for irradiation of the periaortic and pelvic lymph nodes in carcinoma of the prostate. **B,** Separate portals used for irradiation of the periaortic lymph nodes when large fields are not available. Gap separation must be calculated for each patient. (From Perez CA: Prostate. In Perez CA, Brady LW, editors: *Principles and practice of radiation oncology,* ed 2, Philadelphia, 1992, JB Lippincott.)

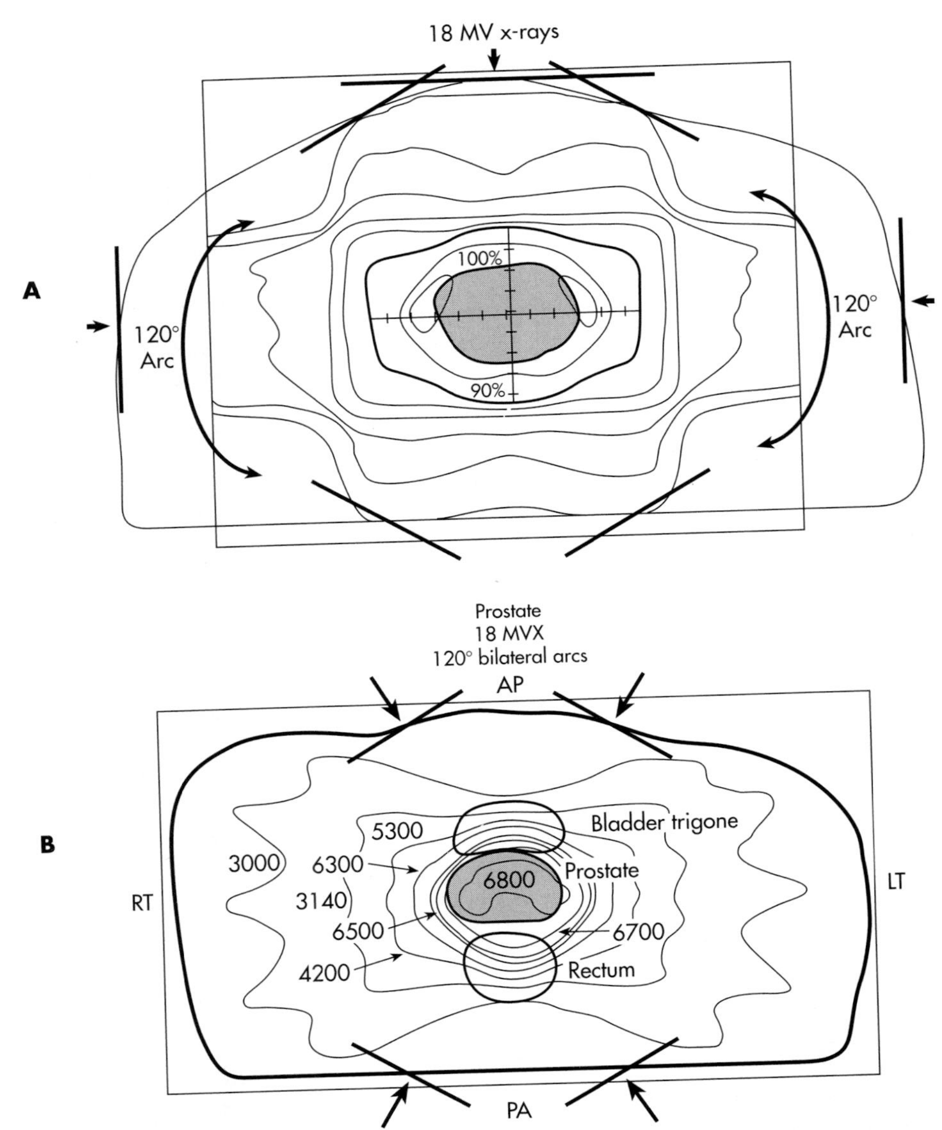

Fig. 12-8 **A,** Isodose curves with 18-MV photons delivering 4500 cGy to the whole pelvis through AP, PA, and lateral portals and 2500 cGy with reduced fields to the prostate through bilateral 120-degree arcs. **B,** Bilateral arcs alone.

a pelvic lymphadenectomy with negative nodes, or after a postradical prostatectomy with positive margins.

The total tumor dose to the prostate for Stages A2 and B tumors is 6800 cGy, and for stage C it is 7100 cGy (Fig. 12-9). For Stage D1 lesions treatment is usually palliative, and the minimal tumor dose can be held at 6000 to 6500 cGy to decrease morbidity. Daily fractions are 180- to 200-cGy tumor dose given in five fractions per week.

Three-dimensional conformal radiation therapy. With the advent of three-dimensional (3-D) treatment planning and **conformal radiation therapy** (the delivery of higher tumor doses to selected target volumes without increased morbidity), the probability of tumor control is improved. Improved dose distribution and lower rectal and bladder volumes receiving higher doses have been reported with conformal irradiation. Fewer acute urinary and rectal sequelae have been described with 3-D treatment planning and conformal therapy.[97] The patient's age, volume treated, and dose of irradiation have been considered important factors influencing acute Grade 2 morbidity in patients treated with conformal therapy.[92]

Of patients with prostate carcinoma irradiated with 3-D conformal therapy to the prostate, seminal vesicles, and adjacent tissues, only 32% had Grade 2 or 3 acute morbidity, requiring short-term medication. In addition, only one patient has developed a severe Grade 4 late complication.[55] The 4-year actuarial clinical tumor-free survival rate was 91%. Hanks et al.[39] observed 93% normal PSA levels 12 months after treatment with conformal irradiation, in contrast to only 38% in patients treated with conventional techniques.

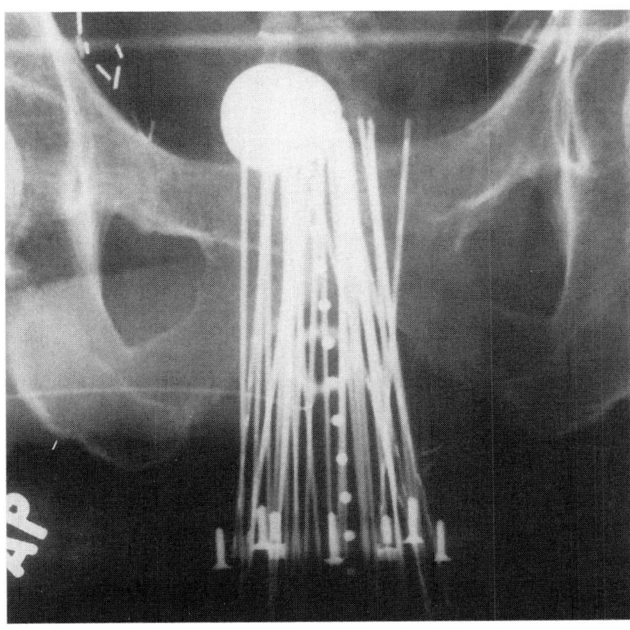

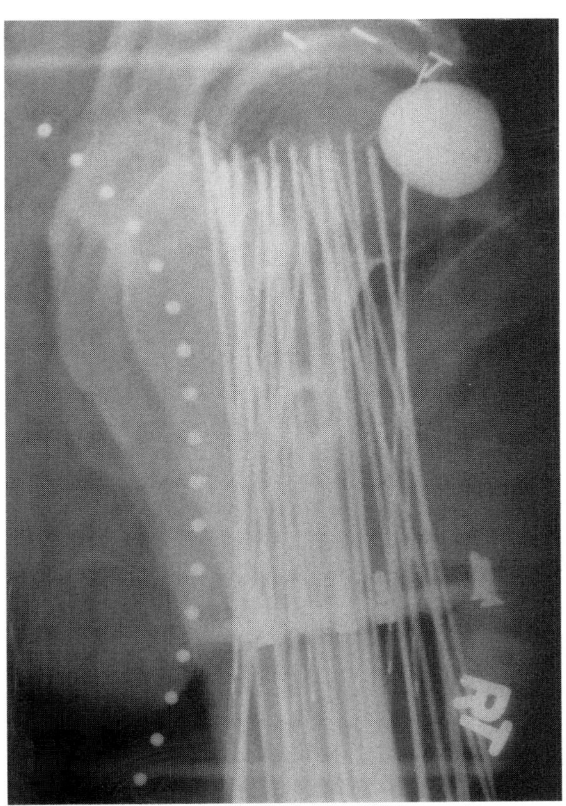

Fig. 12-9 **A** and **B,** Radiographs of the implantation of metallic guides in the prostate for the placement of Iridium 192 wires and seeds.

Interstitial brachytherapy. Whitmore, Batata, and Hilaris[108] popularized retropubic implantation of iodine 125 for clinical Stages A2 and B disease. They concluded that interstitial irradiation is probably unsuitable for patients with locally advanced tumors, those with grossly involved regional lymph nodes, those with poorly differentiated tumors, or those who have had a TURP. A limited staging lymphadenectomy is initially performed. Radioactive sources are implanted into patients who have negative nodes and selected patients who have fewer than three positive lymph nodes. An adequate seed implant delivers a minimum tumor dose of 8000 cGy, with higher doses given to the central portion of the prostate. The rectum and bladder receive 5000 to 6000 cGy.

Radioactive gold (^{198}Au) grains have been combined with external irradiation. After staging pelvic lymphadenectomy, gold grains are implanted into the prostate gland through a suprapubic incision to deliver 3000 to 3500 cGy, followed by external irradiation to the pelvis (approximately 4000 cGy). Recently, some authors have advocated permanent implants with Palladium 103 seeds. Others have described a perineal approach with afterloading techniques for the implantation of removable iridium 192 implants under fluoroscopic or ultrasound guidance[18] (Fig. 12-9).

Irradiation after prostatectomy. Sometimes patients are referred for radiation therapy after a suprapubic prostatectomy for benign hyperplasia in which carcinoma beyond Stage A1 is found incidentally in the specimen. Also, with some patients a radical retropubic prostatectomy is performed and a tumor is found at the margins of the resection, or PSA levels rise after the prostatectomy. In addition, some patients initially treated surgically develop pelvic recurrences that require radiation therapy. In these patients the treatment of smaller volumes limited to the prostate and periprostatic tissues (8 × 10 cm or 10 × 12 cm portals) is customary. Rotational techniques with 120-degree bilateral arcs (skipping of the bladder and rectum) are used to deliver doses of 6000 to 6500 cGy, depending on the tumor's extent.[69] In some patients the pelvic lymph nodes are treated to a 4500-cGy tumor dose, and a boost of 1500 to 1800 cGy is delivered to the prostatic bed with techniques similar to those described.

Results of treatment

Surgery. Survival rates after a classic radical prostatectomy are approximately 80% to 85% at 5 years, 70% at 10 years, and 50% at 15 years. The pelvic recurrence rate ranges from 5% to 15%. Long-term results from a nerve-sparing radical prostatectomy have not been published but are expected with great anticipation. Although the overall survival rate may be comparable to that with the classic operation, the local failure rate may be higher with the nerve-sparing operation because of the smaller amount of tissue removed and the number of patients with positive margins.

External irradiation. Several institutions have become quite experienced in the use of external irradiation to treat carcinoma of the prostate. The disease-free survival rates for patients with tumors localized to the prostate are about 75% to 80% at 5 years and 65% to 70% at 10 years. In patients with extracapsular extension the 5-year survival rate is 55% to 60%, and the 10-year rate is 35% to 45%.

Results obtained with external irradiation in prostatic carcinoma are summarized in Tables 12-4 and 12-5. Survival rates in Stages A2 and B patients with radical prostatectomy or external or interstitial irradiation are compared in Fig. 12-10.

Periaortic lymph node metastases result in a poor prognosis, although some patients survive for extended periods. In 23 patients with periaortic lymph node metastases treated with 5000 cGy and irradiation to the prostate and pelvic lymph nodes, the actuarial survival rates were 80% at 5 years and 60% at 10 years, and the disease-free survival rates were 65% and 52%, respectively.[54]

Postirradiation biopsies. A decreasing incidence of positive specimens has been reported with more time after the completion of radiation therapy; only about 20% of patients continue to have positive specimens after 18 to 24 months.[15] A close correlation exists between the digital examination

Table 12-4 Survival with external beam irradiation in patients with Stage T_{1b} and T_2 carcinoma of the prostate

	Number of patients			Survival (%)		
Study	**Stage A**	**Stage B**	**Stages A and B**	**5 years**	**10 years**	**15 years**
Aristizabal et al.	17			100	(100)*	
		101		82	(65)	
Asbell et al.	84			79 (66)	60 (45)	
		361				
Bagshaw et al.	308			85 (90)	65 (70)	40 (65)
		218		83 (87)	55 (65)	35 (50)
Forman et al.			113	(63)		
Hanks	116			85 (74)	63 (52)	
Hanks		415		75 (53)	46 (34)	
Hanks			60	84 (76)	54 (53)	41 (39)
Hanks	84			86	64	
Hanks		312		74 (56)	43 (27)	22 (15)
Hanks et al.	313			77 (87)	(52)	
Hanks et al.			104†	87 (96)	63 (86)	
Harisiadis et al.		25		87		
	13			88		
Kurup et al.	24			(95)		
		65			(76)	
Perez et al.	48			85 (78)	70 (60)	
		252		82 (76)	65 (56)	
Rangala et al.	10			100 (56)		
		25		90 (59)		
Rosen et al.	25			96 (84)	80 (68)	
		85		77 (68)	43 (60)	
Rounsaville et al.	37			81 (82)	67 (69)	
		50		84(71)	53 (52)	
Sagerman et al.	34			91 (77)		
		100			86 (72)	
Shipley et al.	307‡			85 (85)	66 (70)	50
van der Werf-Messing et al.		24		78 (61)	78 (61)	
Zagars et al.	32			74 (90)	68	
		82		93 (89)	70 (85)	
Zeitman		164		94 (92)	66 (70)	(52)

Modified from Perez CA: Prostate. In Perez CA, Brady LW, editors: *Principles and practice of radiation oncology,* ed 2, Philadelphia, 1992, JB Lippincott; Perez CA et al: Localized carcinoma of the prostate (stages T1B, T1C, and T3): review of management with external beam radiation therapy, *Cancer* 72:3156-3173, 1993.

*Open numbers indicate overall survival; numbers in parentheses indicate disease-free survival.

†Surgically staged patients.

‡Includes T_{2a} tumors.

and pathological findings. Lower survival rates have been described in patients with positive postirradiation biopsy specimens.[90] Positive biopsy results have been correlated with the initial stage: 10% for Stage A2, 18% for Stage B, and 21% for Stage C lesions.[50] After 10 years clinical local failure developed in 75% of patients with positive biopsy results. The disease-free survival rate was 19%, compared with 62% in patients with negative biopsy results.

Palliative irradiation. Irradiation doses of 5000 to 6000 cGy may be effective in the treatment of massive pelvic extensions of prostatic carcinoma or extensive pelvic lymph node involvement, which may produce pain or hematuria, urethral obstruction, or leg edema because of lymphatic obstruction.

Irradiation is frequently used in the treatment of distant metastases from carcinoma of the prostate. Marked symptomatic relief is noted in over 80% of patients treated with doses of 3000 to 3500 cGy in 2 to 3 weeks. Large portals that include the entire bone, such as in the extremities or pelvis, must be used. Brain metastases may be successfully treated with doses of 3000 to 3500 cGy in 2 or 3 weeks to the entire cranial contents (75% of patients have multiple lesions). Hemibody irradiation has been used for the palliation of disseminated bony metastases.

If multiple bones of the body are involved by the tumor and produce symptoms, radioactive phosphorus (^{32}P) may be administered systemically after priming with testosterone or parathormone for the palliation of pain. Strontium 89 (^{89}Sr) has been administered intravenously for diffuse bone metastases, with relief of pain occurring in 80% of patients.[76]

Yttrium 90 (^{90}Y) hypophysectomy has been used in the palliative treatment of patients with widespread, painful bony metastases.[103] About half a small group of patients had good responses, including some patients who had not responded to orchiectomy or estrogen therapy.

Side effects

Surgery. With improved anesthesia and surgical techniques, as well as the availability of antibiotics and other supportive care, operative mortality has been reduced to 1% or less. The most significant morbidity, which is related to the type of radical prostatectomy and whether a lymphadenectomy is performed, is sexual impotence. This problem was reported in over 98% of patients treated with a classic radical prostatectomy but in only 30% to 40% of patients treated with a nerve-sparing operation. The preservation of potency is related to the tumor stage, unilateral or bilateral resection of the neurovascular bundle, and patient's age.[11] Urinary incontinence has been reported in 2% to 10% of patients. A wound infection, hematoma, or pelvic abscess occurs in less than 5% of patients. If a lymphadenectomy is done, patients may develop lymphocele (5%) or penile, scrotal, or lower extremity edema (less than 5%). Thrombophlebitis and pulmonary emboli rarely occur (less than 5%).

Table 12-5 Survival with external beam irradiation in patients with Stage T_3 carcinoma of the prostate

Study	Number of patients	Survival (%) 5 years	10 years	15 years
Aristizabal et al.	82	60	—	—
Bagshaw et al.	385	68 (70)	38 (50)	20 (35)
Del Regato	372	66 (77)	38 (63)	17 (50)
Forman	125	(45)	—	—
Hanks	296	56 (38)	32 (26)	23 (17)
	228	65	—	—
Hanks	197	66 (45)	33 (14)	—
Hanks	503	70	38	—
Harisiadis et al.	112	58	35	—
Neglia	97 (C1)	72	—	—
	53 (C2)	59	—	—
Perez et al.	412	65 (58)	42 (38)	—
Rangala et al.	93	78 (69)	—	—
Rosen et al.	88	61 (53)	35 (35)	—
Rounsaville et al.	140 (C1)	63 (67)	42 (44)	
	12 (C2)	32 (0)	11 (0)	
van der Werf-Messing	247	62 (52)	61 (25)	—
Zagars et al.	551	72 (59)	47 (46)	27 (40)

Modified from Perez CA: Prostate. In Perez CA, Brady LW, editors: *Principles and practice of radiation oncology*, ed 2, Philadelphia, 1992, JB Lippincott; and Perez CA et al: Localized carcinoma of the prostate (stages T1B, T1C, and T3): review of management with external beam radiation therapy, *Cancer* 72:3156-3173, 1993.

C, Clinical stage.

*Open numbers indicate overall survival; numbers in parentheses indicate disease-free survival.

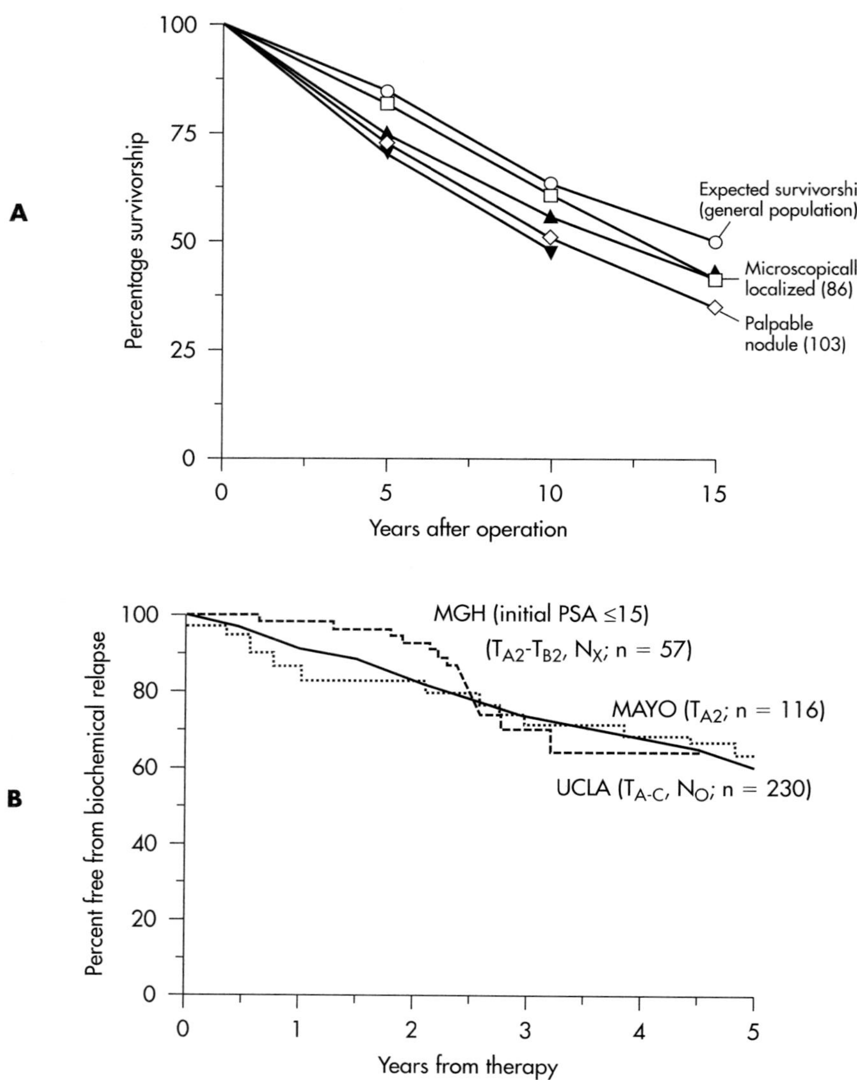

Fig. 12-10 **A,** Survival with histologically localized carcinoma of the prostate and nonlocalized disease for patients treated with surgery (Jewett) or with radiation therapy (Bagshaw, Stanford University, and Perez, Washington University). **B,** Relapse-free survival for $T_{1\text{-}2}$ patients treated with radical surgery or irradiation at Massachusetts General Hospital (Boston) the Mayo Clinic (Rochester, Minnesota), and the University of California (Los Angeles). (From Perez CA et al: Localized carcinoma of the prostate [stages T1B, T1C, and T3]: review of management with external beam radiation therapy, *Cancer* 72:3156-3173, 1993.)

Radiation therapy. Acute gastrointestinal side effects of irradiation include diarrhea, abdominal cramping, rectal discomfort, and occasionally rectal bleeding, which may be caused by transient enteroproctitis. Patients with hemorrhoids may develop discomfort earlier than other patients, and aggressive symptomatic treatment should be instituted promptly.

Severe late sequelae of treatment include persistent proctitis or proctosigmoiditis. The incidence rate of Grade 2 proctitis and rectal ulcers is 5%. A greater incidence of bowel sequelae occurs if larger volumes of the pelvis are irradiated.

In a British study of 10 men with symptomatic chronic radiation proctitis, rectal manometry showed significantly lower maximum resting anal canal pressure and physiological sphincter length than in nonirradiated controls. This indicates that dysfunction of the internal anal sphincter may contribute to anal rectal discomfort after pelvic irradiation.[107]

Genitourinary symptoms secondary to cystourethritis are dysuria, frequency, and nocturia. The urine is usually clear, although microscopic or even gross hematuria may be present. Infections of the urinary tract may occur, and therapy should be promptly instituted.

Table 12-6 Sequelae correlated with the central axis dose in carcinoma of the prostate (MIR 1967-1988)

Sequela	Dose (cGy)		
	<6000 n = 52	6500 n = 92	7000 n = 594
Rectosigmoid and small bowel			
Moderate (Grade 2)			
Proctitis	1 (2%)	5 (6%)	30 (5%)
Enteritis			8 (1%)
Rectal fibrosis and stricture			3 (0.5%)
Rectal ulcer			3 (0.5%)
Anal stricture and fissure			3 (0.5%)
Perianal abscess			1 (0.2%)
Severe (Grade 3)			
Perianal abscess			1 (0.2%)
Proctitis			1 (0.2%)
Small-bowel obstruction			3 (0.5%)
Fatal (Grade 4)			
Radiation-induced ileitis*			1 (0.2%)
Urinary			
Moderate (Grade 2)			
Urethral stricture	1 (2%)		27 (5%)
Cystitis (± hematuria)	1 (2%)	2 (2%)	11 (2%)
Urinary incontinence	1 (2%)	1 (1%)	3 (0.5%)
Ureteral stricture			1 (0.2%)
Severe (Grade 3)			
Vesicosigmoid fistula†			1 (0.2%)
Rectovaginal fistula			1 (0.2%)
Cystitis (hemorrhagic)			1 (0.2%)
Ureteral stricture			2 (0.3%)
Other			
Moderate (Grade 2)			
Subcutaneous fibrosis			2 (0.3%)
Scrotal ulcer			1 (0.2%)
Leg, scrotal, and penile edema	1 (2%)		11 (2%)
Impotence‡	2 (4%)		81 (14%)
Severe (Grade 3)			
Pubic bone necrosis	1 (2%)		
Pelvic soft tissue necrosis			1 (0.2%)

Modified from Perez CA et al: Technical factors affecting morbidity in definite irradiation for localized carcinoma of the prostate, *Int J Radiat Oncol Biol Phys* 28:811-819, 1994.
* History of aortic aneurysm and aortoiliac graft.
† Sigmoid diverticulitis.
‡ Only patients who were potent at the time of radiation therapy.

Less than 5% of patients develop chronic cystitis. Occasionally, with doses over 7500 cGy to the bladder, hemorrhagic cystitis may occur, necessitating a **cystectomy** (surgical removal of the bladder) in less than 1% of patients. Urethral stricture has been reported in approximately 4% of patients and occurs most frequently in those who had TURP before or during radiation therapy.

Erythema and dry or moist desquamation occasionally develop in the perineum or intergluteal fold. Proper skin hygiene and the topical application of Aquaphor, or lanolin should relieve these symptoms. USP zinc oxide ointment or Desitin and intensive skin care may be needed for severe cases.

Treatment sequelae in 738 patients treated at Washington University are summarized in Table 12-6. An overall complication rate of about 5% was reported in 1293 patients treated at institutions participating in the Patterns of Care Study.[38]

Sexual impotence (erectile dysfunction) has been observed in 35% to 40% of formerly potent patients treated with external irradiation but in only 15% of those treated with interstitial iodine 125.[4,72] Age may influence this difference because implants are usually performed in younger patients. In a prospective study of 100 patients treated with external irradiation, sexual potency was preserved in 73% of potent patients who admitted to more than three sexual intercourses per month and 43% of those who had intercourse less frequently.[6]

PENIS AND MALE URETHRA

Epidemiology

Carcinoma of the penis is relatively rare in the United States; the estimated incidence is 1 per 100,000 each year, accounting for 0.03% to 1% of cancers in men. This tumor is extremely rare in circumcised Jewish men; circumcision performed early in life protects against carcinoma of the penis, but this is not true if the operation is done in adult life. The higher incidence in some areas of South America, Africa, and Asia and in African-Americans seems to be related to the absence of the practice of neonatal circumcision. Phimosis (narrowing of the opening of the prepuce) is common in men suffering from penile carcinoma. **Smegma** (a white secretion that collects under the prepuce of the foreskin) is carcinogenic in animals, although the component of the smegma responsible for its carcinogenic effect has not been identified.[16]

Carcinoma of the male urethra is also rare. There are no recognized racial or geographical predisposing factors. Although the etiology remains unknown, some correlation exists between the incidence of carcinoma of the urethra and chronic irritation (infections, venereal diseases, and strictures). The average age at the time of presentation is 58 to 60 years, although 10% of these tumors occur in men younger than 40 years.

Prognostic indicators

The principal prognostic factors in carcinoma of the penis are the extent of the primary lesion and status of the lymph nodes. The incidence of nodal involvement is related to the extent and location of the primary lesion. Tumor-free regional nodes imply an excellent long-term disease-free survival rate (85% to 90%).[17] Patients with involvement of the inguinal nodes do considerably worse, and only 40% to 50% experience long-term survival. Pelvic lymph node involvement implies an even worse prognosis; less than 20% of these patients survive. Tumor differentiation is another important prognostic factor.[31]

The overall prognosis for carcinoma of the urethra in males varies considerably with the location of the primary lesion. The prognosis for distal lesions is generally similar to that for carcinoma of the penis. Lesions of the bulbomembranous urethra are usually extensive and associated with a dismal prognosis. Tumors of the prostatic urethra have prognostic features similar to those of bladder carcinoma. Superficial lesions have a good prognosis and may be managed with a transurethral resection, whereas deeply invasive tumors have a greater tendency to develop inguinal or pelvic lymph node and distant metastases.

Anatomy and lymphatics

The basic structural components of the penis include two corpora cavernosa and the corpus spongiosum (Fig. 12-11, *A*). These are encased in a dense fascia (Buck's fascia), which is separated from the skin by a layer of loose connective tissue. Distally, the corpus spongiosum expands into the glans penis, which is covered by a skin fold known as the *prepuce.*

Composed of a mucous membrane and the submucosa, the male urethra extends from the bladder neck to the external urethral meatus (Fig. 12-11, *B*). The posterior urethra is subdivided into the membranous urethra, the portion passing through the urogenital diaphragm, and the prostatic urethra, which passes through the prostate. The anterior urethra passes through the corpus spongiosum and is subdivided into fossa navicularis (a widening within the glans), the penile urethra (which passes through the pendulous part of the penis), and the bulbous urethra (the dilated proximal portion of the anterior urethra).

The lymphatic channels of the prepuce and the skin of the shaft drain into the superficial inguinal nodes located above the fascia lata. For practical purposes lymphatic drainage may be considered bilateral. Some disagreement exists regarding whether the glans and deep penile structures drain into the superficial or deep inguinal lymph nodes. The sentinel nodes (located above and medial to the junction of the epigastric and saphenous veins) are the primary drainage sites in carcinoma of the penis. The lymphatics of the fossa navicularis and penile urethra follow the lymphatics of the penis to the superficial and deep inguinal lymph nodes. The lymphatics of the bulbomembranous and prostatic urethra may follow three routes: (1) Some lymphatics pass under the pubic symphysis to the external iliac nodes, (2) some go to the obturator and internal iliac nodes, and (3) others end in the presacral lymph nodes. The pelvic (iliac) lymph nodes are rarely involved in the absence of inguinal lymph node involvement.

Clinical presentation

The presence of phimosis may obscure the primary lesion. Secondary infection and an associated foul smell are quite common, whereas urethral obstruction is unusual. Inguinal lymph nodes are palpable at the time of presentation in 30% to 45% of patients.[17,24] However, the lymph nodes contain a tumor in only half the patients; enlargement of the lymph nodes is often related to inflammatory (infectious) processes. Conversely, 20% of patients with clinically normal inguinal lymph nodes have occult metastases.

Patients with urethral carcinoma may exhibit obstructive symptoms, tenderness, dysuria, urethral discharge, and occasionally initial **hematuria** (the abnormal presence of blood in the urine). Lesions of the distal urethra are often

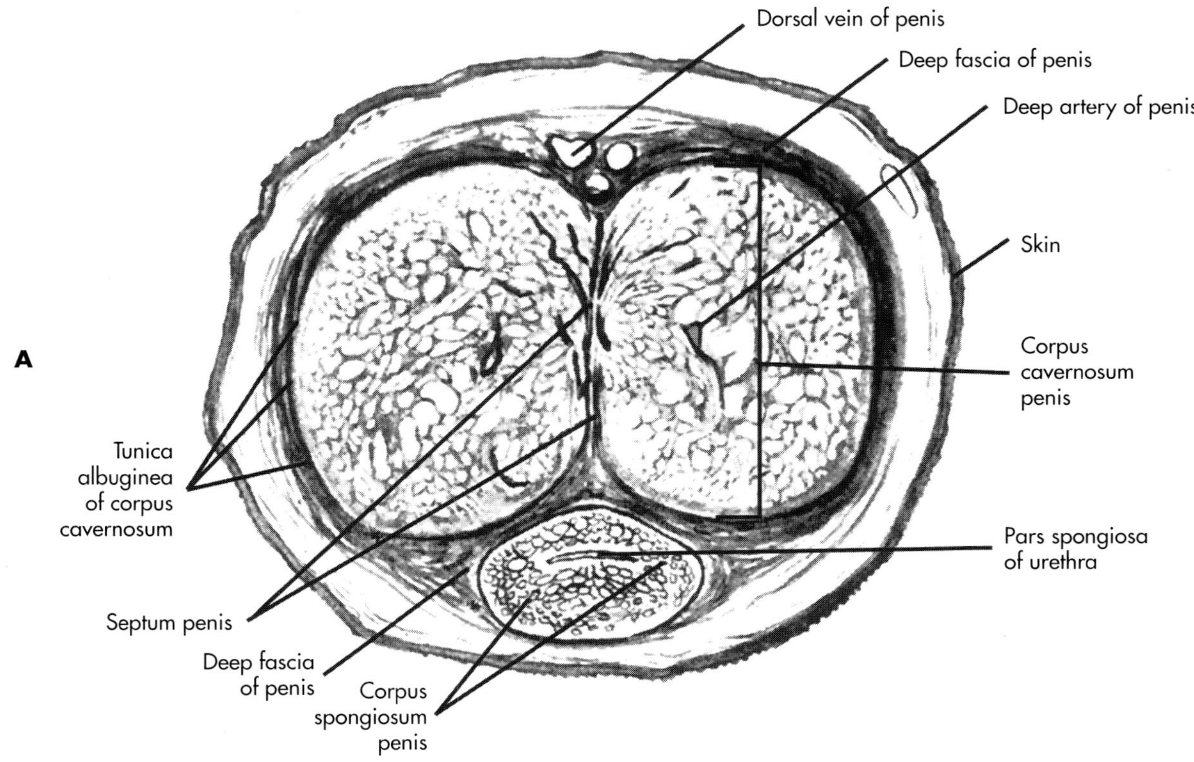

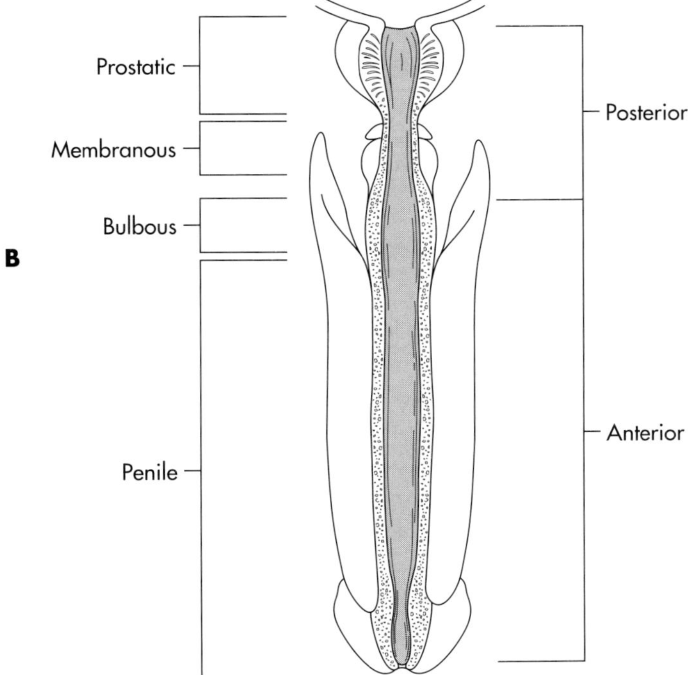

Fig. 12-11 **A,** A cross section of the penis shaft. **B,** Anatomical subdivisions of the male urethra. (**A** from Figge FHJ, editor: Sobotta/Figge: *atlas of human anatomy,* vol 2, ed 9, Baltimore, 1977, Urban & Schwarzenberg; **B** from Perez CA, Pilepich MV: Penis and male urethra. In Perez CA, Brady LW, editors: *Principles and practice of radiation oncology,* ed 2, Philadelphia, 1992, JB Lippincott.)

associated with palpable inguinal lymph nodes at the time of presentation.

Detection and diagnosis

A careful examination of the penis may reveal small lesions. A urethroscopy and cystoscopy are essential. Inguinal lymph nodes should be thoroughly evaluated. Chest radiographs and an intravenous pyelogram are routinely obtained.

Radiographic assessment of the regional lymphatics is of questionable value because of the extensive inflammatory changes often present in the lymph nodes. CT is useful in the identification of enlarged pelvic and periaortic lymph nodes in patients with involved inguinal lymph nodes.

Pathology and staging

Most malignant penile tumors are well-differentiated squamous cell carcinomas. No significant correlation between the histological grade and survival time has been found.

Bowen's disease is squamous cell carcinoma in situ that may involve the shaft of the penis and hairy skin of the inguinal and suprapubic area.

Erythroplasia of Queyrat is an epidermoid carcinoma in situ that involves the mucosal or mucocutaneous areas of the prepuce or glans. This carcinoma appears as a red, elevated, or ulcerated lesion. Some patients with erythroplasia of Queyrat have invasive squamous cell carcinoma at the time of the diagnosis.

Extramammary Paget's disease is a rare intraepithelial apocrine carcinoma. The most common sites are the scrotum, inguinal folds, and perineal region.

Primary lymphoma of the penis is extremely rare. Five cases of secondary involvement of the penis by lymphoma have been reported in the literature.[110]

Cancers metastatic to the penis are rare. The most common neoplasms metastasizing to the penis are carcinomas from the genitourinary organs, followed by carcinomas from the gastrointestinal and respiratory systems. Priapism as an initial presenting feature or later development occurs in 40% of these patients.[77]

About 80% of urethral carcinomas in males are well- or moderately differentiated squamous cell carcinomas.[64] Others include transitional cell carcinomas (15%), adenocarcinomas (5%), and undifferentiated or mixed carcinomas (1%). Over 90% of carcinomas of the prostatic urethra are of the transitional cell type. Adenocarcinomas occur only in the bulbomembranous urethra.

The AJCC staging systems for carcinoma of the penis and male urethra are shown in the boxes below.[7]

Routes of spread

Most carcinomas of the penis start in the preputial area, arising in the glans, the coronal sulcus, or the prepuce itself. Extensive primary lesions may involve the corpora cavernosa or even the abdominal wall. The inguinal lymph nodes are the most common site of metastatic spread. About 20% of patients with clinically nonpalpable inguinal nodes have micrometastases. Pathological evidence of nodal metastases is reported in about 35% of all patients and in approximately 50% of those with palpable lymph nodes.[17,24] Distant metastases are uncommon (about 10%), even in patients with advanced locoregional disease. They usually occur in patients who have inguinal lymph node involvement.[45]

The natural history of carcinoma of the male anterior urethra is similar to that of carcinoma of the penis. Most tumors are low grade and progress slowly at primary and regional sites rather than spread to distal areas. Tumors of the penile urethra spread to the inguinal lymph nodes, and tumors of the bulbomembranous and prostatic urethra metastasize first to the pelvic lymph nodes.[71]

American Joint Committee on Cancer Staging System for Carcinoma of the Penis

Primary tumor (T)

TX	Primary tumor cannot be assessed
T_0	No evidence of primary tumor
Tis	Carcinoma in situ
T_a	Noninvasive verrucous carcinoma
T_1	Tumor invasion of subepithelial connective tissue
T_2	Tumor invasion of corpus spongiosum or cavernosum
T_3	Tumor invasion of urethra or prostate
T_4	Tumor invasion of other adjacent structures

Regional lymph nodes (N)

NX	Regional lymph nodes cannot be assessed
N_0	No regional lymph node metastasis
N_1	Metastasis in a single superficial inguinal lymph node
N_2	Metastasis in multiple or bilateral superficial inguinal lymph nodes
N_3	Metastasis in deep inguinal or pelvic lymph node(s) (unilateral or bilateral)

Distant metastasis (M)

MX	Distant metastasis cannot be assessed
M_0	No distant metastasis
M_1	Distant metastasis

Modified from Beahrs OH et al, editors: *AJCC manual for staging of cancer,* ed 4, Philadelphia, 1992, JB Lippincott.

American Joint Committee on Cancer Staging System for Carcinoma of the Urethra

Primary tumor (T) (male and female)

TX	Primary tumor cannot be assessed
T_0	No evidence of primary tumor
Tis	Carcinoma in situ
Ta	Noninvasive papillary, polypoid, or verrucous carcinoma
T_1	Tumor invasion of subepithelial connective tissue
T_2	Tumor invasion of corpus spongiosum, prostate, or periurethral muscle
T_3	Tumor invasion of corpus cavernosum or beyond the prostatic capsule, anterior vagina, or bladder neck
T_4	Tumor invasion of other adjacent organs

Regional lymph nodes (N)

NX	Regional lymph nodes cannot be assessed
N_0	No regional lymph node metastasis
N_1	Metastasis in a single lymph node (2 cm or less in greatest dimension)
N_2	Metastasis in a single lymph node (more than 2 cm but not more than 5 cm in greatest dimension) or multiple lymph nodes (none more than 5 cm in greatest dimension)
N_3	Metastasis in a lymph node (more than 5 cm in greatest dimension)

Distant metastasis (M)

MX	Distant metastasis cannot be assessed
M_0	No distant metastasis
M_1	Distant metastasis

Modified from Beahrs OH et al editors: *AJCC manual for staging of cancer,* ed 4, Philadelphia,1992, JB Lippincott.

Treatment techniques

Carcinoma of the penis. Therapy is usually performed in two phases: initial management of the primary tumor and later treatment of the regional lymphatics. Surgery for the primary tumor ranges from local excision or chemosurgery in a small group of highly selected patients (particularly those with small lesions of the prepuce) to a partial or total penectomy. Although surgical resection is usually a highly effective and expedient treatment modality, it may not be acceptable to sexually active patients.

Bowen's disease and erythroplasia of Queyrat can be treated with topical 5-FU (5% cream), a local excision, or superficial x-rays (4500 to 5000 cGy in 4 to 5 weeks). The principal advantage of radiotherapeutic management of the primary lesion in penile carcinoma is organ preservation. Many different techniques, doses, and fractionation schemes have been used.[24,45] Interstitial implants, molds, and contact orthovoltage and megavoltage irradiation have improved tumor control in some modern series and decreased the incidence of treatment-related sequelae. Most patients who experience local failure after radiation therapy can be salvaged surgically.

Nodal management by observation with delayed intervention when signs of nodal involvement appear has replaced elective nodal dissection for the following reasons: (1) the 1% to 3% surgical mortality rate, (2) the morbidity associated with lymphadenectomy, and (3) the relatively low incidence of metastatic disease (10% to 20%) in patients with clinically normal lymph nodes. Survival rates are high with this treatment.[89] Patients with clinically negative lymph nodes who are at risk for microscopic nodal metastases because of a primary tumor above Stage I or a less than well-differentiated histology can receive elective irradiation to the inguinal lymph nodes (5000 cGy at 3 cm in 5 weeks) with a high probability of tumor control and low morbidity. Generally, involved and resectable regional lymph nodes are managed by radical lymphadenectomy. Some patients can be treated with combined irradiation and lymphadenectomy, and if necessary, pelvic lymph node dissection.

Carcinoma of the male urethra. Noninvasive carcinoma of the proximal urethra can be treated with a transurethral resection. For lesions of the distal urethra, results with penectomy or radiation therapy are similar to those for carcinoma of the penis, and the 5-year survival rates are comparable (50% to 60%).[80] Involved regional lymph nodes are treated with lymphadenectomy. Most patients, however, exhibit advanced invasive lesions, which are difficult to manage with radical surgery or radiation therapy.

Radiation therapy techniques. If indicated, circumcision must be performed before the start of radiation therapy to minimize radiation therapy-associated morbidity.

External irradiation. External beam therapy requires specially designed accessories (including bolus) to achieve homogeneous dose distribution to the entire organ involved. One device consists of a plastic box with a central circular opening that can be fitted over the penis. The space between the skin and box must be filled with tissue-equivalent material (Fig. 12-12). This box can be treated with parallel-opposed megavoltage beams. An ingenious alternative to the box technique is the use of a water-filled container to envelop the penis while the patient is in a prone position.

A more complex device consists of a Perspex tube attached to a baseplate resting on the skin. This device is placed as close as possible to the base of the penis, and a flexible tube is connected to a vacuum pump. The suction effect keeps the penis in a fixed position during treatment. Appropriate bolus is placed outside the tube. The patient can also be treated in the prone position, with the penis hanging through a small hole placed in the Perspex's cylinder.

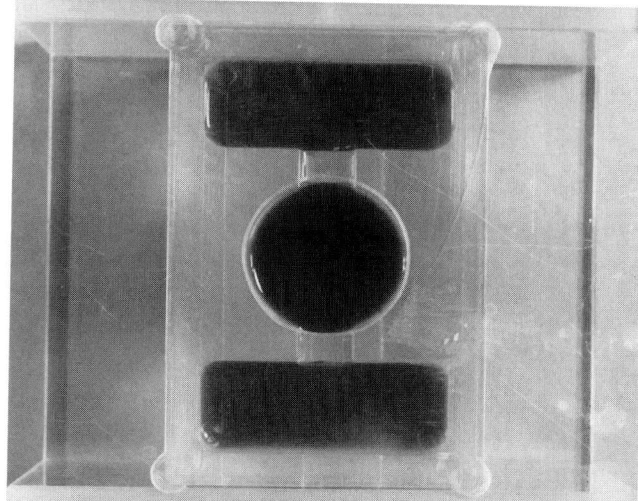

A

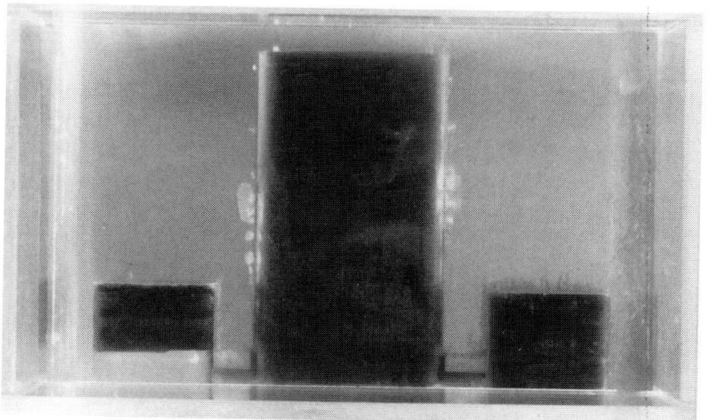

B

Fig. 12-12 **A,** A view from above of a plastic box with a central cylinder for external irradiation of the penis. The patient is treated in the prone position. The penis is placed in the central cylinder, and water is used to fill the surrounding volume in the box. The depth dose is calculated at the central point of the box. **B,** A lateral view. (From Perez CA, Pilepich MV: Penis and male urethra. In Perez CA, Brady LW, editors: *Principles and practice of radiation oncology*, ed 2, Philadelphia, 1992, JB Lippincott.)

A well-established association exists between large fraction size and late tissue damage. The daily fraction in most reported series is 250 to 350 cGy for a total dose of 5000 to 5500 cGy, although a smaller daily fraction size (180 to 200 cGy) and a higher total dose are preferable. A total dose of 6500 to 7000 cGy, with the last 500 to 1000 cGy delivered to a reduced portal, should result in a reduced incidence of late fibrosis.

Regional lymphatics can be treated with external beam megavoltage irradiation. The fields should include bilateral inguinal *and* pelvic (external iliac and hypogastric) lymph nodes (Fig. 12-13). The posterior pelvis may be partially spared by anterior loading of the beams. Depending on the extent of nodal disease and proximity of the detectable tumor to the skin surface or presence of skin invasion, the application of a bolus to the inguinal area should be considered. If clinical and radiographic evaluations show no gross enlargement of the pelvic lymph nodes, the dose to these nodes may be limited to 5000 cGy. In patients with palpable lymph nodes, the doses of 6500 to 7000 cGy in 7 to 8 weeks (180 to 200 cGy per day) with reduced fields after 5000 cGy are advised.

Brachytherapy. A mold is usually built in the form of a box or cylinder with a central opening and channels for the placement of radioactive sources (needles or wires) in the periphery of the device. The cylinder and sources should be long enough to prevent underdosage at the tip of the penis. A dose of 6000 to 6500 cGy at the surface and approximately 5000 cGy at the center of the organ is delivered in 6 to 7 days. The mold can be applied continuously, in which case an indwelling catheter should be in place, or intermittently. Single- or double-plane implants can also be used to deliver 6000 to 7000 cGy in 5 to 7 days. In extensive lesions involving the shaft of the penis (Stage III), obtaining an adequate margin with brachytherapy procedures is difficult, similar to the situation seen in attempting a partial penectomy.

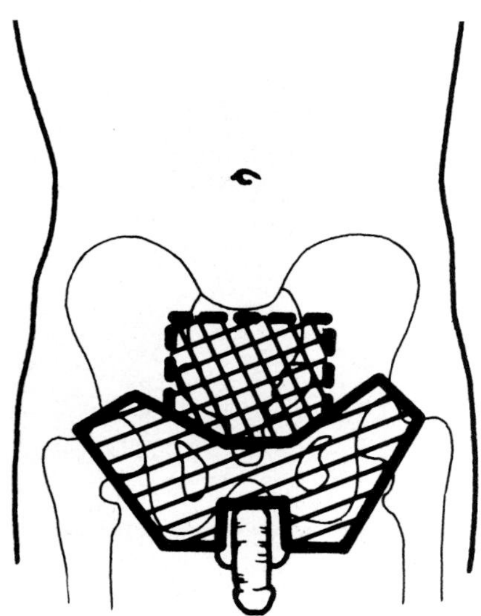

Fig. 12-13 Portals encompassing the inguinal and pelvic lymph nodes. (From Perez CA, Pilepich MV: Penis and male urethra. In Perez CA, Brady LW, editors: *Principles and practice of radiation oncology,* ed 2, Philadelphia, 1992, Lippincott.)

Results of treatment

Carcinoma of the penis. Reports of treatment results are scarce because cancer of the penis is uncommon in the western world. A significant proportion of patients have been treated surgically, with 5-year rates ranging from 25% to 80%, depending on the stage of the primary tumor and inguinal lymph node involvement.

A summary of tumor control rates achieved with irradiation is presented in Table 12-7. In patients 41 to 57 years old treated with various irradiation techniques (mold, interstitial, and external x-ray) 5-year survival rates range from 45% to 68%. A 5-year survival rate of 66% and tumor control rate of 86% have been reported in patients with Stage I carcinoma of the penis treated with irradiation, compared with a 5-year survival rate of 70% and tumor control rate of 81% in surgically treated patients.[49] Survival and local control rates were only slightly affected by the treatment modality in Stage II but were lower in Stage III patients treated surgically. If irradiation did not control the primary lesion after 6 months, the penis was amputated and a significant number of patients were salvaged. Of patients initially treated surgically and initially treated with irradiation, 8% and 20% (respectively) developed inguinal lymph node metastases. Overall, 8% of patients treated surgically and 10% of those irradiated died of inguinal lymph node metastases and tumor spread.

In one study 80% of patients treated with radiation therapy had tumor control and conservation of the penis.[37] Although irradiation alone or combined with a lymph node dissection controlled lymph node metastases smaller than 2 cm in four patients, radiation therapy was successful in controlling lymph node metastases in only one of seven patients who had N_2 or N_3 disease.

Duncan and Jackson[20] observed 3-year tumor-control rates of 90% with external beam irradiation and only 47% with mold therapy. Other authors have reported a 5-year survival rate of 92% in patients with Stages I and II tumors treated with radium 226 or iridium 192 molds, compared with 77% in patients treated with partial penectomy.[89]

Table 12-8 shows a summary of treatment results correlated with the tumor stage, preservation of the organ, and morbidity.

Carcinoma of the male urethra. Most patients with male urethral carcinoma are treated surgically. In 11 patients with tumors at or anterior to the penoscrotal junction, 3 of 4 patients treated with total penectomy and perineal urethrostomy had tumor control.[9] Partial penectomy controlled the local tumor in two patients. Two patients were treated with radiation therapy and a third with a combination of preoperative irradiation (4500 cGy) and total penectomy. In four

Table 12-7 Overall control of primary carcinoma of the penis with radiation therapy

Author	Number of Patients	Treatment method	Dose	Local control (%)
Almgard and Edsmyr	16	Radium implant and external beam therapy		
Engelstad	72	Mold therapy and teleradium	3500-3700 R (500-700 R/day)	50
Jackson	39	Mold (most patients) and external beam therapy (some patients)	?	49
Marcial et al.	25	External beam, interstitial, and mold therapy	4000 R in 2 weeks 5000 R in 4 weeks	
		Mold	5000-6000 R in 5-6 days	64
Murrell and Williams	108	External beam therapy	3000-6700 cGy (200 cGy/day)	52
Kelley et al.	10	External beam therapy (electrons)	5100-5400 cGy (300 cGy/day)	100
Knudson and Brennhovd	145	Mold therapy	3500-3700 cGy in 3-5 days	32
Haile and Delclos	20	Mold therapy, implant, and External beam therapy	? 6000 cGy	90
Mazeron et al.	23	Iridium 192 implant	6000-7000 cGy	78
Pointon	32	External beam therapy	5250-5500 cGy (16 Fx in 22 days)	84.4
Sagerman et al.	15	External beam therapy	4500 cGy (15 Fx in 3 weeks) to 6400 cGy (32 Fx in 6.5 weeks)	60
Salaverria et al.	41	Iridium mold therapy	6000 cGy over several days	84.3

Modified from Perez CA, Pilepich MV: Penis and male urethra. In Perez CA, Brady LW, editors: *Principles and practice of radiation oncology,* ed 2, Philadelphia, 1992, JB Lippincott.
R, Roentgen; *Fx,* fractions.

Table 12-8 Results of radiation therapy for carcinoma of the penis

Author	Modality	Tumor Control: Stages I - II	Tumor Control: Stages III - IV	Complications	Penis preservation
Duncan and Jackson	Teletherapy	16/20 (80%)		2/20 (10%)	16/20 (80%)
Jackson	Mold therapy	20/45 (44%)		2/45 (4%)	20/45 (44%)
Haile and Delclos	External beam therapy	6/6 (100%)	2/2 (100%)	16/20 (80%)	
	Brachytherapy	7/7 (100%)			
Kaushal and Harma	Cobalt 60	14/16 (88%)		2/16 (12%)	13/14 (93%)
Kelley et al.	Electron beam	10/10 (100%)			10/10 (100%)
Pierquin et al.	Iridium implant	14/14 (100%)	12/31 (39%)	3/45 (6.7%)	
Sagerman et al.	External beam therapy	9/12 (75%)	1/3 (33%)		2/15 (13%)
Salaverria et al.	Mold brachytherapy	12/13 (92%)			10/13 (77%)

Perez CA, Pilepich MV: Penis and male urethra. In Perez CA, Brady LW, editors: *Principles and practice of radiation oncology,* ed 2, Philadelphia, 1992, JB Lippincott.

patients with inguinal lymph node metastases the regional disease was controlled with bilateral lymphadenectomy. All six patients in whom local and regional tumors were controlled were alive and disease free 1 to 20 years later. Urethral tumors arose posterior to the penoscrotal junction in 16 patients. A penectomy was performed in five of those patients, all of whom had tumor control and no evidence of recurrence 5 to 29 months after therapy. Two patients treated with a local excision died of disease within 18 months after surgery. Irradiation was used in three patients unsuccessfully, and all died of cancer 13 to 31 months after therapy.

Chemotherapy. The use of chemotherapy for carcinoma of the penis is quite limited. Occasional tumor regression has been described with some antineoplastic agents, such as bleomycin, 5-FU, and methotrexate. For some patients chemotherapy has been combined with irradiation or surgery, making an assessment of the response more difficult. A response to cisplatin has been reported in a few patients.[323]

Side effects. Irradiation of the penis produces brisk erythema, dry or moist desquamation, and swelling of the subcutaneous tissue of the shaft in almost all patients. Although they are quite uncomfortable, these reversible reactions subside within a few weeks with conservative treatment. Telangiectasia and some fibrosis are usually asymptomatic, common, late consequences of radiation therapy.

Most strictures after radiation therapy are at the meatus. Meatal-urethral strictures occur with a frequency of up to 40%.[24,59] This incidence rate compares favorably with that of urethral strictures after penectomy.

Ulceration, necrosis of the glans, and necrosis of the skin of the shaft are rare complications. Lymphedema of the legs has occurred after inguinal and pelvic radiation therapy, but the role of irradiation in the development of this complication remains controversial. Many patients with this symptom have active disease in the lymphatics that may be responsible for lymphatic blockage.

URINARY BLADDER

Epidemiology

Approximately 51,200 new cases and about 10,600 deaths from bladder cancer are reported in the United States each year.[2] The incidence peaks in the seventh decade, and in men this cancer is the fourth most prevalent malignant disease. It occurs about three times more often in men than in women.

Prognostic indicators

The tumor extent (stage) and depth of muscle invasion are important factors affecting the tumor's behavior and outcome of therapy. Tumor morphology is also important because papillary tumors are usually low grade and superficial with a favorable prognosis. Infiltrating lesions tend to be higher grade, sessile, and nodular; they invade muscle, vascular, and lymphatic spaces and generally have a worse prognosis. The degree of histological differentiation must also be considered because well-differentiated tumors are less aggressive and have a better prognosis than poorly differentiated tumors, which are usually more invasive.

Anatomy and lymphatics

The urinary bladder, when empty, lies entirely within the true pelvis. The empty bladder is roughly tetrahedral; each of its four surfaces is shaped like an equilateral triangle. The base of the superior surface (the only surface covered with the peritoneum) is behind, and the apex is in front. The apex of the bladder is directed toward the upper part of the pubic symphysis and is joined to the umbilicus by the middle umbilical ligament, the urachal remnant. The sigmoid colon and coils of the small intestine rest on the superior surface.

In the male the rectovesical pouch separates the upper part of the bladder base from the rectum. The seminal vesicles and deferent duct separate the lower part of the base from the rectum.

The parietal peritoneum of the suprapubic region of the abdominal wall is displaced so that the bladder lies directly against the anterior abdominal wall without any intervening peritoneum.

The ureters pierce the wall of the bladder base obliquely. During contraction of the muscular bladder wall the ureters are compressed, preventing reflux. The orifices of the ureters are posterolateral to the internal urethral orifice, and with the urethral orifice they define the **trigone** (the triangular portion of the bladder formed by the openings of the ureters and urethra orifice). The sides of the trigone are approximately 2.5 cm in length in the contracted state and up to 5 cm in the distended state (Fig. 12-14). In the male the bladder neck rests on the prostate.

The epithelium, or urothelium, is transitional. The mucous membrane is only loosely attached to the subjacent (detrusor) muscle layer by a delicate vascular submucosa (lamina propria), except over the trigone, where the mucosa is firmly attached.

The lymphatics of the bladder form two plexuses, one in the submucosa and one in the muscular layer. They accompany the blood vessels into the perivesical space and ultimately terminate in the internal iliac lymph nodes. Some lymphatics may find their way into the external iliac lymph nodes. From the pelvic lymph nodes the lymphatics progress to the common iliac and periaortic lymph nodes.

Clinical presentation

Most patients with bladder cancer (75% to 80%) have gross, painless, total (throughout urination) hematuria. Clotting and urinary retention may occur. Approximately 25% of patients have symptoms of vesical irritability, although almost all patients with carcinoma in situ experience frequency, urgency, dysuria, and hematuria.

Detection and diagnosis

In addition to a complete history and physical examination (including rectal and pelvic), each patient should have a chest x-ray examination, urinalysis, complete blood cell count, liver function test, cystoscopic evaluation, and bimanual examination performed under anesthesia before and after endoscopic surgery (biopsy or transurethral resection). An intravenous pyelogram should be obtained before a cystoscopy is done so that the upper tracts can be evaluated (by a retrograde pyelogram, with a cytology, brush biopsy, or ureteroscopy at the time of cystoscopy if indicated). CT or MRI is used to evaluate bladder-wall thickening and detect extravesical extension and lymph node metastases. Bone scans are obtained for patients with T_3 and T_4 disease and those with bone pain.

Pathology and staging

Most bladder cancers (98%) are epithelial in origin. In the western hemisphere approximately 92% of epithelial tumors

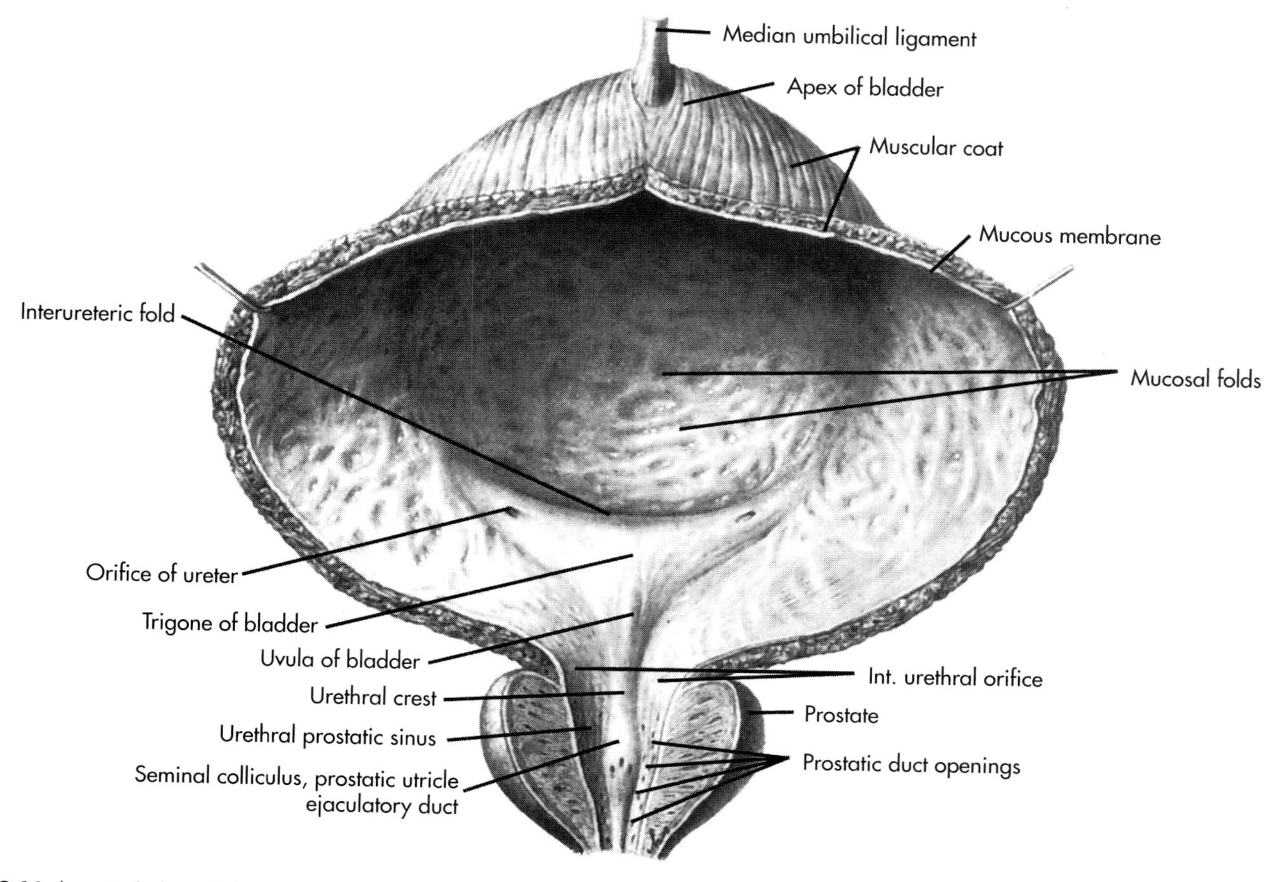

Fig. 12-14 A ventral view of the urinary bladder and prostate, illustrating the location of the trigone of the bladder. (From Figge FHJ, editor: *Sobotta/Figge: atlas of human anatomy*, vol 2, ed 9, Baltimore, 1977, Urban & Schwarzenberg.)

are transitional cell carcinomas, 6% to 7% are squamous cell carcinomas, and 1% to 2% are adenocarcinomas. Squamous or glandular differentiation can be seen in 20% to 30% of transitional cell carcinomas. Patients whose bladders are chronically irritated by long-term catheter drainage (e.g., paraplegics) or bladder calculi are at risk of developing squamous cell carcinoma.

Morphologically, bladder cancers can be separated into the following four categories: (1) papillary; (2) papillary infiltrating; (3) solid infiltrating; and (4) nonpapillary, noninfiltrating, or carcinoma in situ. At the time of diagnosis, 70% of these cancers are papillary, 25% show papillary or solid infiltration, and 3% to 5% indicate carcinoma in situ.

Two clinical staging systems, the Marshall modification of the Jewett-Strong system and the AJCC staging system, are widely used (see the box on p. 268).[7] Both systems combine histological (from transurethral resection specimens) and clinical (from bimanual examination under anesthesia) findings. Pathological staging is based on histological findings from cystectomy specimens. In the AJCC system these stages are preceded by the prefix *p* (e.g., pT_3).

The presence of muscle invasion categorizes the lesion as Stage B1, B2, C, D1, or D2 (T_2 to T_{4b}). Although a bimanual examination with the patient under anesthesia and radiography are helpful in further separating the various stages, understaging is common. Overstaging is infrequent.

Routes of spread

Bladder cancer spreads by direct extension into or through the wall of the bladder. In a small proportion of cases the tumor spreads submucosally under intact, normal-appearing mucosa. Intraepithelial involvement of the distal ureters, prostatic urethra, and periurethral prostatic ducts is frequently found with multifocal or diffuse carcinoma in situ. Approximately 75% to 85% of new bladder cancers are superficial (Tis, T_a, or T_1), and about 15% to 25% have evidence of muscle invasion at the time of the diagnosis. Other patients with superficial disease develop muscle invasion when tumors recur after conservative therapy. Of all patients with muscle-invasive bladder cancer, approximately 60% have evidence of muscle invasion at the time of the initial diagnosis, and the remaining 40% initially exhibit more

Comparison of the Marshall and American Joint Committee on Cancer Staging Systems for Bladder Cancer

	Marshall modification of Jewett-Strong classification	AJCC classification
Tumor extent		
Confined to mucosa	O	
Nonpapillary, noninvasive		Tis
Papillary, noninvasive		T_a
Not beyond lamina propria (no mass palpable after complete TUR)	A	T_1
Invasion of superficial muscle (no induration present after complete TUR)	B1	T_2
Invasion of deep muscle (induration present after complete TUR)	B2	T_{3a}
Invasion into perivesical fat (mobile mass present after TUR)	C	T_{3b}
Invasion of neighboring structures; muscle invasion present		
Substance of prostate, vagina, and uterus	D1*	T_{4a}
Pelvic sidewall fixation or invading abdominal wall	D1*	T_{4b}

AJCC staging system for regional lymph nodes (N)†

NX	Regional lymph nodes cannot be assessed
N_0	No regional lymph node metastasis
N_1	Metastasis in a single lymph node (2 cm or less in greatest dimension)
N_2	Metastasis in a single lymph node (more than 2 cm but not more than 5 cm in greatest dimension) or multiple lymph nodes, (none more than 5 cm in greatest dimension)
N_3	Metastasis in a lymph node (more than 5 cm in greatest dimension)

AJCC staging system for distant metastases (M)

MX	Distant metastasis cannot be assessed
M_0	No distant metastasis
M_1	Distant metastasis

Modified from Parsons JT, Million RR: Bladder. In Perez CA, Brady LW, editors: *Principles and practice of radiation oncology,* ed 2, Philadelphia, 1992, JB Lippincott; and Beahrs OH et al, editors: *AJCC manual for staging of cancer,* ed 4, Philadelphia, 1992, JB Lippincott.
*In the Marshall modification of the Jewett-Strong staging system, D1 disease may involve lymph nodes below the sacral promontory (bifurcation of the common iliac artery). D2 disease implies distant metastases or more extensive lymph node metastases.
†Regional lymph nodes are those within the true pelvis; all others are distant nodes.
TUR, Transurethral resection; *AJCC,* American Joint Committee on Cancer.

superficial disease that later progresses. Perineural invasion and lymphatic or blood vessel invasion are common after the tumor has invaded muscle.

Lymphatic drainage occurs via the external iliac, internal iliac, and presacral lymph nodes. Published data correlate the incidence of pelvic lymph node metastases with the depth of tumor invasion in the bladder wall (Table 12-9).[96] The most common sites of distant metastasis are the lung, bone, and liver.

Treatment techniques

For carcinoma in situ a radical cystectomy is usually curative. However, most patients and urologists prefer more conservative initial management. For lesions that are smaller than 5 cm, reasonably well delineated, and without involvement of the bladder neck, prostatic urethra, or ureters, treatment consists of electrofulguration followed by intravesical chemotherapy or Calmette-Guérin bacillus (BCG).

T_a and T_1 disease is usually treated with a transurethral resection and fulguration. Patients with diffuse Grade 3, T_1 disease or involvement of the prostatic urethra or ducts are difficult to treat locally and are sometimes initially treated with a cystectomy.

Intravesical chemotherapy is often administered after a transurethral resection for T_1, Grade 2 or 3 lesions. Most physicians withhold intravesical treatment for patients with T_1, Grade 1 tumors. Some commonly used agents are thiotepa, mitomycin, doxorubicin, and BCG. Patients require a close follow-up with cystoscopy, cytology, and resection as indicated.

Definitive treatment with transurethral resection is not applicable to most patients with muscle-invasive disease. Failure to completely eradicate high-grade disease, progression to muscle invasion, or involvement of the prostatic urethra or prostatic periurethral ducts usually signals the need for radical cystectomy.

Table 12-9 Incidence of histologically positive lymph nodes correlated with pathological stage in bladder cancer

Pathological stage	Number of Patients	Positive Lymph Nodes (%)
pT_1	41	5
pT_2	20	30
pT_{3a}	13	31
pT_{3b}	28	64
pT_4	8	50

Modified from Skinner DG, Tift JP, Kaufman JJ: High dose, short course preoperative radiation therapy and immediate single stage radical cystectomy with pelvic node dissection in the management of bladder cancer, *J Urol* 127:671-674, 1982.

Partial cystectomy. Carefully chosen patients with solitary, well-defined lesions, muscle-invasive disease, or superficial disease not suitable for transurethral resection may be treated by segmental resection (partial cystectomy). Many patients who are disease free 5 years after partial cystectomy owe their survival to salvage treatment with total cystectomy, irradiation, or transurethral resection. In the Stanford series, radical cystectomy was the most successful salvage treatment.[26]

Circumferential submucosal tumor extensions and lymphatic vessels in the muscularis deep to adjacent normal mucosa and the fact that most recurrences occur at the margins of resection rather than elsewhere in the bladder justify the use of preoperative irradiation or an interstitial implant adjacent to the bladder suture line at the time of segmental resection. Preoperative irradiation does not adversely affect bladder capacity.

Radical cystectomy with or without preoperative irradiation. Radical cystectomy without preoperative irradiation is recommended for superficial disease (Tis, T_a, T_1) in which all attempts at conservative management have proved unsuccessful. Patients are included whose recurrences after each successive transurethral resection and/or intravesical chemotherapy treatment increase in frequency or grade or progress to muscle invasion. Cystectomy is also indicated for patients with recurrent tumors in whom bladder capacity has been so reduced by repeated transurethral resections and intravesical chemotherapy treatments that the successful eradication of the tumor by conservative means (repeat fulguration or irradiation) would still produce an unsatisfactory functional result.

For clinical Stage T_2 disease, radical cystectomy with or without preoperative irradiation is commonly used. Preoperative irradiation is recommended for large tumors ($\geq$4 cm) or high-grade lesions because the risk of understaging is high.[60] In the University of Iowa series, patients with stage B cancers measuring greater than 3 cm experienced a 5-year survival rate of 50% when they were treated with preoperative irradiation and cystectomy, versus 16% after radical cystectomy alone.[41]

For T_3 and resectable T_{4a} disease there are clear indications for the use of preoperative irradiation before radical cystectomy.[66] Doses of 2000 cGy (five fractions of 400 cGy) to 4000 to 4500 cGy (180 to 200 cGy daily fractions) have been used with comparable pelvic tumor control and survival rates.

Full-dose external beam irradiation with surgery reserved for salvage. Patients treated with radical irradiation ideally should have adequate bladder capacity without substantial voiding symptoms or incontinence. The completeness of transurethral resection before irradiation significantly influenced local control in some studies but not in others.[95,106]

After irradiation, patients undergo a cystoscopy every 3 months for 2 years and every 6 months thereafter. Some persistent or recurrent lesions (particularly low-grade tumors) that were downstaged with radiation therapy have been successfully managed with endoscopic resection. If a local tumor persists 3 months after resection, a cystectomy is indicated.[79]

Neoadjuvant chemotherapy plus irradiation. Because of the high rate of local recurrence after irradiation alone, several investigators have administered chemotherapy concurrently with irradiation in an attempt to sensitize the tumor to the effects of irradiation.[86] Because of toxicity and the lack of proven benefit, neoadjuvant MVAC (methotrexate, vincristine, Adriamycin, and cyclophosphamide) and CMV (cyclophosphamide, methotrexate, and vincristine) should be used only in clinical trials.

Interstitial implants. Interstitial treatment may be used alone, with low- or moderate-dose external beam irradiation, or to treat the suture line in patients undergoing partial cystectomy. Suitable patients are those with solitary T_1 to T_{3a} lesions measuring less than 5 cm whose general medical condition permits suprapubic cystotomy.

Radiation therapy

Initial target volume. Portals should include the total bladder and tumor volume, prostate and prostatic urethra, and pelvic lymph nodes. Fields extend 1 cm inferiorly to the caudal border of the obturator foramen and superiorly to just below the sacral promontory or just below the S1-L5 disk interspace on the AP projection. These fields include the perivesical, obturator, external iliac, and internal iliac lymph nodes but clearly not the common iliac lymph nodes. The anterior and posterior fields should be shaped with inferior corner blocks (usually 3 to 4 cm on a side), which should shield the medial border of the femoral heads when possible. The field widths should extend 1.5 cm laterally to the bony margin of the pelvis at its widest point. The irradiation portals should be at least 12 × 12 cm to include the empty bladder.[25] The anterior boundary of the lateral fields should be 1 cm anterior to the most anterior portion of the bladder mucosa seen on an air contrast cystogram or 1 cm anterior to the anterior tip of the symphysis, whichever is more anterior. Posteriorly, the fields should extend at least 2.5 cm posterior to the most posterior portion of the bladder or 2.5 cm posterior to the tumor mass if it is palpable or present on a pelvic CT scan. The posterior border is usually at or posterior to the S1-2 junction on the anterior surface. The heights of such lateral fields are usually 13 to 14 cm at the isocenter. The lateral fields should be shaped with corner blocks inferiorly to shield the tissues outside the symphysis and block the entire anal canal (Fig. 12-15).

Boost target volume. The contour of the primary bladder tumor volume is obtained from findings gathered via a bimanual examination and other diagnostic radiographic or surgical information. If the radiation oncologist is satisfied that all initial sites of the tumor are limited to one section of the bladder (usually in the trigone or posteriorly), the high-dose volume should exclude the uninvolved areas of the bladder (Fig.12-15). This can be done with 120-degree bilateral arcs or a 270- to 360-degree rotation for linear accelerators of lower beam energy (6 MV). The same rotation techniques or two or four parallel-opposed fixed isocentric field

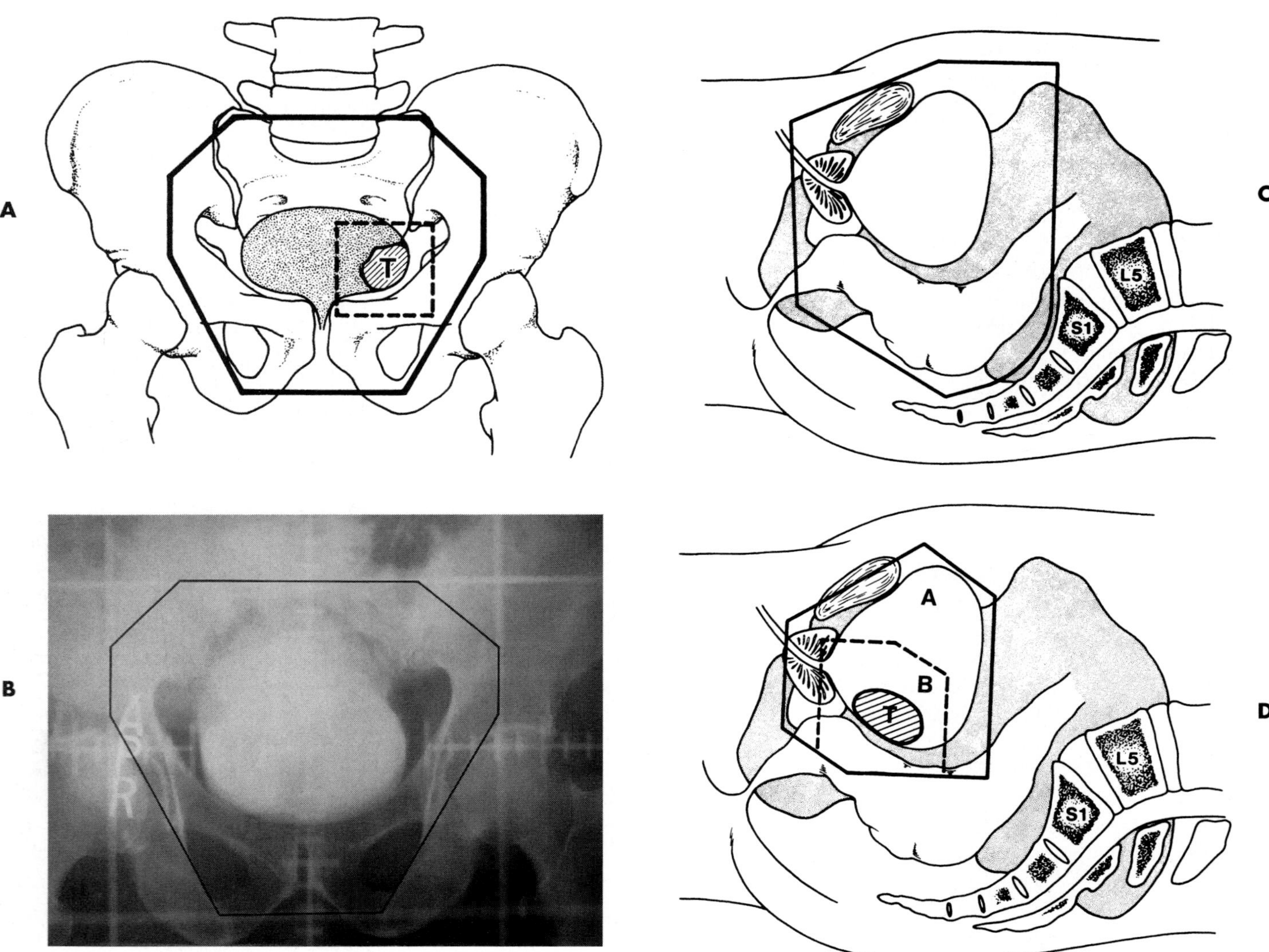

Fig. 12-15. **A,** A diagram of the AP pelvic field used for carcinoma of the bladder. The boost volume is outlined with dashed lines. *T* stands for the residual primary tumor. **B,** Simulation film of the AP portal. **C,** A diagram of the lateral pelvic field encompassing the bladder and pelvic lymph nodes. **D,** Reduced portals after 5000 cGy *(A)* and 5500 or 6000 cGy *(B)*.

plans may be used for linear accelerators with 10 MV or greater beam energy.

Simulation is performed with the patient in the supine position. A Foley catheter is inserted in the bladder through the use of sterile techniques, and 150 to 250 ml of iodinated contrast material (20% concentration) is injected to outline the posterior portion of the bladder. For visualization of the anterior wall of the bladder on lateral (crosstable) radiographs, 100 to 150 ml of air is injected.

Doses. If the patient requires treatment according to Radiation Therapy Oncology Group (RTOG) protocol 89-03, the preliminary radiation therapy course consists of 3960 to 4500 cGy to the bladder and adjacent pelvic lymph nodes in 22 to 25 fractions (180 cGy per day) in 4½ to 5 weeks. After the initial irradiation is delivered to the entire bladder and adjacent tissues, an additional dose is delivered to the initial volume with a 1-cm reduction of portals to complete a 5400-cGy total dose. The boost volume, which encompasses the initial gross tumor volume with a 1-cm margin, receives an additional 1080 cGy, excluding uninvolved portions of the bladder.

In patients treated with irradiation alone, total doses of 6500 to 7000 cGy are administered with techniques that use progressively decreasing portals as described earlier.

Results of treatment

The rate of complete response at the first follow-up cystoscopy after the delivery of 5500 to 5750 cGy in 20 fractions over 4 weeks reported in the Edinburgh series was approximately 45% for all T stages.[21] About 40% to 50% of patients who achieved complete remission developed local recurrence later, yielding 5-year local control rates of approximately 25% to 30% for T_1, T_2, and T_3 lesions. The 5- and 10-year local control rates for T_4 cancers are 16%.[84] For T_2 to T_4 disease a complete response is associated with significantly improved survival rates.

Within each T stage, 5-year survival rates for patients with papillary, solid, or mixed tumors do not differ significantly after external beam irradiation alone.[79]

After salvage cystectomy, 5-year survival rates are 40% to 45%. The rate for superficial disease (Tis, T_1, T_2) is approximately 60%.

The results of "sandwich" irradiation—in which patients with clinical B2, C, or D disease sequentially received a single fraction of 500 cGy preoperatively, radical cystectomy, and 4500 cGy postoperatively—showed 5-year disease-free survival rates of only 20%.[62,99] An 18% incidence of small-bowel obstruction occurred in patients receiving complete sandwich therapy.[99] The incidence of small-bowel obstruction or peritonitis was 15%.[62]

Stein and Kaufman[101] noted a "significant benefit" after concomitant 5-FU and irradiation compared with irradiation alone. Other authors report high complete-response rates for T_2 to T_4 cancers after 6000 to 6500 cGy plus cisplatin.[47,94] Although the 4-year survival rate (64%) for clinical T_2 patients was as high as that after cystectomy (with or without irradiation), the 4-year rates for T_3 and T_4 tumors were only 24%.[94] RTOG Phase III trials have not yet shown an effect of neoadjuvant chemotherapy on survival rates, although single-agent chemotherapy was used in all studies, each of which had a fairly small number of patients. A modest but significant difference in survival rates has been documented in an international randomized trial comparing cisplatin and MVAC (methotrexate, vinblastine, doxorubicin, and cisplatin). Well-designed, prospective randomized trials using effective neoadjuvant combination chemotherapy that assess survival as the primary end point are needed.

Several randomized trials of adjuvant chemotherapy (5-FU, doxorubicin and 5-FU, or cisplatin) following conventional therapy have not demonstrated increased survival rates.[82]

TESTIS

Epidemiology

The American Cancer Society estimates that 7400 new cases of testicular cancer and 370 deaths from the disease occurred in 1996.[2] The incidence of this tumor has been reported to be 3.8 per 100,000 in the United States. Although testicular tumors are relatively rare, they are the most common malignancy in men between 20 and 34 years of age.[105] The incidence is lowest in Asians, Africans, Puerto Ricans, and North American blacks. Higher rates are reported among whites in the United States, United Kingdom, and Denmark. The origin of testicular tumors may be related to gonadal dysgenesis, as strongly suggested by a higher incidence in men with undescended testes. (About 10% of patients have such a history.) **Cryptorchidism** (undescended testes) also increases the risk of intraabdominal testicular tumors. Patients with one testicular tumor are at increased risk for developing a contralateral malignancy; about 5% may develop a contralateral lesion within 5 years. Patients with carcinoma in situ also have a significantly higher risk.

Prognostic indicators

In seminoma the tumor stage is a significant prognostic factor. The histological subtype and elevation of serum beta human chorionic gonadotropin (HCG) have no prognostic implications. In Stages II and III the outcome is related to the bulk of the retroperitoneal tumor, which is associated with an increased propensity for distant metastasis. Patients with Stages III and IV disease have a worse prognosis because of the possibility of mediastinal supraclavicular lymph node involvement or distant metastasis.

The prognosis of nonseminoma tumors is related to the stage of the disease. Most patients with Stage I or II disease survive with modern multiagent chemotherapy. In these patients the levels of tumor markers and the volume of metastasis have some prognostic value. Patients with choriocarcinoma have a poor prognosis.

Anatomy and lymphatics

The testes are contained in the scrotum and suspended by the spermatic cords. The left testis is usually longer than the right. The testis is invested by the tunica vaginalis, tunica albuginea, and tunica vasculosa. The functioning testis lodges the spermatozoa in different stages of development.

A close network of anastomosing tubes in a fibrous stroma at the upper end of the testis constitutes the rete testis and vasa efferentia. These small tubes converge in the vas deferens, a continuation of the epididymis, which is a hard, cordlike structure about 2 feet in length and 5 mm in diameter. The vas deferens enters the pelvis along the spermatic cord and empties into the **seminal vesicles** (two lobulated membranous pouches located between the base of the bladder and the rectum). The ejaculatory ducts, one on each side, begin at the base of the prostate, run forward and downward between its middle and lateral lobes, and end in the verumontanum after entering the prostate.[36]

The lymphatics from the hilum of the testes accompany the spermatic cord up to the internal inguinal ring along the cords of the testicular-spermatic veins. These lympatics drain into the retroperitoneal lymph nodes between the level of T11 and L4 but are concentrated at the level of the L1 and L3 vertebrae. They drain to the left renal hilum on the left side and to the pericaval lymph nodes on the right. Crossover from the right to the left side is constant, but crossover from the left to the right is rare. From the retroperitoneal lumbar nodes, drainage occurs through the thoracic duct to lymph nodes in the mediastinum and supraclavicular fossa and occasionally to the axillary nodes.

Clinical presentation

Usually, a testicular tumor appears as a painless swelling or nodular mass in the scrotum and is sometimes noted incidentally by the patient or a sexual partner. Occasionally, patients complain of a dull ache, heaviness, or pulling sensation in the scrotum or an aching sensation in the lower abdomen. Approximately 10% of patients have acute and severe pain, which may be related to torsion of the spermatic cord. Frequently, patients relate the appearance of the mass to a previous trauma, although this is coincidental rather than etiological. Rarely, patients exhibit metastatic disease, such as a neck mass, respiratory symptoms, or low back pain. Gynecomastia occurs in approximately 5% of patients with testicular germ cell tumors.[22]

Detection and diagnosis

A complete history and physical examination are mandatory. If a testicular tumor is suspected, a testicular ultrasound should be performed. The appropriate surgical procedure to make the diagnosis and remove the primary tumor is radical orchiectomy through an inguinal incision. Beta HCG levels may be slightly elevated in 17% of patients with pure **seminomas** (the most common malignant testicular tumors).[22] However, any elevation of alpha-fetoprotein (AFP) signals nonseminomatous disease. Beta HCG and/or AFP levels are elevated in 80% to 85% of patients with disseminated nonseminomatous disease. Serum markers (i.e., beta HCG and AFP) should be assayed before *and* after orchiectomy, can be used to document persistent or recurrent cancer, and may predict the responsiveness of nonseminomas to surgery or chemotherapy.

A chest radiograph and, if clinically warranted, an evaluation of the retroperitoneal lymphatics by CT or a pedal lymphangiogram are critical components of the staging process. A semen analysis and sperm banking should be considered for patients in whom treatment is likely to compromise fertility or who intend to have children in the near future.

Pathology and staging

A representation of the dual origin of testicular tumors is shown in Fig. 12-16. About 95% of testicular neoplasms originate in germinal elements. The most common type of testicular tumor is seminoma, which has three histological subtypes: classical, anaplastic, and spermatocytic. The prognosis is not significantly different for the various subtypes. The nonseminomatous tumors include embryonal carcinoma, teratoma carcinoma, choriocarcinoma, and yolk sac tumor (embryonal adenocarcinoma in the prepubertal testis). The most common single-cell type is embryonal seminoma. Yolk sac tumors are the most common in children. Sometimes nonseminomatous tumors contain more than one element; the most common combination is teratocarcinoma (teratoma and embryonal carcinoma). Choriocarcinoma accounts for about 1% of these tumors.

For testicular seminoma the modified Royal Marsden Hospital staging system (see the box on p. 273), which closely resembles the Walter Reed staging system, was adopted for use at the Leeds Consensus Conference in 1989[104] (see the box on p. 274).

Routes of spread

Although the routes of dissemination are similar for seminomas and nonseminomas, the propensity for involvement of various sites differs. Pure seminoma has a much greater tendency to remain localized or involve only lymph nodes, whereas nonseminomatous germ cell tumors of the testes more frequently spread by the hematogenous route.

Seminoma spreads orderly, initially to the lymph nodes in the retroperitoneum. From the retroperitoneal nodes, the seminoma spreads to the next echelon of drainage lymphatics in the mediastinum and supraclavicular fossa (Stage III disease). Only rarely and late does pure seminoma spread hematogenously to involve the lung parenchyma, bone, liver, or brain (stage IV disease). Less than 5% of patients have Stage III or IV disease at the time of presentation.[105] The orderly route of spread for pure seminoma has been confirmed by surveillance studies. A total of 255 patients participated in postorchiectomy surveillance studies. Of 33 patients with relapses, 29 had disease in the retroperitoneal

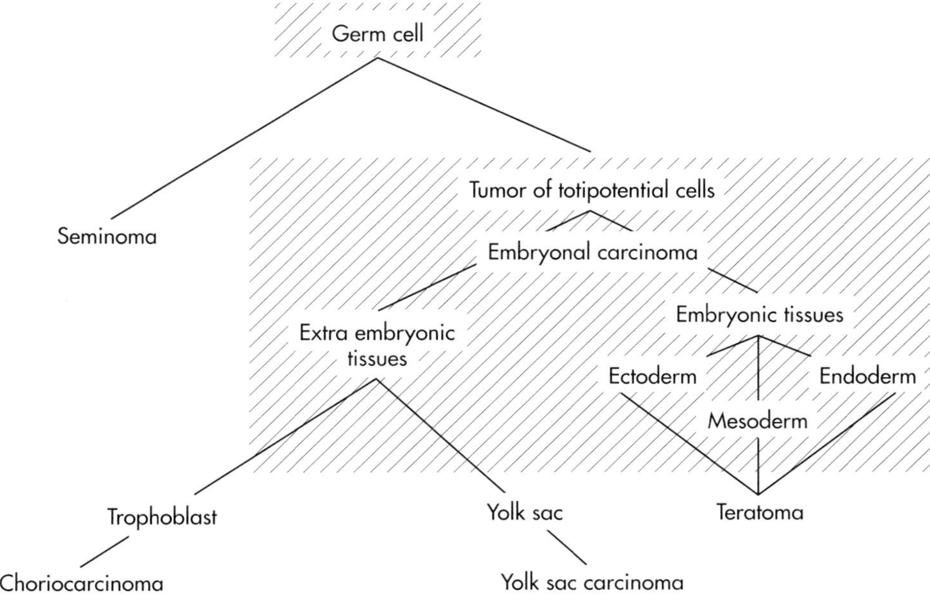

Fig. 12-16 Dual origin for derivation of testes tumors.

Royal Marsden Hospital Staging System for Testicular Seminoma

Stage

Stage	
I	No evidence of metastases
II	Metastases confined to abdominal nodes
	A Maximum diameter of metastases <2 cm
	B 2-5 cm
	C 5-10 cm
	D >10 cm
III	Involvement of supradiaphragmatic and infradiaphragmatic lymph nodes
	No extralymphatic metastases
	Abdominal status: A, B, C, and D, as for Stage II
IV	Extralymphatic metastases
	Abdominal status: 0, A, B, C, and D, as for Stage II
	Lung status
	L1 <3 metastases
	L2 multiple <2 cm diameter
	L3 multiple >2 cm
	Liver status
	H + liver involvement

lymph nodes. The site of the second relapse when infradiaphragmatic irradiation was used for the first relapse was the supradiaphragmatic nodes.[19]

When they metastasize, nonseminomatous tumors usually involve the lungs and liver.

Treatment techniques

The initial management goal for a suspected malignant germ cell tumor of the testis is to obtain serum AFP and beta HCG measurements and, after staging procedures, to perform a radical (inguinal) orchiectomy with high ligation of the spermatic cord. Further management depends on the pathological diagnosis of the stage and extent of the disease.

Seminoma. The standard treatment for patients with Stage I seminoma is radical orchiectomy and postoperative irradiation of the periaortic and ipsilateral pelvic nodes (2500 cGy in 160- to 180-cGy fractions) (Fig. 12-17).[51] Surveillance studies performed in Canada and the United Kingdom of patients receiving no further treatment after an orchiectomy have indicated recurrence rates of 20% to 28%.[105]

For patients with Stage IIA disease (<2 cm diameter mass) the radiation dose and portals for the periaortic and ipsilateral pelvic lymph nodes are identical to those used for Stage I disease. For Stage IIB disease (>5 cm diameter mass) the periaortic and ipsilateral pelvic lymph nodes should be irradiated with appropriate modification of the treatment field and doses to encompass the larger mass. The dose to the entire nodal volume is 2500 to 3000 cGy in 160- to 180-cGy fractions, with an additional boost of 500 to 1000 cGy in 180- to 200-cGy fractions with reduced portals to the residual gross tumor.

The optimal therapy for patients with Stage IIC retroperitoneal disease (5 to 10 cm in transverse diameter) must be individualized. If the mass is centrally located and does not overlap most of one kidney or significantly overlap the liver, primary radiation therapy is the treatment of choice, with cis-

Testis Staging Systems

EORTC UICC/AJCC

Primary tumor (T) (pathological classification)

Stage I	pT_1	Tumor limited to testis (including rete)
	pT_2	Tumor invasion beyond tunica albuginea or into epididymis
	pT_3	Tumor invasion of spermatic cord
	pT_4	Tumor invasion of scrotum

Lymph nodes (N)

Stage II		
IIA	N_1	Metastasis in single node (<2 cm maximum diameter)
IIB	N_2	Metastasis in a single node (2 to 5 cm in maximum diameter)
IIC, D	N_3	Metastasis in a lymph node (>5 cm in maximum diameter)
Stage III		Supradiaphragmatic and infra-diaphragmatic nodes: abdominal sites A, B, C, and D

Distant metastasis (M)

	M_0	No distant metastasis
Stage IV	M_1	Distant metastases (specific site)

Stage groupings

I	T_1, T_2, N_0, M_0
II	T_3, T_4, N_0, M_0
III	Any T, N_1, M_0
IV	Any T, N_2 or N_3, M_0
	Any T, any N, M_1

EORTC, European Organization for Research on Treatment of Cancer; UICC, International Union Against Cancer; AJCC, American Joint Committee on Cancer.

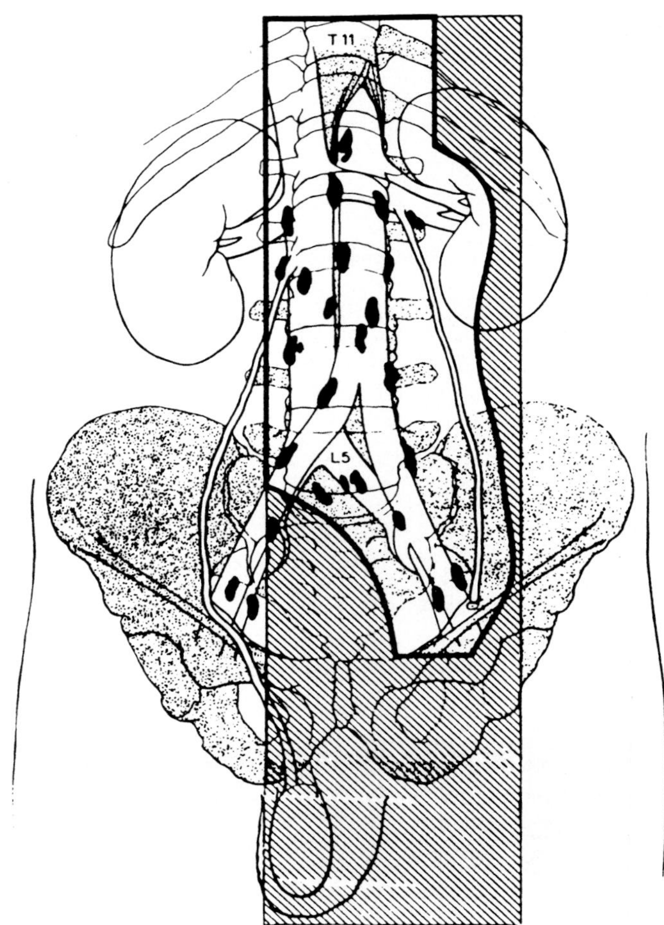

Fig. 12-17 Contoured anterior and posterior radiation treatment fields for clinical stage I or IIA left testicular cancer. The diagonally shaded area is an individually made, 8-cm thick Ostalloy block (shield 2). (From Kubo H, Shipley WU:Reduction of the scatter dose to the testicle outside the radiation treatment fields, *Int J Radiat Oncol Biol Phys* 8:1741-1745, 1982.)

platin-containing combination chemotherapy reserved for a relapse. However, if the location of the mass is such that the radiation volume covers most of one kidney or significant volumes of the liver, the potential morbidity of radiation therapy can be avoided by the use of primary cisplatin-containing combination chemotherapy.

Stage IID is rare. Patients in this stage should be treated with primary cisplatin-containing combination chemotherapy.

The current standard therapy for Stages III and IV disease is four courses of cisplatin-containing combination chemotherapy. Often, residual masses may exist in the abdominal or mediastinal area after four cycles of chemotherapy. The 1989 Germ Cell Consensus Conference in Leeds, England, concluded from the available data that patients should be observed after appropriate chemotherapy and that further exploratory surgery or consolidative irradiation should be given only for overt disease progression.[104]

Nonseminoma. The initial treatment for nonseminoma is radical inguinal orchiectomy, followed by cisplatin-based chemotherapy. The most commonly accepted standard regimens include four courses of PVB (cisplatin, vinblastine, and bleomycin) or BEP (bleomycin, VP-16, cisplatin). Several investigators are exploring the use of fewer courses of cisplatin-containing combination chemotherapy and the use of single-agent cisplatin, carboplatinum, or ifosfamide. One third of chemotherapy-treated patients have a radiographically apparent residual mass or masses after chemotherapy. In general, these masses should be excised because approximately 40% are teratomas and another 10% to 15% are carcinomas. Presumptive evidence exists indicating that unresected teratomas may give rise to later relapse or progression and that they have a lower risk of recurrence after surgical excision. Patients with persistent carcinoma require additional chemotherapy but generally do well with these treatments.

Irradiation has no role in the management of patients with disseminated nonseminoma, except in the palliation or management of brain metastasis in some patients. Although rare, newly diagnosed brain metastases are still potentially curable.

Radiation therapy. Patients with Stage I testicular seminoma should receive megavoltage irradiation to the periaortic and ipsilateral pelvic lymph nodes. The top of the portal should be at the T9-10 interface, the inferior border should be at the top of the obturator foramen, and the lateral border must include the periaortic lymph nodes and ipsilateral renal hilum (usually 10 to 12 cm wide). However, the left hilar should be cut where it may be wider. A shaped field with 2-cm margins on the visualized lymph nodes should encompass the ipsilateral iliac and pelvic lymph nodes. Testicular shielding for decreasing primary and, to a lesser degree, scattered irradiation should be applied if the patient wants to preserve fertility.

Recommended doses to retroperitoneal and pelvic lymphatics for Stages I and IIA disease are 2500 and 3000 cGy, respectively, in fractions of 160 to 180 cGy with AP/PA fields given 5 days per week and both fields treated daily. For Stages IIB and IIC tumors the portals are the same as those in Stages I and IIA, except the fields should be modified to cover the palpable or radiographic mass with an adquate margin. The first 2500 to 3000 cGy is delivered in fractions of 160 to 180 cGy. A boost of 500 to 1000 cGy in 180- to 200-cGy fractions is given to a reduced field to encompass the mass with an adequate margin of at least 2 cm.

If the primary radiation therapy field encompasses most of one kidney, care must be taken to protect at least two thirds of the kidney from receiving doses higher than 1800 cGy. The initial shrinkage of large masses is often rapid, and the abdominal CT scan should be repeated after the first 3 weeks of radiation therapy to determine possible field reduction. Care should also be taken to limit the radiation dose to a significant volume of the liver to less than 3000 cGy.

Controversial issues

Scrotal or inguinal irradiation. A standard recommendation has been to modify the treatment volume to include the inguinal regions if there has been previous inguinal surgery and to include the scrotum if it has been violated. Reports from the Princess Margaret Hospital and Royal Marsden Hospital demonstrated that previous inguinal or scrotal interferences without scrotal irradiation result in no increased risk of relapse. The 1989 Consensus Conference in Leeds, England, recommended that inguinal or scrotal irradiation be omitted even if scrotal interference has occurred.[104]

Mediastinal irradiation. In the 1960s and early 1970s, using prophylactic mediastinal irradiation to treat patients who had Stage I or II testicular seminoma was common. Compiled data from six series suggest that supradiaphragmatic relapse is extremely rare (even for relatively poorly staged patients with Stage IIA or IIB disease) if prophylactic mediastinal irradiation is withheld. Mediastinal relapse occurred in only 8 of 250 patients, and 7 of 8 patients were salvaged with irradiation. Because the possible survival benefit of elective mediastinal irradiation is only 0.4%, most radiation oncologists have abandoned its use for Stages IIA and IIB disease.[88]

Periaortic versus iliac and periaortic irradiation. There is growing interest in Europe and the United Kingdom in reducing the radiation volumes for the treatment of Stage I disease by omitting irradiation of the pelvic lymph nodes. Less than 2% of patients have involved pelvic nodes, and it is unlikely that the reduction of the irradiated volume will cause a significant increase in relapses. The delivery of periaortic nodal irradiation only, without ipsilateral pelvic irradiation, is considered nonstandard practice.

Results of treatment

Rates of disease-free survival, overall survival, and survival corrected for intercurrent disease for 95 patients with Stage I testicular seminoma treated at Mallinckrodt Institute of Radiology were 96%, 100%, and 100%, respectively. No patient had died of testicular seminoma 5 years after treatment. These results are comparable to those reported by many authors.[105,111,112]

For 33 patients with Stages IIA and B disease treated at Mallinckrodt Institute of Radiology, rates of disease-free survival, overall survival, and survival corrected for intercurrent illness were 93%, 89%, and 97%, respectively. These rates are comparable to those from other institutions.[91,112] Only one patient with initial Stage IIA and IIB disease died of seminoma.

Survival for patients with Stages IIC, IID, and III disease depends on the initial bulk of the tumor and the therapeutic approach. With irradiation alone, tumor-free survival rates range from 30% to 50%, and primary chemotherapy yields a progression-free survival rate of 91%. More than half the patients receive consolidation irradiation or surgery for an initial bulky tumor.

Side effects. Subdiaphragmatic irradiation was well tolerated in a study of 128 patients. One patient developed an intestinal obstruction after receiving 150 mCi of intraperitoneal colloidal gold 198 for a ruptured seminoma in an undescended testis, in addition to a midplane dose of 3363 cGy with external beam therapy.[53] Three other patients had mild, late complications that were managed conservatively. Severe dyspepsia or a peptic ulcer occurs in 3% to 5% of irradiated patients.[29]

A significant increase occurred in late complications with wide-field irradiation for seminoma and Hodgkin's disease with doses over 2500 cGy. However, no late complications were reported with lower doses.[14] The complication rate increased to 2% with 3500 cGy and to 6% with 4000 to 4500 cGy.

About 50% of patients have some decreased sperm count at the time of diagnosis. Further decreases are noted after pelvic and periaortic irradiation, even if gonadal shielding is used. (The dose remains 1% to 2% of the prescription because of scattered irradiation through the body tissues.[30]) Spermatogenesis may be affected by doses as low as 50 cGy, and cumulative doses above 200 cGy will probably induce permanent sterility.[93]

Second primary malignancy. A 5% to 10% incidence rate of second malignancy has been reported in patients treated with radiation therapy for testicular seminoma. These second malignancies arise from inside and outside the radiation treatment portal. Whether they result from radiation treatment, a predisposition of patients with testicular seminoma to develop a second primary, or a combination of both is not clear. The incidence of second malignancies among patients in surveillance studies is invaluable in clarifying this issue. However, because of the relatively short duration of follow-ups for surveillance studies, the true relative risk of second malignancies in patients with testicular seminoma remains unknown.

KIDNEY

Epidemiology

Renal cell carcinoma. The estimated number of new cases of kidney and other urinary cancers in the United States in 1996 was 30,600, resulting in more than 12,000 deaths, representing approximately 2% of all new cancers and cancer deaths.[2] The average age at the time of diagnosis is 55 to 60 years, with a male-to-female ratio of 2 to 1.

Several environmental, occupational, hormonal, cellular, and genetic factors are associated with the development of renal cell carcinoma.[57] Cigarette and tobacco use, obesity, and analgesic abuse (i.e., phenacetin-containing analgesics) have been correlated with an increased risk and incidence of kidney cancer. A higher incidence of renal cell carcinoma has also been reported among leather tanners, shoe workers, and asbestos workers. Exposure to cadmium, petroleum products, or thorium dioxide (a radioactive contrast agent used in the 1920s) causes renal cell carcinoma in humans. Renal cell cancer has been reported after diethylstilbestrol therapy given for prostate cancer.

The association of renal cell cancer and von Hippel-Lindau disease has long been established. Various tumor-produced growth factors have been described in the initiation or progression of renal cell carcinoma.[57]

Renal pelvic and ureteral carcinoma. About 7% of all renal neoplasms and less than 1% of all genitourinary tumors are transitional cell carcinomas of the upper urinary tract.[81] The incidence rate of bilateral upper urinary tract tumors is 1.5% to 2% for synchronous and 6% to 8% for metachronous presentations.[43] For renal pelvic tumors the incidence ratio of men to women is 3 to 1, and the peak incidence is in the fifth and sixth decades of life. About one third of patients with upper urinary tract tumors develop bladder carcinoma. Etiological factors for renal pelvic and ureteral cancer are similar to those for tumors of the urinary bladder. Urban residency, cigarette and tobacco use, aminophenol exposure (e.g., benzidine, β-naphthylamine), renal stones, and analgesics (e.g., chronic phenacetin abuse) have been associated with an increased risk of developing upper urinary tract tumors.

Prognostic indicators

Renal cell carcinoma. The major prognostic factors for the survival of patients with renal cell carcinoma are the stage and histological grade of the tumor. Reported 5-year survival rates are 88% for Stage I, 67% for Stage II, 40% for Stage III, and 2% for Stage IV.[35] Renal vein or vena cava involvement (without corresponding regional lymph node metastasis) is not a poor prognostic sign if the entire tumor thrombus is removed. The mean survival time for patients with metastasis at the time of diagnosis is approximately 4 months, and only about 10% of patients survive 1 year.[78]

Renal pelvic and ureteral carcinoma. Stage *and* grade are important prognostic factors in carcinoma of the renal pelvis and ureter. One report noted that 54 patients with transitional cell carcinoma of the renal pelvis and ureter had a median survival time of 91.1 months for low-stage tumors and 12.9 months for high-stage tumors.[45] When patients were stratified according to the low or high tumor grade the median survival time was 66.8 months and 14.1 months, respectively.

Anatomy and lymphatics

The kidneys and ureters, as well as their vascular supply and lymphatics, are located in the retroperitoneal space between the parietal peritoneum and the posterior abdominal wall. The kidneys are located at a level between the eleventh rib and the transverse process of the third lumbar spine. The renal axis is parallel to the lateral margin of the psoas muscle. Each kidney is about 11 to 12 cm in length, with the right kidney usually 1 to 2 cm lower than the left. Gerota's fascia envelopes the kidney in its fibrous capsule and the perinephric fat.

The caliceal collecting system lies on the anteromedial surface of the kidney and forms a funnel-shaped system that is continuous with the ureter. The ureters course posteriorly, parallel to the lateral border of the psoas muscle, until they curve anteriorly in the pelvis to join the base of the bladder.

The lymphatic drainage of the kidney and renal pelvis occurs along the vessels in the renal hilum to the periaortic and paracaval nodes. The lymphatic drainage of the ureter is segmented and diffuse, involving any of the following: renal hilar, abdominal periaortic, paracaval, common iliac, internal iliac, or external iliac nodes.

The topographical relationship of the kidneys, renal pelvis, and ureters to other abdominal organs is illustrated in Fig. 12-18.

Clinical presentation

Renal cell carcinoma. Renal cell carcinoma may appear as an occult primary tumor or with signs and symptoms. In one report the classic triad of gross hematuria, a palpable abdominal mass, and pain occurred in only 9% of patients.

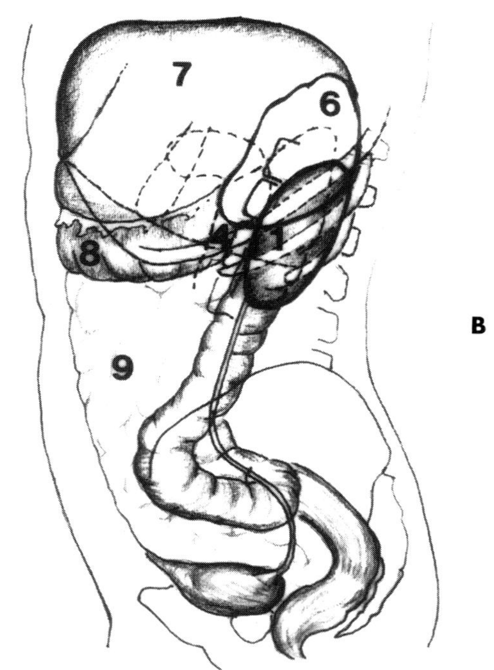

Fig. 12-18 Anatomical relationships of the kidneys, renal pelvis, and ureters to the abdominal viscera. The surrounding structures as numbered (*1*, right kidney; *2*, left renal pelvis; **3**, left ureter; *4*, pancreas; *5*, stomach; *6*, spleen; *7*, liver; *8*, transverse colon; *9*, small bowel) become dose-limiting factors in the planning of abdominal or retroperitoneal irradiation. **A**, An anteroposterior view. **B**, A lateral view. (Courtesy Peter P. Lai, M.D.)

Two of the three components of the triad occurred in 36% of patients, whereas hematuria (gross or microscopic) was noted in 59% of patients.[78] Several paraneoplastic syndromes or systemic symptoms of renal cell carcinoma have been described, and the tumor may masquerade as a variety of symptom patterns.

Renal pelvic and ureteral carcinoma. Gross or microscopic hematuria is the most common sign in patients who have a renal pelvic or ureteral tumor (70% to 95% incidence).[81] The other less common symptoms include pain (8% to 40%), bladder irritation (5% to 10%), and other constitutional symptoms (5%). About 10% to 20% of patients have a flank mass secondary to the tumor or associated hydronephrosis. Otherwise, physical findings are otherwise unremarkable.

Detection and diagnosis

Renal cell carcinoma. The diagnosis of renal cell carcinoma is established clinically and radiographically in most patients. After a radiographic diagnosis is made a thorough staging work-up is performed to determine resectability. A metastatic work-up that includes a bone scan, chest radiograph, and CT or MRI scan of the abdomen and pelvis should be performed before surgery. If metastatic lesions are detected, a histological confirmation of the most easily accessible lesion should be obtained.

An intravenous pyelogram is essential in identifying the tumor, determining its location, and showing the function of the contralateral kidney when surgery is contemplated. However, an intravenous pyelogram is not sensitive or specific for small to medium tumors. Ultrasonography provides accurate anatomical detail of extrarenal extension of the tumor. In addition, it differentiates solid from cystic renal lesions. If the lesion is cystic, a percutaneous cyst puncture should be done (if no echinococcosis is suspected) via ultrasound or CT guidance to rule out malignancy. Renal arteriography detects neovascularity, arteriovenous fistula, and pooling of a contrast medium, and it accentuates capsular vessels. Contrast-enhanced or dynamic CT provides extremely accurate information about the location and size of the tumor, as well as lymph node enlargement. CT plus digital subtraction angiography provides adequate diagnostic and anatomical details with much less morbidity than arteriography. Inferior venacavography is sometimes used to detect the extent of the tumor thrombus' involvement with the vena cava. MRI provides a 3-D picture of renal cell carcinoma. If indicated, a bone or CT scan of the brain or lung should be performed to rule out metastasis.

Renal pelvic and ureteral carcinoma. Excretory urography is frequently used to evaluate patients with renal pelvic carcinoma. The most common finding is a filling defect in the renal pelvis or collecting system. Retrograde pyelography accurately delineates upper-tract filling defects and defines the lower margin of the ureteral lesion. CT or MRI of the abdomen and pelvis before and after contrast gives useful information regarding tumor extension. Angiography is not often used. Endoscopic ureteroscopy with percutaneous nephroscopy is a recently developed technique. A brush cytology or biopsy from such an endoscopic and retrograde procedure has a diagnostic accuracy of 80% to 90%.[57]

Pathology and staging

The proximal tubular epithelium is the tissue of origin for renal cell carcinoma. Clear cell carcinoma is the most predominant subtype. Some reports indicate that spindle cell (or sarcomatoid variant) carcinoma is associated with a poor prognosis. A tumor's high nuclear grade is associated with an increased incidence of lymph node involvement and a poor survival time.[78]

Transitional cell carcinoma accounts for more than 90% of malignant tumors of the renal pelvis and ureter, and squamous cell carcinoma accounts for 7% to 8%.[57] Adenocarcinoma of the upper urothelial tract is rare. Squamous cell carcinoma of the renal pelvis is often deeply invasive and is associated with a worse prognosis than transitional cell carcinoma. High-grade renal pelvic or ureteral tumors are associated with poor survival rates.[45]

The staging system used for renal cell carcinoma in the United States is the Robson[85] modification of the system proposed by Flocks and Kadesky.[27] The drawback of this staging system is the subgrouping of Stage III patients with vastly different prognoses.

The AJCC system for the classification of renal cell carcinoma of the kidney is shown in the box on p. 279. Compared with the previous AJCC system, the T categories have been redefined and simplified. T_1 and T_2 refer to cancers that are intrarenal and have not invaded through the capsule. T_3 and T_4 cancers are based on the local extension of the primary tumor. The N classification depends on the size and number of involved lymph nodes and not on laterality.

The AJCC staging classification for renal pelvic and ureteral carcinoma is shown in the box on p. 280. The grouping of the T categories depends on the tumor's extent (i.e., depth of penetration of the lesion).

Routes of spread

Renal cell carcinoma. A tumor may spread in the following ways: (1) by local infiltration through the renal capsule to involve the perinephric fat and Gerota's fascia; (2) by direct extension in the venous channels to the renal vein or inferior vena cava; (3) by retrograde venous drainage to the testis; and (4) by lymphatic drainage to the renal hilar, periaortic, and paracaval nodes and eventually to any part of the body, including the lung, liver, central nervous system, thyroid, eye, larynx, intestines, or other organs. The incidence rate of lymph node metastasis is 12% to 23%.

Approximately 45% of patients with renal cell carcinoma have localized disease, 25% have advanced disease, and 30% have radiographic evidence of metastasis at the time of the diagnosis.[57] About 50% of patients with renal cell carcinoma eventually develop metastasis. Common metastatic sites include the lung (75%), soft tissue (36%), bone (20%), liver (18%), cutaneous areas (8%), and central nervous system (8%).[58]

Spontaneous regression of metastatic renal cell carcinoma after nephrectomy has been reported but is extremely rare.

Renal pelvic and ureteral carcinoma. Upper urinary tract carcinoma is a multifocal process; patients with cancer at one site in the upper urinary tract are at a greater risk of developing tumors elsewhere.

Transitional cell carcinoma of the upper urothelial tract may spread by direct extension or blood and lymphatics. The implantation of tumor cells in the bladder has been demonstrated, especially in previously traumatized areas.[83]

Regional lymph nodes are commonly involved before other sites of metastasis. The incidence of lymph node metastasis ranges from 37% to 82% in patients with renal pelvic tumors and 22% to 41% in patients with ureteral tumors. Distant metastases are common and occur most frequently in the lungs, liver, and peritoneal cavity.

Treatment techniques

Renal cell carcinoma. Standard treatment for patients with localized renal cell carcinoma (T_1 and T_2) is radical nephrectomy, which consists of the complete removal of the intact Gerota's fascia and its contents, including the kidney, adrenal gland, and perinephric fat. Regional lymphadenectomy is often performed at the time of radical nephrectomy.

The role of preoperative radiation therapy before nephrectomy has not been defined. Tumor shrinkage and increased resectability have been reported in patients who received preoperative irradiation, but no survival benefit has been noted.[52]

Definitive radiation treatment is indicated if the patient is not a candidate for surgical resection. Definitive irradiation for renal cell carcinoma is limited by the inability to deliver high doses of radiation to the upper abdomen, where most surrounding structures are dose limiting.

Chemotherapy, as adjuvant therapy or as treatment for unresectable or metastatic disease, does not increase the survival rate over that achieved with treatment not including chemotherapy.

Patients with a solitary bony metastasis are at risk of developing multiple metastases, but these patients also have a 30% to 40% chance of surviving for 5 years.[49] Thus high-dose palliative radiation therapy to metastatic bony lesions should be performed to ensure a long disease-free survival time for these patients.

Hormonal therapy of metastatic renal cell carcinoma results in an overall objective response of 6% to 33%. Nearly all responses are partial and short and primarily affect pulmonary metastases. At the National Cancer Institute, biological therapy trials, such as adoptive cellular therapy with lymphokine-activated cells plus interleukin-2, are in progress.

American Joint Committee on Cancer Staging Classification for Kidney Cancer

Primary tumor (T)

TX	Primary tumor cannot be assessed
T_0	No evidence of primary tumor
T_1	Tumor 2.5 cm or less in greatest dimension (limited to the kidney)
T_2	Tumor more than 2.5 cm in greatest dimension (limited to the kidney)
T_3	Tumor extension into major veins or invasion of adrenal gland or perinephric tissues but not beyond Gerota's fascia
T_{3a}	Tumor invasion of adrenal gland or perinephric tissues but not beyond Gerota's fascia
T_{3b}	Tumor grossly extends into renal vein(s) or vena cava below the diaphragm
T_{3c}	Tumor gross extension into the vena cava above the diaphragm
T_4	Tumor invasion beyond Gerota's fascia

Regional lymph nodes (N)

NX	Regional lymph nodes cannot be assessed
N_0	No regional lymph node metastasis
N_1	Metastasis in a single lymph node (2 cm or less in greatest dimension)
N_2	Metastasis in a single lymph node (more than 2 cm but not more than 5 cm in greatest dimension) or multiple lymph nodes (none more than 5 cm in greatest dimension)
N_3	Metastasis in a lymph node (more than 5 cm in greatest dimension)

Distant metastasis (M)

MX	Distant metastasis cannot be assessed
M_0	No distant metastasis
M_1	Distant metastasis

Stage grouping

Stage I	T_1	N_0	M_0
Stage II	T_2	N_0	M_0
Stage III	T_1	N_1	M_0
	T_2	N_1	M_0
	T_{3a}	N_0, N_1	M_0
	T_{3b}	N_0, N_1	M_0
	T_{3c}	N_0, N_1	M_0
Stage IV	T_4	Any N	M_0
	Any T	N_2, N_3	M_0
	Any T	Any N	M_1

Histopathological grade

GX	Grade cannot be assessed
G1	Well differentiated
G2	Moderately well differentiated
G3-4	Poorly differentiated or undifferentiated

Modified from Beahrs OH et al, editors: *AJCC manual for staging of cancer,* ed 4, Philadelphia, 1992, JB Lippincott.

Renal pelvic and ureteral carcinoma. Management of renal pelvic or ureteral carcinoma consists of nephroureterectomy with the excision of a cuff of bladder and bladder mucosa. Less aggressive surgery, such as nephrectomy and partial ureterectomy, is accompanied by a ureter stump recurrence rate of 30%. More conservative surgical excision has been advocated for patients with low-stage, low-grade, and solitary lesions. The survival rate of patients with solitary, well-differentiated tumors after surgical resection is greater than 90%.[64]

Combination chemotherapy consisting of MVAC (methotrexate, vinblastine, Adriamycin [doxorubicin], and cisplatin) produces an objective response of more than 70% in limited groups of patients who have metastatic transitional cell carcinoma of the bladder, ureter, and renal pelvis.[102] For patients who have high-stage and high-grade tumors with local extension or patients with regional lymph node metastases, MVAC combination chemotherapy and irradiation offer the best chance of disease control.

American Joint Committee on Cancer Staging Classification for Renal Pelvic and Ureteral Cancer

Primary tumor (T)

TX	Primary tumor cannot be assessed
T_0	No evidence of tumor
Tis	Carcinoma in situ
T_a	Papillary noninvasive carcinoma
T_1	Tumor invasion of subepithelial connective tissue
T_2	Tumor invasion of muscularis
T_3	Tumor invasion beyond muscularis into periureteric-peripelvic fat or renal parenchyma
T_4	Tumor invasion of adjacent organs or through the kidney into perinephric fat

Regional lymph nodes (N)

NX	Regional lymph nodes cannot be assessed
N_0	No regional lymph node metastasis
N_1	Metastasis in a single lymph node (2 cm or less in greatest dimension)
N_2	Metastasis in a single lymph node (more than 2 cm but not more than 5 cm in greatest dimension) or multiple lymph nodes (none more than 5 cm in greatest dimension)
N_3	Metastasis in a lymph node (more than 5 cm in greatest dimension)

Distant metastasis (M)

MX	Distant metastasis cannot be assessed
M_0	No distant metastasis
M_1	Distant metastasis

Stage grouping

Stage 0	Tis	N_0	M_0
	T_a	N_0	M_0
Stage I	T_1	N_0	M_0
Stage II	T_2	N_0	M_0
Stage III	T_3	N_0	M_0
Stage IV	T_4	N_0	M_0
	Any T	N_1, N_2, N_3	M_0
	Any T	Any N	M_1

Histopathological grade

GX	Grade cannot be assessed
G1	Well differentiated
G2	Moderately well differentiated
G3-4	Poorly differentiated or undifferentiated

Modified from Beahrs OH et al, editors: *AJCC manual for staging of cancer,* ed 4, Philadelphia, 1992, JB Lippincott.

Radiation therapy techniques.

Renal cell carcinoma. Except for the total dose, the radiation therapy technique and time-dose fractionation are similar in most curative (adjuvant) or palliative situations. The usual treatment volume includes the entire kidney (if the renal cell carcinoma is left in place), renal fossa, and periaortic and paracaval lymph nodes. For preoperative irradiation a CT scan should be used to delineate the tumor's extent and for treatment planning. For postoperative irradiation a postnephrectomy, preirradiation baseline CT should be obtained for later comparison.

The preoperative radiation doses reported in the literature range from 3000 to 4800 cGy.[60,72] Postoperative radiation doses range from 4500 to 5500 cGy; the usual recommended dose that can be safely given to the upper abdomen with an acceptable complication rate is 5040 cGy at 180 cGy per fraction over 5 to 6 weeks. A boost of 540 cGy in three fractions to a smaller volume may be added with special care to bring the total tumor dose to 5580 cGy. The remaining kidney should not receive doses above 1800 cGy. For a right-sided tumor a field reduction may be needed at 3600 to 4000 cGy to ensure that no more than

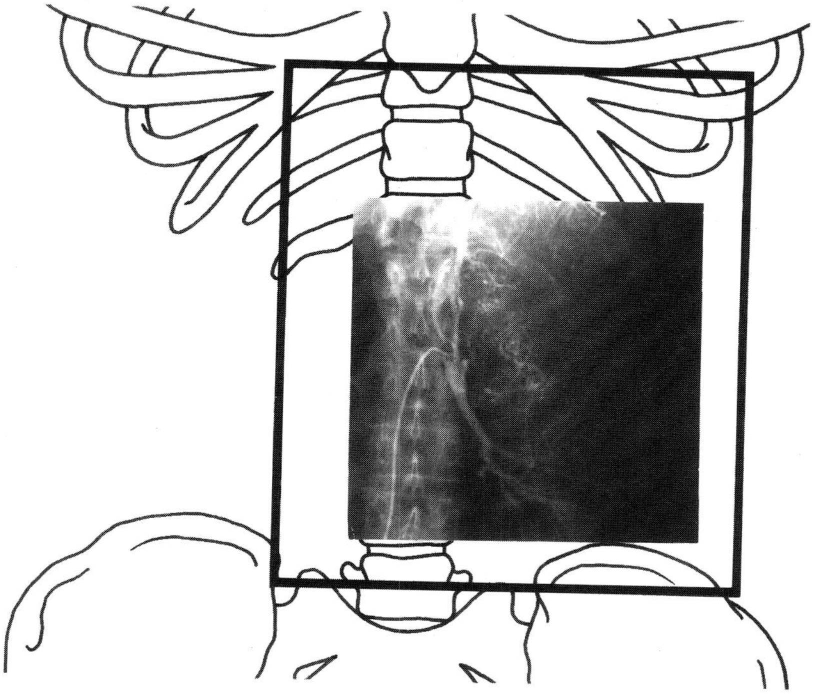

Fig. 12-19 A radiation portal for large, left-sided renal cancer. The primary tumor and bilateral lymph nodes are included. (From Lai PP: Kidney, renal pelvis, and ureter. In Perez CA, Brady LW, editors: *Principles and practice of radiation oncology,* ed 2, Philadelphia, 1992, JB Lippincott.)

30% of the liver parenchyma is irradiated to a higher dose. The nominal dose for the spinal cord should be limited to 4500 cGy (180-cGy fractions). No attempt is made to include the entire surgical incision in the treatment field for patients who receive postnephrectomy irradiation, unless specific knowledge exists of significant wound contamination by tumor spillage.[52]

The patient is usually treated via isocentric and parallel-opposed AP/PA-shaped fields (Figs. 12-19 and 12-20). Treatment plans include (1) a single posterior oblique field, (2) equal weighting of parallel-opposed AP/PA fields, (3) bias loading (i.e., 3:1 or 2:1 posterior loading), and (4) other rotating or wedge pair techniques.[87] A shrinking-field technique should be used to reduce exposure to dose-limiting adjacent structures. High-energy photons (10 MV or higher) from linear accelerators should be used.

Renal pelvic and ureteral carcinoma. Preoperative radiation doses of 2000 cGy in five fractions or postoperative irradiation has been used to treat patients with carcinoma of the renal pelvis and ureter. The treatment portal usually includes the entire renal fossa, entire ureteral bed, and ipsilateral bladder trigone. The extent is dictated by clinical information obtained at the time of surgery and a pathological analysis of the resected specimen (Fig. 12-21). Because of the high incidence of lymph node involvement, the treatment portal should also include the periaortic and paracaval areas. As in renal cell carcinoma of the kidney, the postoperative radiation dose is limited by the tolerance of the normal tissues in the treatment field (usually 5040 cGy in 180-cGy fractions, with a boost of an additional 540 cGy in three fractions to a reduced volume for a total of 5580 cGy). Techniques are similar to those just described.

Results of treatment

Results of studies of preoperative or postoperative radiation therapy and nephrectomy for renal cell carcinoma are summarized in Tables 12-10 and 12-11. Future studies should (1) select patients who may benefit from adjuvant radiation therapy (i.e., patients with advanced-stage and high-grade renal cell carcinoma) and (2) stratify patients according to the stage, grade, and uniformity of the technique and radiation dose.

In renal pelvic and ureteral carcinoma, less than 30% of patients with poor prognostic factors are cured by surgery alone, and about 45% of these patients develop distant metastases.

Side effects. The side effects and complications from radiation treatment of cancer of the kidney, renal pelvis, and ureters are similar to those expected from irradiation of the abdomen and pelvis. Acute side effects include nausea, vomiting, diarrhea, and abdominal cramping, which usually respond to conservative medical management.[52] The complication rate is related to the total dose and fraction size. With careful attention given to the treatment technique and dose-volume distribution, some complications can be eliminated.

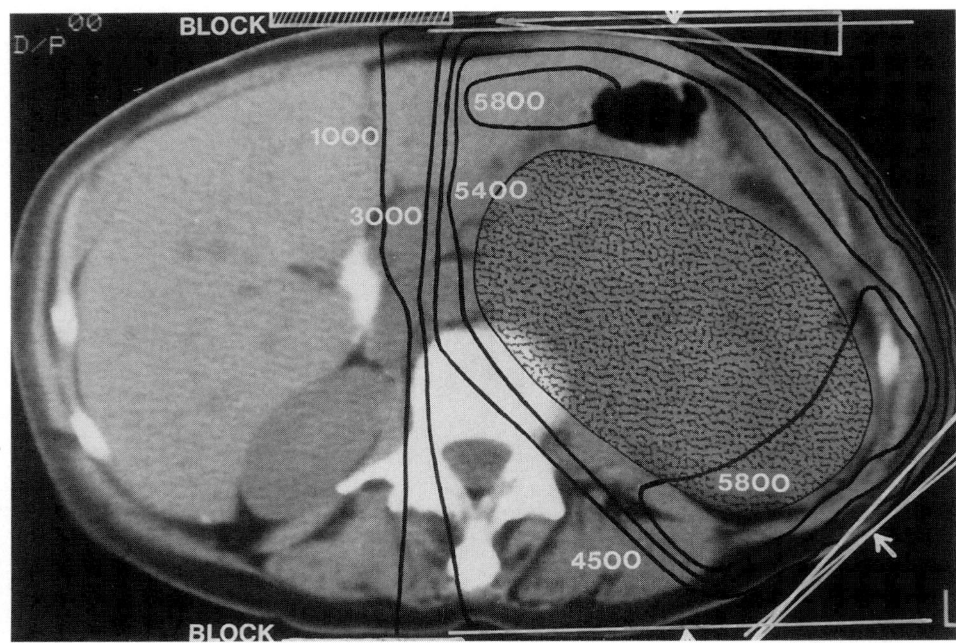

Fig. 12-20 Radiation dose distribution corresponding to the treatment portal in Fig. 12-19. Notice that a combination of AP/PA plus oblique portals with wedges is used to encompass the entire lesion with an isodose curve of 5400 cGy. The spinal cord dose is less than 4150 cGy. (From Lai PP: Kidney, renal pelvis, and ureter. In Perez CA, Brady LW, editors: *Principles and practice of radiation oncology,* ed 2, Philadelphia, 1992, JB Lippincott.)

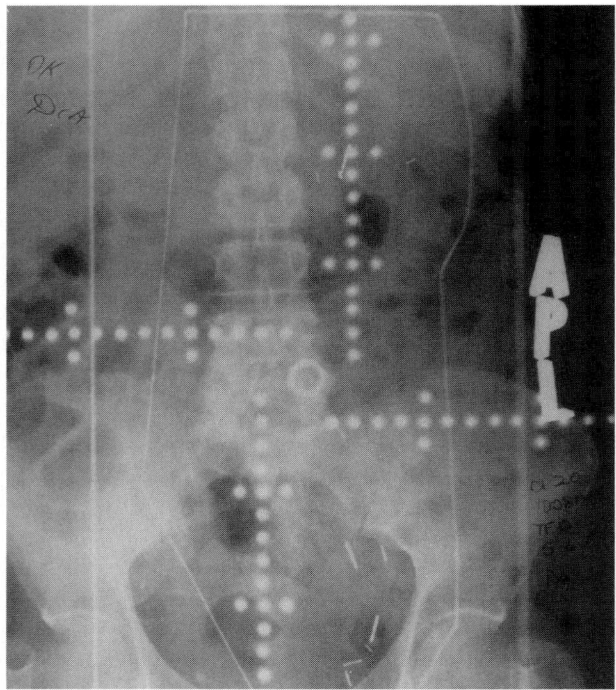

Fig. 12-21 A postoperative radiation portal for cancer of the renal pelvis and ureter. Usually, the entire renal fossa, ureteral bed, and ipsilateral trigone are included; the exact extent is determined by pathological information. (From Lai PP: Kidney, renal pelvis, and ureter. In Perez CA, Brady LW, editors: *Principles and practice of radiation oncology,* ed 2, Philadelphia, 1992, JB Lippincott.)

Table 12-10 Renal cell carcinoma: 5-year survival rates after nephrectomy or preoperative irradiation and nephrectomy

Author	Stage	Number of patients	Radiation dose/fraction size (cGy)	Treatment	5-year survival	Local recurrence (%)
van der Werf-Messing 1973*	P1	21		N	88%	0
		22	3000/200	RT + N	85%	0
	P2	19		N	64%	1
		12	3000/200	RT+N	62%	0
	P3	22		N	29%	3
		30	3000/200	RT+N	27%	3
van der Werf-Messing et al. (1978)†		85			No difference	
		89	3000-4000/200	RT+N		
Juusela et al. (1977)‡		50		N	63%	
		38	3300/220	RT+N	47%	
Rubin et al. (1975)§	II			N	52%	
			4500-4800/200	RT+N	68%	
	I			N	No difference	
			4500-4800/200	RT+N		

Modified from Lai PP: Kidney, renal pelvis, and ureter. In Perez CA, Brady LW, editors: *Principles and practice of radiation oncology*, ed 2, Philadelphia, 1992, JB Lippincott.

N, Nephrectomy; RT, preoperative radiation therapy.

*The 5-year actuarial survival rates were interpolated from a graph. Higher survival rates during the first 18 months were noted for P3 patients who received irradiation. Complete resectability was noted for 73% (22 of 30) of P3 patients who received irradiation, versus 50% (11 of 22) for those who did not receive radiation therapy. About 34% (43 of 126 patients) had P1 tumors and probably would not have benefited from radiation therapy anyway.

†The 126 patients reported in the 1973 study are apparently also included in this article. The radiation dose had apparently been changed to 4000 cGy for patients treated after 1973. The 5-year survival rate was about 50%, and the authors stated that "preoperative irradiation had no bearing on survival." The incidence of local recurrences was not reported.

‡Subgroup analysis by histological grade and pathological stage indicated no survival advantage for patients who received radiation therapy. However, there was no mention of local control or resectability.

§The 2-year survival rates were interpolated from a graph. In the study 155 patients were randomized to receive irradiation; the number of nephrectomy patients was not specified. Details of the radiation therapy technique were provided for only 101 of 155 patients; however, only 21 patients were adequately treated to the regional lymph nodes (>4000 cGy). Better survival rates (15% to 20% in the first 2 years) were noted in Stage II patients who received irradiation. No difference in surivival rates was detected in Stage I patients. The exact number in each subgroup was not specified.

ROLE OF RADIATION THERAPIST

Treatment-plan implementation

Accurate dose delivery, daily observation of the patient's tolerance to therapy, and psychological needs of the patient are important aspects of the radiation therapist's role. Reproducibility of the daily treatment is of prime importance because the patient's outcome depends on accurate dose delivery to the target volume and the sparing of critical structures. A positive outcome, however, can be overshadowed if the patient is unhappy because of a lack of appropriate psychological support and understanding of potential side effects during the course of treatment.

Treatment information and psychological support

Accurate dose delivery is important for the control of disease. However, patients are just as concerned with potential side effects of radiation treatments and the way they affect their daily routine and interactions with family and friends. The potential side effects of treatment to the abdomen and pelvis are similar to those of other sites treated with radiation, including skin reactions, fatigue, weight loss, nausea and vomiting, diarrhea, and hair loss in the area being treated.

Skin changes caused by radiation exposure depend on the beam energy and dose. Because most tumors in the abdomen and pelvis (>85%) are treated with a beam energy greater than 6 MV, skin reactions are usually not more severe than dry desquamation or slight tanning.[33] Single or parallel-opposed treatment fields given with beam energies less than 4 MV may produce more severe skin reactions because of higher surface doses for low-energy beams and the thick body parts involved. Patients should be instructed to avoid the use of harsh creams or soaps in the irradiated area.

Many patients are more easily fatigued during radiation treatments because much of the body's energy is being used to fight the disease process or repair the effects of radiation

Table 12-11 Renal cell carcinoma: 5-year survival rates after nephrectomy or postoperative irradiation and nephrectomy

Author	Stage	Number of patients	Radiation dose/fraction size (cGy)	Treatment	5-year survival rate	Local recurrence (%)
Peeling et al. (1969)*		96		N	52% (50/96)	
		68		N+RT	25% (17/68)	
Rafla (1970)†	All	96		N	37% (35/94)	
		94		N + RT	57% (46/81)	
	Renal vein	36		N	30% (11/36)	
	± others	40		N + RT	40% (14/35)	
	Renal pelvis	50		N	32% (16/49)	
	± others	60		N + RT	60% (30/50)	
	Renal capsule	52		N	28% (15.52)	
	± others	69		N + RT	57% (34/59)	
Rafla and Parikh (1984)‡		135		N	18% (24/135)	
		105	4500	N + RT	38% (40/105)	
Finney (1973)§		48		N	47% (17/35)	7
		52	5500/204	N + RT	36% (14/39)	7
Kjaer et al. (1987)‖		33		N	63%§	1
		32	5000/250	N + RT	38%‖	0

Modified from Lai PP: Kidney, renal pelvis, and ureter. In Perez CA, Brady LW, editors: *Principles and practice of radiation oncology,* 1992, JB Lippincott.

N, Nephrectomy; RT, postoperative radiation therapy.

*This is a retrospective study with incomplete staging information and no description of the radiation dose or technique. The endpoint was 5-year survival, with no mention of local recurrence.

†This is the only report that described the benefits of irradiation with survival *and* local recurrence as endpoints. Unfortunately, there was no description of the radiation dose or technique. The study was performed in the pre-CT era; therefore local recurrence is an underestimate. Subgroup analysis (involvement of renal vein, renal pelvis, renal capsule + others) indicated an effect of radiation therapy on survival.

‡The authors also showed some data attesting to the benefits of radiation therapy in patients with renal capsular, renal vein, and regional lymphatic involvement.

§This is a randomized study, but no staging information is available. The incidences of local recurrence and distant metastasis are similar. However, there are four fatal liver complications among the patients who received radiation therapy.

‖In this randomized study 27 or 32 patients assigned to the irradiation arm completed treatment; 12 of 27 (44%) reported significant complications, with five fatal complications related to irradiation.

on normal tissues. The therapist should counsel patients not to be alarmed if they are more easily tired during the course of treatment; patients should be told to maintain good nutrition and get plenty of rest to minimize weight loss and fatigue. If the patient encounters problems with nausea, vomiting, or diarrhea, the physician can prescribe medications to alleviate these symptoms.

Hair loss can occur in the irradiated field because of the sensitivity of the follicles to radiation. This hair loss may be permanent, depending on the dose of radiation.

The therapist should encourage the patient and family to discuss with the physician any problems concerning treatment. Problems dealing with transportation, work, or financial concerns should be referred to social service personnel to minimize the patient's emotional stress. A pleasant, friendly, and helpful attitude can also provide good emotional support.

Treatment planning and delivery

The basic steps in the planning and delivery of the physician's treatment plan generally apply to all sites. However, some issues that improve the daily reproducibility of the treatment apply specifically to abdominal and pelvic treatments. Procedures should be developed and followed to improve consistency in the setup between simulation and treatment units.

Simulation

Immobilization. The construction of immobilization devices (an important part of the treatment-planning process) should be accomplished during the initial simulation. The patient's treatment position must be established, and appropriate immobilization and repositioning devices should be constructed before any simulation films are taken or treatment-planning CT data are obtained. This helps ensure agreement in the transfer of information between the simulator and treatment unit.

Reproducibility of the patient setup can be improved with a treatment position that the patient can maintain through proper immobilization and repositioning devices. The method most commonly used for the immobilization of treatments to the abdomen and pelvis is the polyurethane foam mold with the patient in the supine position. However, thermal plastic molds are also being used at a few facilities with the patient in the prone position. Thermal plastic and foam devices that extend from the lower chest to the midthigh provide some improved reproducibility over those supporting only the area of interest because of a larger area for indexing the patient to the repositioning device.

Simulation and treatment variations. Daily isocenter variation in the AP/PA direction can be reduced by setting the isocenter based on the digital couch height or lateral lasers rather than using the optical distance indicator projected on the patient's skin surface. The depth of the isocenter should be checked daily for consistency and verification that the depth of calculation is not changing as a result of weight loss or bloating. Daily fluctuations of 1 to 2 cm in the skin's isocenter depth for an anterior abdominal or pelvic field are not uncommon. If the depth of calculation is consistently off in one direction, the physicist and physician should be notified so that the resulting change in dose may be evaluated for a new monitor unit calculation. Differences in the skin's isocenter depth on lateral or posterior fields are generally less than 1 cm when patients are carefully aligned with the sagittal lasers and the vertical height is set with a digital readout or lateral lasers. Variations in laser marks placed on the lateral aspect of the pelvis can also be reduced by placing a rubber band around the feet to hold them together.

Systematic errors can also occur from differences in the alignment of lasers and optical distance indicators from the simulator and the treatment unit. A tolerance of ±2 mm on the laser alignment or optical distance indicator can result in a 4-mm discrepancy in the setup from the simulator to the treatment unit. Similar discrepancies can occur from differences in the alignment of blocking trays from machine to machine caused by worn or damaged parts.

A study of variations in the daily setup of portals relative to bony landmarks in treatment of the prostate shows a maximum variation of 7 mm for patients with foam-mold immobilization and 15 mm without the immobilization device.[98] Average errors with and without the immobilization devices were 3.3 mm and 8 mm, respectively.

Treatment verification

Portal images of the treatment fields should be taken before treatment on the first day and compared with the simulation films for correct field placement. The first-day films serve as a guide for subsequent films taken during the course of therapy. Both portals for parallel-opposed beams should be filmed on the same day with a fiducial grid in place to distinguish block-mounting errors from patient-positioning or patient-movement errors. The fiducial grid provides a means for determining the magnification factor on the portal image so that required adjustments can be made easily. Interpreting anatomical changes resulting in a magnification change of corresponding anatomy on each of the images is also much easier with a fiducial grid in place.

Most conformal treatment techniques use multiple oblique beam arrangements, which are difficult to interpret for anatomical coverage and positional accuracy of the isocenter. For these reasons conformal beam arrangements are best evaluated from a set of orthogonal films that allow vertical and horizontal shifts in the isocenter position to be viewed separately. A set of portal images taken with the exact treatment angles may still be useful for documentation and comparison with the simulation films for anatomical coverage.

Dose-verification measurements can also be taken on all photon portals through the use of diode detector or thermoluminescent dosimeter. The dose measurements are meant to discover large-dose errors greater than ±5% resulting from incorrect or missing wedges, compensating filters, or incorrect monitor unit calculations.

Record-and-verify systems are also highly recommended to ensure that daily setups are consistent and correct.

Site-specific instructions

Some type of immobilization or repositioning device is always used for patients treated with conformal techniques. Immobilization is not always used in treatments to the whole pelvis or abdomen with parallel-opposed techniques. However, lasers are always used to aid in repositioning of the patient. Typical simulation procedures are listed in the simulation section.

Prostate. Patients should be treated when they have a full bladder to minimize the amount of bladder in the treatment portals.

Bladder. Patients should be treated when they have an empty bladder to maintain an adequate margin around the bladder during daily treatment.

Kidney. Considerations relative to abdominal treatments should be applied to treatment of the kidney.

Penis. The treatment approach depends on the need to treat only the penis or the penis and regional lymphatics. External beam therapy requires specially designed accessories (including bolus) to achieve homogeneous dose distribution to the entire organ involved.

Review Questions

Multiple Choice

1. What is the most common pathology of malignant tumors of the prostate?
   a. Squamous cell carcinoma
   b. Adenocarcinoma
   c. Transitional cell carcinoma
   d. Burkitt's cell carcinoma
2. What is the most common type of testicular tumor?
   a. Transitional cell lymphoma
   b. Choriocarcinoma
   c. Adenocarcinoma
   d. Seminoma
3. Which of the following has the highest incidence rate for males?
   a. Prostate cancer
   b. Penile cancer
   c. Kidney and ureteral cancer
   d. Lung cancer
4. Which of the following are common immobilization-repositioning devices used in the treatment of prostate cancer?
   I. Polyurethane molds
   II. Plaster casts
   III. Contrast media
   IV. Rubber bands around the feet
      a. I and III only
      b. I and IV only
      c. II and III only
      d. I, II and IV only

Fill in the Blank

5. For patients with bladder cancer the bladder should be _________ during radiation treatment.
   a. Empty
   b. Partially full
   c. Full
   d. Localized with contrast material
6. ______________ is a side effect associated with the treatment of prostate cancer, in which the adult male is unable to obtain an erection or ejaculate after achieving an erection.
   a. Benign Prostatic Hypertrophy
   b. Transurethral resection of the prostate
   c. Impotence
   d. None of the above

Questions to Ponder

1. Discuss the role of a digital rectal examination, prostate-specific antigen (PSA), and prostatic acid phosphatase in the screening of prostate cancer.
2. Compare and contrast the following prognostic indicators related to carcinoma of the prostate: age, race, PSA level, lymph node status, and method of biopsy.
3. Examine the following specific treatment options for carcinoma of the prostate: surgery, chemotherapy, hormones, external beam radiation therapy, and brachytherapy.
4. Discuss the general management of cancer (surgery versus radiation therapy) of the urinary bladder.
5. Compare the treatments for testicular seminoma and non-seminoma.
6. Analyze the role of the radiation therapist in the treatment of patients with genitourinary tumors.

REFERENCES

1. Adolfsson J, Steineck G, Whitmore WF Jr: Recent results of management of palpable clinical localized prostate cancer, *Cancer* 72:310-322, 1993.
2. American Cancer Society: *Cancer facts and figures—1996,* Atlanta, GA, 1996, The Society.
3. Aziz H et al: Radiation-treated carcinoma of prostate: Comparison of survival of black and white patients by Gleason's grading system, *Am J Clin Oncol* 11:166-171, 1988.
4. Bagshaw MA, Cox RS, Ray GR: Status of radiation therapy of prostate cancer at Stanford University, *NCI Monogr* 7:47-60, 1988.
5. Bagshaw MA, Ray GR, Cox RS: Radiotherapy of prostatic carcinoma: long- or short-term efficacy (Stanford University Experience), *Urology* 25:17-23, 1985.
6. Banker FL: The preservation of potency after external beam irradiation for prostatic cancer, *Int J Radiat Oncol Biol Phys* 15:219-220, 1988.
7. Beahrs OH et al, editors: *AJCC manual for staging of cancer,* ed 4, Philadelphia, 1992, JB Lippincott.
8. Benson MC: Fine-needle aspiration of the prostate, *NCI Monogr* 7:19-24, 1988.
9. Bracken RB, Henry R, Ordonez N: Primary carcinoma of the male urethra, *South Med J* 73:1003-1005, 1980.
10. Byar DP, Veterans Administration Cooperative Urological Research Group: Survival of patients with incidentally found microscopic cancer of the prostate: results of a clinical trial of conservative treatment, *J Urol* 108:908-913, 1972.
11. Catalona WJ, Bigg SW: Nerve-sparing radical prostatectomy: evaluation of results after 250 patients, *J Urol* 143:538-544, 1990.
12. Catalona WJ et al: Measurement of prostate-specific antigen in serum as a screening test for prostate cancer, *N Engl J Med* 324:1156-1161, 1991.
13. Chodak GW et al: Comparison of digital examination and transrectal ultrasonography for the diagnosis of prostate cancer, *J Urol* 135:951-954, 1986.
14. Coia LR, Hanks GE: Complications from large field intermediate dose infradiaphragmatic radiation: an analysis of the Patterns of Care Outcome Studies for Hodgkin's disease and seminoma, *Int J Radiat Oncol Biol Phys* 15:29-35, 1988.
15. Cox JD, Kline RW: Do prostate biopsies 12 months or more after external irradiation for adenocarcinoma, stage III, predict long-term survival? *Int J Radiat Oncol Biol Phys* 9:299-303, 1983.
16. Crawford ED, Dawkins CA: Cancer of the penis. In Skinner DG, Lieskovsky G, editors: Diagnosis and management of genitourinary cancer, Philadelphia, 1988, WB Saunders.
17. deKernion JB et al: Carcinoma of the penis, *Cancer* 32:1256-1262, 1973.
18. Drzymala RE et al: A system for ultrasound-guided transperineal interstitial implants of the prostate with iridium-192, *Endocurie Hypertherm* 9:69-76, 1993.
19. Duchesne GM et al: Orchiedectomy alone for stage I seminoma of the testis, *Cancer* 65:1115-1118, 1990.
20. Duncan W, Jackson SM: The treatment of early cancer of the penis with megavoltage X-rays, *Clin Radiol* 23:246-248, 1972.
21. Duncan W, Quilty PM: The results of a series of 963 patients with transitional cell carcinoma of the urinary bladder primarily treated by radical megavoltage x-ray therapy, *Radiother Oncol* 7:299-310, 1986.
22. Einhorn LH, Richie JP, Shipley WU: Cancer of the testis. In DeVita VJ Jr, Hellman S, Rosenberg SA, editors: *Cancer: principles and practice of oncology,* ed 4, Philadelphia, 1993, JB Lippincott.
23. Eisenberger MA: Chemotherapy for prostate cancer, *NCI Monogr* 7:151-163, 1988.
24. Ekstrom T, Edsmyr F: Cancer of the penis: a clinical study of 229 cases, *Acta Chir Scand* 115:25-45, 1958.
25. Emami BE, Pilepich MV: Anatomic considerations in radiotherapeutic management of bladder cancer, *Am J Clin Oncol (CCT)* 6:593-597, 1983.
26. Faysal MH, Freiha FS: Evaluation of partial cystectomy for carcinoma of bladder, *Urology* 14:352-356, 1979.
27. Flocks RH, Kadesky MC: Malignant neoplasms of the kidney: an analysis of 353 patients followed five years or more, *J Urol* 79(2):196, 1958.
28. Fossa SD, Aass N, Kaalhus O: Radiotherapy for testicular seminoma stage I: treatment results and long-term post-irradiation morbidity in 365 patients, *Int J Radiat Oncol Biol Phys* 16:383-388, 1989.
29. Fraas BA et al: Peripheral dose to the testes: the design and clinical use of a practical and effective gonadal shield, *Int J Radiat Oncol Biol Phys* 11:609-615, 1985.
30. Fraley EE et al: Cancer of the penis: prognosis and treatment plans, *Cancer* 55:1618-1624, 1985.
31. Gagliano RG et al: Cis-diamminedichloroplatinum in the treatment of advanced epidermoid carcinoma of the penis: a Southwest Oncology Group study, *J Urol* 141:66-67, 1989.
32. Gerber RL et al: Patterns of Care Survey results: treatment planning for carcinoma of the prostate. Presented at the AAPM Meeting, Anaheim, California, July 24-28, 1994.
33. Gleason DF, Veterans Administration Cooperative Urological Research Group: Histologic grading and clinical staging of prostatic carcinoma. In Tannenbaum M, editor: Urologic pathology: the prostate, Philadelphia, 1977, Lea & Febiger.
34. Golimbu M et al: Renal cell carcinoma: survival and prognostic factors, *Urology* 27(4):291-301, 1986.
35. Gray HG: *Anatomy, descriptive and surgical, 1901 ed.,* Philadelphia, 1974, Running Press.
36. Haile K, Delclos L: The place of radiation therapy in the treatment of carcinoma of the distal end of the penis, *Cancer* 45:1980-1984, 1980.
37. Hanks GE: External-beam radiation therapy for clinically localized prostate cancer: Patterns of Care Studies in the United States, *NCI Monogr* 7:75-84, 1988.
38. Hanks GE: Conformal radiation in prostate cancer: reduced morbidity with hope of increased local control, *Int J Radiat Oncol Biol Phys* 25:377-378, 1993
39. Hanks GE et al: Outcome for lymph node dissection negative T-1b, T-2 (A-2,B) prostate cancer treated with external beam irradiation therapy in RTOG 77-06, *Int J Radiat Oncol Biol Phys* 21:1099-1103, 1991.
40. Hanks GE et al: The outcome of treatment of 313 patients with T-1 (UICC) prostate cancer treated with external beam irradiation, *Int J Radiat Oncol Biol Phys* 14:243-248, 1988.
41. Heaney JA et al: Prognosis of clinically undiagnosed prostatic carcinoma and the influence of endocrine therapy, *J Urol* 118:283-287, 1977.
42. Henry K et al: Comparison of transurethral resection to radical therapies for stage B bladder tumors, *J Urol* 140:964-967, 1988.
43. Hilaris BS et al: Behavioral patterns of prostate adenocarcinoma following an ^{125}I implant and pelvic node dissection, *Int J Radiat Oncol Biol Phys* 2:631-637, 1977.
44. Huben RP, Mounzer AM, Murphy GP: Tumor grade and stage as prognostic variables in upper tract urothelial tumors, *Cancer* 62:2016-2020, 1988.
45. Hudson MA, Bahnson RR, Catalona WJ: Clinical use of prostate specific antigen in patients with prostate cancer, *J Urol* 142:1011-1017, 1989.
46. Huggins C, Stevens RE, Hodges CV: Studies on prostatic cancer. II. The effects of castration on advanced carcinoma of the prostate gland, *Arch Surg* 43:209-223, 1941.
47. Jakse G, Frommhold H, Nedden DZ: Combined radiation and chemotherapy for locally advanced transitional cell carcinoma of the urinary bladder, *Cancer* 55:1659-1664, 1985.
48. Johansson JE et al: High 10-year survival rate in patients with early, untreated prostatic cancer, *JAMA* 267:2191-2196, 1992.
49. Kjaer M: The treatment and prognosis of patients with renal adenocarcinoma with solitary metastasis 10 year survival results, *Int J Radiat Oncol Biol Phys* 13:619-621, 1987.

50. Kuban DA, El-Mahdi AM, Schellhammer PF: The significance of postirradiation prostate biopsy with long-term follow-up, *Int J Radiat Oncol Biol Phys* 24:409-414, 1992.
51. Kubo H, Shipley WU: Reduction of the scatter dose to the testicle outside the radiation treatment fields, *Int J Radiat Oncol Biol Phys* 8:1741-1745, 1982.
52. Lai PP: Kidney, renal pelvis, and ureter. In Perez CA, Brady LW, editors: *Principles and practice of radiation oncology,* ed 2, Philadelphia, 1992, JB Lippincott.
53. Lai PP et al: Radiation therapy for stage I and IIA testicular seminoma, *Int J Radiat Oncol Biol Phys* 28:373-379, 1993
54. Landmann C, Hunig R: Prostatic specific antigen as an indicator of response to radiotherapy in prostate cancer, *Int J Radiat Oncol Biol Phys* 17:1073-1076, 1989.
55. Lawton CA et al: Extended-field radiation therapy for prostatic carcinoma with paraaortic lymph node metastasis, *Am J Clin Oncol* 9:302-306, 1986.
56. Leibel SA et al: Three-dimensional conformal radiation therapy in locally advanced carcinoma of the prostate: preliminary results of a phase I dose-escalation study, *Int J Radiat Oncol Biol Phys* 28:55-65, 1994
57. Linehan WM, Shipley WU, Longo DL: Cancer of the kidney and ureter. In DeVita VT, Hellman S, Rosenberg SA, editors: *Cancer: principles and practice of oncology,* ed 3, Philadelphia, 1989, JB Lippincott.
58. Maldazys JD, deKernion JB: Prognostic factors in metastatic renal carcinoma, *J Urol* 136:376-379, 1986.
59. Mandler JI, Pool TL: Primary carcinoma of the male urethra, *J Urol* 96:67-72, 1966.
60. McGowan DG: The effect of transurethral resection on prognosis in carcinoma of the prostate: real or imaginary? *Int J Radiat Oncol Biol Phys* 15:1057-1064, 1988.
61. Mettlin C, Natarajan N: Epidemiologic observations from the American College of Surgeons' survey on prostate cancer, *Prostate* 4:323-331, 1983.
62. Mohiuddin M et al: Combined preoperative and postoperative radiation for bladder cancer: results of RTOG/Jefferson study, *Cancer* 55:963-966, 1985.
63. Mufti GR et al: Transitional cell carcinoma of the renal pelvis and ureter, *Br J Urol* 63:135-140, 1989.
64 Narayana AS et al: Carcinoma of the penis: analysis of 219 cases, *Cancer* 49:2185-2191, 1982.
65. Onik GM et al: Transrectal ultrasound-guided percutaneous radical cryosurgical ablation of the prostate, *Cancer* 72:1291-1299, 1993.
66. Parsons JT, Million RR: Planned preoperative irradiation in the management of clinical stage B2-C (T3) bladder carcinoma, *Int J Radiat Oncol Biol Phys* 14:797-810, 1988.
67. Partin AW et al: The use of prostate specific antigen, clinical stage and Gleason score to predict pathological stage in men with localized prostate cancer, *J Urol* 150:110-114, 1993.
68. Pearse HD: The kidney. In Moss WT, Cox JD, editors: *Radiation oncology: rationale, technique, results,* St Louis, 1989, Mosby.
69. Perez CA, Eisbruch A: Role of postradical prostatectomy irradiation in carcinoma of the prostate, *Semin Radiat Oncol* 3:198-209, 1993.
70. Perez CA et al: Factors influencing outcome of definitive radiotherapy for localized carcinoma of the prostate, *Radiother Oncol* 16:1-21, 1989.
71. Perez CA, Pilepich MV: Penis and male urethra. In Perez CA, Brady LW, editors: *Principles and practice of radiation oncology,* ed 2, Philadelphia, 1992, JB Lippincott.
72. Perez CA et al: Definitive radiation therapy in carcinoma of the prostate localized to the pelvis: experience at the Mallinckrodt Institute of Radiology, *NCI Monogr* 7:85-94, 1988.
73. Perez CA, Pilepich MV, Zivnuska FR: Tumor control in definitive irradiation of localized carcinoma of the prostate, *Int J Radiat Oncol Biol Phys* 12:523-531, 1986.
74. Pilepich MV et al: Correlation of pretreatment transurethral resection and prognosis in patients with stage C carcinoma of the prostate treated with definitive radiotherapy: RTOG experience, *Int J Radiat Oncol Biol Phys* 13:195-199, 1987.
75. Pilepich MV et al: Prognostic factors in carcinoma of the prostate: analysis of RTOG Study 75-06, *Int J Radiat Oncol Biol Phys* 13:339-349, 1987.
76. Porter AT et al: Results of randomized phase III trial to evaluate the efficacy of strontium-89 adjuvant to local external beam irradiation in the management of endocrine metastatic prostate cancer, *Int J Radiat Oncol Biol Phys* 25:805-813, 1993.
77. Powell BL, Craig JB, Muss HB: Secondary malignancies of the penis and epididymis: a case report and review of the literature, *J Clin Oncol* 3:110-116, 1985.
78 Pritchett TR, Lieskovsky G, Skinner DG: Clinical manifestations and treatment of renal parenchymal tumors. In Skinner DG, Lieskovsky G, editors: *Diagnosis and management of genitourinary tumors,* Philadelphia, 1988, WB Saunders.
79. Quilty PM et al: Results of surgery following radical radiotherapy for invasive bladder cancer, *Br J Urol* 58:396-405, 1986.
80. Raghavaiah NV: Radiotherapy in the treatment of carcinoma of the male urethra, *Cancer* 41:1313-1316, 1978.
81. Reitelman C et al: Prognostic variables in patients with transitional cell carcinoma of the renal pelvis and proximal ureter, *J Urol* 138:1144-1145, 1987.
82. Richards B et al: Adjuvant chemotherapy with doxorubicin (Adriamycin) and 5-fluorouracil in T3, NX, M0 bladder cancer treated with radiotherapy, *Br J Urol* 55:386-391, 1983.
83. Richie JP: Carcinoma of the renal pelvis and ureter. In Skinner DG, Lieskovsky G, editors: Diagnosis and management of genitourinary tumors, Philadelphia, 1988, WB Saunders.
84. Rifkin MD et al: Comparison of magnetic resonance imaging and ultrasonography in staging early prostate cancer: results of a multi-institutional cooperative trial, *N Engl J Med* 323:621-626, 1990.
85. Robson CJ, Churchill BM, Anderson W: The results of radical nephrectomy for renal cell carcinoma, *J Urol* 101:297, 1969.
86. Rotman M et al: Treatment of advanced transitional cell carcinoma of the bladder with irradiation and concomitant 5-fluorouracil infusion, *Int J Radiat Oncol Biol Phys* 18:1131-1137, 1990.
87. Rubin P et al: Preoperative irradiation in renal carcinoma: evaluation of radiation treatment plans, *Am J Roentgenl Radium Ther Nucl Med* 123(1):114-121, 1975.
88. Sagerman RH et al: Stage II seminoma: results of postorchiectomy irradiation, *Radiology* 172:565-568, 1989.
89. Salaverria JC et al: Conservative treatment of carcinoma of the penis, *Br J Urol* 51:32-37, 1979.
90. Scardino PT, Wheeler TM: Local control of prostate cancer with radiotherapy: frequency and prognostic significance of positive results of postirradiation prostate biopsy, *NCI Monogr* 7:95-103, 1988.
91. Schnall MD et al: Prostate cancer: local staging with endorectal surface coil MR imaging, *Radiology* 178:797-802, 1991.
92. Schultheiss TE et al: Factors influencing incidence of acute grade II morbidity in conformal therapy and standard radiation treatment of prostate cancer: univariate and multivariate analysis, *Int J Radiat Oncol Biol Phys (*in press).
93. Shapiro E et al: Effects of fractionated irradiation on endocrine aspects to testicular function, *J Clin Oncol* 3:1232-1239, 1985.
94. Shipley WU et al: Treatment of invasive bladder cancer by cisplatin and radiation in patients unsuited for surgery, *JAMA* 258(7):931-935, 1987.

95. Shipley WU et al: Full-dose irradiation for patients with invasive bladder carcinoma: clinical and histological factors prognostic of improved survival, *J Urol* 134:679-683, 1985.
96. Skinner DG, Tift JP, Kaufman JJ: High dose, short course preoperative radiation therapy and immediate single stage radical cystectomy with pelvic node dissection in the management of bladder cancer, *J Urol* 127:671-674, 1982.
97. Soffen EM et al: Conformal static field radiation therapy treatment of early prostate cancer versus non-conformal techniques: a reduction in acute morbidity, *Int J Radiat Oncol Biol Phys* 24:485-488, 1992.
98. Soffen EM et al: Conformal static field therapy for low volume low grade prostate cancer with rigid immobilization, *Int J Radiat Oncol Biol Phys* 20:141-146, 1991.
99. Spera JA et al: A comparison of preoperative radiotherapy regimens for bladder carcinoma: The University of Pennsylvania experience, *Cancer* 61:255-262, 1988.
100. Stamey TA, Kabalin JN, Ferrari M: Prostate specific antigen in the diagnosis and treatment of adenocarcinoma of the prostate. III. Radiation treated patients, *J Urol*141:1084-1087, 1989.
101. Stein JJ, Kaufman JJ: The treatment of carcinoma of the bladder with special reference to the use of preoperative radiation therapy combined with 5-fluorouracil, *Am J Roentgenol Radium Ther Nucl Med* 102:519-529, 1968.
102. Sternberg CN et al: Preliminary results of M-VAC (methotrexate, vinblastine, doxorubicin and cisplatin) for transitional cell carcinoma of the urothelium, *J Urol* 133:403-407, 1985.
103. Straffon RA et al: Yttrium hypophysectomy in the management of metastatic carcinoma of the prostate gland in 13 patients, *J Urol* 99:102-105, 1968.
104. Thomas G et al: Consensus statement on the investigation and management of testicular seminoma 1989, *EORTC Genitourinary Group Monogr* 7:285-294, 1990.
105. Thomas GM, Williams SD: Testis. In Perez CA, Brady LW, editors: *Principles and practice of radiation oncology,* ed 2, Philadelphia, 1992, JB Lippincott.
106. Timmer PR, Hartlief HA, Hooijkaas JAP: Bladder cancer: Pattern of recurrence in 142 patients, *Int J Radiat Oncol Biol Phys* 11:899-905, 1985.
107. Varma JS, Smith AN, Busuttil A: Function of the anal sphincters after chronic radiation injury, *Gut* 27:528-533, 1986.
108. Whitmore WF Jr, Batata MA, Hilaris BS: Prostate irradiation: iodine-125 implementation. In Johnson DE, Samuels ML, editors: *Cancer of the genitourinary tract,* New York, 1979, Raven Press.
109. Worgul TJ, et al: Clinical and biochemical effect of aminoglutethimide in the treatment of advanced prostatic carcinoma, *J Urol* 129:51-55, 1983.
110. Yu GSM, Nseyo UO, Carson JW: Primary penile lymphoma in a patient with Peyronie's disease, *J Urol* 142:1076-1077, 1989.
111. Zagars GK: Stage I testicular seminoma following orchidectomy: to treat or not to treat, *Eur J Cancer* 14:1923-1924, 1993.
112. Zagars GK,Babaian RJ: The role of radiation in stage II testicular seminoma, *Int J Radiat Oncol Biol Phys* 13:163-170, 1987.

BIBLIOGRAPHY

Fleming C et al: A decision analysis of alternative treatment strategies for clinically localized prostate cancer, *JAMA* 269:2650-2659, 1993.

Jackson SM: The treatment of carcinoma of the penis, *Br J Surg* 53:33-35, 1966.

Marshall VF: The relation of preoperative estimate to the pathologic demonstration of the extent of vesical neoplasms, *J Urol* 68:714-723, 1952.

C H A P T E R

13

Breast Cancer

Cheryl R. Glisch
Susan Barber-Derus

Outline

Key terms

Adjuvant therapy
Aneuploid
Atypical hyperplasia
Carcinoma in situ
Coplanar
Fibrosis
Hyperpigmentation
Menarche
Menopause
Necrosis
Oophorectomy
Ploidy
Specificity
Telangiectasia

HISTORICAL PERSPECTIVE

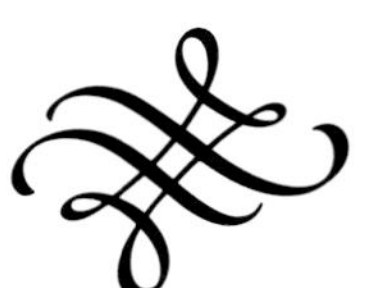

The recorded history of the treatment of breast cancer dates back 5000 years to a document known as the *Edwin Smith Papyrus.* Written between 3000 and 2500 BC, the papyrus discusses surgical and other treatments for illnesses afflicting the ancient Egyptians. A translation of the document, first published in 1930, reveals that, at the time, there was believed to be no treatment for what were most likely malignant tumors of the breast.

Several millennia later, Hippocrates (460-370 BC), the revered Greek physician who gave the name *carcinoma* to malignant disease, referred only twice to breast cancer. Both references describe advanced disease that resulted in the patient's death. He felt that it was better not to treat deep-seated cancer, because in his experience, treatment only hastened death. Hippocrates taught that cancer was caused by an excess or imbalance of "black bile" in the body.[31] Therefore medical belief of the day was that cancer is a systemic disease and essentially incurable.

During the Roman Empire, physicians performed surgery for breast cancer, sometimes using an extremely aggressive approach that included removal of the pectoralis muscles. This approach was discouraged by Aulus Celsus, an important scholar of the early first century AD, who wrote that cancer of the breast is "irritated" by the surgeon's intervention and thus results more rapidly in the patient's death than treatment with "mild medicines."

Leonidus, a Greek physician from the first century AD, described the surgical procedure he used for breast cancer.

He removed the breast with a margin of normal-appearing tissue and was careful to stop the bleeding during surgery through the use of cautery (heat).

Claudius Galen (138-201 AD), a physician who was educated in Greece and practiced in Rome, became the authority on medicine for the next 1000 years. Galen subscribed to Hippocrates' black bile theory of the systemic nature of cancer, and he recommended no intervention in the course of the disease.

During the 1000 years that comprised the Medieval period, or Dark Ages, which followed the fall of the Roman Empire, essentially no advances were made in the scientific understanding of cancer or any human illnesses. This was a period of political and religious activity, to the exclusion of scientific endeavor. Restrictions placed on the study and practice of medicine by religious authorities and adherence to the teachings of Galen as all encompassing left the world of medicine basically unchanged for a millennium. Despite the lack of advancement between 500 and 1500 AD, knowledge of medicine and an appreciation for learning were kept alive in monasteries. Eventually, the foundations of future progress were laid in the eleventh century, when several medical schools came into existence in cities such as Paris and Oxford.

In the middle of the sixteenth century, Andreas Versalius published *De Humani Corporis Fabrica,* the work that established the science of human anatomy. Humans were no longer bound by religious dictum and centuries of tradition. Increasingly, extensive surgical techniques were developed. The seventeenth century saw the treatment of breast cancer evolve to include the excision of enlarged axillary lymph nodes at the time of mastectomy. However, in the days before anesthesia and asepsis, surgery of any kind was fraught with danger for patients, many of whom died of overwhelming infection.

A revolution in thinking relative to the nature of breast cancer occurred in the mideighteenth century, when French surgeons Henri Le Dran and Jean Louis Petit theorized that the disease originated locally in the breast and was not initially systemic. They believed the malignancy spread from its primary site in the breast to involve regional lymph nodes and ultimately to disseminate widely via the circulatory system. As a result, physicians of the day realized an opportunity to cure patients if the cancer could be removed early in its course and if local control could be established. Therefore wide surgical excision with axillary dissection and removal of the pectoralis muscle was advised.

With the advent of anesthesia, antisepsis, and the ability to examine tissue microscopically in the midnineteenth century, radical breast surgery evolved rapidly. William Stewart Halsted perfected the technique of radical mastectomy shortly before the turn of the century. For the first time a dramatic improvement in local recurrence and overall survival rates could be demonstrated. The Halstedian approach remained preeminent until the midtwentieth century.

Current concepts in the treatment of breast cancer include a much less radical role for surgery and the emergence of radiation therapy and systemic drug treatment, all of which have permitted a conservative, breast-preserving approach in women with relatively early disease. However, although great strides have been made in the detection and treatment of breast cancer, it remains a disease that defies complete control. Approximately 20% of women who have breast cancer die of the disease.[17] Therefore the need exists for continued research into improved treatment modalities, earlier diagnoses, and ultimately, the prevention of breast cancer.

EPIDEMIOLOGY

Incidence

According to American Cancer Society statistics, breast cancer is the most common malignant disease in American women, affecting an estimated 184,300 new patients in 1996. In addition, breast cancer was diagnosed in about 1400 men during the same year. Current data indicate that every woman has approximately a one in eight chance of developing breast cancer over her lifetime.[1] The incidence rate has steadily risen since the 1980s, correlating with diagnostic advances and the increased use of mammography.

Fig. 13-1 shows 1996 estimates for leading sites of cancer incidence and death. Approximately 44,300 women and 240 men will die of breast cancer in 1996.[1] In women, breast cancer is the second major cause of cancer death, preceded only by lung cancer. Despite a rise in incidence, early detection and treatment advances have maintained stable mortality rates over the past 50 years.

Risk factors

Gender. The most significant risk factor for breast cancer is gender. The female-to-male incidence ratio is approximately 100 to 1.[1] In men, breast cancer represents less than 1% of all malignancies.[18] Major risk factors for women are listed in the box below.

Major Risk Factors for Breast Cancer

- Gender
- Age
- Family history
- Hormonal factors
- History of other malignancies
  - Previous breast cancer
  - Colon, thyroid, uterus, ovary, and salivary gland
- History of benign breast disease
  - Atypical hyperplasia
  - Lobular carcinoma in situ

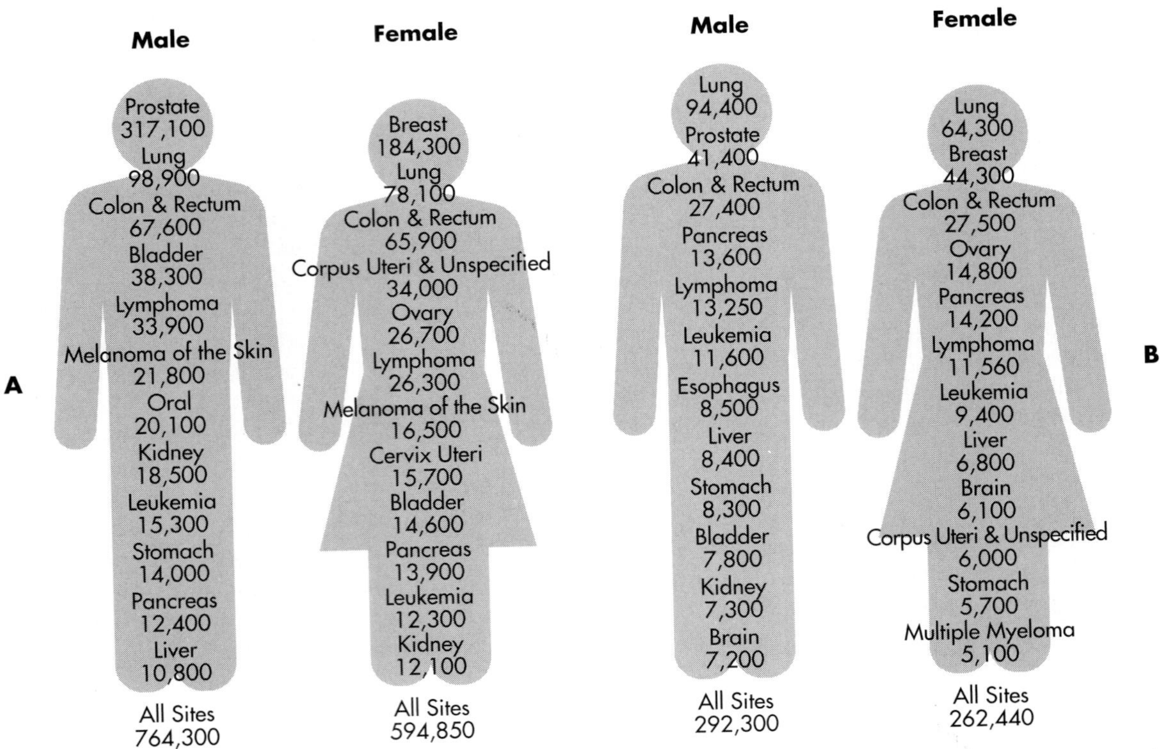

Fig. 13-1 Leading sites of new cancer cases and deaths, 1996 estimates. **A,** This illustration shows cancer cases by site and gender (excluding basal and squamous cell skin cancer and carcinoma in situ). **B,** This illustration shows cancer deaths by site and gender. (From the American Cancer Society: *Cancer facts and figures,* Atlanta, 1996, The Society.)

Age. Older women have the highest probability of developing breast cancer. Women 80 to 84 years old have an incidence rate of 435 per 100,000. This is double the rate for women 50 to 54 years old, whose incidence rate is 212 per 100,000.[27] Although incidence rates are high for older persons, these patients represent only a small number of the total cases.

Incidence rises steadily during the reproductive years after age 30. The median age of onset is approximately 55 years, with the predominant age group between 40 and 70 years.[11] A slight decrease in incidence occurs in the perimenopausal years, followed by a gradual rise during postmenopausal years. The decrease in incidence is attributed to hormonal changes that occur during menopause.

Family history. Genetic associations and racial differences in breast cancer rates suggest inherited tendencies toward development of the disease. Although hereditary patterns may be partially attributed to shared risk factors such as dietary and environmental factors, a genetic association is strongly suggested. Family history appears to be significant because female relatives of women with breast cancer have a higher incidence than the general population. However, despite the influence of hereditary patterns, less than 20% of new breast cancer cases diagnosed each year are associated with a significant family history.

The probability of developing breast cancer is highest for women whose mothers and/or sisters (first-degree relatives) have the disease, especially if the family members were premenopausal. Overall, these women have two to three times the usual risk of developing breast cancer.[23] Women with a strong family history of breast cancer must follow a good breast health program.

The gene BRCA 1-2 is associated with a 100% likelihood of breast cancer development. This particular type of heritable breast cancer comprises less than 4% of all cases. In the future, women of families with multiple cases of breast cancer may be tested for this gene so that the risk will be known.

Hormonal factors. Risk factors for breast cancer are influenced by hormonal variables, as listed in the box on p. 293. These risk factors appear to reflect menstrual and childbearing history. Early **menarche** (the beginning of menstruation) and late **menopause** (the ending of menstruation) increase breast cancer risk. **Oopherectomy** (removal of one or both ovaries) before age 50 appears to reduce risk.[17] These facts lead to a general assumption that the overall length of ovarian function is related to breast cancer risk.

Women who have given birth to a child (parous women) have less risk than women who have never been pregnant (nulliparous women). Pregnancy later in life increases the

Hormonal Influences on Breast Cancer Risk

- Ovarian function
  - Age at menarche
  - Age at menopause
  - Oophorectomy
- Parity
- Hormonal manipulation

risk more than nulliparity. Women who give birth to their first child after age 35 are twice as likely to develop breast cancer as women who give birth to their first child before age 20.[17]

Hormonal manipulation, relative to progesterone and estrogen, has also been associated with an increased incidence of breast cancer. Women taking estrogens (used to alleviate menopausal symptoms) and those taking oral contraceptives (used to prevent ovulation) continue to be studied for hormonal causation of or protection from the development of breast cancer. Although information to date is inconclusive, the magnitude of alteration in risk caused by hormonal manipulation, if any, appears to be quite small.

History of malignancy. A history of breast cancer, either invasive or ductal **carcinoma in situ** (cancer confined to the breast), in one breast increases the risk for development of cancer in the opposite breast. The greatest risk is for women treated curatively for breast cancer at a relatively young age. Breast cancer patients must be closely monitored for the development of a contralateral breast malignancy.

Women with a history of malignant tumors of the colon, thyroid, uterus, ovary, or major salivary glands have also demonstrated an increased risk for breast cancer. Patients with these malignant diagnoses may share some of the dietary and hormonal factors that appear to influence breast cancer risk.

History of benign breast disease. Benign breast disease encompasses a variety of histological subcategories associated with varying degrees of cancer risk. Women with **atypical hyperplasia** or lobular carcinoma in situ have an increased risk of developing breast cancer. These abnormal findings, in association with a family history of breast cancer, may increase the risk between 20% and 25% at 15 years.[37]

Dietary and environmental factors. International differences in breast cancer rates have been well documented. Incidence rates are higher in Europe, Canada, and the U.S. and lower in the Orient and developing countries such as Mexico. Caucasian women have a higher incidence of breast cancer than non-Caucasian women. Increased incidence has been observed for women who migrate from low-incidence areas to high-incidence areas, indicating that environmental and dietary factors influence the level of risk.

Total caloric intake and obesity are less relevant than fat intake. Risk from fat intake is relative to the type and amount of fat in the diet. Animal fat is the type associated with the highest risk.

Moderate consumption of alcohol (more than two drinks per day) appears to increase the risk of breast cancer development. The exact level of consumption relative to risk remains controversial. Alcohol consumption appears to have the greatest effect on breast cancer risk in women under the age of 30.[36]

Radiation exposure. Radiation exposure causes breast cancer. However the issue is complicated by numerous variables, including the type and quality of radiation, frequency of exposure, and magnitude of dose. Retrospective studies of women exposed to low levels of radiation for the monitoring of tuberculosis or treatment of benign conditions such as postpartum mastitis or fibroadenomas of the breast indicate increased breast cancer incidence. Subsequently, the treatment of nonmalignant conditions with radiation has been almost completely abandoned.

Much information on cancer induction by radiation exposure has been gained from the study of Hiroshima and Nagasaki atomic bomb survivors. A series of reports have been prepared by the National Research Council's committees on the Biological Effects of Ionizing Radiations (BEIR). The BEIR V report indicates that radiation-induced cancer is dose and time dependent and that the latent period appears to be relatively long (between 20 and 30 years).[8] The risk of breast cancer resulting from radiation appears to be greatest for women exposed at a relatively young age.

A threshold dose for breast cancer induction by radiation has not been determined. It is possible that exposure at levels similar to that of natural background radiation carries no risk. Based on current knowledge, the risk of radiation-induced breast cancer rarely contraindicates medically necessary radiation exposure.

PROGNOSTIC INDICATORS

The box on p. 294 lists prognostic indicators for breast cancer; however, the list continues to expand through clinical and laboratory research. The pathological staging system incorporates the most important factors, including the lymph node status, extent of the tumor, and presence of distant metastasis.

Lymph node status

The number of axillary lymph nodes involved by a tumor is the most important prognostic indicator and is a significant aspect of staging. A higher number of involved nodes correlates with an increased recurrence rate and a decreased survival rate. At least 10 axillary nodes must be evaluated to separate low risk (fewer than three positive nodes) from high risk (four or more positive nodes). The prognosis for patients with more than 10 positive axillary lymph nodes is extremely poor.

The involvement of internal mammary lymph nodes by cancer, with or without axillary lymph node involvement,

Prognostic Indicators for Breast Cancer

- Lymph node status
- Tumor extent
- Histology
- Estrogen and progesterone receptor status
- Flow cytometry
- Other laboratory studies

further reduces disease-free survival rates. Similarly, supraclavicular lymph node involvement implies a poor prognosis.

Tumor extent

The size of the primary tumor is another aspect of the staging system that serves as a prognostic indicator. Larger tumors increase the likelihood of involvement of the skin, muscle, chest wall, and regional lymph nodes, resulting in a worse overall prognosis. The 5-year survival rate for patients with lesions less than 0.5 cm is 99%, whereas the rate associated with lesions over 5 cm is 82%. With regional lymph node metastasis, 4.5-cm tumors have a 70% incidence rate of nodal involvement, whereas 1.5-cm tumors have a 38% incidence rate.[36]

Although tumor location by quadrant influences the pattern of lymph node metastasis, no evidence indicates that the location of the primary tumor directly affects the prognosis. The fixation of a mass to the chest wall involves significant negative staging and prognostic implications.

Histology

Infiltrating ductal carcinoma is the most common histological type of breast malignancy, accounting for 70% of all breast cancers. Infiltrating lobular carcinoma is the next most common type, comprising about 5% to 10% of breast cancers.[17]

There are several other relatively rare types of infiltrating cancer, such as mucinous or colloid, tubular, and papillary carcinoma. These lesions have distinct histological characteristics and tend to yield a more favorable prognosis.

Inflammatory carcinoma

Tumors classified as inflammatory carcinoma yield an extremely poor prognosis. The diagnosis of inflammatory cancer is based on pathological evidence of malignancy and clinical findings of breast tenderness and enlargement, Peau d' orange appearance, erythema, warmth, and diffuse induration of the skin.

Estrogen and progesterone receptor status

Samples of tumor tissue should be analyzed to determine the effect of estrogen and progesterone on the cells. This information and other factors indicate the potential response to hormonal therapy. Patients who are receptor positive are more likely to respond to hormonal therapy. However, a receptor-negative status does not automatically indicate a lack of response to hormonal therapy. In general, patients with receptor-positive tumors have a better outcome than those with receptor-negative tumors.

Flow cytometry

Deoxyribonucleic acid (DNA) from breast cancer cells is routinely evaluated for prognostic information. The content of the DNA is studied for **ploidy** status because **aneuploid** tumors are associated with a poorer prognosis than diploid tumors. Cell-cycle indicators are an even more sensitive marker for prognosis than ploidy status. Tumors with a high proportion of cells in the S phase of the cell cycle tend to be much more aggressive.

Other laboratory studies

Thymidine labeling indices, growth regulators, oncogene amplification, protein levels, and the use of monoclonal antibodies are under investigation for their prognostic and predictive value. These laboratory tests indicate the tumor cell proliferation, DNA content (ploidy), and fraction of tumor cells in the S phase of the cell cycle. Knowledge of such predictive factors influences treatment-management decisions.

Survival

Advancements in methods of detection and treatment of breast cancer have resulted in improved survival rates at all stages. The overall 5-year survival rate, indicated by women surviving 5-years after the initial diagnosis (regardless of disease status), is 96%. The 5-year survival rate decreases to 75% if evidence exists of regional spread and to 20% if distant metastasis is present at the time of the diagnosis.[1] Survival rates correlate with early detection, tumor characteristics, the treatment approach, and the patient's general condition.

However, 5-year survival is not the best indicator of survival for breast cancer patients. Because of breast cancer's systemic nature, patients may relapse up to 20 years or more after treatment, and few options are available for cure after relapse. According to 1996 American Cancer Society statistics, the 10-year breast cancer survival rate is 65%, and the 15-year survival rate is 56%.

ANATOMY

Embryology

The breast evolves from sudoriferous (sweat) gland tissue. Early in human fetal development the galactic band or milk streak develops, extending bilaterally from the axilla to the inguinal region. The portion of the band located on the thoracic trunk continues to develop, with the appearance of cells that form the nipple, areola, and ultimately all tissues of the breast. The remainder of the band regresses and disappears.

Location and extent

The protuberant portion of the adult breast is located between the second and sixth ribs in the sagittal plane and extends from the sternochondral junctions to the midaxillary line in the axial plane. Additional breast tissue is often present beyond these margins, particularly medially and superiorly. Breast tissue is also in the axilla, which is referred to as the *axillary tail of Spence.* The average diameter of the gland at its base is 10 to 12 cm, and the average central thickness is 5 or 6 cm.

Structure

The breast parenchyma consists of 15 to 20 sections or lobes that are embedded in adipose (fat) tissue. Each lobe is drained by a system of ducts that open at the nipple. In each lobe are numerous lobules that contain the milk-producing alveoli. The subcutaneous tissues of the breast also include fat, connective tissue, circulatory and lymphatic vessels, and nerve supply (Figs. 13-2 and 13-3).

The skin overlying the breast is thin and contains sweat glands, hair follicles, and sebaceous (oil) glands. The circular, pigmented area surrounding the nipple is the areola. The nipple and areola are largely composed of smooth muscle tissue and contain sweat and sebaceous glands.

Musculature

The breast is contiguous with or in close proximity to several functionally important muscles. These include the pectoralis major and minor, serratus anterior, and latissimus dorsi. The breast lies over the pectoralis major and serratus anterior muscles and is attached to them by a layer of connective tissue, the deep pectoral fascia. The superficial pectoral fascia encompasses the breast tissue and is attached to the deep fascia by bands of connective tissue called *Cooper's suspensory ligaments,* which support the breast. Surgical approaches to breast cancer have historically involved the removal of several of these muscles, at times producing significant disfigurement and functional deficit.

Blood supply

Arteries. The major arterial supply to the breast is via the branches of the internal mammary artery. Several branches of the axillary artery provide blood to the lateral aspect of the breast, most notably the lateral thoracic artery.

Veins. The deep venous drainage of the breast lies along three major routes that play significant roles in the development of blood-borne metastasis from breast cancer. The internal mammary vein, axillary vein, and intercostal veins empty into the pulmonary capillaries via the superior vena cava, allowing metastatic spread into the lung.

In addition, the intercostal veins communicate with the vertebral plexus of Batson, a system of small veins running vertically through and around the vertebral column. This system drains the proximal humeri, shoulders, skull, vertebral bodies, bony pelvis, and proximal femurs. Venous blood can flow in both directions in this system because of the

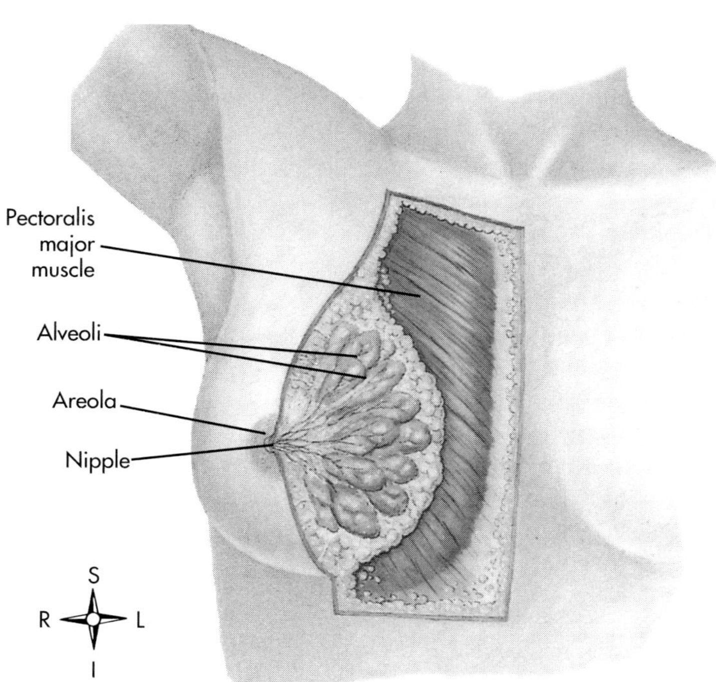

Fig. 13-2 Dissected view of the breast. (From Thibodeau GA, Patton KT: *Anatomy and Physiology,* ed 3, St Louis, 1996, Mosby.)

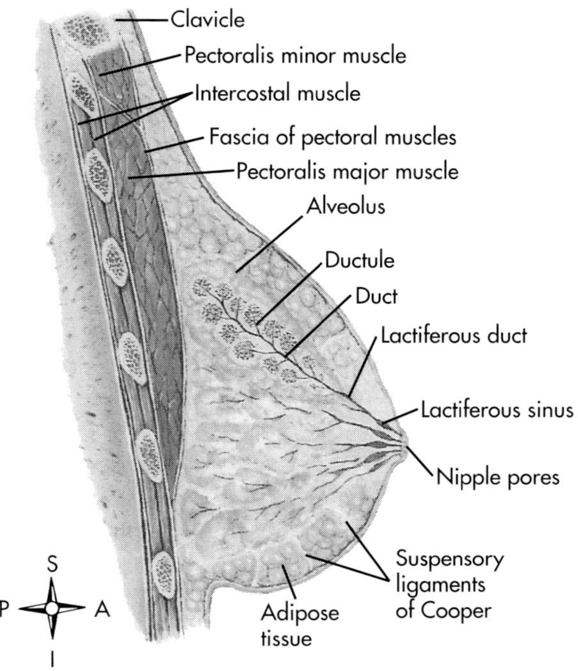

Fig. 13-3 Sagittal section of the breast. (From Thibodeau GA, Patton KT: *Anatomy and Physiology,* ed 3, St Louis, 1996, Mosby.)

absence of valves and low pressure in the channels. Malignant cells in the blood draining through the intercostal veins from the breast can therefore enter the axial skeleton, resulting in metastatic disease.

Lymphatic drainage

Lymph vessels. Two sets of lymphatic channels are associated with the breast. These were first delineated in the late eighteenth century by Cruikshank and Mascagni, who used injections of mercury on cadavers to visualize the lymphatics of this area.[10,25] The first group of lymphatics is superficial and drains the skin covering the breast. The second is a deep group that drains the internal breast tissues. The superficial and deep groups of lymphatics communicate with each other extensively, a fact that has implications for the management of breast cancer.[16] Fig. 13-4 illustrates lymphatic channels of the breast.

Axillary lymph nodes. Primary deep lymphatic drainage of the breast occurs to the ipsilateral axilla. Between 10 and 38 lymph nodes are in each axilla. These can be divided into three major sections (Levels I, II, and III) based on location and sequential drainage patterns. Nodes in Level I are located lowest, or most superficially, in the axilla and represent the first station of drainage from the breast. These are followed by nodes in Levels II and III, which are positioned at increasing height in the axilla.[18] Studies in the 1800s first demonstrated that 70% of the lymphatic drainage of the breast occurs to the axilla, with 30% going to the internal mammary nodes.

Internal mammary lymph nodes. The internal mammary lymph nodes are located near the edge of the sternum, embedded in fat in the intercostal spaces. The majority of internal mammary nodes are in the first, second, and third intercostal spaces, with the average person having approximately eight small nodes (four per side).[18]

Supraclavicular lymph nodes. In addition to direct drainage to the previously mentioned nodal groups, lymphatic drainage occurs from the breast to the supraclavicular nodes, liver, and contralateral internal mammary nodes.

NATURAL HISTORY

Sites of origin

The location of a primary breast tumor is best described by dividing the breast into quadrants. As shown in Fig. 13-5, approximately 48% of breast cancers arise in the upper-outer quadrant, 15% in the upper-inner quadrant, 11% in the lower-outer quadrant, 6% in the lower-inner quadrant, and 17% in the subareolar area (around the nipple, where the ducts converge); an additional 3% are multicentric.[17] The higher frequency of cancers in the upper-outer quadrant is explained

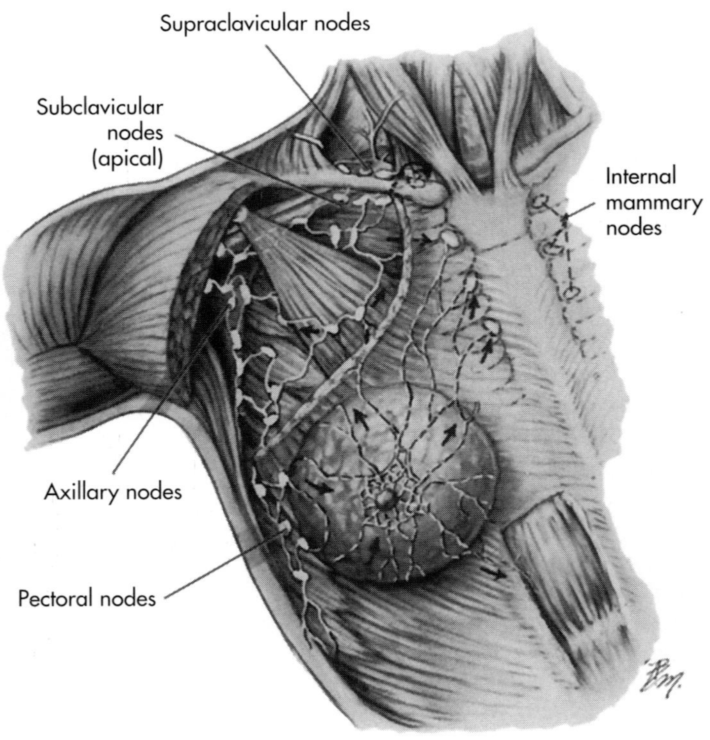

Fig. 13-4 Lymph drainage and lymph node groups of the breast. (From Cox JD, editor: *Moss' radiation oncology: rationale, technique, results,* ed 7, St Louis, 1994, Mosby.)

by the fact that more breast tissue is contained in this area. Breast cancer rarely appears in both breasts (bilaterally).

The term *multicentric* describes tumors that appear in several areas of the breast. Multifocal breast cancer denotes a situation in which elements of a tumor are contained in tissue near the primary lesion in the same quadrant. Multifocal breast cancer is more common than multicentric cancer and is prognostically more favorable.[17]

Tumor progression

Breast cancer tends to grow locally, involving the ducts and adjacent tissues, and may spread to local and regional lymphatics. Left untreated, the cancer can become fixed in position, and the overlying skin may become infiltrated by the tumor, eventually causing ulceration. Disease involving the dermal lymphatics is a sign of inflammatory cancer.

The involvement of axillary lymph nodes occurs orderly and progressively. Large tumor size and multicentricity are highly associated with axillary lymph node involvement. Lesions of the upper-outer quadrant more frequently metastasize to the axillary lymph nodes, whereas lesions of the medial quadrants and central area have a tendency to metastasize to the internal mammary lymph nodes. Progressive involvement of supraclavicular lymph nodes may also occur.

Recurrence

Breast cancer can recur in the breast (local recurrence), in the lymphatics (regional recurrence), or at distant metastatic sites. Patients with local recurrence after conservative treatment can be treated with additional surgery. Patients who experience regional recurrence are usually treated with systemic therapy and, if possible, surgical resection.

Distant metastasis

Breast cancer can spread to distant sites via invasion of the blood vessels, followed by hematogenous spread to other sites. Distant metastatic sites include bone, brain, liver, lung, eyes, ovaries, and adrenal and pituitary glands.

CLINICAL PRESENTATION

With early detection, breast cancer is one of the most curable malignant diseases. A three-step breast health program is recommended for all women. This program includes a monthly self-examination, an annual clinical examination by a qualified medical professional, and a routine mammographic examination as defined by established guidelines. Women must pay careful attention to breast cancer warning signs. Presenting symptoms of breast cancer are listed in the box on p. 298.

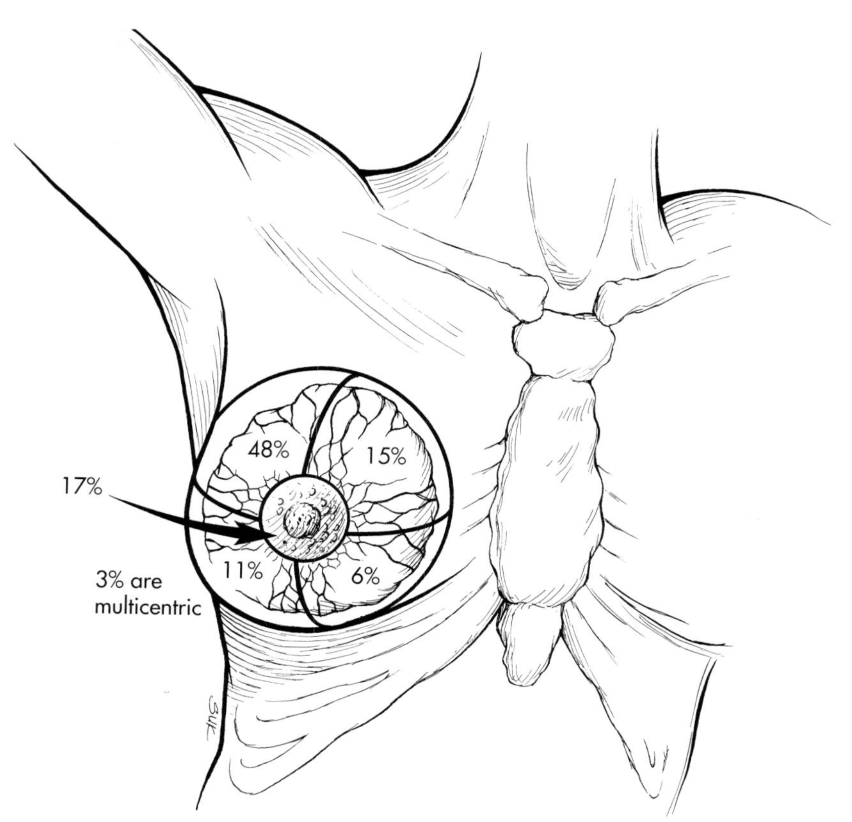

Fig. 13-5 Frequency of breast lesions by location in the breast.

Although most changes of the breast are benign, 20% of all masses are malignant. The potential for a malignant diagnosis, combined with the shortness of breast tumor doubling time, warrants immediate attention and close follow-up of women with breast complaints. Women who follow a good breast health program and seek medical attention promptly after the detection of breast changes may benefit from an early diagnosis and treatment, ultimately leading to a better outcome.

Breast mass

The most common presentation of breast cancer is a painless lump. Unfortunately, by the time a breast lesion is palpable it has already grown to about 0.5 cm. Small lesions can be quite difficult to detect, especially if they are deep within breast tissues. The assessment of a breast mass must address the size, shape, consistency, mobility, pain or tenderness, location in the breast, and relation to skin and surrounding tissues. The opposite breast should be compared for asymmetry. A clinical history relative to known risk factors, a physical assessment of the mass, and a biopsy of a suspicious lesion are critical to the proper management of a patient who has a breast mass.

In premenopausal women, glandular breast tissues tend to change throughout the menstrual cycle. For this reason the evaluation of a breast mass over one or two menstrual cycles may be necessary. An aspiration, biopsy, or both may be recommended for a persistent mass.

Because benign breast conditions (including cysts) are more rare postmenopausally, the finding of palpable breast masses in postmenopausal women tend to be highly suspicious. In these instances a biopsy is strongly recommended.

Nipple discharge or retraction

The sudden onset of nonlactational serous discharge from one breast is the second most common symptom of breast cancer. Nipple retraction and tenderness or pain in the nipple may also suggest cancer. Nipple changes must also be investigated for benign diagnoses, including cystic mastopathy, intraductal papilloma, and Paget's disease.

Clinical Presentation of Breast Cancer

- Breast mass
- Nipple discharge or retraction
- Skin changes
- Alteration in breast contour
- Lymphadenopathy
- Mammographic abnormality
- Distant metastasis

Skin changes and alterations in breast contour

Changes in skin texture, dimpling, irritation, increased warmth, scaling, pain, and ulceration of the skin are breast cancer symptoms requiring careful evaluation. Other types of symptomatic changes include distortion of the normal breast contour, swelling, and thickening of subcutaneous tissues. Peau d' orange, a condition in which the skin develops an orange peel appearance, is a clinical sign of inflammatory breast cancer.

Lymphadenopathy

Occasionally, the first sign of breast cancer is the enlargement of an axillary lymph node. Cervical, supraclavicular, and axillary lymph nodes drain breast tissues and require careful assessment. Arm edema may also be a sign of lymph node involvement.

Mammographic abnormality

A mammogram and a clinical examination of the breast can detect small, discreet lesions and chest wall involvement. On a mammogram, breast cancer typically appears as an ill-defined, opacified lesion with or without spiculated margins, as demonstrated in Fig. 13-6.

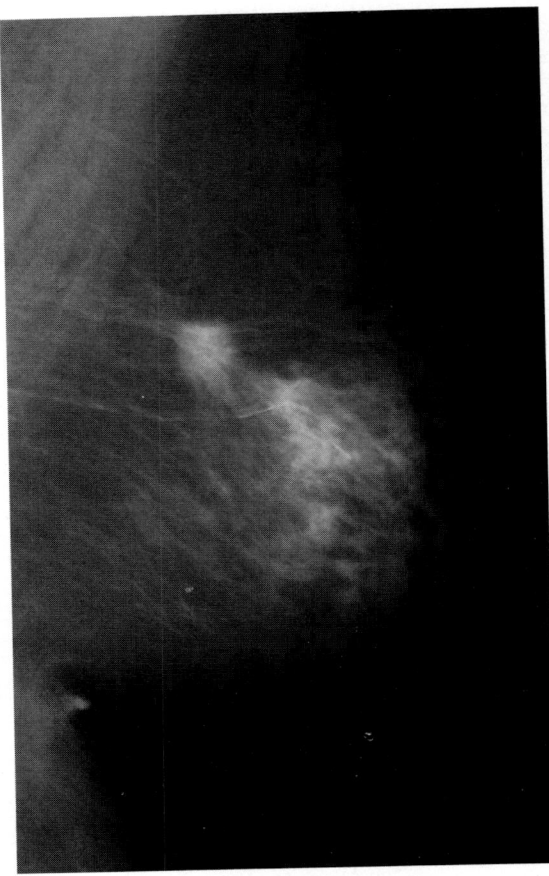

Fig. 13-6 Mammogram demonstrating a malignant lesion.

Mammographic breast cancer screening is recommended for improving survival rates through early detection. Patients with an incidental finding of breast cancer through a mammography tend to have the best prognosis.

Distant metastasis

Distant metastasis (most commonly in the form of bone, brain, lung, or liver involvement) may be present at the time of the diagnosis. Patients with distant metastasis (Stage IV disease) have an extremely poor prognosis. Discomfort from the metastatic site is usually not the patient's only symptom; however, it provides the patient with the impetus for seeking medical attention. As a result of improvements in health education, awareness, detection, and diagnosis, fewer patients exhibit distant metastasis at the time of the diagnosis.

DETECTION AND DIAGNOSIS

As the most common malignancy in women, cancer of the breast affects one in every eight women in the U.S.[1] Such a widespread disease merits the continued development of screening and detection methods that provide the earliest possible diagnosis because early lesions can be highly curable.[21,30] Important features of breast cancer screening and detection methods include cost effectiveness, accuracy, **specificity,** safety, and availability.

The medical community has come far already in this regard. As recently as several decades ago the majority of breast cancer patients were first treated in an advanced stage of disease. Fear and ignorance played a large role in preventing earlier diagnoses. Women were not cognizant of the need to examine their own breasts and thus were often not aware of any change until it became obtrusive. In addition, women were not anxious to hear that they needed a radical mastectomy, and they often delayed seeking medical attention. Surgical treatment for breast cancer was perceived as disfiguring and defeminizing and was often psychologically traumatic for the patient.

Detection

As a result of public education campaigns by the American Cancer Society and other groups, many breast cancers are being diagnosed early (i.e., at a smaller size and before involvement of the lymph nodes). Such tumors can often be successfully treated without removal of the breast.

The ACS periodically publishes updated recommendations for the detection of breast cancer. The current cornerstones of breast cancer detection are breast self-examination (BSE), clinical breast examination, and mammographic screening.

Breast self-examination. BSE is widely regarded as a simple and effective means of familiarizing women with the consistency and feel of their breasts, thereby allowing them to detect changes. The ACS recommends that women examine their breasts monthly; however, an ACS survey in 1987 indicated that only one quarter of the women who responded were adhering to this schedule.

Varying reports describe the effectiveness of BSE in terms of its influence on the stage of disease at the time of the diagnosis and on survival rates. Some retrospective studies found a lower mortality rate among women who had breast cancer and practiced BSE. One reported that women who had been given a brochure on BSE had somewhat smaller tumors at the time of diagnosis.

BSE can be effective only if performed correctly. Educational materials are available that describe the technique, the frequency of examinations, the position of the body during an examination, and the way to palpate the breast and axillary tissue.

Clinical breast examination. A clinical breast examination is an important aspect of breast cancer detection. Physicians and other health professionals perform this procedure, which can detect tumors as small as 0.5 cm in diameter. The skin over the breast is evaluated for color and textural changes. With the patient in the sitting and supine positions, the breast is examined visually and by palpation for mobility and the presence of a mass. The presence of chest wall fixation is assessed through a series of muscle-tensing maneuvers by the patient. Dimpling of the skin, nipple discharge, and axillary lymph node enlargement are evaluated during the clinical examination.

Mammographic screening. Mammography is a powerful tool in the quest for early detection of breast cancer. However, aspects of mammographic screening remain controversial. One of the major sources of contention is disagreement concerning the ideal interval for mammographic screening. The ACS and American College of Radiology (ACR) recommend that a baseline mammogram be obtained between ages 35 and 39 in asymptomatic women who are at an average risk for developing breast cancer. Women between 40 and 49 years of age should have a mammogram every other year, and women over the age of 50 are advised to get annual mammograms.

Numerous prospective, randomized trials have demonstrated the efficacy of mammography in the screening of asymptomatic women for breast cancer. In addition, mammography remains the only modality that routinely detects breast cancer if the lesion is too small to feel during a clinical examination.

Mammography is not without limitations. Mammograms miss 10% to 15% of small and moderate-size breast cancers. This is often due to radiographic overlap between glandular and tumor tissue, rendering the tumor difficult to discern. Because of the relative radiographic similarity of glandular and tumor tissue, mammographic findings are often not specific for malignancy, resulting in numerous invasive diagnostic procedures (biopsies) that are negative. Several studies have shown as few as one positive biopsy for every seven performed. Other series show that approximately one out of three and one half biopsies are positive for cancer. Most centers today have similar results.

Another problem affecting the efficacy of mammography as a screening tool is the lack of its access for many women. Not all insurance policies cover mammographic screening, and uninsured women in lower socioeconomic strata are often unable to pay the cost of screenings. Through the efforts of many individuals and organizations, low-cost screening programs have been made available, but a pressing need for services remains for millions of economically disadvantaged women.

Many factors are involved in the production of an optimal mammographic study. These include the age, upkeep, and type of equipment, as well as the competency of the radiographer and radiologist. Proper positioning of the breast is essential to produce a useful mammogram. Even the film processor must be appropriately maintained to avoid the appearance of artifacts and to optimize the quality of the mammogram. For many years the ACR conducted a voluntary program that granted accreditation to mammographic facilities meeting their quality standards. Since October of 1994 the U.S. Food and Drug Administration (FDA) has required the certification of all mammographic facilities. At this time the FDA authorizes only two agencies to grant mammography accreditation, the ACR and the state of Iowa.

The two primary modalities of mammography are low-dose film and screen mammography and xerography. The standard low-dose film mammogram involves exposures in two views, a cranio-caudad and medial-lateral view. Although the current maximum acceptable radiation dose from a two-view mammogram is 0.01 Gy, the average optimally performed procedure delivers 0.002 Gy. With radiation doses at this level, mammography presents a favorable risk-benefit ratio to patients.

Xerography is a technique of mammography that provides greater visualization of the area close to the chest wall but lacks the detail of good quality film mammography. As a result, xerography is reserved for obtaining additional detail in the patient whose lesion is adjacent to the chest wall.

Ultrasound. Ultrasound (US) has been used fairly extensively in breast cancer detection. US is currently used as an adjunct to mammography for its ability to distinguish between cystic and solid masses and to guide biopsy procedures. US is not a suitable screening modality for breast cancer for several reasons. It cannot detect microcalcifications, it is not sensitive enough to detect small breast cancers, and it can miss subtle structural irregularities indicative of breast malignancy.

Thermography. Thermography is a procedure that uses one of several methods to produce an image of the temperature of the skin overlying the breast. In theory, a malignant lesion radiates heat, which is then detected by one of these techniques. The image produced corresponds to the location of cancer cells in the breast. However, there is a high incidence of false-positive and false-negative results with this modality. Therefore it is not currently recommended as a breast cancer screening tool.

Transillumination. Transillumination, or diaphanography, is a procedure that involves the transmission of light of various wavelengths through breast tissue for detecting masses. Theoretically, a malignant tumor absorbs more of the light passing through the breast than the surrounding normal tissue, thereby casting a shadow on the opposite skin surface. The technique, first described about 60 years ago, has evolved to include computer enhancement but has not demonstrated accuracy or specificity in the detection and/or differentiation of breast malignancies. Transillumination is not currently accepted as a screening method for breast cancer.

Magnetic resonance imaging. Magnetic resonance imaging (MRI) of the breast has been used for approximately a decade. It has been of some value in women with silicone breast implants, extremely dense breast tissue, or changes in the breast secondary to radiation treatment. MRI of the breast has several significant limitations, including its inability to detect microcalcifications and its high cost. Recent advances in the development of surface coils have resulted in several studies on the efficacy of MRI for breast cancer, but additional clinical trials are necessary to further define its role.

Computed tomography. The expense of computed tomography (CT) is sufficiently high to rule out its use as a screening method. However, it is an important tool for the evaluation of local and regional disease in selected patients who have an established diagnosis of breast cancer.

Diagnosis

A definitive diagnosis of breast cancer can only be made through a microscopic examination of tissue removed from the breast. This tissue is obtained from a biopsy through one of several techniques.

Fine-needle biopsy. Fine-needle biopsy involves the careful placement of a relatively small gauge needle into the suspicious tissue in the breast. The needle is attached to a syringe in which the evacuated blood and/or tissue is collected. This material is prepared on slides for cytological evaluation.

Core-needle biopsy. Core-needle biopsy is similar to fine-needle biopsy in that a syringe and a larger gauge needle are used to aspirate a core of tissue from the breast mass. The pathologist then examines this tissue histologically.

Incisional biopsy. An incisional biopsy involves the partial removal of a breast mass to make a histological diagnosis. This procedure is usually performed if the mass is too large to be completely removed without compromising subsequent surgical treatment.

Excisional biopsy. Excisional biopsy, sometimes referred to as *lumpectomy,* removes the mass in its entirety with or without a portion of surrounding normal tissue. This has become the method of choice for removing small breast masses. The placement of the surgical incision is extremely important. Cosmetic effect and treatment considerations (radiotherapeutic and surgical) are directly related to the type and placement of the incision. Curvilinear rather than radial incisions must be used.[16] The incision should be placed directly over the mass to avoid tunneling through breast tissue (a situation with implications for the placement of the boost field during radiation treatment).

PATHOLOGY

Two basic methods are used for obtaining pathological information. Gross examination is performed to record the dimensions of the specimen, the size of the tumor, and the tumor's relationship to the excisional margin. Microscopic examination is performed through an analysis of the specimen under a microscope whereby tumor margins are assessed to evaluate the adequacy of the excision. In addition, the pathologist determines the tumor histology and presence of associated ductal carcinoma in situ and lymphatic invasion, if any.

Histopathological types of breast cancer are listed in the box to the right. Most breast cancers arise in the terminal ductal lobular units of the breast and are classified as ductal or lobular, depending on the specific site of origin. The specific type is defined based on cytological features and growth patterns. Carcinoma in situ (CIS) is also classified as ductal or lobular and is characterized by a proliferation of malignant epithelial cells that do not invade the basement membrane.

Over 70% of invasive breast cancers are infiltrating ductal carcinoma. These tumors usually contain some component of ductal carcinoma in situ (DCIS) and tend to spread to the axillary lymph nodes. Infiltrating lobular carcinoma comprises about 5% to 10% of breast cancers.[17] The prognosis and likelihood of lymph node involvement is similar to that of ductal carcinoma.

Inflammatory breast cancer can be composed of any histological cell type. However, its clinical features are quite distinct. Comprising less than 1% of all breast cancer, it is characterized by obvious skin changes such as Peau d' orange, erythema, thickening, increased warmth, and diffuse induration caused by dermal lymphatic involvement. The entire breast may be tender and enlarged. Inflammatory cancer involves a grave prognosis, with a survival time of less than 2 years. It tends to be aggressive and fast growing. Therefore combined-modality treatment (including surgery, chemotherapy, and radiation therapy) is used for these patients.

In addition to defining the histological type of breast cancer, the pathologist can assess the tumor grade. The degree of differentiation is coded as indicated in the box on this page.

Histopathology of Breast Cancer

Histopathological types of breast cancer

- Cancer, NOS
- Ductal
  - Intraductal (in situ)
  - Invasive with predominant intraductal component
  - Invasive, NOS
  - Comedo
  - Inflammatory
  - Medullary with lymphocytic infiltrate
  - Mucinous (colloid)
  - Papillary
  - Scirrhous
  - Tubular
  - Other
- Lobular
  - In situ
  - Invasive with predominant in situ component
  - Invasive
- Nipple
  - Paget's disease, NOS
  - Paget's disease with intraductal carcinoma
  - Paget's disease with invasive ductal carcinoma
- Other
  - Undifferentiated carcinoma

Histopathological grade (G)

GX	Grade cannot be assessed
G1	Well differentiated
G2	Moderately differentiated
G3	Poorly differentiated
G4	Undifferentiated

NOS, Not otherwise specified.

STAGING

Patients with breast cancer are staged for a variety of reasons. Staging aids in the selection of the treatment technique, allows the evaluation of treatment methods, and indicates the prognosis. The two methods of staging breast cancer are clinical and pathological. Clinical staging involves all physical, operative, and gross pathological findings used to establish the diagnosis, including the primary tumor, breast, skin, chest wall, lymph nodes, and any sites of metastasis. Pathological staging includes all these factors plus microscopic assessment of the tumor margin. If gross involvement of the tumor margin is present, the true extent of the primary tumor cannot be assessed and is therefore coded as TX. Level I axillary lymph nodes should also be pathologically assessed for staging purposes.

The currently accepted staging system is that of the American Joint Committee on Cancer (AJCC), which is based on TNM (tumor, node, metastasis) definitions and stage groupings (see the box on p. 302). The primary tumor, regional lymph node status, pathological classification status, and distant metastasis are parameters used to place patients into four main groups. With simultaneous bilateral breast cancers the tumors are staged separately.

American Joint Committee on Cancer Staging System for Breast Cancer

Primary tumor (T)

- TX Primary tumor cannot be assessed
- T_0 No evidence of primary tumor
- Tis Carcinoma in situ (intraductal carcinoma, lobular carcinoma in situ, or Paget's disease* of the nipple with no tumor)
- T_1 Tumor (2 cm or less in greatest dimension)
  - T_{1a} Tumor (0.5 cm or less in greatest dimension)
  - T_{1b} Tumor (more than 0.5 cm but not more than 1.0 cm in greatest dimension)
  - T_{1c} Tumor (more than 1 cm but not more than 2 cm in greatest dimension)
- T_2 Tumor (more than 2 cm but not more than 5 cm in greatest dimension)
- T_3 Tumor (more than 5 cm in greatest dimension)
- T_4 Tumor of any size with direct extension to the chest wall or skin
  - T_{4a} Extension to the chest wall
  - T_{4b} Edema (including peau d' orange), ulceration of the skin of the breast, or satellite skin nodules confined to the same breast
  - T_{4c} Both T_{4a} and T_{4b}
  - T_{4d} Inflammatory carcinoma

Regional lymph node involvement (N)

- NX Regional lymph nodes cannot be assessed (e.g., previously removed)
- N_0 No regional lymph node metastasis
- N_1 Metastasis to movable ipsilateral axillary lymph node(s)
- N_2 Metastasis to ipsilateral axillary lymph node(s) fixed to one another or the other structures
- N_3 Metastasis to ipsilateral mammary lymph node(s)

Pathological classification (pN)

- pNX Regional lymph nodes cannot be assessed (e.g., previously removed or not removed for pathological study)
- pN_0 No regional lymph node metastasis
- pN_1 Metastasis to movable ipsilateral axillary lymph nodes(s)
  - pN_{1a} Only micrometastasis (none larger than 0.2 cm)
  - pN_{1b} Metastasis to lymph node(s) (any larger than 0.2 cm)
    - pN_{1bi} Metastasis in one to three lymph nodes (any more than 0.2 cm and all less than 2 cm in greatest dimension)
    - pN_{1bii} Metastasis to four or more lymph nodes (any more than 0.2 cm and all less than 2 cm in greatest dimension)
    - pN_{1biii} Extension of tumor beyond the capsule of a lymph node (metastasis less than 2 cm in greatest dimension)
    - pN_{1biv} Metastasis to a lymph node (2 cm or more in greatest dimension)
- pN_2 Metastasis to ipsilateral axillary lymph nodes that are fixed to one another or to other structures
- pN_3 Metastasis to ipsilateral internal mammary lymph nodes(s)

Distant metastasis (M)

- MX Distant metastasis cannot be assessed
- M_0 No distant metastasis
- M_1 Distant metastasis (includes metastasis to ipsilateral supraclavicular lymph node[s])

Stage grouping

Stage 0	Tis	N_0	M_0
Stage I	T_1	N_0	M_0
Stage IIa	T_0	N_1	M_0
	T_1	N_1†	M_0
	T_2	N_0	M_0
Stage IIb	T_2	N_1	M_0
	T_3	N_0	M_0
Stage IIIa	T_0	N_2	M_0
	T_1	N_2	M_0
	T_2	N_2	M_0
	T_3	N_1, N_2	M_0
Stage IIIb	T_4	Any N	M_0
	Any T	N_3	M_0
Stage IV	Any T	Any N	M_1

Modified from Beahrs OH et al, editors: *AJCC manual for staging of cancer,* ed 4, Philadelphia, 1992, JB Lippincott.
*Paget's disease associated with a tumor is classified according to the size of the tumor.
†The prognosis for patients with N_{1a} is similar to that of patients with pN_0.

ROUTES OF SPREAD

Cancer of the breast is a relatively slow disease process, with distant metastases sometimes occurring decades after definitive treatment of the primary tumor.[18] Some researchers believe that cancer of the breast is a systemic disease, even in the earliest clinical stages, based on the following facts: (1) Little change has occurred in long-term survival rates since the radical mastectomy was developed, and (2) late distant metastases continue to appear, even with the use of advanced treatment techniques.[20]

Extension in the breast

A basic therapeutic tenet of this disease is that all ipsilateral breast tissue is at risk and requires treatment. This is due to the fact that extension throughout the breast is possible as a result of the following mechanisms:

1. Direct invasion into surrounding breast tissue
2. Extension via the duct system
3. Spread along the lymphatic channels in the breast

Direct extension of a primary breast lesion can be demonstrated mammographically. The tumor has fingerlike projections that extend into the parenchyma of the breast (Fig. 13-7). Without treatment, such lesions ultimately involve the skin of the breast and/or the chest wall.

Cancer also spreads in the breast by progressive involvement of the ducts. Whether this process represents actual direct extension along the ducts or a more generalized development of cancer in multiple ducts simultaneously is not fully understood.

The extensive lymphatic system of the breast provides an avenue for the primary spread of tumor cells in breast tissue. Cells can migrate via lymphatic channels deep into the chest wall or central portion of the breast beneath the nipple-areola complex.

Regional lymph node involvement

Lymph nodes in the axillary and internal mammary areas are the most likely sites of regional involvement of breast cancer. The supraclavicular nodes are only occasionally involved. The presence or absence of disease in these nodal groups is an important factor in treatment decisions and as an indicator of the prognosis.

Axillary lymph node involvement. Lymph nodes located in the axilla represent the primary lymphatic drainage of the breast. Half of all patients with breast cancer have microscopic involvement of the axillary nodes.[16] The incidence of axillary lymph node involvement is a function of several factors, including the following:

1. Size of the primary tumor—As tumor size increases, so does the likelihood of axillary node involvement.[7]
2. Quadrant location of the primary tumor—Lesions located in the upper-outer, or lower-outer quadrants have a greater chance of axillary node involvement.[13]

Lymph nodes in the axilla can be divided into three subsections. Because of the sequential drainage pattern, the lowest (Level I) nodes are the first and most likely to be involved, followed by Levels II and III. Occasionally, lymph nodes in a higher level may be involved while the nodes in the lower level(s) are negative, a situation referred to as *skip metastasis*. The two largest series studying this process demonstrated a 3.5% rate of skip metastasis in patients with axillary lymph node involvement.[28,33]

Internal mammary lymph node involvement. Internal mammary (IM) lymph nodes are the second most common site of involvement from breast cancer. Of all breast cancer patients, 20% have positive IM nodes.[16] The incidence of IM involvement is directly related to axillary node involvement and the size of the primary tumor. The age of the patient also influences IM node involvement, with younger patients demonstrating a higher incidence.[34] Most studies also show that the primary tumor location in the medial quadrants or center of the breast increases the incidence of IM involvement.

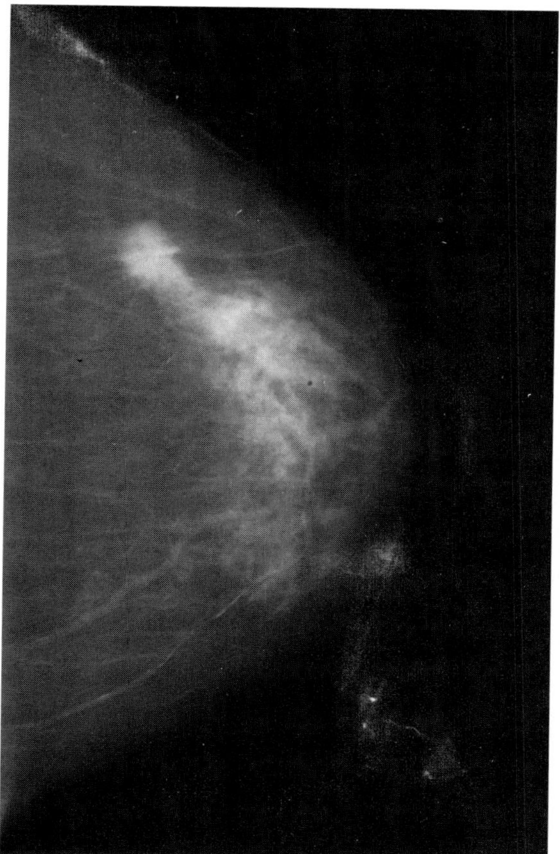

Fig. 13-7 Mammographic demonstration of a primary breast lesion.

Assessing the status of IM nodes as a result of their intrathoracic location, which is relatively inaccessible for a biopsy, can be difficult. CT and lymphoscintigraphy are used to image the IM nodes.

Supraclavicular lymph node involvement. Supraclavicular lymph node involvement from breast cancer is correlated with extensive axillary metastasis and medial quadrant location.[18] The involvement of IM and supraclavicular nodes is considered a grave prognostic indicator in breast cancer.

Distant metastasis

Breast cancer has a propensity to metastasize to distant sites, most commonly bone, lung, and liver.[4,29,35] The mechanism of this type of dissemination is embolization (i.e., spread via tumor cells entering the circulatory system and traveling to a distant organ). The length of time between the initial diagnosis and discovery of distant metastasis varies widely in this disease but can be extremely long, measured sometimes in decades. The development of distant metastasis is linked to the size and histology of the primary tumor and extent of lymph node involvement.

TREATMENT MANAGEMENT

A multidisciplinary approach that includes surgery, radiation therapy and chemotherapy is required for breast cancer treatment. Historically, breast cancer was treated quite aggressively via radical mastectomy with or without radiation therapy. In addition to single-institution studies, large national cooperative groups, such as the National Surgical Adjuvant Breast and Bowel Project (NSABP) and the Radiation Therapy Oncology Group (RTOG), contribute to continuing breast cancer research and the development of its treatment. The research of these and other groups (carried out over the last 25 years) indicates that breast cancer appears to be quite systemic in its progression. Historically, aggressive local treatment via radical mastectomy has not improved survival rates. Therefore current surgical and radiation treatment techniques are more conservative. Chemotherapy has been used increasingly to address microscopic, lymphatic, and systemic disease. When indicated, radiation therapy is usually delivered postoperatively.

Decisions regarding treatment are influenced by the extent of the primary tumor, the patient's general medical condition, and the patient's personal preference. Although limited surgery (breast conservation) with or without radiation treatment is quite popular, it is not appropriate for all patients. If the breast is small relative to the tumor or multicentric tumor involvement is present, a mastectomy may be the best treatment choice. In addition, limited surgery is not an option for patients with advanced breast cancer.

Surgery

Radical mastectomy. Introduced by William S. Halsted in the late 1800s, the Halsted radical mastectomy was the treatment of choice for breast cancer through the 1970s. Before this, patients were more likely to have large, bulky tumors, and early, limited surgical techniques were ineffective in reducing the incidence of chest wall recurrence. To address the high incidence of chest wall recurrence and lymph node involvement, Halsted devised the radical mastectomy, which involves the removal of the breast with its overlying skin, all the axillary lymph nodes, and the pectoral muscles (Fig. 13-8).

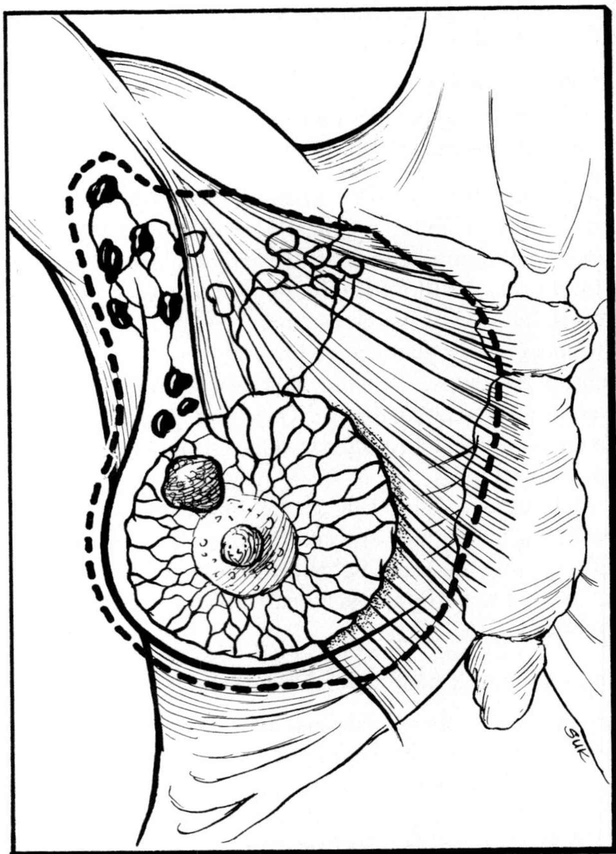

Fig. 13-8 Radical mastectomy: removal of the breast with its overlying skin, the axillary lymph nodes, and the pectoralis major and minor muscles.

Although the Halsted radical mastectomy did not lead to improved long-term survival rates, chest wall recurrences were reduced, and hence the procedure's initial popularity. Unfortunately, the complication rate from radical mastectomy is high and complications can be severe, often leaving the patient with a concave chest wall, arm weakness, shoulder stiffness, and lymphedema (arm swelling). Eventually, the extent of surgery was reduced because radical mastectomy did not reduce the incidence of metastatic disease and because of the high risk of complications. Currently, radical mastectomy is rarely performed, comprising less than 2% of all breast surgeries in the U.S.

Modified radical mastectomy. Radical mastectomy was subsequently modified to preserve muscle, some skin, lymphatics, and blood vessels, thereby improving cosmetic results, reducing arm edema, and improving arm strength. Modified radical mastectomy involves removal of the breast and some or all of the axillary lymph nodes. It may also include removal of the pectoralis minor muscle, while preserving the pectoralis major (Fig. 13-9). Sometimes the lymph nodes are sampled through a separate axillary incision. The use of modified radical mastectomy resulted in survival rates similar to those for radical mastectomy, therefore this modified procedure eventually replaced the more extensive operation.

Lumpectomy. The excisional biopsy of a breast mass is sometimes referred to as *lumpectomy, tylectomy,* or *tumorectomy.* This procedure involves removal of the tumor with a margin of normal-appearing tissue (Fig. 13-10). Overlying skin and underlying tissue are left intact. Lymph nodes are sampled through a separate axillary incision.

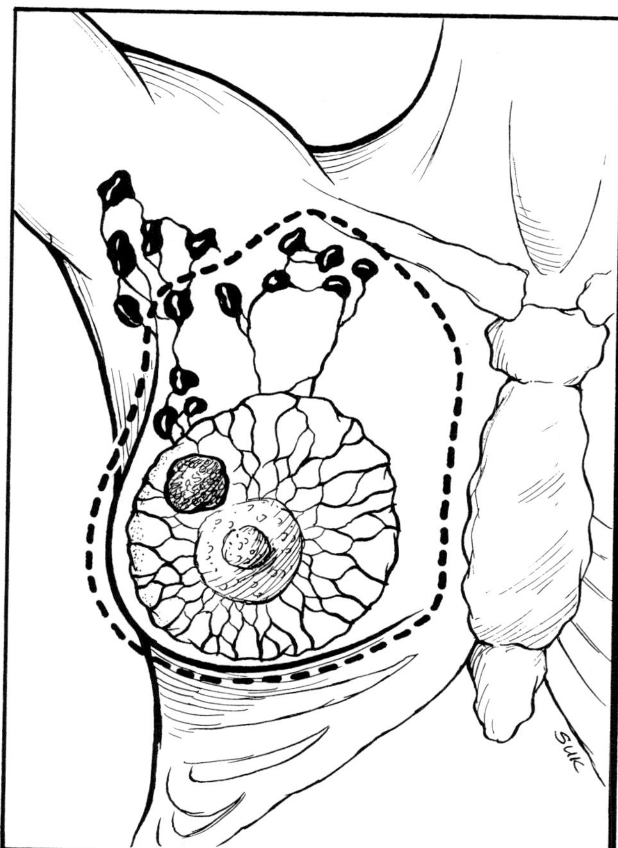

Fig. 13-9 Modified radical mastectomy: removal of the breast with its overlying skin, some or all of the axillary lymph nodes. The pectoralis minor muscle may be removed, leaving the pectoralis major muscle intact.

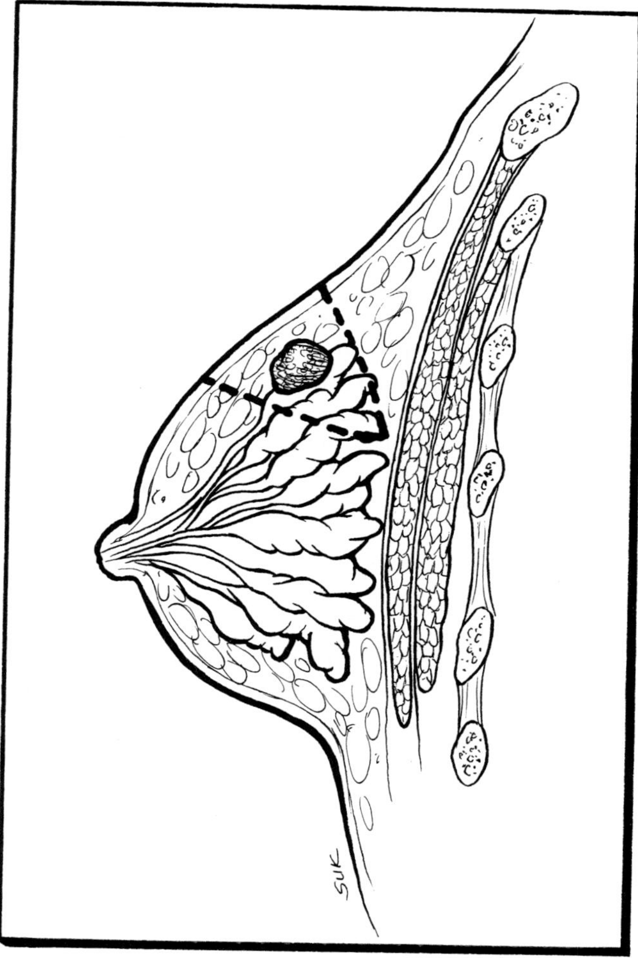

Fig. 13-10 Lumpectomy: removal of the tumor with a margin of normal-appearing tissue.

Axillary dissection. Removal of a sample of axillary lymph nodes in the axilla on the side of the involved breast (ipsilateral) is necessary for staging the patient's disease. The pathological status of axillary lymph nodes influences the selection of the treatment technique and helps indicate the prognosis.

Breast reconstruction. Breast reconstruction, which may be an option for women who have undergone a mastectomy, is achieved through the gradual expansion of existing skin and muscle and the subsequent placement of an artificial breast implant. If remaining tissues are inadequate for expansion after a mastectomy, skin and muscle may be transferred to the chest area from other parts of the body. A normal breast contour may be obtained by matching the size and shape of the implant with that of the opposite breast. It is possible to reconstruct just the contour of the breast or, in some patients, the entire breast, including the nipple and areola. A plastic surgeon performs the procedure, which may require several operations over 6 to 12 months.

Systemic therapy

Systemic therapy may be combined with surgery and/or radiation therapy and consists of chemotherapy or endocrine therapy (hormonal manipulation). The goal of systemic treatment is the destruction, prevention, or delay of tumor spread to distant sites in the body. When systemic therapy is used with surgery or radiation, it is referred to as **adjuvant therapy.**

Chemotherapy. Chemotherapy consists of the following cancer-killing agents (used alone or in combination): cyclophosphamide (C); 5-fluorouracil (F); methotrexate (M); Adriamycin, also known as *doxorubicin* (A); vinblastine; mitoxantrone; and mitomycin C. Combination chemotherapy is the use of several agents together. For example, combination chemotherapy consisting of CMF means that cyclophosphamide, methotrexate, and 5-fluorouracil are used together.

A treatment regimen is defined according to the order of administration, specific agent(s), dosages, routes of administration, and exact administration schedule. Drugs can be administered through the patient's mouth or via an injection into a vein or muscle. A schedule of administration indicates whether the drugs are given daily, weekly, or monthly. The duration of treatment is expressed in terms of months or years. Chemotherapy may be administered before or after surgery, before or after radiation therapy, or with radiation treatment. The sequence of chemotherapy, surgery, and radiation therapy continues to be studied for its effect on local control and survival. In addition, a variety of adjuvant treatment regimens are under investigation.

Endocrine therapy. Current endocrine therapy consists of a variety of drugs used to deprive cancer cells of the hormones needed for growth. The most commonly used agents are tamoxifen and megace (megestrol acetate). Tamoxifen is frequently a component of adjuvant therapy for postmenopausal women. It is used alone or with other chemotherapeutic agents. The estrogen receptor status also plays a role in the selection of hormonal therapy as an element of treatment.[22]

Treatment approach. Each patient is considered unique, and management depends on the patient's stage of disease, lymph node status, estrogen receptor and progesterone receptor (ER/PR) status, and menopausal status. Although no single treatment exists that is best for any group of patients, some general comments can be made. In general, Stage I breast cancer patients have a low incidence of relapse; therefore chemotherapy is reserved for high-risk patients in this group. For Stages II and III breast cancer patients, systemic therapy is useful in reducing relapse rates and increasing overall survival rates. Multiagent chemotherapy is the present treatment of choice for premenopausal women with ipsilateral lymph node involvement, whereas tamoxifen alone or with chemotherapy is beneficial for postmenopausal women.[15,20,22] A combination of systemic and local treatment is usually required for patients with advanced disease (Stage IV).[22] For patients with unresectable tumors chemotherapy is frequently sequenced first to achieve a systemic effect and to potentially downstage the tumor. Although data suggest that delaying irradiation during chemotherapy increases the risk of local failure, this risk may be acceptable for patients with locally advanced disease because distant metastasis is a predictor of overall survival. Optimal sequencing of chemotherapy, surgery, and radiation therapy has not yet been determined.

Treatment of advanced breast cancer. For metastatic breast cancer, current chemotherapy can often prolong the survival time or inhibit progression of the disease. For some patients chemotherapy is used as a palliative measure.

Treatment efforts involving high-dose chemotherapy and autologous bone marrow transplantation for patients with advanced breast cancer (more than 10 involved lymph nodes) are under investigation. Initial results of several institutions indicate that the 2-year relapse-free survival rate for patients with advanced disease treated with this approach appears to be superior to results for similar patients treated with adjuvant chemotherapy. Continued research efforts involving randomized clinical trials and longer follow-up evaluations contribute to determining the optimal treatment management of advanced breast cancer.

Side effects. Endocrine and chemotherapeutic agents can also affect healthy tissues, causing side effects such as nausea and vomiting, loss of appetite, fatigue, change in menstruation, mouth ulcers, and hair loss. The type of side effects the patient experiences depends on the agent(s) used and the patient's response to the drugs. For example, some patients may experience hot flashes (a short-term side effect of tamoxifen) as a result of lowered levels of estrogen. Most side effects are acute, resolving after the completion of treatment. A few side effects are permanent. For example, Adriamycin may cause cardiac damage. In addition, a small chance exists that the chemotherapy will cause a second cancer.

Radiation therapy

Conservative breast cancer management. Current methods for conservative breast cancer management have been well established. The ACR adopted "Standards for Breast Conservation Treatment" in 1992. The American College of Surgeons, the College of American Pathologists, and the Society of Surgical Oncology have endorsed this document. A variety of research efforts have provided the evidence necessary to conclude that mastectomy and breast conservation treatment (lumpectomy, ipsilateral axillary lymph node dissection, and radiation therapy) are equally effective for selected patients with early-stage breast cancer (Stages I and II). In addition, these studies revealed no difference in the rate of development of metastasis or contralateral breast cancer.[10]

As defined by ACR standards, the four critical elements used to select patients for breast conservation are as follows:

1. The patient's history and a physical examination are used to establish familial patterns and assess physical findings.
2. A mammographic evaluation is used to define the extent of the tumor, investigate the potential presence of multicentric or multifocal disease, and evaluate the contralateral breast.
3. A pathological evaluation of the tumor, including a gross and microscopic examination is used, as well as additional data such as estrogen and progesterone receptor analysis, extent of carcinoma in situ, DNA ploidy, S phase fraction, and mitotic grade.
4. An assessment of the patient's needs and expectations is a difficult but essential consideration. Long-term survival, possibility and consequences of local recurrence, treatment options for potential local recurrence, follow-up procedures, physical and cosmetic outcomes, psychological adjustment, and quality of life are factors requiring careful consideration.

Although properly staged and selected patients may be eligible for conservative treatment, some contraindications have been identified. First- and second-trimester pregnancy, multicentric disease, and a history of prior breast irradiation of significant dosage are absolute contraindications of breast conservation treatment. A history of vascular disease, a large tumor in a small breast, an extremely large or pendulous breast, and the specific location of the tumor in the breast are factors requiring special consideration and potentially contraindicating the use of a conservative approach to treatment.

Total gross removal of the tumor and a margin of surrounding tissue with maintenance of good cosmesis is the main goal of conservative breast surgery. A separate axillary dissection is performed, which minimally involves the removal of Level I lymph nodes. Based on the size and histology of the tumor, removal of Level II or III lymph nodes may be appropriate.

After a 2- to 4-week surgical recovery, radiation therapy may begin. Proper simulation and treatment planning are critical factors in establishing an appropriate treatment technique. Special attention to physical and technical considerations substantially reduces the risk of complications. Specific techniques are addressed in the following section. Generally, however, lower megavoltage beam energies (4 to 8 MV) and tissue compensators are used to improve dose homogeneity. Tangential fields are used to encompass the entire breast and chest wall. The amount of lung projected at the center of the tangential fields should be limited to between 1.0 and 3.4 cm, thereby reducing the risk of radiation pneumonitis. If peripheral lymphatic irradiation is required, overlapping or excessive gapping between fields must be avoided. If the axillary dissection includes Level III, axillary irradiation should be avoided so that lymphedema does not result.

Fields are treated daily with standard fractionation (180 to 200 cGy per fraction) to a total dose of 4500 to 5000 cGy. A boost dose may be delivered with an electron beam or interstitial technique, increasing the total dose to the primary tumor site to 6000 to 6600 cGy. Although precise indications for performing the boost remain controversial, patients with positive or close margins of surgical resection usually receive boost irradiation.

Follow-up assessment of patients receiving conservative breast treatment is carefully scheduled to evaluate new or recurrent disease status, treatment sequelae, and cosmetic outcome. The patient's medical history, physical examination, and follow-up mammograms contribute to the evaluation process. The RTOG and European Organization for Research on Treatment of Cancer Acute and Late Radiation Morbidity Scoring Schemes are provided in Tables 13-1 and 13-2. An assessment of the cosmetic result is based on the physician's evaluation (using a four-point scoring index) and the patient's perception.

Postoperative management of breast cancer. Currently, the role of radiation therapy in postoperative breast cancer treatment is not well defined. Radiation therapy was initially used in breast cancer management as an adjuvant to radical mastectomy for the purpose of prophylaxis. The main goal was to reduce the local recurrence rate, thereby improving survival. The risk of radiation-induced cardiac damage and the evolution of the role of chemotherapy have reduced the use of radiation therapy in postoperative patients. The tumor size and location, number of positive axillary lymph nodes, tumor involvement of the skin or supraclavicular lymph nodes, and hormone receptor status may be indications for adjuvant radiation therapy.

If radiation therapy is indicated, the chest wall is treated via tangential fields with lower megavoltage beam energies, using tissue compensators as necessary. Peripheral (supraclavicular and/or axillary) lymphatic irradiation may also be required. Fields are treated daily with standard fractionation (180 to 200 cGy per fraction) to a total dose of 4500 to 5000 cGy. Patients with positive internal mammary lymph nodes are usually treated with chemotherapy. However, if radiation therapy is indicated, wider tangential ports that extend across the midline may be used. Another technique for treating the internal mammary nodes combines photon and electron treatment, helping to limit the cardiac dose. Adjoining fields must be carefully planned to avoid overdosage or underdosage of tissues in these areas, leading to potential matchline **fibrosis** or local recurrence, respectively.

Radiation treatment technique

Radiation treatment for primary breast malignancy is one of the more technically challenging and relatively high-volume procedures performed in a radiation oncology department. Therefore straightforward, reproducible techniques are advantageous, affording optimal target-volume-dose homogeneity and acceptable dose limits for normal structures.

There are almost as many techniques for breast irradiation as there are radiation oncology centers. Many techniques are only slight variations on a theme. Current standard of practice incorporates several essential elements in the treatment of breast cancer. This section presents these elements and details one specific technique.

Positioning and immobilization. Radiation treatment of breast cancer is demanding, requiring stringent positioning and immobilization techniques. One of the key elements involves the mobility of the patient's arm. Many postoperative patients (whether the surgery involved a mastectomy or an axillary dissection) experience initial difficulty in raising the arm to an acceptable position for radiation treatment. Most patients who encounter this problem can correct it with exercise in several days. Therefore the simulation and start of therapy should be delayed until the patient's arm moves appropriately. If the patient is simulated before mobility is restored, the shoulder girdle will assume a different position for treatment than for simulation, leading to poor reproducibility of the treatment fields. At the time of consultation, before the simulation appointment, the radiation oncologist can give the patient a handout detailing exercises and explaining their necessity.

Table 13-1 RTOG Acute radiation morbidity scoring criteria

Organ tissue	Grade 0	Grade 1	Grade 2	Grade 3	Grade 4
Skin	No change over baseline	Follicular, faint, or dull erythema; epilation; dry desquamation; decreased sweating	Tender or bright erythema and patchy, moist desquamation; moderate edema	Confluent, moist desquamation other than skin folds and pitting edema	Ulceration; hemorrhage; necrosis
Mucous membrane	No change over baseline	Injection; possible experience of mild pain not requiring analgesic	Patchy mucositis that may produce an inflammatory serosanguineous discharge; possible experience of moderate pain requiring analgesia	Confluent fibrinous mucositis; possibility of severe pain requiring narcotic	Ulceration; hemorrhage; necrosis
Eye	No change over baseline	Mild conjunctivitis with or without scleral injection; increased tearing	Moderate conjunctivitis with or without keratitis requiring steroids and/or antibiotics; dry eye requiring artificial tears; iritis with photophobia	Severe keratitis with corneal ulceration; objective decrease in visual acuity or in visual fields; acute glaucoma; panophthalmitis	Loss of vision (unilateral or bilateral)
Ear	No change over baseline	Mild external otitis with erythema and pruritis secondary to dry desquamation not requiring medication; audiogram unchanged from baseline	Moderate external otitis requiring topical medication; serous ototis medius; hypoacusis on testing only	Severe external otitis with discharge or moist desquamation; symptomatic hypoacusis; tinnitus, not drug related	Deafness
Salivary gland	No change over baseline	Mild mouth dryness; slightly thickened saliva; possibility of slightly altered taste, such as metallic taste (these changes not reflected in alteration in baseline feeding behavior, such as increased use of liquids with meals)	Moderate to complete dryness; thick, sticky saliva; markedly altered taste	—	Acute salivary gland necrosis
Pharynx and esophagus	No change over baseline	Mild dysphagia or odynophagia; possible requirement of topical anesthetic or nonnarcotic analgesics and soft diet	Moderate dysphagia or odynophagis; possible requirement of narcotic analgesics and puree or liquid diet	Severe dysphagia or odynophagia with dehydration or weight loss (>15% from pretreatment baseline) requiring N-G feeding tube, intravenous fluids, or hyperalimentation	Complete obstruction; ulceration; perforation; fistula
Larynx	No change over baseline	Mild or intermittent hoarseness; cough not requiring antitussive; erythema of mucosa	Persistent hoarseness but ability to vocalize; referred ear pain, sore throat, patchy fibrinous exudate or mild arytenoid edema not requiring narcotic; cough requiring antitussive	Whispered speech and throat pain or referred ear pain requiring narcotic; confluent fibrinous exudate and marked arytenoid edema	Marked dyspnea; stridor or hemoptysis with tracheostomy or intubation necessary
Upper gastrointestinal system	No change	Anorexia with $\leq 5\%$ weight loss from pretreatment baseline; nausea not requiring antiemetics; abdominal discomfort not requiring parasympatholytic drugs or analgesics	Anorexia with $\leq 15\%$ weight loss from pretreatment baseline; nausea and/or vomiting requiring antiemetics; abdominal pain requiring analgesics	Anorexia with >15% weight loss from pretreatment baseline or requiring N-G tube or parenteral support. Nausea and/or vomiting requiring tube or parenteral support; abdominal pain (severe despite medication; hematemesis or melana; abdominal distention (flat plate radiograph demonstrates distended bowel loops)	Ileus, subacute or acute obstruction, perforation, and bleeding requiring transfusion; abdominal pain requiring tube decompression or bowel diversion

Table 13-2 RTOG and EORTC late radiation morbidity scoring scheme

Organ tissue	Grade 0	Grade 1	Grade 2	Grade 3	Grade 4
Skin	None	Slight atrophy; pigmentation change, some hair loss	Patch atrophy; moderate telangiectasia; total hair loss	Market atrophy; gross telangiectasia	Ulceration
Subcutaneous tissue	None	Slight induration (fibrosis) and loss of subcutaneous fat	Moderate fibrosis but asymptomatic; slight field contracture; <10% linear reduction	Severe induration and loss of subcutaneous tissue; field contracture >10% linear measurement	Necrosis
Mucous membrane	None	Slight atrophy and dryness	Moderate atrophy and telangiectasia; little mucous	Marked atrophy with complete dryness; severe telangiectasia	Ulceration
Salivary glands	None	Slight dryness of mouth; good response on stimulation	Moderate dryness of mouth; poor response on stimulation	Complete dryness of mouth; no response on stimulation	Fibrosis
Spinal cord	None	Mild Lhermitte's sign	Severe Lhermitte's sign	Objective neurological findings at or below cord level treated	Mono; paraquadraplegia
Brain	None	Mild headache; slight lethargy	Moderate headache; great lethargy	Severe headaches; severe central nervous system dysfunction (partial loss of power or dyskinesia)	Seizures or paralysis; coma
Eye	None	Asymptomatic cataract; minor corneal ulceration or keratitis	Symptomatic cataract; moderate corneal ulceration; minor retinopathy or glaucoma	Severe keratitis; severe retinopathy or detachment; severe glaucoma	Panopthalmitis; blindness
Larynx	None	Hoarseness; slight arytenoid edema	Moderate arytenoid edema; chondritis	Severe edema; severe chondritis	Necrosis
Lung	None	Asymptomatic or mild symptoms (dry cough); slight radiographic appearances	Moderate symptomatic fibrosis or pneumonitis (severe cough); low-grade fever; pathy radiographic appearances	Severe symptomatic fibrosis or pneumonitis; dense radiographic changes	Severe respiratory insufficiency; continuous O2; assisted ventilation
Heart	None	Asymptomatic or mild symptoms; transient T wave inversion and ST changes; sinus tachychardia >110 (at rest)	Moderate angina on effort; mild pericarditis; normal heart size; persistent abnormal T wave and ST changes; low ORS	Severe angina; pericardial effusion; constrictive pericarditis; moderate heart failure; cardiac enlargement; electrocardiogram abnormalities	Tamponade; severe heart failure; severe constrictive pericarditis
Esophagus	None	Mild fibrosis; slight difficulty in swallowing solids; no pain on swallowing	Inability to take solid food normally; swallowing semisolid food; possible indication of dilatation	Severe fibrosis; ability to swallow only liquids; possibility of pain on swallowing; dilation required	Necrosis; perforation; fistula
Small and large intestine	None	Mild diarrhea; mild cramping; bowel movement five times daily; slight rectal discharge or bleeding	Moderate diarrhea and colic; bowel movement >5 times daily; excessive rectal mucus or intermittent bleeding	Obstruction of bleeding requiring surgery	Necrosis; perforation; fistula
Liver	None	Mild lassitude; nausea, dyspepsia; slightly abnormal liver function	Moderate symptoms; some abnormal liver function tests; serum albumin normal	Disabling hepatic insufficiency; liver function tests grossly abnormal; low albumin; edema or ascites	Necrosis; hepatic coma or encephalopathy
Kidney	None	Transient albuminuria; no hypertension; mild impairment of renal function; urea 25-35 mg%; creatinine 1.5-2.0 mg% creatinine clearance >75%	Persistent moderate albuminuria (2+); mild hypertension; no related anemia; moderate impairment of renal function; urea >36-60 mg%; creatinine clearance (50-74%)	Severe albuminuria; severe hypertension; persistent anemia (<10%); severe renal failure; urea >60 mg%; creatinine >4.0 mg%; creatinine clearance<50%	Malignant hypertension; uremic coma ; urea > 100%
Bladder	None	Slight epithelial atrophy; minor telangiectasia (microscopic hematuria)	Moderate frequency; generalized telangiectasia; intermittent macroscopic hematuria	Severe frequency and dysuria; severe generalized telangiectasia (often with petechiae); frequent hematuria; reduction in bladder capacity (<150 cc)	Necrosis; contracted bladder (capacity >100 cc); Severe hemorrhagic cystitis
Bone	None	Asymptomatic; no growth retardation; reduced bone density	Moderate pain or tenderness; growth retardation; irregular bone sclerosis	Severe pain or tenderness; complete arrest of bone growth; dense bone sclerosis	Necrosis; spontaneous fracture
Joint	None	Mild joint stiffness; slight limitation of movement	Moderate stiffness; intermittent or moderate joint pain; moderate limitation of movement	Severe joint stiffness; pain with severe limitation of movement	Necrosis; complete fixation

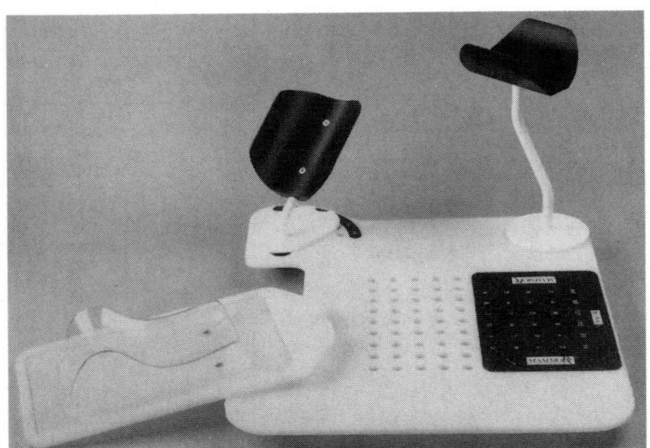

Fig. 13-11 Diacor immobilization device used to assist in patient positioning for radiation treatment. (Courtesy Diacor.)

Many commercially available devices are available to assist in patient positioning for treatment of breast cancer. These range from custom-molded foam casts to boards with adjustable head and arm supports. One such device is illustrated in Fig. 13-11. An important element of reproducibility in immobilization is the ability to index the patient to the immobilization device exactly the same way daily.

For this type of treatment the patient should, at minimum, disrobe from the waist up. The patient lies supine in the selected positioning device on the simulator-treatment table. The patient's body must be straight (in the sagittal plane) and level from side to side. Laser triangulation points are marked on the patient's anterior and side surfaces in the area between the waist and inframammary fold to assist in the daily positioning process.

The arm on the uninvolved (contralateral) side should rest on the table top with the hand palm down. Patients must not place the contralateral hand on the abdomen or grasp the belt or waistband of their clothing. Such a position of the contralateral hand and arm (particularly in large-breasted women) can result in distortion of the thoracic anatomy, including rotation and/or displacement of the uninvolved breast into the treatment field.

The ipsilateral arm is raised and supported far enough in a cephalad direction to allow the tangential radiation beam to treat the breast or chest wall while avoiding the patient's upper arm. Adjustment of the patient's arm position can help reduce or eliminate skin folds in the axilla and supraclavicular areas.

The patient's head should be straight if treatment is limited to the breast or chest wall. If the peripheral lymphatics also require irradiation, the head should be turned slightly to the contralateral side. Identical daily positioning of the patient's arm and head is extremely important for the accuracy of the treatment process.

The feet should be held together with a band or masking tape around the toes. This helps eliminate rotation of the patient's lower abdomen, thereby enhancing setup reproducibility. A triangular sponge or bolster may be placed under the patient's knees to relieve pressure on the lumbar region. The same immobilization devices must be used each time the patient is treated.

When lying supine, patients with large and/or pendulous breasts often have breast tissue displaced up into the infraclavicular area. These patients can be positioned on an incline board so that their head and thorax are elevated relative to their pelvis and lower extremities. This position can be useful in keeping the breast tissue in a more normal location, which is necessary to adequately irradiate the breast and avoid treating the upper arm. This position can also help alleviate the problem of deep skin folds in the supraclavicular area. Care must be taken, however, to avoid overtilting the patient and causing redundancy of the skin in the inframammary area.

The patient position should be well documented and explained in the setup instructions. For patients with unusual conditions or situations in which the setup needs further clarification, Polaroid photographs of the patient in the treatment position are essential.

Intact breast or chest wall treatment technique. Women who require only breast or chest wall irradiation are treated with tangential (glancing) fields. The purpose of this field arrangement is to maximize coverage of the tissues at risk and minimize the radiation dose to underlying structures, primarily the lung and heart. Radiation beams produced by lower-energy linear accelerators (4 to 6 MV) and cobalt units are ideally suited to this type of treatment. Considerations for field margins for tangential fields are as follows:

Superior, at the most cephalad of the following points:
- First intercostal space
- As far cephalad as possible without including the arm
- Superior extent of the palpable breast tissue
- Cephalad (>2 cm) to original location of the mass

Inferior
- Caudad (1 to 2 cm) to the inframammary fold
- In postmastectomy patient this can be extrapolated from inframammary fold of contralateral breast

Medial
- At midline of patient, as determined by palpation of suprasternal notch and xyphoid process
- Exceptions include patient whose mass or incision extends to or beyond midline and patient who will receive internal mammary lymphatic irradiation

Lateral
- Corresponding to midaxillary line (a line drawn from the center of the patient's axilla in a caudad direction)
- Including drain sites or incisions considered at risk, original tumor bed, and appropriate amount of lung margin

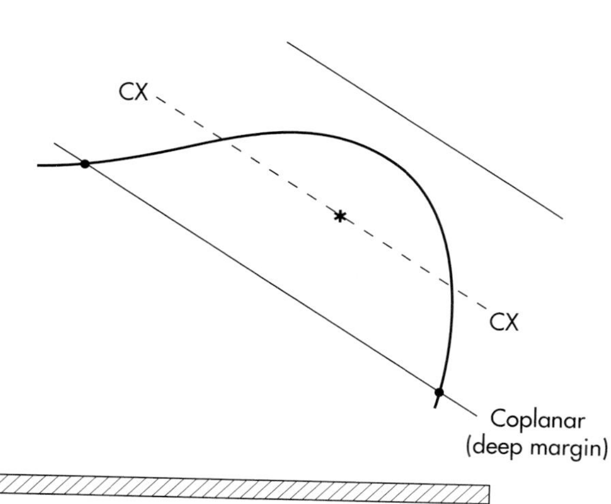

Fig. 13-12 Tangential breast irradiation field arrangement features a coplanar deep margin.

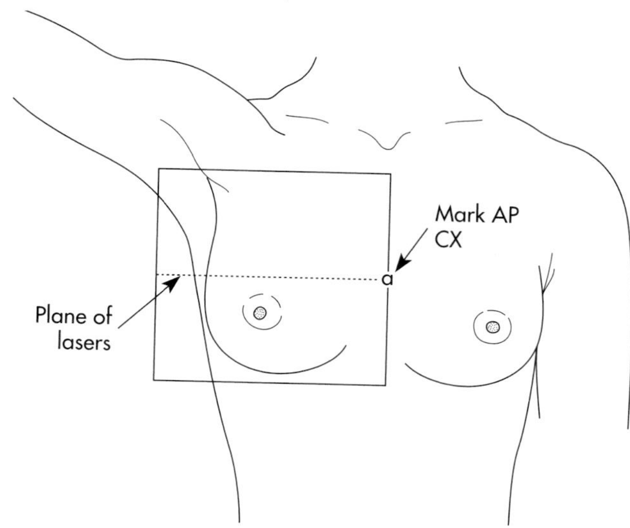

Fig. 13-13 Anterior setup point for tangential breast fields.

Most current techniques use an isocentric method of tangential field irradiation. In these techniques the isocenter is placed at some depth in the patient's breast or chest wall. At many institutions the isocenter is placed approximately halfway between the ribs and skin, at a point approximately midway between the medial and lateral entrance points of the beam. Other techniques place the isocenter at the deep edge of the tangential field and split the radiation beam in half, blocking the deep half of the beam.

An important feature of the tangential field arrangement is the **coplanar** nature of the deep (or posterior) margin of the ports (Fig. 13-12). In coplanar fields the deep border of the medial tangent and the deep border of the lateral tangent form a single plane. This is important in ensuring a dose as homogeneous as possible throughout the treatment volume. Coplanar tangential fields may be achieved with a split-beam technique, as just mentioned, or an unblocked technique.

Asynchronous jaws or multileaf collimation provides the best result with a split-beam technique. Suspended blocks are least desirable because of transmission through the block and scatter that reaches the contralateral breast. Unintended irradiation of the contralateral breast is of concern, especially in younger patients. Several investigators have demonstrated a small but finite incidence of radiation-induced cancer in the contralateral breast of women who received radiation treatment for breast cancer.[5,9]

Perhaps the most desirable method of treating coplanar tangential fields (from the standpoint of limiting dose to the contralateral breast) is the unblocked isocentric technique. Coplanar tangential fields are not parallel opposed. The number of degrees from parallel opposition is a function of field size and may be calculated.

Planning tangential fields can be a relatively complex process. Several techniques described in the literature over the past 10 to 12 years have become well-established methods for planning comprehensive radiation treatment of the breast or chest wall and peripheral lymphatic areas.[25,29,32,34] Techniques used at many institutions today are exact replicas or variations of these themes. Several commercial vendors market systems that include immobilization devices and programmable calculators capable of performing the necessary mathematical calculations. Other techniques use factors that are derived empirically.

The following empirical isocentric method is reproducible, satisfies all essential criteria, and incorporates the advantage of a stable setup point. Tangential fields are set up with a mark on the anterior chest overlying the sternum. The table is then raised to a specified source-skin distance (SSD) and shifted laterally to place the isocenter at the appropriate location in the breast or chest wall. Steps in patient simulation with this technique are as follows:

1. Mark superior, inferior, medial, and lateral margins on the patient.
2. Set the field center at the midline of the chest, halfway between the superior and inferior borders, and mark this point on the patient. This is identified as point a on the contour and is the anterior setup point (Fig. 13-13). Measure the separation at this point by raising the table top to the isocenter, reading the SSD and subtracting this number from the SAD, (e.g., an SSD of 78 subtracted from an SAD of 100 results in a separation of 22).
3. Measure the height of the lateral border relative to the table top. This is identified as point b on the contour.

4. Measure the separation between the medial and lateral margins with a caliper.
5. Obtain a contour through the plane of the field center, marking the medial (point a) and lateral (point b) borders on the contour material.
6. Indicate the patient's separation (step 2) and height of the lateral border from the table top (step 3) as horizontal planes on the graph paper. These will correlate with points a and b.
7. Draw line ab, which is equal in length to the separation measured in step 4 (Fig. 13-14).
8. Trace the contour outline onto the paper, taking care to align points a and b of the contour material with points a and b on the graph paper.
9. Draw a perpendicular line from the midpoint of line ab, extending approximately 2 cm above the apex of the breast. This 2-cm extension allows for flash of the tangential field and accommodates tissue swelling during treatment. The length of the perpendicular line equals the field width (Fig. 13-15).
10. Measure the perpendicular line, and mark point c at the midpoint.
11. Draw a line parallel to ab, through point c (Fig. 13-16).
12. Mark point d on the parallel line at the midpoint between the contour of the medial and lateral skin surfaces. Point d is the isocenter of the tangential fields (Fig. 13-17).
13. The horizontal distance between point a (the anterior setup point) and point d (the isocenter) is the distance the table is shifted laterally (Fig. 13-18).
14. The vertical distance between point a and point d is subtracted from the SAD (100 or 80 cm) and is the setup SSD.
15. Align the patient to the anterior setup point. Apply the vertical and horizontal adjustments from steps 13 and 14 by shifting the table.
16. Place lead markers on the medial and lateral field borders, as marked on the patient.
17. To align the medial tangent field, rotate the gantry via fluoroscopy until the two lead markers are superimposed (coplanar). There should be 1 to 3 cm of lung in the field.

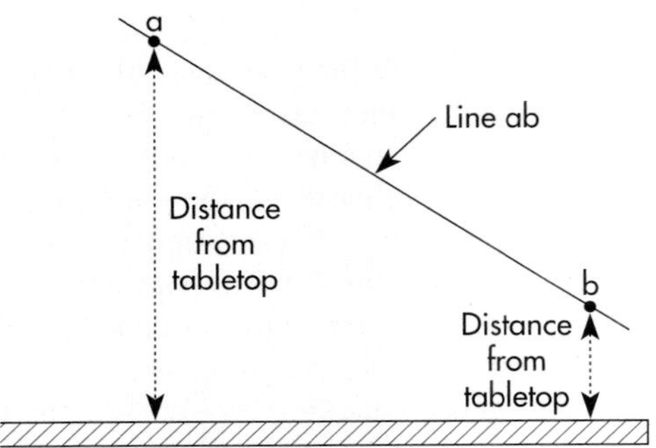

Fig. 13-14 Line a,b, which is equal in length to the oblique separation at the deep (coplanar) edge of the tangential fields.

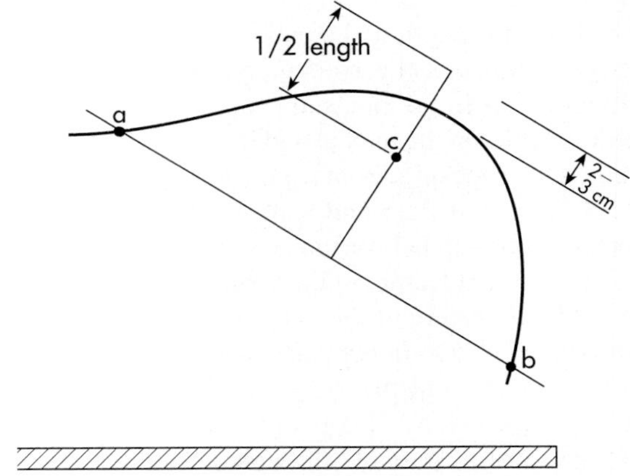

Fig. 13-16 A line is drawn parallel to line a, b through point c.

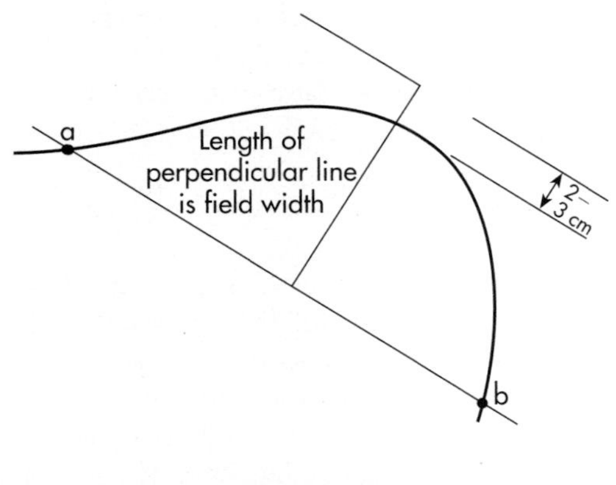

Fig. 13-15 The length of a perpendicular line, drawn from the midpoint of line a, b, and extending approximately 2 to 3 cm above the apex of the breast, is the field width.

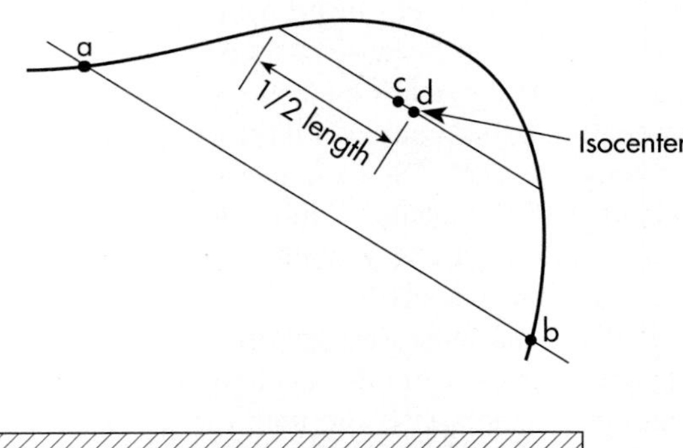

Fig. 13-17 Based on the anterior setup point, vertical and horizontal table shifts are determined with reference to point d.

18. Rotate the collimator so that the medial field edge is parallel to the chest wall. Film this field (Fig. 13-19).
19. To align the lateral tangent field, rotate the gantry approximately 180 degrees, and confirm via fluoroscopy that the two lead markers are superimposed (coplanar). Adjustment of the gantry may be necessary to obtain superimposition. There should be 1 to 3 cm of lung in the field. Rotate the collimator the same number of degrees in the opposite direction of that used in step 18. Radiograph this field (Fig. 13-20).
20. The amount of lung included in the tangential fields should be carefully considered. If insufficient lung is in the field, adjust the lateral border in a posterior direction (if clinically allowable). If there is too much lung, move the lateral border anteriorly (if clinically allowable). It may also be possible to adjust the medial border, depending on the location of the lesion. If adjustments are necessary, return to step 3 and continue.
21. Mark the setup points and field borders on the patient for accurate realignment of the fields for treatment.
22. Complete the setup documentation form.

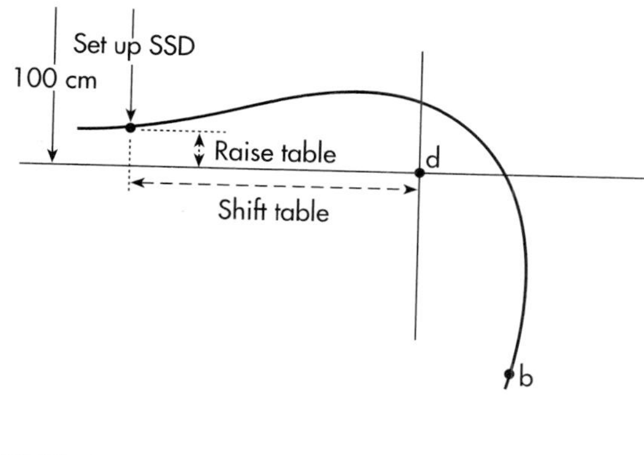

Fig. 13-18 Based on the anterior setup point, vertical and horizontal table shifts are determined with reference to point d.

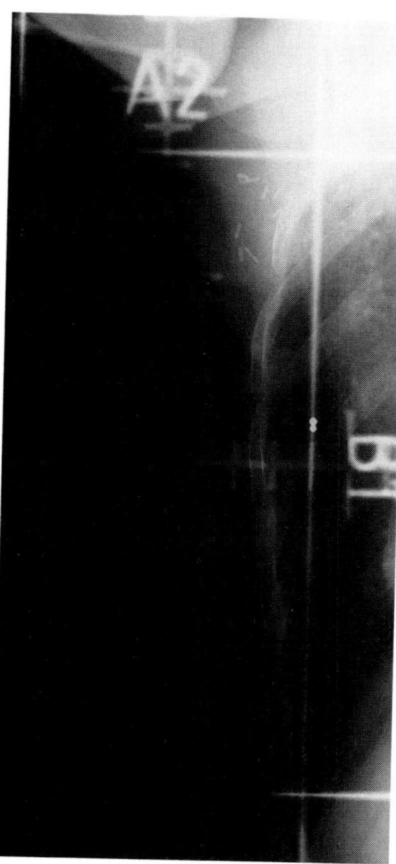

Fig. 13-19 Simulation radiograph of the medial tangential field.

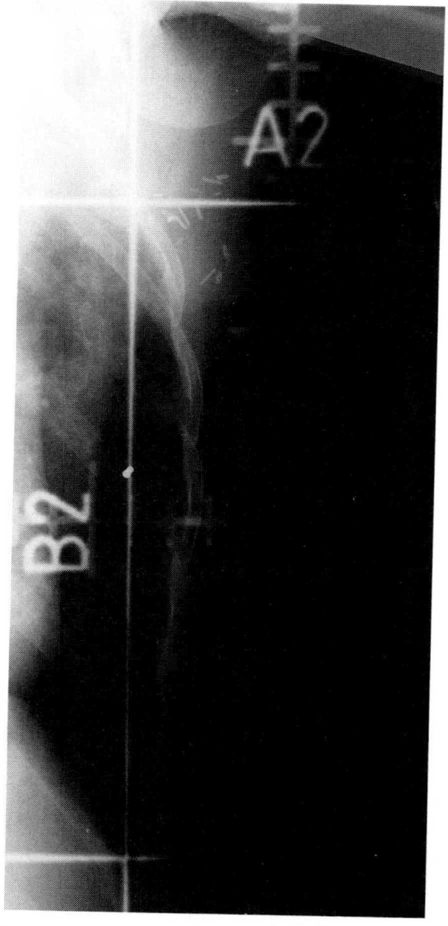

Fig. 13-20 Simulation radiograph of the lateral tangential field.

Computerized treatment planning of the tangential field pair is necessary to visualize the dose distribution throughout the treatment volume. Based on the isodose plot, a decision is made regarding the use of wedges to improve dose homogeneity. In the conservatively managed patient, it may be advantageous to obtain computer-generated isodose plots in up to three planes (one at the central ray or widest part of the breast and one each closer to the superior and inferior field margins). This assists in evaluating dose variation in the breast as a result of the changing contour. Skin doses are adequate because of their inherent reduction from tangentially configured radiation beams; therefore bolus is not usually required.

Comprehensive breast or chest wall and peripheral lymphatics-treatment technique. One critical aspect of comprehensive irradiation for breast cancer is the avoidance of junctional inconsistency between the peripheral lymphatic fields (i.e., supraclavicular-axillary and tangential fields). If overlap occurs, hot or overdosed areas result from a combination of divergence and geometrical distortion of the radiation beams. Such excess dose can lead to matchline fibrosis and a poor cosmetic result. Conversely, a cold or underdosed area provides the potential for tumor recurrence. Avoidance of junctional irregularities can be achieved through the establishment of a vertical straight edge in the axial plane, perpendicular to the floor where the fields meet.

Supraclavicular field. When used, the supraclavicular field is planned before the tangential fields. Considerations for field margins for the supraclavicular field are as follows:

Superior
- Approximately 5 cm above the suprasternal notch (SSN)
- Avoidance of flash over the skin of the supraclavicular area

Medial
- Midpoint of the SSN

Lateral
- Approximately 2 to 3 cm of the humeral head

Inferior, at one of the following:
- Approximately at the angle of Louis
- Just above the superior extent of the palpable breast tissue
- A point >2 cm cephalad to the original location of the mass

The central ray of the supraclavicular field is placed at the inferior margin of the volume to be treated. The inferior half of the beam is blocked by multileaf collimation, an asymmetrical jaw, or a suspended block, creating a vertical straight edge at the inferior border of the supraclavicular field. The gantry is angled 10 to 15 degrees mediolaterally to avoid exiting through the spinal cord. A simulation film of the supraclavicular field is provided in Fig. 13-21.

Posterior axillary boost field. A posterior axillary boost (PAB) field is sometimes used to increase the midaxillary dose to the prescribed level in a subset of patients who have not had dissection of the Level III lymph nodes. This is done because at midplane the radiation dose from an anterior supraclavicular field alone may be insufficient. A simulation film of the PAB field is provided in Fig. 13-22.

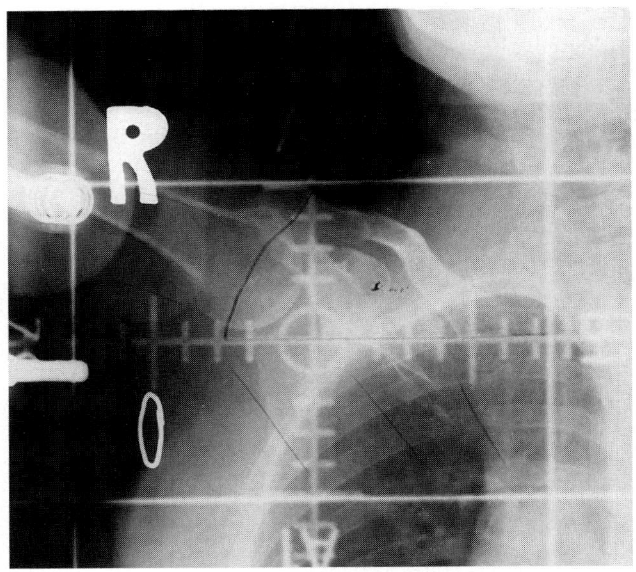

Fig. 13-21 Simulation radiograph of the supraclavicular field.

The PAB field should be parallel opposed to the supraclavicular field and uses the identical inferior margin, preserving the vertical straight edge. Considerations for field margins of the PAB field are as follows:

Superior
- Mid- to upper-clavicle

Medial
- A strip of lung approximately 1 cm wide

Lateral
- Approximately 1 to 2 cm of the humeral head, which is subsequently blocked

Inferior
- Corresponding to the inferior border of the supraclavicular field

Its relatively small total dose notwithstanding, the PAB should be treated with the same fractionation scheme as the supraclavicular field. Considering larger boost fractions (about 1.8 or 2.0 Gy delivered over a few days) may be tempting. However, this dose must be considered as additive to that being delivered via the supraclavicular field, and it results in an extremely large daily dose to the PAB site.

Tangential breast or chest wall fields. The tangential photon fields in comprehensive irradiation for breast cancer are planned in the same way as those described in the section on tangential breast or chest wall irradiation, with several notable additions necessary for an appropriate junction with the supraclavicular-axillary fields. To establish a vertical straight edge at the superior border of the tangential fields, correction must be made for the divergence of the tangential

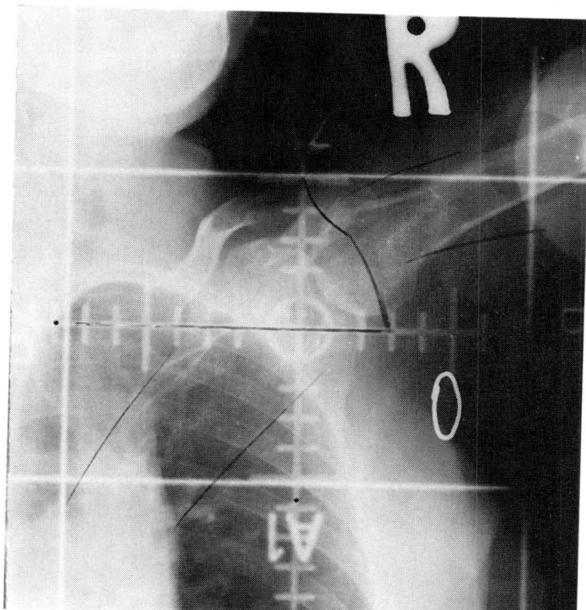

Fig. 13-22 Simulation radiograph of the posterior axillary boost field.

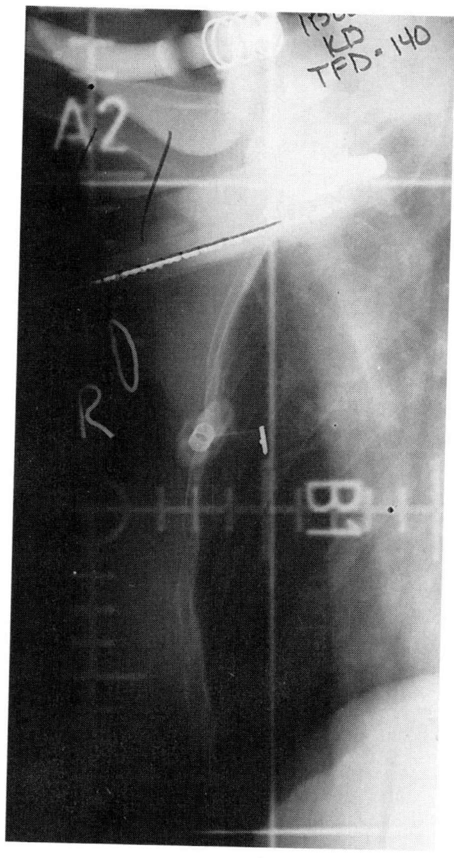

Fig. 13-23 Simulation radiograph of the medial tangential field, illustrating the use of the rod and chain.

fields into the supraclavicular-axillary field and for geometrical distortion of the radiation beam. The couch assembly is rotated in such a way that the patient's feet are directed away from the collimator and a block is placed at the superior edges of the tangential fields. This is done to force correspondence to the vertical straight edge created by the inferior border of the supraclavicular-axillary field pair. The exact location of the block can be determined by placing a rod with a dependent chain on the patient's skin at the level of the supraclavicular field's inferior border. Steps in comprehensive breast irradiation are as follows:

1. After filming the supraclavicular-axillary fields, follow steps 1 through 17 of the previously described tangential technique with some modification. A device composed of a metal rod with an attached chain is used to help define the inferior border of the supraclavicular-axillary field. The metal rod is taped to the patient's skin at the level of the inferior border of the supraclavicular-axillary field, allowing the dependent chain to hang freely over the patient's side. In step 1, add approximately 3 cm to the superior edge of the tangential field. This overlap into the supraclavicular field will be blocked for treatment.
2. Rotate the collimator so that the medial field edge is parallel to the chest wall.
3. Rotate the couch until fluoroscopic images of the rod and chain are superimposed. Film this field (Fig. 13-23).
4. To align the lateral tangent field, rotate the gantry approximately 180 degrees, and confirm via fluoroscopy that the two lead markers are superimposed (coplanar). Adjustment of the gantry angle may be necessary to obtain superimposition. There should be 1 to 3 cm of lung in the field (Fig. 13-24). Rotate the collimator the same number of degrees in the opposite direction of that used in step 2.
5. Mark the edge of the lateral tangential light field on the patient's skin.
6. Rotate the couch in the opposite direction from that in step 3 until fluoroscopic images of the rod and chain are superimposed.
7. Readjust the gantry and collimator angles to match the line marked on the patient in step 5.
8. Verify superimposition of the medial field edge markers and the rod and chain via fluoroscopy. Film this field.
9. Mark the setup points and field borders on the patient for accurate realignment of the fields for treatment.
10. Complete a setup documentation form.

Internal mammary lymph nodes. A relatively small proportion of patients with breast cancer may be at risk for involvement of the internal mammary lymph nodes.[14,35]

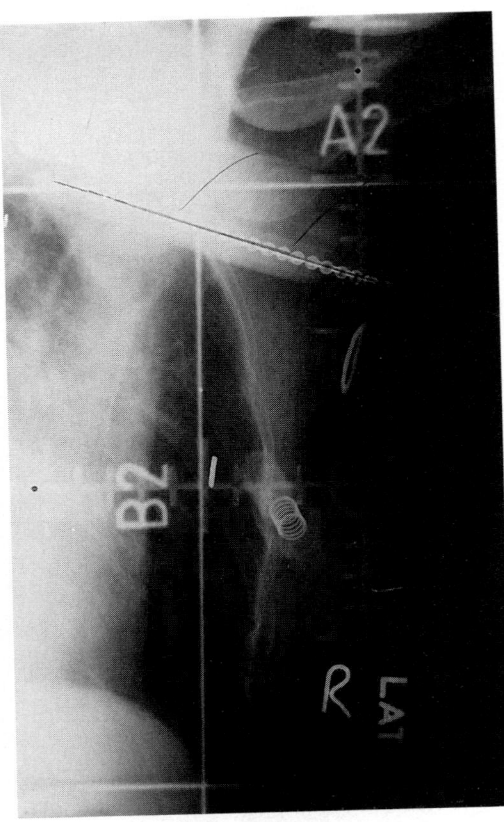

Fig. 13-24 Simulation film of the lateral tangential field, illustrating the use of the rod and chain.

Whether to irradiate the IM nodes remains controversial, partly because current techniques are potentially damaging to normal tissues. One method of irradiating the IM nodes is the extended or deep tangential field configuration. Rather than placing the edge of the medial tangential field at the patient's midline, the field is extended beyond the midline to the contralateral side by approximately 3 cm. Although this arrangement is usually successful in encompassing the ipsilateral IM nodes, it results in a significant increase in the volume of lung irradiated. The extended tangential field also encroaches on the contralateral breast tissue, causing an increase in scattered dose to the breast. Furthermore, in the treatment of left-sided lesions a fairly large portion of the heart is often included in the extended tangential field.

An alternative method of irradiating the IM nodes involves the use of an en face (perpendicular to the skin surface) IM field with a combination of electrons and photons. This field arrangement is subject to the difficulties of matching en face and tangential fields, as well as the problems of joining photon and electron ports, and may result in a hot or cold spot at the junctional area. In addition, an increased volume of cardiac tissue is included in the en face configuration. The photon portion of the IM node treatment contributes exit dose to the vertebral bodies and spinal cord. Conversely, if electrons are used for most or all of the IM treatment, the skin dose may be unacceptably high, contributing to acute and chronic sequelae and potentially a less acceptable cosmetic result.

Breast boost. Patients with conservatively managed breast cancer usually receive additional radiation treatment to the tumor bed immediately after the completion of tangential irradiation. This boost may be delivered with electron teletherapy or radioactive implantation. Electrons are the technique of choice at most institutions because of patient convenience, cost, and cosmetic considerations. In planning the electron boost, care must be taken to ensure that the treatment volume adequately encompasses the tumor bed. The assumption that the location and length of the scar accurately reflect the position and size of the tumor bed may be inaccurate.[2,26,32] If the surgeon places clips on the tumor bed at the time of resection, the position and size of the electron field can be optimized via fluoroscopy and/or radiographs obtained in the simulator room.

Occasionally, the tumor-bed boost is delivered via radioactive implantation. Potential indications for this method include the presence of a gross residual tumor at the time of resection, a deep-seated lesion in an extremely large breast, and rarely, patient preference. Because implantation is invasive, relatively expensive, and labor intensive, and because it requires anesthesia and sometimes inpatient admission, current practice does not routinely include boosting the tumor bed with a radioactive implant.

Special problems. Occasionally, patients requiring radiation therapy for breast malignancy have special circumstances that render planning and treatment difficult. These include a lack of arm mobility, extreme breast size, and very pendulous breasts.

Lack of arm mobility. When planned appropriately in terms of energy selection, field placement, and junction considerations, electron beams offer a viable method of treating postmastectomy patients who have severely compromised arm mobility, as in instances of brachial plexopathy. Because electron fields are treated en face as opposed to tangentially, the problem of avoiding the patient's arm is circumvented. The ideal candidate for this technique has a relatively flat chest wall of uniform thickness. The patient's arm can rest on the treatment table, at her side, and in as abducted a position as the patient can manage. Typically, a minimum of two electron fields are used to encompass the chest wall margins listed previously. One field treats the anterior-medial chest wall, and the other covers the lateral chest wall. The precise matching of adjacent electron field edges can be difficult, so care must be taken to shift the matchline or use junctional wedges or some other means of enhancing dose uniformity where the fields meet.

Some postoperative patients are completely unable to abduct the arm, usually as a result of advanced disease. These individuals can be treated with their arm in an abducted position through the use of an anterior photon field that encompasses the supraclavicular, axillary, and lateral chest wall regions in a single field. The anterior chest wall can be treated with an en face electron field.

Extreme breast size and pendulous breasts. Patients with extremely large and/or pendulous breasts are particularly challenging to treat. Numerous devices and techniques have been developed to stabilize the breast and position it on the chest, permitting a reasonably accurate setup and treatment. Elastic netting can be placed over the breasts; however, this works best on smaller breasts because the material is not strong enough to support an extremely large breast on the chest wall. Systems that use thermoplastic materials to mold the breast into an appropriate position are available commercially. Thermoplastic sheets may also be molded to the patient and fastened around the patient's back with bandage material. A simple ring can be placed around the breast to immobilize and retain the breast in position on the anterior chest.[3] A Styrofoam crutch can also be fashioned and positioned to support pendulous breast tissue located far to the patient's lateral chest.

Side effects. The aim of radiation therapy to the breast is the complete eradication of tumor cells with minimal structural and functional damage to normal tissue. A compromise accepting a certain degree of acute and chronic tissue damage in return for a potential cure is necessary. In every situation, careful planning and treatment delivery are essential to minimize side effects.

Combining radiation treatment and chemotherapy may intensify toxicity. In breast cancer patients the use of Adriamycin is of particular concern. When used concomitantly, radiation and Adriamycin may be hazardous. If Adriamycin is given after radiation therapy, a recall phenomenon may occur in previously treated areas, displayed by exacerbation of reactions of the esophagus, skin, lungs, and heart.

Skin changes. Skin and subcutaneous tissue changes are expected in the irradiated treatment volume. The skin dose depends on the exact treatment technique used for each patient. Variables in the treatment plan that affect the skin dose include the type of radiation (photons or electrons), beam energy, boost technique (external beam or brachytherapy), wedge, bolus, fraction size, total dose, and physical conformation of the patient.

Special consideration must be given to the physical conformation of the patient. Skin folds tend to intensify skin reactions as a result of bolus effect and are therefore the most sensitive areas. Proper positioning is necessary to help minimize folds in potential problem areas. Axillary folds may be minimized by adjusting arm abduction. Skin folds in the inframammary, supraclavicular, and neck areas may be altered or eliminated by increasing or decreasing the cephalocaudad incline of the patient. Obese patients or those with large, pendulous breasts may require netting or thermoplastic material for the immobilization and reduction of skin folds.

During a standard radiation treatment schedule, skin reaction intensifies according to the escalating dose. The RTOG categorizes acute and chronic skin reactions, as shown in Tables 13-1 and 13-2. Dryness and redness (erythema) of the skin are common after a skin dose of about 3000 cGy (3 to 4 weeks into treatment). Dry desquamation, which involves flaking of superficial layers of the epidermis, may appear after the delivery of about 4000 cGy to the skin. Moist desquamation, involving the loss of superficial and deep epidermal layers, occurs when doses to the skin exceed 5000 cGy. Moist desquamation may arise earlier in treatment in areas where skin folds or bolus intensify the prescribed dose. Treatment of the large breast is more difficult secondary to such acute effects and can result in a less acceptable cosmetic outcome.

Care of irradiated skin varies according to the type and severity of the reaction. Patients should be advised regarding measures that protect the skin from further irritation and damage. The treatment area must be kept clean through normal, gentle cleansing, and sun exposure should be avoided. Cornstarch is often recommended as a soothing agent for early skin reactions and as a substitute for commercial deodorant. The use of lotions, creams, deodorants, or powders in the treatment area should be discouraged because they may contain irritating agents such as perfumes, alcohol, or metals. Shaving under the arm is not recommended, and clothing should be soft and loose fitting. Extreme temperatures from hot water bottles, heating pads, and ice packs should also be avoided over the skin of the treated area.

Patients experiencing moist desquamation may require daily skin care to help prevent infection and minimize fluid loss. Gentle cleansing may be performed with a solution of hydrogen peroxide diluted by sterile water and dabbed carefully onto the affected area. Proper wound dressing using nonstick bandaging techniques is essential to promote healing. Care must be taken to avoid placing bandage adhesives or tape in the treatment area. Cornstarch should never be used in areas of moist desquamation because it may promote fungal growth and increase the risk of wound infection.[19]

Severe acute reactions may result in a longer healing time and higher incidence of chronic skin changes. Such skin changes progress slowly and can persist for months or years after irradiation. Most chronic skin changes are cosmetic and rarely problematic, and they include **hyperpigmentation,** (excessive coloration), hair loss, epidermal thinning, **telangiectasia** (permanent dilation of vessels, producing small, red lesions), and subcutaneous fibrosis. Rare cases of delayed wound healing, ulceration, and **necrosis** (death of skin cells) may occur after skin doses of over 70 Gy.[12]

Fatigue. Most patients receiving radiation therapy complain of generalized fatigue. The incidence appears to be related to the radiation dose, treatment volume, and site of involvement. Breast cancer patients may experience a comparatively minor degree of fatigue. Other factors (such as a history of recent surgery or chemotherapy, the patient's general medical and psychological condition, current medications, pain, or anemia) may contribute to fatigue.

Cardiac effects. Portions of the heart are sometimes necessarily included in the radiation fields used in breast cancer treatment. Tangential fields used to treat the left chest wall may include a small to moderate volume of the heart, depending on the patient's anatomy and physical configuration. A larger volume of the heart may be included during irradiation of the internal mammary lymph nodes. Although the myocardia (heart muscle) is relatively radioresistant, the risk of promoting arteriosclerosis, leading to pericarditis, is of concern. The incidence of pericarditis is less than 5% for small heart volumes treated to 60 Gy with standard fractionation or for large heart volumes treated to 40 Gy.[6,12] In addition, larger fraction sizes may intensify cardiac damage.

Pulmonary effects. Tangential fields used to irradiate the breast and/or chest wall always include a small volume of lung tissue. Peripheral lymphatic fields may also irradiate lung tissue. Some degree of radiation pneumonitis and fibrosis can be expected after the administration of over 2500 cGy to any portion of lung via standard fractionation.[24] These effects are directly related to the total dose, fraction size, and irradiated lung volume. The incidence of pulmonary damage grows as the volume, dose, and fraction size increase. The time of onset and degree of severity also vary depending on the volume, dose, and fraction size of lung irradiated.

Although initial morphological changes are not clinically manifested, symptoms may appear after a latent period of 1 to 3 months.[24] These symptoms may include coughing, dyspnea, sputum production, fever, and night sweats and may subside after several months. Scarring or fibrosis may begin 3 to 7 months after irradiation, and depending on its severity, chronic respiratory distress may develop. The degree of severity can be monitored via a chest radiograph, CT scan, and pulmonary function tests. Fortunately, the incidence of chronic pulmonary effects is rare in breast cancer patients because of the small volume of lung irradiated.

Lymphedema. Lymphedema of the arm may occur as a result of axillary lymphatic obstruction. Some acute lymphedema usually occurs immediately after breast surgery and axillary dissection. The severity and risk of lymphedema are directly related to the extent of the axillary dissection and may be further complicated by radiation and chemotherapy. Approximately 25% to 30% of patients receiving radiation therapy after Level III axillary lymph node dissection experience arm edema. Tumor infiltration, infection, inflammation, scarring of the lymph nodes, and radiation-induced fibrosis (alone or in combination) may cause lymphatic obstruction. If a collateral circulatory pathway develops in response to the obstruction, allowing for lymphatic drainage, the edema will resolve. Where the obstruction is severe or the damage is irreparable, lymphatic circulation may be permanently compromised, resulting in chronic edema of the arm.

Radiation-induced lymphedema is relatively rare and similar to other chronic effects in that the incidence and severity are directly related to the radiation dose and treatment volume. Depending on the degree of edema, this condition may be disfiguring and uncomfortable and may impair mobility and function of the arm.

Brachial plexopathy. The brachial plexus (a network of nerves supplying the upper extremities) originates between C-5 and T-1 and extends downward over the first rib, behind the middle of the clavicle, and into the axilla. Damage to these nerves in the form of fibrosis is termed *brachial plexopathy.* High doses of radiation (5500 to 6000 cGy) may lead to this condition.[3,19] Fortunately, standard dose levels prescribed for breast cancer treatment do not exceed 4500 to 5400 cGy and rarely result in this complication. The incidence of brachial plexopathy may also be related to surgery and chemotherapy. Symptoms include a loss of motor function (paresthesia of the arm and hand), weakness, and pain, for which the only treatment is symptomatic pain relief.

Myelopathy. Although the spine is usually avoided entirely during breast irradiation, portions of the cervical and thoracic spine may need to be included in the internal mammary and supraclavicular fields. Care must be taken not to exceed the spinal cord's tolerance dose to avoid delayed complications of chronic progressive myelopathy (ranging from severe to fatal). The $TD_{5/5}$ (minimal tolerance dose) is 4500 to 5000 cGy for instances in which portions of the spinal cord are irradiated with standard fractionation.[3,12]

The supraclavicular field may be angled 10 to 15 degrees mediolaterally to avoid the spinal cord completely. The internal mammary chain field may be treated via expanded tangential fields that entirely avoid the spinal cord or with a combination of en face photons and electrons to reduce the spinal cord dosage. Any adjoining of fields over the spinal cord must be planned carefully to avoid overlap, which can result in an overdose of radiation to the spinal cord.

Osteoradionecrosis. Tangential treatment fields of the chest wall may incidentally deliver a relatively high dose of radiation to the ribs. The incidence of a resulting rib fracture is relatively low (less than 1%), and the ribs appear to heal on their own.

SUMMARY

Breast cancer represents an enigmatic yet fascinating challenge in cancer management. The incidence of breast cancer is widespread and often fatal, recurring sometimes 2 or 3 decades after the initial diagnosis and treatment. Breast cancer is especially important because it affects a part of the female anatomy that is functionally and culturally associated with beauty, femininity, sexuality, and nurturing. With recorded history dating back several millennia, the pendulum of breast cancer treatment has swung between extremes of belief that breast cancer is an incurable systemic disease and the notion that it is a local, therefore curable, problem. This debate continues today, with many researchers occupying a rational middle ground in which each patient is evaluated against the backdrop of multiple prospective and retrospective analyses to maximize survival potential.

Review Questions
Multiple Choice

1. The pathological staging system for breast cancer incorporates which of the following?
   I. Lymph node status
   II. Tumor extent
   III. Distant metastasis
   a. I and II
   b. II and III
   c. I and III
   d. I, II, and III
2. What is the most common presenting symptom of early-stage breast cancer?
   a. Nipple discharge
   b. Pain
   c. Palpable mass
   d. Ulceration
3. Which of the following is proper advise for a patient receiving radiation treatment to the breast?
   I. Do not wear restrictive clothing.
   II. Avoid using commercial deodorant.
   III. Avoid sun exposure to the skin of the treated area.
   a. I and II
   b. II and III
   c. I and III
   d. I, II, and III
4. To what does TD $_{5/5}$ refer?
   a. Minimal tolerance dose
   b. Maximum tolerance dose
   c. Tumor dose of 5 Gy in 5 days
   d. Tumor dose of 5 cGy in 5 days
5. What is the $TD_{5/5}$ for the spinal cord delivered through standard fractionation?
   a. 1500 cGy
   b. 3000 cGy
   c. 4500 cGy
   d. 6000 cGy
6. Which of the following is *not* currently a standard technique for breast surgery?
   a. Radical mastectomy
   b. Modified radical mastectomy
   c. Lumpectomy
   d. Tyelectomy
7. Chemotherapy for breast cancer may consist of which of the following?
   I. Drug therapy
   II. Endocrine therapy
   III. Immunotherapy
   a. I and II
   b. II and III
   c. I and III
   d. I, II, and III
8. In treating a breast cancer patient via tangential fields plus an electron field boost, what is the usual total dose to the tumor bed delivered through a standard fractionation schedule?
   a. 4000 to 4600 cGy
   b. 5000 to 5600 cGy
   c. 6000 to 6600 cGy
   d. 7000 to 7600 cGy
9. Which of the following techniques may be used to adequately irradiate the internal mammary lymph nodes on a patient with left breast cancer and simultaneously deliver the least cardiac dose?
   a. Anterior photon field, 50 Gy in 5 weeks
   b. Anterior photon-electron fields, equally weighted, 50 Gy in 5 weeks
   c. Wide tangential fields, extending 5 cm across the midline, 50 Gy in 5 weeks
   d. Anterior electron field, 50 Gy in 5 weeks

Matching (The skin usually reacts in a pattern that is dose dependent. Match the skin dose to the expected reaction for radiation administered by a standard fractionation schedule.)

10. Dry desquamation
11. Erythema
12. Moist desquamation
    a. 30 Gy
    b. 40 Gy
    c. 50 Gy

Questions to Ponder

1. Discuss the significant prognostic indicators for breast cancer.
2. Describe the signs of inflammatory breast cancer.
3. Describe the acute effects experienced by patients undergoing radiation treatment to the breast.
4. Define the three elements of treatment in conservative management of early-stage breast cancer.
5. Describe the field arrangements most commonly used for patients receiving conservative management of breast cancer.
6. Discuss important considerations for positioning the conservatively managed patient for breast irradiation.
7. Describe the methods for detection and diagnosis of breast cancer.
8. Identify the common presenting symptoms of breast cancer.
9. Discuss the importance of staging breast cancer.
10. Describe the primary lymphatic drainage of breast tissue.

REFERENCES

1. American Cancer Society: *Cancer facts and figures —1996,* Atlanta, 1996, The Society..
2. Bedwinek J: Breast conserving surgery and irradiation: the importance of demarcating the excision cavity with surgical clips, *Int J Radiat Oncol Biol Phys* 26:675-679, 1993.
3. Bentel GC, Nelson CE, Noell KT: *Treatment planning & dose calculation in radiation oncology,* ed 4, Elmsford, New York, 1989, Pergamon Press.
4. Boag JW et al: The number of patients required in a clinical trial, *Br J Radiol* 44:122-125, 1971.
5. Boice JD et al: Risk of breast cancer following low dose radiation exposure, *Radiology* 131:589-597, 1979.
6. Byhardt RW, Moss WT: The heart and blood vessels. In Cox JD, editor: *Moss' radiation oncology rationale, technique, results,* ed 7, St Louis, 1994, Mosby.
7. Carter C, Allen C, Henson D: Relation of tumor size, lymph node status, and survival in 24,740 breast cancer cases, *Cancer* 63:181-187, 1989.
8. Committee on the Biological Effects of Ionizing Radiations; Board on Radiation Effects Research; Commission on Life Sciences; National Research Council: *Health effects of exposure to low levels of ionizing radiation BEIR V,* Washington, DC, 1990, National Academy Press.
9. Cruikshank WC: *The anatomy of the absorbing vessels of the human body,* London, 1786, G. Nicol.
10. Cumberlin RL, Dritchilo A, Mossman KL: Carcinogenic effects of scattered dose associated with radiation therapy, *Int J Radiat Oncol Biol Phys* 17:623-629, 1989.
11. Donegan WL, Spratt JS: *Cancer of the breast,* ed 3, Philadelphia, 1988, WB Saunders.
12. Emami B et al: Tolerance of normal tissue to therapeutic radiation, *Int J Radiat Oncol Biol Phys* 22:109-122, 1991.
13. Fisher B et al: Location of breast carcinoma and prognosis, *Surg Gynecol Obstet* 129:705-716, 1969.
14. Fox MS: On the diagnosis and treatment of breast cancer, *JAMA* 241:489-494, 1979.
15. Goldhirsch A, Gelber RD: Understanding adjuvant chemotherapy for breast cancer, *N Engl J Med* 330(18): 1308-1309, 1994.
16. Haagensen CD: *Diseases of the breast,* ed 3, Philadelphia, 1986, WB Saunders.
17. Harris JR, Morrow M, Bonadonna G: Cancer of the breast. In DeVita VT, Hellman S, Rosenberg SA, editors: *Cancer principles and practice of oncology,* ed 4, Philadelphia, 1993, JB Lippincott.
18. Harris JR et al: *Breast diseases,* ed 2, Philadelphia, 1991, JB Lippincott.
19. Hassey Dow K, Hilderley L: *Nursing care in radiation oncology,* Philadelphia, 1992, WB Saunders.
20. Henderson IC: Adjuvant systemic therapy for early breast cancer, *Cancer* (Suppl) 74(1):401-408, 1994.
21. Henderson IC, Canellos GP: Cancer of the breast: the past decade, *N Engl J Med* 302:17-30, 1980.
22. John MJ et al: *Chemoradiation: an integrated approach to cancer treatment,* Malvren, Pennsylvania, 1993, Lea & Febiger.
23. Kelsey JL: A review of the epidemiology of human breast cancer, *Epidemiol Rev* 1:74-109, 1979.
24. Komaki R, Cox JD: The lung and thymus. In Cox JD, editor: *Moss' radiation oncology: rationale, technique, results,* ed 7, St Louis, 1994, Mosby.
25. Mascagni P: *Vasorum lymphaticorum corporis humani historia et ichnographia,* Siena, 1787, P. Carli.
26. Regine WF et al: Computer-CT planning of the electron boost in definitive breast irradiation, *Int J Radiat Oncol Biol Phys* 20:121-125, 1991.
27. Ries LAB, Hankey BR, Edwards BK, editors: *Cancer statistics revew, 1983-87,* Bethesda, Maryland, 1988, National Cancer Institute Division of Cancer Prevention and Control Surveillance Program.
28. Rosen PP et al: Discontinuous or "skip" metastases in breast carcinoma: analysis of 1228 axillary dissections, *Ann Surg* 276-283, 1983.
29. Saphillo O, Parker MI: Metastases of primary carcinoma of the breast with special reference to spleen, adrenal glands and ovaries, *Arch Surg* 42:1003, 1941.
30. Schottenfeld D et al: Ten-year results of the treatment of primary operable breast carcinoma, *Cancer* 38:1005, 1976.
31. Shinkin MB: *Contrary to nature,* Washington, DC, 1977, United States Printing Office.
32. Solin LJ et al: A practical technique for the localization of the tumor volume in definitive irradiation of the breast, *Int J Radiat Oncol Biol Phys* 11:1215-1220, 1985.
33. Veronesi U et al: Distribution of axillary node metastases by level of invasion: an analysis of 539 cases, *Cancer* 59:682-687, 1987.
34. Veronesi U et al: Prognosis of breast cancer patients after mastectomy and dissection of internal mammary nodes, *Ann Surg* 202:702-707, 1985.
35. Warren S, Wittman EM: Studies on tumor metastases: the distribution of metastases in cancer of the breast, *Surg Gynecol Obstet* 57:81, 1937.
36. Wilson JF: The breast. In Cox JD, editor: *Moss' radiation oncology: rationale, technique, results,* ed 7, St. Louis, 1994, Mosby.
37. Wise L, Johnson H: *Breast cancer: controversies in management,* Armonk, New York, 1994, Futura Publishing.

BIBLIOGRAPHY

Bentel GC, Marks LB: A simple device to position large/flaccid breasts during tangential breast irradiation, *Int J Radiat Oncol Biol Phys* 29:879-882, 1994.

Breasted JH: *The Edwin Smith Surgical Papyrus,* Chicago, 1930, University of Chicago Press.

Cox JD, Winchester DP, editors: Standards for breast conservation treatment. Adopted by the Board of Chancellors, American College of Radiology, and endorsed by the Board of Regents, American College of Surgeons, 1992.

Fowble B et al: Frequency, sites of relapse, and outcome of regional node failures following conservative surgery and radiation for early breast cancer, *Int J Radiat Oncol Biol Phys* 17:703-710, 1989.

Halsted WS: The results of operations for the cure of cancer of the breast performed at Johns Hopkins Hospital from June 1889 to January 1894, *Johns Hopkins Hospital Bull* 4:297, 1894-1895.

Hanke BF, Steinhorn SC: Long term patient survival for some of the more frequently occurring cancers, *Cancer* 50:1904-1912, 1982.

Harness JK et al: *Breast cancer, collaborative management,* Chelsea, Michigan, 1988, Lewis Publishers.

Harris JR, Hellman S: Observations on survival curve analysis with particular reference to breast cancer treatment, *Cancer* 57:925-928, 1986.

Lichter AS et al: A technique for field matching in primary breast irradiation, *Int J Radiat Oncol Biol Phys* 9:263-270, 1982.

Rosenow UF, Valentine ES, Davis LW: A technique for treating local breast cancer using a single set-up point and asymmetric collimation, *Int J Radiat Oncol Biol Phys* 19:183-188, 1990.

Siddon RL et al: Three field technique for breast irradiation using tangential field corner blocks, *Int J Radiat Oncol Biol Phys* 9:583-588, 1983.

Svensson GK et al: A modified three-field technique for breast treatment, *Int J Radiat Oncol Biol Phys* 6:689-694, 1980.

Veronesi U, Vallagussa P: Inefficacy of internal mammary node dissection in breast cancer surgery, *Cancer* 47:170-175, 1981.

CHAPTER

14

Pediatric Solid Tumors

Jeffrey Young

Outline

Key terms

Astrocytomas
Autologous bone marrow transplantation (ABMT)
Craniospinal irradiation (CSI)
Ependymomas
Germ cell tumors
Histiocytosis X
Medulloblastoma
Neuroblastoma
Oncogene
Palliation
Retinoblastoma
Rhabdomyosarcomas
Second malignant neoplasm (SMN)
Wilms' tumor

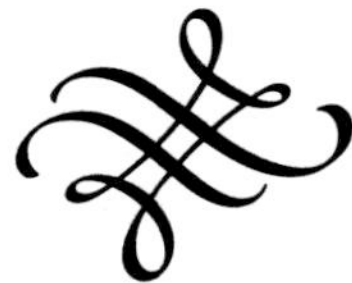

Although older groups dominate the patient population of radiation oncology centers, childhood cancer (age 18 or under) is a significant problem. Almost 7000 new cases occur annually in the U.S., and cancer is the second leading cause of death (behind accidents) in children. The treatments, cure rates, and types of cancers that develop in children are distinctively different than those of the adult population (Table 14-1). Predisposing genetic conditions include xeroderma pigmentosa, ataxia telangiectasia, Bloom and Fanconi's syndromes, neurofibromatosis, and gene abnormalities such as p53.[31] Acute leukemias and lymphomas account for about 40% of pediatric cancers. Central nervous system tumors are the most frequent solid tumors, and radiation has a critical role in their treatment. Although a shift toward other effective therapies has taken place, radiation is still involved with patients who have soft tissue sarcoma, Wilms' tumor, neuroblastoma, and other benign and malignant conditions.

The treatment of childhood malignancies is always multidisciplinary and requires close attention to the physical and emotional needs of the child and family. Care is coordinated with medical, surgical, and nursing oncological colleagues and supported from social services, physical therapists, nutritionists, educators, and others. This team approach usually requires referral to a specialized children's cancer program. (This is especially true outside the U.S.) Over 50% of patients are involved in clinical trial investigations led by the Pediatric Oncology Group (POG) and Children's Cancer Group (CCG) in the U.S. and Societe Internationale d'Oncologie Pediatrique (SIOP) in Europe. Therapists have special demands for such protocol patients. Because many

Table 14-1 Cancer incidence, peak age, and survival rate in children under 15 years old—1991 estimates

Site or type of cancer	New cases	Peak age	Survival rate (%)
All sites	7000	—	75
Leukemia	2150	2-5	70
Brain and nervous system	1700	5-10	60
Lymphoma	700	6-16	80
Kidney and Wilms' tumor	400	5	88
Neuroblastoma	500	<3	55
Bone and soft tissue	750	10-18	60
Retinoblastoma	200	<3	90
Other sites	600	—	—

Data from Pizzo PA et al: Solid tumors of childhood. In Devita VT, Hellman S, Rosenburg SA, editors: *Cancer: principles and practice of oncology,* ed 4, Philadelphia, 1993, Lippincott; and Ries LAG et al: *SEER cancer statistics review, 1973-1991: tables and graphs,* NIH Publication number 94-2789, Bethesda, Maryland, 1994, National Cancer Institute.

Table 14-2 Relative incidence of brain tumors in children

Type of tumor	Percentage of total
Supratentorial (45%-50%)	
Low-grade astrocytoma	25
Anaplastic astrocytoma, glioblastoma, and PNET	10
Ependymoma	3
Pineal and germ cell tumors	4
Pituitary and craniopharyngioma	5
Infratentorial (50%-55%)	
Medulloblastoma	25
Low-grade astrocytoma	15
Ependymoma	5
Brain stem glioma	10

Data from Duffner PK et al: Survival of children with brain tumors: SEER program, 1973-1980, *Neurology* 36:597-601, 1986.
PNET, primitive neuroectodermal tumor.

radiation therapists do not see pediatric patients, the remainder of this chapter highlights selected childhood cancers and their unique treatments.

BRAIN TUMORS

Epidemiology

The nearly 2000 central nervous system (CNS) cancer cases annually involve a wide spectrum of lesions histologically and anatomically. In children (compared with adults) low-grade and infratentorial (posterior fossa) tumors are more frequent, metastatic lesions from non-CNS primaries are rare, and late effects of treatment are a major concern. Table 14-2 illustrates relative incidences from a combination of patient series. Neurofibromatosis is linked to low-grade glioma risk, and retinoblastoma suppressor gene defects on chromosome 13 can be inherited, leading to a high risk of bilateral disease. However, most benign and high-grade tumors occur sporadically. Because the disease and its treatment can have major long-term side effects for children, individualized multidisciplinary care involving neurosurgery, endocrinology, pediatric and radiation oncology, rehabilitation, and other services is a must.

Low-grade astrocytomas

Astrocytomas are tumors originating from the nonneuronal-supporting cells of the brain. These tumors can be histologically similar to normal glial cells but continue slow, relentless growth. They occur about equally in the cerebrum and posterior fossa. A long history of mild symptoms dependent on the area of brain involved is the usual course. Headaches, degenerating coordination, visual impairment, or poor school performance can worsen subtly for months or years, and seizures can eventually develop. Radiologically, a cystic component may be present, and there is less surrounding edema than with high-grade lesions (Fig. 14-1, *A*).

If discovered in an extremely young child without major neurological deficits, a low-grade brain tumor can be followed with serial physical and radiologic examinations. After the child reaches an age at which the brain is more mature (usually 3 to 5 years old), neurosurgery is the primary treatment. If the lesion can be completely removed, the long-term prognosis is excellent. A recurrence-free survival rate of 90% to 100% has been achieved.[42]

Radiation therapy has been reserved for surgically inaccessible or recurrent lesions and those with postsurgical residua. A dose of 5000 to 5500 cGy at 180 cGy per day is routinely used. Because infiltration of surrounding brain is limited, only a 2-cm margin around the lesion is necessary. Radiation has enhanced the long-term control of residual tumors in most series,[4] but progression may occur years later. Stereotactic radiosurgery has been used for focal lesions, and the POG is investigating carboplatin chemotherapy, with some early encouraging results.

High-grade astrocytomas

In contrast to their low-grade counterparts, high-grade astrocytomas definitely behave malignantly. They grow rapidly, invade and destroy adjacent brain tissues, and can spread through the CNS or distantly. Neuropathologists commonly classify high-grade gliomas in order of escalating malignancy as *anaplastic astrocytoma, glioblastoma multiforme,* and *malignant primitive neuroectodermal tumor (PNET).* High-grade gliomas are usually supratentorial, with neurological symptoms progressing quickly. Headaches and lethargy are followed by motor or sensory loss, seizures, and intracranial hemorrhage. Radiologically, these lesions have indistinct borders, areas of necrosis, and much surrounding edema (Fig. 14-1, *B*). Steroids are used to reduce edema before surgery. Staging has been proposed according to tumor size, ventricle or brainstem invasion, and metastases; however, staging is not routinely used.

Neurosurgery is the important first step of multidisciplinary treatment for high-grade brain tumors. Surgery yields the histological diagnosis, removes the gross tumor, and decompresses adjacent structures, but residual tumor invariably remains. Chemotherapy and radiation are standardly used postoperatively. The optimal sequencing is still uncertain, but cooperative research groups have demonstrated improvements in survival rates with various combinations.[17] Chemotherapy is especially vital in infants for delaying the need for radiation while the brain matures to reduce late sequelae.

The radiation technique requires large fields. Anaplastic astrocytomas may be treated with a margin of 3 cm or more. Glioblastoma and PNET usually receive whole-brain radiation therapy to a dose of 3000 cGy or more, followed by a tumor boost of 6000 cGy and higher. Because of the occasional occurrence of cerebrospinal fluid (CSF) seeding, some pediatric radiation oncologists recommend **craniospinal irradiation (CSI)** initially. CSI involves irradiation of all CNS and CSF regions from behind the eye down to the midsacrum. The overall prognosis is poor, even with aggressive treatment. The survival rate at 5 years is 20% to 35% in many series.[19] Local control is still a major problem. Hyperfractionated radiation to doses over 7000 cGy is under study without excessive early toxicity, but results are pending.

Optic gliomas

Optic tract and hypothalamic gliomas are usually extremely low-grade astrocytomas and some authors argue they are benign. Children with neurofibromatosis are at a much higher risk. Because visual and hormonal functions can be impaired, they frequently require treatment. The POG has an ongoing study with observation for asymptomatic patients. Those who progress radiologically or develop symptoms receive carboplatin chemotherapy or radiation. Potential bilateral, chiasmatic, and distal optic tract involvement must be considered during radiation therapy. In such instances larger tailored fields with about 2-cm margins are required, and the prognosis is worse. Long-term follow-up is required before any conclusions can be made about the treatment of this indolent disease.

Benign tumors of the central nervous system

Pituitary adenomas usually occur in adolescents and adults but can also be seen in young children. These patients can have excessive hormone production, visual disturbance from pressure on the optic chiasm, or diabetes insipidus (DI). Transphenoidal hypophysectomy or medical management with bromocriptine used to counteract hormone production usually supplants radiation in the treatment of children. Localized radiation therapy with multiple fields or stereotactic radiation therapy with a dose of 4500 cGy can be given if other methods fail and can control over 70% of tumors.[9]

Craniopharyngiomas arise from embryological remnants of pharyngeal pouch tissues. These tumors eventually enlarge (usually with a prominent cystic component) and disrupt the hypothalamic pituitary axis (DI or precocious puberty), impair vision, or induce seizures. Surgery and focal radiation can be effective with the goal of reducing visual or late side effects. External radiation portals and doses are similar to those for pituitary adenomas. Because subsequent panhypopituitarism almost always develops, a pediatric endocrinologist must be included on the management team for these patients. Some physicians have injected

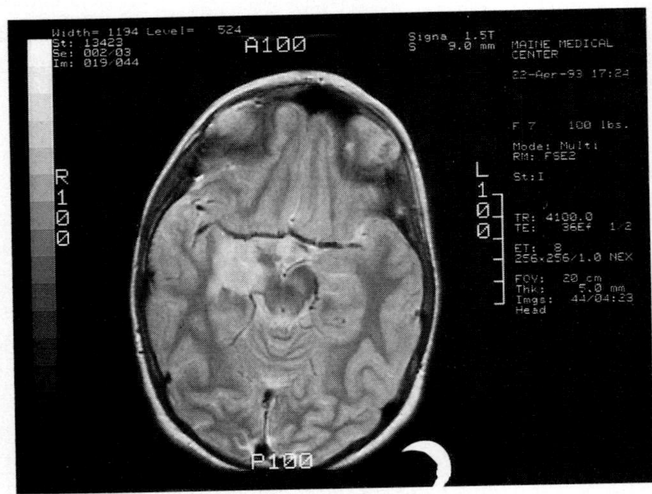

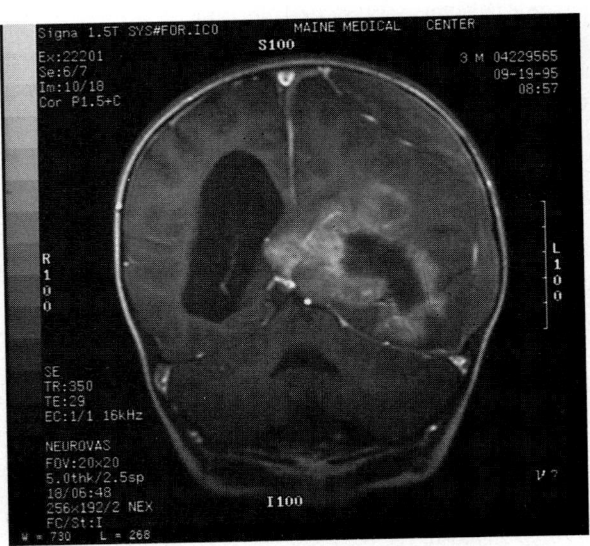

Fig. 14-1 **A,** Low-grade astrocytoma. Note the regular border and minimal edema. **B,** Glioblastoma multiforme. Invasive borders, edema, and shift of normal structures.

radionuclides into the cysts, with good results in selected patients.[54] Meningiomas and acoustic neuromas are histologically benign lesions that occur far more often in patients who have neurofibromatosis. These lessons are treated by observation or surgery if they progress and cause neurological symptoms. Arteriovenous malformations in surgically difficult regions were treated with proton beam therapy many years ago. Now they are the predominant lesions treated in some stereotactic radiosurgery programs. Usually 1500 to 2000 cGy is delivered in a single fraction, with control of potentially deadly rebleeding in 80% of patients.[20]

Medulloblastomas

Epidemiology. Medulloblastoma is the prototype posterior fossa malignancy and constitutes about 25% of all childhood brain tumors. It usually occurs in children 2 to 12 years old, with a peak at 5 years.[10] It rarely occurs in adults. Medulloblastoma is believed to arise from primitive neuroepithelial cells and histologically appears as small, round, blue cells forming pseudorosettes.[46] The tumor usually arises in the midline of the cerebellum, can invade the fourth ventricle and brain stem, and has a high propensity to spread throughout the CSF.

Diagnosis and staging. The presenting symptoms of medulloblastoma usually occur over a period of weeks to a few months. Several symptoms develop as a result of the invasion and compression of the fourth ventricle, thus stopping the inferior flow of CSF with resultant hydrocephalus. Headaches and early-morning vomiting occur intermittently at first and then become more steady. Later findings are ataxia and cranial nerve abnormalities from invasion of the brain stem. Computed tomography (CT) and magnetic resonance imaging (MRI) scans show a round, central cerebellar-enhancing mass (Fig. 14-2), and hydrocephalus is often noted. Steroids and a ventriculostomy can be used to reduce pressure in the acute situation. Because of the propensity for

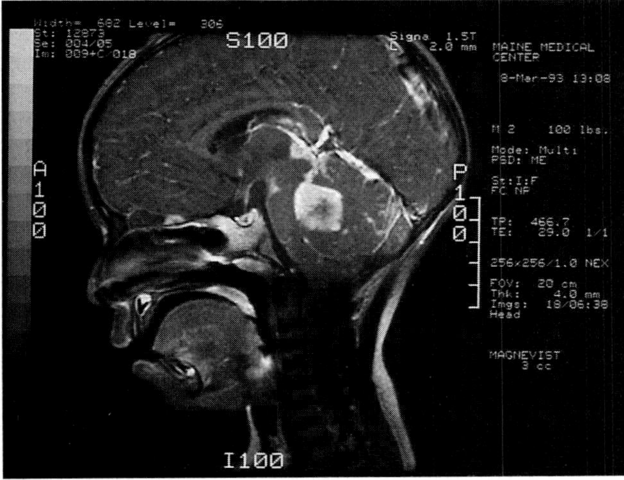

Fig. 14-2 MRI scan of medulloblastoma. Pressure on the brain stem and CSF obstruction are evident. Diffuse CFS seeding is present.

CSF seeding, imaging the entire CNS via myelography or MRI is important. Supratentorial and spinal cord drop metastases can be present in up to 25% of patients.[14] CSF cytology for tumor cells can be performed from a ventriculostomy or lumbar puncture preoperatively.

Chang, Housepian, and Herbert[8] initially developed a staging system at Columbia University. This system relates to the tumor size, invasion of the fourth ventricle and brain stem, and amount of CSF spread (see the box below). This staging correlates with survival and has been used to delineate advanced presentations for more aggressive treatment.

Medulloblastoma is one CNS tumor that can develop distant metastases, usually in bone. The intense, technical multidisciplinary therapy necessary for medulloblastomas must be performed in a center with pediatric cancer expertise.

Treatment techniques. After the patient is stabilized neurologically, every attempt should be made for neurosurgical removal of the gross tumor. A posterior occipital craniotomy is used. The purple, friable, bulging tumor is usually quickly evident. Although the central mass is removed easily, it is the anterior extent into the brain stem or into the cervical spinal cord inferiorly that often leads to residua. Most studies have demonstrated a survival benefit with gross total removal, but surgery is not curative. The routine use of ventriculo-peritoneal (VP) shunts is discouraged because of the risk of tumor seeding into the peritoneal cavity.

The Chang Staging System for Medulloblastoma

- T_1 Tumor less than 3 cm in diameter and limited to the classic midline position in the vermis, to the roof of the fourth ventricle, and less frequently to the cerebellar hemispheres
- T_2 Tumor 3 cm or greater in diameter, further invading one adjacent structure or partially filling the fourth ventricle
- T_3
  - T_{3a} Tumor further invading two adjacent structures or completely filling the fourth ventricle with extension into the aqueduct of Sylvius, foramen of Magendie, or foramen of Luschka, producing marked internal hydrocephalus
  - T_{3b} Tumor arising from the floor of the fourth ventricle or brain stem and filling the fourth ventricle
- T_4 Tumor further spreading through the aqueduct of Sylvius to involve the third ventricle or midbrain, or tumor extending to the upper cervical cord
- M_0 No evidence of dissemination beyond the posterior fossa; CSF cytological results negative for tumor cells; myelogram results negative; CT and MRI scan not showing any supratentorial involvement
- M_1 Evidence of dissemination

Modified from Chang CH, Housepian EM, Herbert C: An operative system and a megavoltage radiotherapeutic technique for cerebellar medulloblastoma, *Radiology* 93:1351-1359, 1969.

T, Tumor; *M,* metastasis; *CSF,* cerebrospinal fluid; *CT,* computed tomography; *MRI,* magnetic resonance imaging.

The benefit of postoperative radiation therapy was documented by Patterson and Farr[43] as early as 1953. CSI is a technical challenge, and several methods have been used. The most common technique uses lateral-opposed fields for the brain and CSF spaces from the retroorbital space down through the midcervical cord. Careful shielding must be done for the anterior globe, oropharynx, and neck. The treatment couch is angulated a few degrees to compensate for divergence over the spinal cord. The divergence of the spinal radiation field determines the collimator angle for the brain field. Depending on the height of the child, one or two posterior fields are used to encompass the spine down to the level of the second or third sacral segment. This technique is illustrated in Fig. 14-3.[50] Some centers have used electrons to treat the spinal cord, avoiding radiation exposure to anterior tissues; however, this requires precise physics and extensive tissue compensators. Usually, 4- to 6-MV x-rays are used for each field. Present physics recommendations are for a 0- to 0.5-cm gap between the spinal field and lateral brain fields. Usually, this junction and the one between the two spine fields in taller children are moved up and down 1 cm daily or weekly. This prevents excessive dose gradients at the junctions with the potential for a spinal cord overdose or a cold spot that can allow tumor cells to survive. These children should be immobilized in a prone position unless doing so is deemed unsafe. Custom head holders or body cradles are helpful. Reproducible positioning of the head and careful marking of treatment portal edges are paramount. If sedation is needed, the anesthesia staff members may require some modifications of the previous technique for airway safety and monitoring equipment.

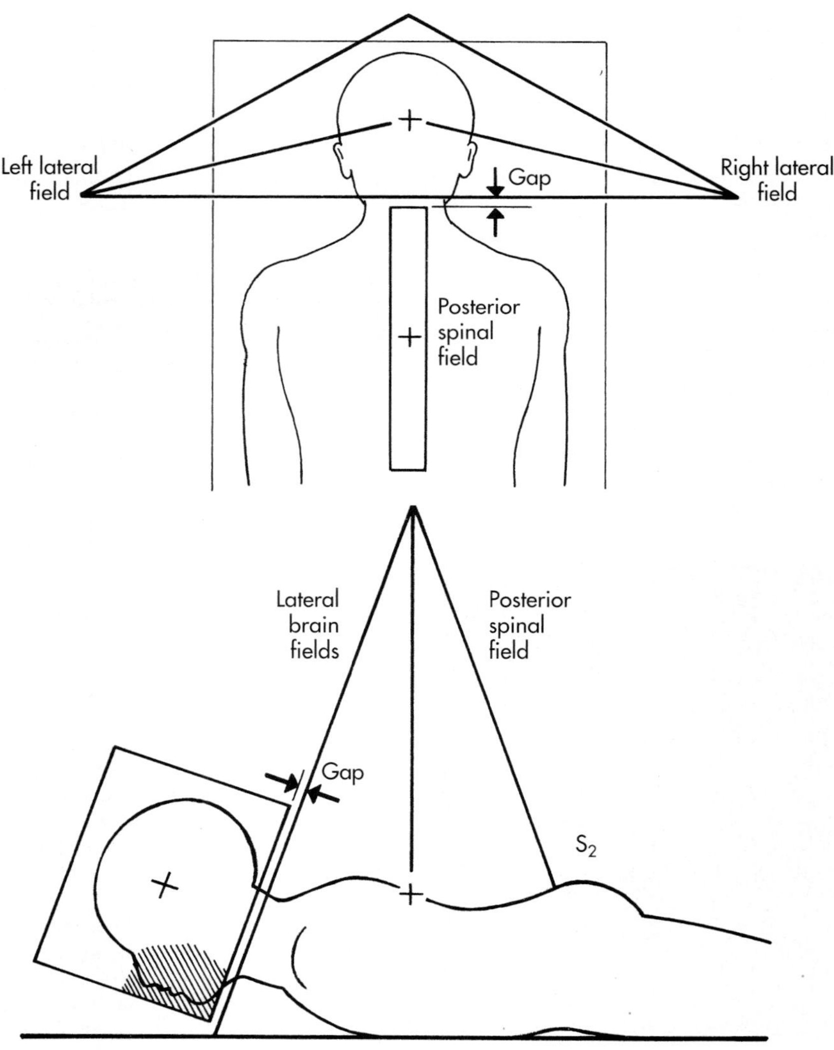

Fig. 14-3 Radiation portal alignment for medulloblastoma. The brain portal collimator angle is adjusted for spinal field divergence. The junction gap is moved 1 cm daily.

CSI can usually proceed at 150 cGy per day. Premedication for nausea is often needed because of the exit beam of the spinal field interacting with the gastrointestinal tract. Because of late sequelae, an attempt has been made to reduce the CSI dose or use chemotherapy as a substitute. However, in the U.S. a recent study by POG and CCG found increasing relapses outside the posterior fossa with a dose of 2340 cGy versus 3600 cGy.[52] Because the primary site of recurrence is still the posterior fossa, that region is boosted with lateral-opposed fields after CSI. This boost field should extend from the posterior clinoids to the back of the skull and from beyond the superior aspect of the tentorium (usually over halfway from the skull's base to its top) down to the level of C2. A midline sagittal MRI scan is helpful in designing this portal. The daily fraction is usually increased to 180 cGy per day up to a total of about 5400 cGy. Dose response in earlier studies noted lower control rates with doses under 5000 cGy.[48] There are some proponents for radiosurgery to an even higher dose if gross residua is present. The entire radiation treatment course for medulloblastoma is 6 to 7 weeks, even without any treatment breaks that are possible due to surgical complications, low blood counts and infection, or gastrointestinal toxicity. In addition to weekly blood counts, nutrition must be carefully monitored in these children. The psychological trauma of alopecia (hair loss) and a daily hospital trip are not insignificant. Despite the rigors of the treatment, the addition of radiation has brought survival rates to over 60%.[30]

Chemotherapy was initially used in relapsed patients, and some lasting responses were seen. Over the last few years cooperative research groups in Europe and the U.S. have added chemotherapy in a randomized fashion to standard surgery and radiation. In most studies a 10% to 20% benefit has been noted with chemotherapy, with most of the improvement in $T_{3,4}$ or M_1 situations.[23] The sequencing of chemotherapy before or after radiation is still being evaluated.

Ependymomas and other cerebrospinal fluid seeding tumors

Ependymomas arise from the ventricular linings and can be cerebral or posteria fossa in location. CSF metastatic seeding is far more likely in infratentorial and anaplastic ependymomas. Although neuropathologists debate the grading of ependymomas, a definite relationship exists with higher rates of CSF seeding and primary tumor relapse in highly malignant histology lesions.[33] Staging of the entire brain and spinal cord is necessary. If CSF seeding is noted or high-risk histology exists, CSI with techniques similar to medulloblastoma are needed. Supratentorial and low-grade tumors can be treated with a 2- to 3-cm margin. Doses of about 5500 cGy to the primary mass are recommended. Chemotherapy is being used in some investigational trials, but the value has yet to be established.

Germ cell tumors (which develop from embryological rests of tissue in the midline from the brain down to the ovaries and testes) and pineal-region tumors may also seed the CSF. Germinomas and pineoblastomas may require CSI. Before neurosurgical biopsy became safe, empirical treatment of the tumor mass with radiation was common. If the tumor regressed after 1500 to 2000 cGy, the assumption was made that the tumor was a germinoma or high-grade pineal lesion, and craniospinal therapy was initiated. In most instances a biopsy can now be performed to guide the radiation oncologist. Although lower CSI doses are reasonable, the primary lesion is best controlled with 5000 cGy. In addition, these histologies are more senstive to chemotherapeutic agents that may supplant the need for CSI.[3]

Brain stem gliomas

Brain stem gliomas typically involve cranial nerve deficits that can affect vision, facial nerves, and swallowing. Most of these lesions are diffuse in the pons and thus are entirely unresectable. Biopsy has been possible lately, and most of these pontine tumors are high-grade astrocytomas. Posterior expansion of the pons can create hydrocephalus.

The mainstay of treatment is radiation therapy. The fields should cover the entire brain stem and midbrain region, reaching from about 4 cm superior to the clinoids down to at least the level of C1. Doses of 180 cGy per day have historically been delivered with lateral-opposed fields, although a truly central lesion can be treated with rotational fields or newer conformal therapy. Doses of 5500 cGy in the past resulted in poor cure rates. In the hope of improvement, hyperfractionation has been used with doses escalated to 7800 cGy delivered at 100 to 117 cGy twice daily. However, the survival rate in diffuse lesions is only 10%.[22] A present study involves cisplatin chemotherapy as a radiation sensitizer with a randomization between radiation once and twice daily.

There is an unusual brain stem glioma that has a better prognosis. This is an exophytic lesion extending from the posterior aspect of the brain stem into the fourth ventricle. These lesions tend to have a low-grade histology and are amenable to surgical resection by select pediatric neurosurgeons. The survival rate for patients with these lesions is over 50%.[29]

Late effects of treatment

The treatment of large areas of the brain and spinal cord can have a variety of devastating late sequalae. These effects are definitely worse the younger the child's age at the time of treatment. Because survival rates were so poor for many decades, only now are these factors being assessed. Postsurgical deficits of motor-sensory loss, poor coordination, or cranial nerve dysfunction can last a lifetime. Parents are always extremely concerned about the child's subsequent intellectual abilities. Whole-brain radiation with high doses for high-grade gliomas and CSF seeding tumors has decreased the median intelligence quotient of survivors.[28] Changes of cortical atrophy and basal ganglia calcifications can occur, even with lower doses used in leukemic CNS prophylaxis, but do not correlate with neurological impairment. The interaction of methotrexate and radiation can cause severe degeneration of the CNS white matter, termed *leukoencephaly.* Cisplatin and radiation can decrease hearing. Doses over 2000 cGy to the pituitary and hypothalamus can cause delayed decreases in pituitary hormones. Thyroid and growth hormone deficits are most likely and with early detection can be reversed via supplemental hormones.[41] CSI can decrease the height of vertebral bodies, leading to a short-waisted adult. The acute hair loss can be psychologically traumatic, and high doses of radiation can lead to permanent hair loss for some children. Second malignancies may develop many years later in the CNS, bones, or bone marrow from the damage that earlier radiation and chemotherapy induces. Careful follow-up and early intervention, medically and educationally, can lessen many of the late effects just mentioned. Although doing so may frighten parents, mentioning the risks for late effects when obtaining informed consent for a child's radiation treatment is necessary. Despite these risks, parents are almost always ecstatic that even an impaired child has survived a life-threatening brain tumor.

RETINOBLASTOMAS

Epidemiology

Although **retinoblastoma** (the primitive neuroectodermal tumor of the retina) is the most common intraocular tumor in young children, it only occurs about 200 times annually in the U.S. Most retinoblastomas occur in children 6 months to 4 years of age.[1] A well-documented hereditary autosomal-dominant pattern is present in 25% to 35% of patients. The retinoblastoma gene is located on chromosome 13 and is a tumor-suppressor gene. Therefore both halves of the chromosome must suffer a deletion of the gene for retinoblastoma to occur. These patients account for the majority of cases of bilateral retinoblastoma and have a significant risk of development of later nonocular cancers. At least 65% of retinoblastomas are unilateral and without evidence of inheritance.[6]

Diagnosis and staging

Retinoblastoma is usually discovered as a result of an abnormal retinal light reflex (white rather than red). This tumor may be noted from a flash photograph or during the pediatrician's routine examination. An ophthalmologist should examine both eyes with the child under anesthesia to document multifocality or bilaterality. Careful retinal mapping is required for treatment and follow-up. A biopsy is not done because of the risk of vitreous seeding. CT or ultrasound of the orbit can detect unusual cases with extraocular extension or simultaneous supratentorial-pineal lesions (trilateral retinoblastoma). With extraocular disease the CSF is assessed by lumbar puncture cytology, and a bone marrow biopsy may be indicated. This author has seen one recurrence in temporal skull soft tissue.

Clinical staging systems have developed to suggest preferred treatments and predict success rates. The foremost system is that of Reese-Ellsworth,[45] which highlights multifocality, tumor size and location, vitreous involvement, and bilaterality (see the box below). Obviously, extraocular disease transcends such clinical staging of local disease.

Treatment techniques

As mentioned, the pediatric ophthalmologist must detail the extent of local disease. With small focal tumors away from the optic disc and macula, photocoagulation or cryosurgery may yield control. With more extensive but unilateral retinoblastoma not involving the optic nerve, enucleation leads to almost certain cure while sacrificing the globe. Surgery is intricately involved in radiation implant procedures, careful follow-up, and salvage after failure of organ-sparing treatments.

Radiation has classically been used in cases of bilateral or inoperable unilateral disease. If both eyes are involved, they must be treated with organ-sparing intent because visual preservation may occur on the side with more advanced initial disease. It is a technical challenge with external beam therapy to treat the entire retina, which extends anterior to the lateral bony canthus, and still spare the cornea and lens. Methods include (1) combined lateral and anterior fields

Reese-Ellsworth Staging System for Retinoblastoma

Group I (quite favorable)

a. Solitary tumor (less than 4 dd at or behind the equator)
b. Multiple tumors (none over 4 dd at or behind the equator)

Group II (favorable)

a. Solitary lesion (4-10 dd at or behind the equator)
b. Multiple tumors (4-10 dd behind the equator)

Group III (doubtful)

a. Any lesion anterior to the equator
b. Solitary lesions (larger than 10 dd behind the equator)

Group IV (unfavorable)

a. Multiple tumors (some larger than 10 dd)
b. Any lesion extending anteriorly to the ora serrata

Group V (quite unfavorable)

a. Massive tumors involving over half the retina
b. Vitreous seeding

Modified from Reese A: *Tumors of the eye,* Hagerstown, Pennsylvania, 1976, Harper & Row.
dd, Disc diameter (equal to 1.6 mm).

with a divergent hanging lens block, (2) a lateral field leaving a small amount of anterior retina will be untreated, or (3) a suction cup to displace the anterior globe (popular in Europe) (Fig. 14-4). Daily general anesthesia is required, with specialized dosimetry verifying doses in such small-shaped radiation portals. The usual dose is 180 to 300 cGy, delivered three to five times weekly. Several series report local control and visual preservation ranging from 30% to 100%, depending on the stage (Table 14-3). If the tumor masses are less extensive, radiation implant plaques can be used. Cobalt 60 and iodine 125 are the most widely used radionuclides. Doses of 4000 to 6000 cGy over 1 week are delivered, with a cure rate of over 80% and visual preservation in most patients.[26] Implants reduce radiation exposure to the bones, contralateral globe, and anterior structures, with a resultant decrease in long-term effects.

Because retinoblastoma is a small blue cell tumor of neuroectodermal origin, a good response to chemotherapeutic agents is expected. Combinations such as VAC (vincristine, Adriamycin, cyclophosphamide) and OPEC (vincristine, cisplatin, etoposide, cyclophosphamide) have been delivered when extraocular or disseminated disease is present. Although it is rarely curative, retinoblastoma may become involved in multidisciplinary treatments in the future.

Late effects of treatment

Long-term sequelae of retinoblastoma therapies are major because of the cosmetics of the face, effect on vision, and risk of a **second malignant neoplasm (SMN),** a new cancer developing years after treatment of the initial tumor. After enucleation is chosen the child will require several prosthetic eyes as growth occurs. Limited orbital growth may continue. Because external radiation uses doses of 4000 cGy or more and occurs in children who are quite young, facial growth will definitely be impaired. As adults, these patients have small orbits, which are narrow between the temples. Cured tumors can leave blind spots. Radiation retinitis or dry eyes from decreased tear gland function can limit useful vision. However, overall survival rates and visual acuity are excellent (Table 14-3). Depending on the radiation technique, cataracts can be a certainty.

As noted earlier, the retinoblastoma gene is a tumor-suppressor gene. If this gene is absent, other cancers (especially osteosarcomas) develop later in life with alarming frequency. In fact, Abramson[2] believes that most retinoblastoma survivors will eventually suffer a second malignancy. Sarcomas can be induced in the radiation therapy portal but occur outside the radiation therapy field more often. When a young adult cured of retinoblastoma develops a facial bone osteosarcoma, it is indeed a tragic late effect.

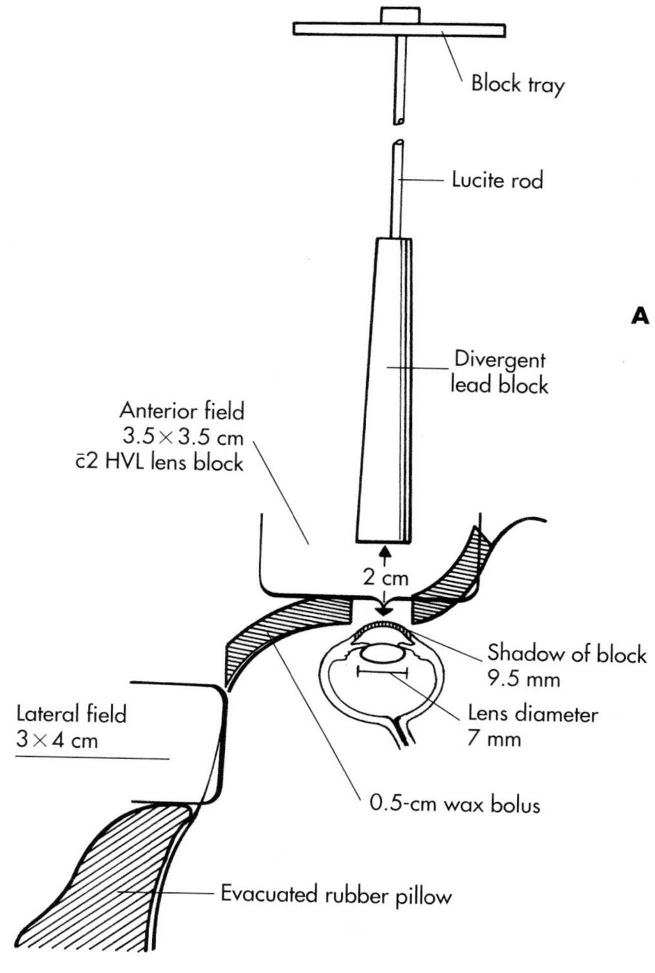

Fig. 14-4 Radiation techniques for retinoblastoma. **A,** Anterior-lateral wedge pair with a hanging eye block.

Continued.

Table 14-3 Visual preservation per Reese group after radiation therapy for retinoblastoma

Institution	Preservation for Group I	Preservation for Groups II and III	Preservation for Groups IV and V
Columbia University	84%	68%	20%
Stanford University	88%	63%	30%
Utrecht University	100%	89%	58%

Data from Cassady JR et al: Radiation therapy in retinoblastoma, *Radiology* 93:405-409, 1969; Egbert PR et al: Visual results and ocular complication following radiotherapy for retinoblastoma, 96:1826-1830, 1978; and Schipper J, Tan KE, Von Peperzeel HA: Treatment of retinoblastoma by precision megavoltage radiation therapy, *Radiother Oncol* 3:117-132, 1985.

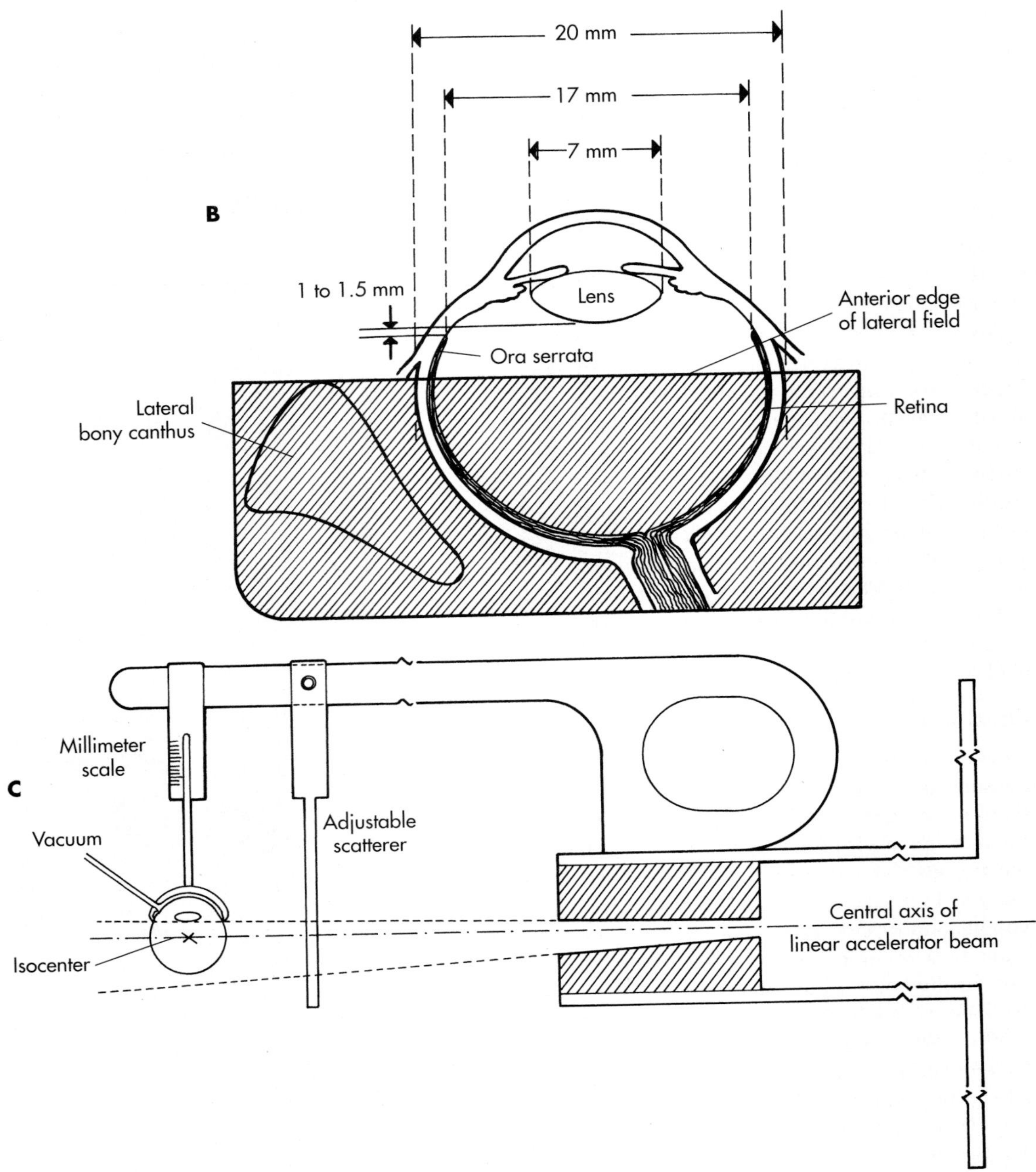

Fig. 14-4—cont'd Radiation techniques for retinoblastoma. **B,** Direct lateral field that misses the most anterior retina. **C,** Vacuum displacement of lens and closely collimated lateral field. This is popular in Europe. (**A,** From Weiss DR et al: Retinoblastoma: a modification in radiation therapy technique, *Radiology* 114:705-708, 1975; **B,** From Cassady JR et al: Radiation therapy in retinoblastoma, *Radiology* 93:405-409, 1969; **C,** From Schipper et al: Treatment of retinoblastoma by precision megavoltage, *Radiother Oncol* 3:117-132, 1985.)

NEUROBLASTOMAS

Epidemiology

Neuroblastoma is a small, round, blue cell tumor derived from cells of neural crest origin. These cells migrate embryologically to form paravertebral sympathetic ganglia and the adrenal medulla. Neuroblastoma-like cells occur in fetal adrenals and in 1% of infant autopsies. Because only about 500 such tumors develop in the U.S. annually, most of these precursor lesions must spontaneously regress. However, neuroblastoma is the second most common solid tumor (after brain tumors). Patients range from newborns to children several years old, with a median age of less than 24 months.[32]

Like the normal adrenal tissues, neuroblastoma cells can manufacture epinephrine-like compounds such as vanilmandelic acid (VMA) and homovanillic acid (HVA), which can be detected in the urine. Molecular genetic studies have demonstrated a deletion on the short arm of chromosome 1 in up to 80% of patients.[6] Surprisingly, neuroblastomas with an excessive or aneuploid number of chromosomes yield a better prognosis. The **oncogene** (a gene regulating the development and growth of cancerous tissues) primarily associated with neuroblastoma is n-myc. This gene occurs on the short arm of chromosome 2 and is a promoter of growth. Thus when excessive copies of this gene are present (called *n-myc amplified tumors),* aggressive growth and poor survival are typical.[7]

Diagnosis and staging

The majority of neuroblastomas occur in the abdomen, with the origin in the adrenal gland or paraspinal ganglia. A lethargic, ill-appearing child less than 2 years of age with an abdominal mass is common. The invasion of the spinal canal in a dumbbell fashion from a paravertebral neuroblastoma can cause symptoms of neurological compromise and spinal cord compression. Even a routine chest radiograph of an ill infant can show a thoracic paraspinal mass. If the upper sympathetic ganglia are disrupted, unilateral Horner's syndrome with meiosis (small pupil), ptosis (droopy eyelid), and anhydrosis (no sweating on one side of the face) may occur. Flushing and diarrhea occur in response to the vasoactive peptides. In the newborn a large abdominal mass or liver metastases usually cause respiratory compromise, necessitating emergency intervention.

Unfortunately, many children present with symptoms of metastatic disease. Patients older than 18 months have a 70% chance of developing metastatic disease.[32] Weakness and anemia from bone marrow invasion, painful bony metastases, blue skin lesions, or massive liver involvement may occur, even with a small primary tumor. In general, these patients are younger and sicker than those with a corresponding-sized **Wilms' tumor** (the childhood embryonal kidney cancer). The radiologic evaluation depends on the presentation in the abdomen or chest. Abdominal ultrasound or CT and chest CT are appropriate. Sometimes calcifications are visible in the mass on a CT scan. The lungs and liver must be assessed for metastases. MRI of the spine is used for paravertebral masses to delineate spinal canal invasion. A bone marrow biopsy is required and a bone scan is done to look for bone cortex lesions. More recently, radioiodinated catecholamine precursors have been used to detect occult metastatic involvement. Staging systems have historically evolved based on radiographic and surgical findings. Initially, Evans and D'Angio developed such a prognostic staging system. The POG and an international staging committee have included surgical guidelines. These systems are summarized in Table 14-4.

As mentioned, the age at the time of presentation is extremely important regarding the prognosis. The special category IV-S predominantly occurs in infants younger than 1 year of age. Many of these patients spontaneously regress, and the cancerous elements turn benign if acute situations can be managed.[13] Increasingly, molecular genetic markers (especially n-myc amplification) are being used to predict clinical behavior. Although this technique has not yet been included in universal staging systems, it is certainly directing the aggressiveness of therapy in most clinical research groups. Less abnormal molecular genetics may explain the differential age prognosis observed clinically. A novel approach to early detection has shown benefits in Japan. Urine samples from diaper pads of infants were analyzed for catecholamine excretions. This led to earlier stage presentations and higher cure rates in initial evaluations.[40]

Treatment techniques

The therapy for neuroblastoma remains an enigma to most pediatric oncologists. Although it may spontaneously regress in the newborn, neuroblastoma often has a progressive metastatic course in older children. Individual masses may regress well with low doses of chemotherapy or radiation, but cure of the usual advanced disease presentation is infrequent. Completely resected localized disease without nodal metastases is often cured with surgery alone. In 1967 Lingley[36] showed 100% local control and long-term survival in 8 of 13 patients after they underwent incomplete surgery followed by radiation. The use of multiagent chemotherapy has supplanted radiation in most resected patients, even with nodal metastases or microscopic residua. More extensive stage III tumors definitely benefit from tumor bed irradiation, usually to doses of 2000 to 3000 cGy.[37] Radiation is directed to residua after surgery and chemotherapy, rather than to all areas of initial disease.

The likelihood of children over 2 years of age developing metastatic disease depends on the use of multiagent chemotherapy. In Europe and the U.S., aggressive regimens involving platinum compounds, vincristine, Adriamycin, etoposide, and cyclophosphamide have been used. Although such treatment has improved the previously almost uniformally fatal Stage IV results, overall survival rates have been disheartening (Table 14-5). Newer efforts involve therapeutic radionuclides and the frequent use of high dose chemotherapy and **autologous bone marrow transplantation (ABMT),** which is the use of a patient's own bone marrow to prevent hematological toxicity.

Radiation therapists can also be called on to palliatively treat patients who have progressive metastatic disease. Low doses of 1000 cGy may achieve pain relief or regression of soft tissue masses, which are important for short-term quality of life. The treatment of orbital or skin metastases that are disfiguring is a major comfort to terminally ill patients and their families.

Late effects of treatment

Because neuroblastoma patients are often infants, the late effects of radiation can be significant. In the acute situation with a newborn, doses of only 500 cGy may be effective and

Table 14-4 Neuroblastoma staging systems

Evans and D'Angio	Pediatric Oncology Group	International
Stage I—Tumor confined to the organ or structure of origin Stage II—Tumor extending in continuity beyond the organ or structure of origin but not crossing the midline; regional lymph nodes on the ipsilateral side Stage III—Tumor extending in continuity beyond the midline; possible involvement of regional lymph nodes bilaterally Stage IV—Remote disease involving the skeleton, bone marrow, soft tissue, and distant lymph node groups, etc. (see Stage IV-S) Stage IV-S—Patients who would otherwise be in Stage I or II but have remote disease confined to the liver, skin, or bone marrow (without radiographic evidence of bone metastases on a complete skeletal survey)	Stage A—Complete gross resection of primary tumor, with or without microscopic residual; intracavitary lymph nodes, not adhered to and removed with primary (nodes adhered to or within tumor resection may be positive for tumor without upstaging patient to Stage C), histologically free of tumor; if primary in abdomen or pelvis, liver histologically free of tumor Stage B—Grossly unresected primary tumor; nodes and liver same as in Stage A Stage C—Complete or incomplete resection of primary; intracavitary nodes not adhered to primary histologically positive for tumor; liver as in Stage A. Stage D—Any dissemination of disease beyond intracavitary nodes (i.e., extracavitary nodes, liver, skin, bone marrow, bone)	Stage 1—Localized tumor confined to area of origin; complete gross excision, with or without microscopic residual disease; identifiable ipsilateral and contralateral lymph nodes negative microscopically Stage 2A—Unilateral tumor with incomplete gross excision; identifiable ipsilateral and contralateral lymph nodes negative microscopically Stage 2B—Unilateral tumor with complete or incomplete gross excision; with positive ipsilateral regional lymph nodes; identifiable contralateral lymph nodes negative microscopically Stage 3—Tumor infiltrating across the midline with or without regional lymph node involvement; unilateral tumor with contralateral regional lymph node involvement; or midline tumor with bilateral regional lymph node involvement Stage 4—Dissemination of tumor to distant lymph nodes, bone, bone marrow, liver, and/or other organs (except as defined in Stage 4S) Stage 4S—Localized primary tumor as defined for Stage 1 or 2, with dissemination limited to liver and skin

Data from Brodeur GM et al: International criteria for diagnosis, staging and response to treatment with neuroblastoma, *J Clin Oncol* 6:1874-1881, 1988; Evans AE: Staging and treatment of neuroblastoma, *Cancer* 45:1799-1802, 1980; and Hayes FA, study coordinator: *Comprehensive care of the child with neuroblastoma: a stage and age oriented study,* Chicago, 1982, Pediatric Oncology Group.

Table 14-5 5-year survival rates in 550 neuroblastoma patients on POG protocols, 1981-1989

Stage	Children less than 1 year old	Children more than 1 year old
A and B	95%	85%
C	80%	60%
D	50%	15%

Modified from Ries LAG et al, editors: *SEER Cancer Statistics Review, 1973-1991: tables and graphs,* NIH Pub. No. 94-2789, Bethesda, Maryland, 1994, National Cancer Institute.
POG, Pediatric Oncology Group.

thus have almost no long-term side effect. In older patients receiving 2000 to 3000 cGy the bones and soft tissues of the treated region will have decreased growth. This may cause asymmetry as the child grows. Kidney and liver tissues must be shielded from the highest doses of radiation to prevent impaired function. Lung fibrosis occurs with thoracic radiation. The intense doses of multiagent chemotherapy and ABMT used for neuroblastoma can adversely affect many organ systems. Although late second malignancies are always a risk after radiation and chemotherapy, the oncogenes associated with neuroblastoma do not exacerbate the risk to an alarming level.

WILMS' TUMORS

Epidemiology

Wilms' tumor is a malignant embryonal cancer of the kidney. It was first described in the German medical literature in 1899. Nearly 400 cases occur annually in the U. S., and about 5% are bilateral. The average age at the time of presentation is 3 or 4, and almost all such tumors occur before the age of 8. A higher risk of Wilms' tumor occurs in patients with multiple genitourinary abnormalities, hemihypertrophy and aniridia, and the facial abnormality syndrome Beckwith-Wiedemann. A Wilms' tumor gene has recently been discovered and represents a deletion on chromosome 11p13.[15] Benign embryonal rests called *nephroblastomatoses* can be associated with malignant Wilms' tumor, especially in bilateral cases. Wilms' tumors can contain renal tubular, glomerular, and connective tissue elements. Unfavorable histologies occur in up to 15% of patients and include highly anaplastic, clear cell sarcomas and rhabdoid tumors. These unfavorable tumors have a cure rate only half that of their usual histological Wilms' tumor counterpart and metastasize to bone or brain.[5]

Diagnosis and staging

Wilms' tumor most often appears as a painless abdominal mass noted at the pediatrician's examination or when parents bathe the child. As the cancers enlarge, they can cause pain and pressure on the gastrointestinal tract. They may even hemmorage and rupture. Despite large tumors, children do not often appear severely ill. A differential diagnosis includes neuroblastomas, lymphomas, sarcomas, and liver tumors.

After the physical examination an abdominal ultrasonogram is usually the first step in making a diagnosis. In the U. S. this is followed by a CT scan of the chest and abdomen because of the tendency for lymph node and pulmonary metastases. Because Wilms' tumor can be bilateral, the contralateral kidney must be carefully examined (Fig. 14-5, *A*). With right-sided tumors, direct liver invasion can mimic liver metastases. The unfavorable histologies of clear cell sarcomas and rhabdoid tumors can metastasize to bone and brain. The initial staging system recommended by Cassady focused on tumor size, tumor spill or postoperative residua, and metastases. The National Wilms' Tumor Study Group (NWTS) was formed in the U.S. to investigate treatment options; members are presently beginning protocol study #5. The staging system of the NWTS is based on operative findings and is listed in the box on p. 334. These stages relate to prognosis and direct the aggressiveness of treatment options.

Treatment techniques

In the U. S. the removal of the malignant kidney via nephrectomy is nearly always the first step. Careful examination of the other kidney for bilateral tumors is done intraoperatively. A biopsy is performed on the lymph nodes, and those suspicious for metastases are removed. Wilms' tumor can track intravascularly to the renal vein, inferior vena cava (IVC), and chest. These tumor thrombi can be removed during surgery. Because large Wilms' tumors are often soft and necrotic, rupture of the mass and tumor spill into the abdominal cavity are risks. Because widespread tumor spill adversely affects the prognosis and demands more subsequent treatment, SIOP studies usually use chemotherapy or radiation preoperatively. In the first SIOP cooperative study this method reduced intraoperative tumor spill from 32% to 4%.[35] In patients with bilateral disease a partial resection can be done on the minimally affected side. Because surgery alone led to cure rates of less than 30% many years ago, radiation therapy by the 1940s and chemotherapy by the 1960s have greatly increased survival rates.

Radiation was initially used to cover the entire tumor bed and abdomen. If tumor spill occurred, the whole abdomen was treated. Doses over 3000 cGy were quite successful but led to significant late effects. The first four NWTS studies have resulted in conclusions for less radiation. With the addition of effective chemotherapy routine radiation for completely removed Stages I and II tumors is not necessary. Data from NWTS 3 indicated no significant difference in local control between 1080 and 2000 cGy.[53] This lower dose is still indicated for residual disease, lymph node metastases, bilateral disease, and pulmonary metastases. All cases of unfavorable histology are treated as high-stage lesions and uniformly irradiated. Known areas of residual disease are usually boosted to at least 2000 cGy.

In designing the radiation portals, it is important to use the preoperative imaging and surgeon's intraoperative findings to delineate the radiation portal. If treating only unilateral disease, it is still important to cover the entire width of the vertebral body plus 1 to 2 cm contralaterally. This allows periaortic nodal coverage and homogeneous irradiation of the vertebral bodies to reduce the risk of scoliosis. At the low dose of 1080 cGy, which is often used now, the risk of bony or visceral toxicity (including the remaining kidney) is minimal. Still, it is wise to shield the growth plates of the femoral heads for whole-pelvis treatment and humeral heads when treating the whole lungs for pulmonary metastases. Fig. 14-5, *B* represents a postoperative radiation portal for a bilateral Wilms' tumor patient whose large left-sided cancer was removed. Because abdominal recurrence is still a major problem in an unfavorable histological Wilms' tumor, the fields are similar but doses are usually 2000 cGy or more.

Farber[18] first reported the encouraging survival improvement associated with Wilms' tumor by using actinomycin-D in 1966. The addition of vincristine and Adriamycin for advanced stages led to cure rates of 80% to 100% in later NWTS studies. Even patients with metastatic disease can be cured over 70% of the time (Table 14-6). Patients with late pulmonary metastases can often be salvaged with chemotherapy, lung irradiation, and lung resections. With the high overall cure rates the present aim of studies is to reduce late effects and find more successful multidisciplinary combinations for patients who have advanced disease and unfavorable histology.

Late effects of treatment

Historically, when doses of 3000 to 4000 cGy of orthovoltage radiation were used, atrophy of soft tissues on the treated side and scoliosis were common. With modification of the technique to include the entire vertebral body plus the mar-

A

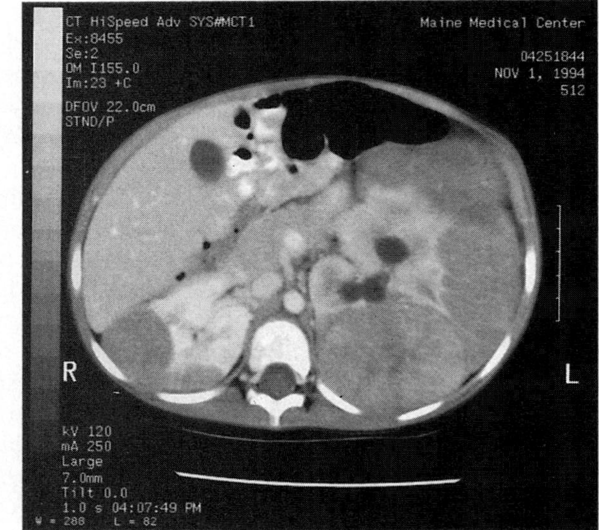

B

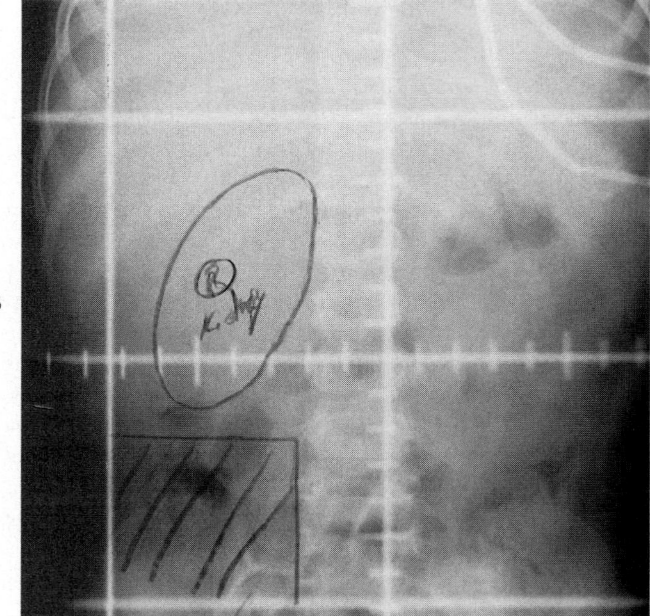

Fig. 14-5 Wilm's tumor. **A,** Preoperative CT scan of a bilateral Wilm's tumor in a 3-year-old girl. **B,** Postoperative radiation portal received 1200 cGy to the left tumor bed and remaining involved right kidney. Note the shielding for the bowel and pelvic structures inferiorly on the right side.

The National Wilm's Tumor Study Staging System

Stage	
I	Tumor limited to kidney and completely excised
II	Tumor beyond kidney but completely excised Local tumor spillage or vessel invasion permitted but resected
III	Residual nonhematogenous tumor confined to abdomen Involved lymph nodes, diffuse tumor spillage, or grossly unresected tumor
IV	Hematogenous metastases Usually lung, liver, bone, or brain
V	Bilateral kidney involvement at time of diagnosis

Table 14-6 4-year survival rates of NWTS-3 patients

Stage	Relapse-free rate (%)	Overall rate (%)
I FH	90	96
II FH	88	92
III FH	79	86
IV FH	75	82
I-III UH	65	68
IV UH	55	55

Modified from Green DM et al: Wilms' tumor. In Pizzo PG, Poplack DG, editors: *Principles and practice of pediatric oncology,* ed 2, Philadelphia, 1993, JB Lippincott.
NWTS-3, National Wilms' Tumor Study Group protocol study #3; *FH,* favorable histology; *UH,* unfavorable histology.

gin and the use of doses less than 2000 cGy, such late effects should rarely occur now. For the treatment of pulmonary metastases, doses must be kept below 1500 cGy to prevent diffuse lung fibrosis. If thoracic radiation is needed for a prepubertal female, breast development can be impaired. High doses of actinomycin-D have resulted in liver damage. SMN's have occurred in a small percentage of long-term survivors. Because these children go through life with only one kidney, any urinary tract symptoms must be addressed quickly to prevent infections, stones, or other diseases from damaging the remaining kidney.

SOFT TISSUE SARCOMAS

Epidemiology

Soft tissue sarcomas arise from mesenchymal tissues and can occur anywhere in the body. At Children's Hospital in Philadelphia a decade of oncology cases were reviewed and 8% were soft tissue sarcomas. A wide variety of histologies can be seen, but **rhabdomyosarcomas** and undifferentiated sarcomas constitute over 60% of cases. No dominant chromosomal abnormality has been noted, but familial cases may be related to the p53 oncogene mutation, as noted by Li and Fraumeni. About 75% of soft tissue sarcomas occur before the age of 10. The rhabdomyosarcoma sites are nearly evenly divided between the head and neck area (including the orbit), genitourinary region, and extremities and trunk.[44]

Rhabdomyosarcoma has distinct histological variants. A more favorable embryonal type tends to occur in the orbit and genitourinary (GU) regions. The alveolar subtype has a worse prognosis and a predilection for extremities and the trunk.[39] Other undifferentiated sarcomas are often treated along guidelines established by the Intergroup Rhabdomyosarcoma Study Group (IRS).

Diagnosis and staging

The presenting symptoms of soft tissue sarcomas depend on the area of involvement. A painless mass can enlarge relatively asymptomatically in an extremity, whereas much growth in the orbit causes pain, tearing, and outward displacement of the globe, known as *proptosis.* The GU occurrences in the prostate and bladder in males cause urinary difficulties. A fleshy, exophytic mass extruding from the vagina in young girls has been called *sarcoma botyroides* because of its resemblance to clusters of grapes.

The staging of rhabdomyosarcomas and other soft tissue sarcomas has historically included size and resectability, nodal involvement, and metastases. The latter are most likely to occur in the lung and bone marrow. The IRS first developed a clinical grouping system based on surgical findings but some experts now favor the TGNM system (Table 14 -7), which also includes the histology (a known prognostic factor). After the histological diagnosis is obtained from an incisional biopsy, staging includes a physical examination and ultrasound, CT, or MRI scans to determine the tumor's size and involvement of adjacent structures. A bone marrow biopsy and chest CT scan are done to detect metastases. The stage and histology dictate the treatment regimen in IRS and other international studies. Metastatic disease is extremely rare with orbital presentations but may be present in about 25% of patients who have tumors in the extremities and trunk.[38]

Table 14-7 Intergroup Rhabdomyosarcoma Study staging systems

Clinical system	TGNM system
I. Localized, completely resected	**Tumor**
II. Grossly resected with microscopic residue or involved lymph nodes	T_1—Confined to site origin
III. Gross residual tumor	T_2—Extension to surrounding tissues
IV. Distant metastases	a. <5 cm
	b. >/= 5 cm
	Histology
	G_1—Favorable: embryonal, undifferentiated, mixed
	G_2—Unfavorable: alveolar
	Nodes
	N_0—Not clinically involved
	N_1—Clinically involved by tumor
	Metastases
	M_0—No distant metastases
	M_1—Metastatic disease at time of diagnosis

Modified from Raney RB et al: Rhabdomyosarcoma and other undifferentiated sarcomas. In Pizzo PA, Poplack DG, editors: *Principles and practice of pediatric oncology,* Philadelphia, 1989, JB Lippincott.
TGNM, Tumor, Grade, Node, Metastases.

Treatment techniques

After the biopsy and staging the surgical possibilities must be assessed. The first choice, if possible, is the complete removal of the mass with appropriate margins without the destruction of precious anatomy. The original approach of removing the entire organ or extremity is no longer necessary because of multidisciplinary treatment including chemotherapy and radiation. The initial IRS study proved that small, fully resected lesions have good curability without additional treatment. In more advanced cases the local relapse rate was extremely high with surgery alone. The removal of a child's eye or GU structures is generally not preferred and has led to organ-sparing combined treatments.

Radiation improves local control and organ preservation in all rhabdomyosarcoma groups, except small and fully excised lesions. Some authors have reported increased local control with doses of 5000 cGy versus less than 4000 cGy. Fortunately, the frequently unresectable areas of the orbit and pelvis are usually the more favorable embryonal histology, and local control rates of 90% or more have been obtained with combinations of chemotherapy and radiation.[51]

Original margins of treatment for radiation fields included the entire muscular compartment. More recently, the IRS has decreased margins to 5 cm or sometimes 2 cm if critical normal tissues can be spared. Around the orbit a wedge pair alignment or mixed beam with electrons can spare the contralateral eye, facial bones, optic chiasm, and most brain tissues. In the pelvis or along extremities the growth plates of the long bones must be shielded. With the routine use of chemotherapy the bone marrow in the pelvic wings should be spared if possible. For locally positive intraoperative margins and some surface gynecological presentations, brachytherapy implants have been used with success.[24] In general, the external beam radiation portals include the prechemotherapy tumor volume with at least a 2-cm margin. Standard doses have been 180 cGy per day to a total of 5040 cGy. IRS-IV included hyperfractionated radiation twice daily at 110 cGy per treatment to a total of 5940 cGy to decrease long-term effects but maintain a high local control rate. Preliminary toxicity data prove this regimen to be feasible, but long-term results are not yet available.

Chemotherapy was initially used only for metastatic disease, but its subsequent use postoperatively led to higher survival rates because of the elimination of occult metastatic disease.[27] In serial IRS studies, vincristine and actinomycin-D have been quite effective. New regimens have combined these agents with etoposide and ifosfamide in IRS-IV. Because of good response rates, chemotherapy is also used for unresectable lesions, with a reevaluation after the response. With good tumor reduction some cancers can be resected or radiation fields greatly reduced. Surgery or radiation therapy must be performed for local control early in the overall treatment because resistant clones of cells can lead to tumor growth and lost opportunities. Local control procedures are usually at 2 to 3 months into the overall treatment program of about 1 year. The tumor's histology, stage, and location affect survival rates (Table 14-8). Although the survival rate for patients with orbital lesions is over 90%, patients with large unresectable pelvic masses or metastatic disease still fare poorly.

Late effects of treatment

The long-term sequelae of rhabdomyosarcoma and other soft tissue sarcoma treatment depends on the tumor's location and treatment modality. Amputations and pelvic exenterations are generally reserved for the salvaging of organ-sparing treatment failures. However, a recent patient's family preferred bladder removal rather than the long-term effects of radiation on their young daughter's reproductive structures. With the high radiation doses, bone and soft tissue growth is affected unless the growth points of bones can be excluded. In the head and neck region, invasion of the cranial contents can occur, necessitating CNS radiation to 3000 cGy or more. (Its well-known side effects are listed in the brain tumor section). Treatment of the orbit and facial structures causes bony growth decreases. Dryness of the treated eye or retinal damage from chemotherapy and radiation sometimes necessitates enucleation, even if the rhabdomyosarcoma is cured. The appropriate use of brachytherapy implants can spare many of the surrounding normal tissues from damage. Chemotherapeutic agents can cause acute and chronic neurological, kidney, heart, and liver damage. The risk of SMNs after cytoxic therapy must be mentioned to parents. This will be especially important if genetic studies can identify patients at high risk for multiple malignancies. As survivors grow to adulthood, fertility is questionable after chemotherapy and highly unlikely for those receiving pelvic radiation.

UNUSUAL CHILDHOOD TUMORS

Germ cell tumors

According to embryological development, benign and malignant germ cell tumors can occur anywhere in the midline, from the CNS through the mediastinum and retroperitoneum, down to the ovaries and testicles. Sacrococcygeal teratomas often occur in newborns. The majority of these

Table 14-8 Actuarial survival rates at 3 years: results of the Intergroup Rhabdomyosarcoma Studies I and II

Prognostic factors	IRS study I (%)	IRS study II (%)
Clinical group		
I	79	88
II	68	77
III	42	68
IV	18	32
Histological type		
Embryonal	—	69
Alveolar	—	56
Other	—	66
Primary site		
Orbit	91	93
GU	74	—
GU (mainly Group III)	—	64
Cranial parameningeal	53	71
Other head or neck areas	59	69
Trunk	53	57
Extremity	53	56
Retroperitoneum and pelvis	39	46

Modified from Pizzo PA et al: Solid tumors of children. In DeVita T, Hellman S, Rosenberg SA, editors: *Cancer: principles and practice of oncology,* ed 4, Philadelphia, 1993, JB Lippincott.
IRS, Intergroup Rhabdomyosarcoma Study Group; *GU* genitourinary.

tumors are histologically benign and are almost always cured by surgery. Tumors affecting older children in this region have a higher risk of malignancy but can usually be controlled with chemotherapy. Radiation is rarely used in this young age group. Ovarian and testicular tumors that occur in adolescents differentiate along seminoma-dysgerminoma or nonseminomatous lines. The latter group includes embryonal carcinoma, choriocarcinoma, and yolk sac tumors. The nonseminomatous tumors often produce alpha-fetaprotein (AFP) or human chorionic gonadotropin (HCG), which can be used as chemical markers for response to therapy. Surgical removal of the testicles or ovaries is done first and is often curative in Stage I disease. Chemotherapy with regimens containing cisplatin, bleomycin, etoposide, and vinblastine have led to a high rate of success. Moderate doses of radiation in the 2000- to 2500-cGy range prevents pelvic and periaortic nodal relapse in seminoma-germinoma patients[34] and is used most often in older adolescent males. CNS germ cell tumors are discussed in the brain tumor section.

Liver tumors

Liver tumors appear as right upper quadrant abdominal masses, much like Wilms' tumor or neuroblastoma. Ultrasound or CT scanning can usually determine the organ of origin. Benign vascular or fetal remnant tumors can be observed if they are small, or if necessary due to their large size, they can be resected with excellent results. Hepatoblastoma is a malignancy usually occuring in patients under the age of 2. Hepatocellular carcinoma occurs in the second decade of life and can be multifocal. AFP can be elevated in both hepatic malignancies.[21]

Primary surgical resection is the goal. If this is not possible or postoperative residua is present, chemotherapy with Adriamycin and cisplatin is often used. Radiation has demonstrated some good response but is rarely used, especially in infants. Still, overall survival rates (usually less than 50%) are poor.[25] The use of injectable radionuclides, which has been helpful in adults, has not been routinely used in children. External radiation can be used for palliation after relapse.

Histiocytosis X syndromes

Histiocytosis X is a spectrum of diseases that involves abnormal proliferation of the histiocytic immune system's Langerhans' cells. Sometimes a single bone is involved with a lytic lesion in a situation called *eosinophilic granuloma.* Infants can have multifocal visceral disease involving the lung, skin, liver, and bone marrow. This is a life-threatening condition known as *Letterer-Siwe.* Individual histiocytosis lesions may wax and wane over time and occasionally spontaneously regress. Focal bony lesions can be treated via surgical curettage with success. If an impending fracture is a concern or the lesion is in a surgically unresectable region such as the base of skull or spinal column, low doses of radiation are usually effective. Although no direct dose-response curve has been substantiated, doses from 400 to 1200 cGy can be effective.[30]

Miscellaneous tumors

Male adolescents may develop nasopharyngeal angiofibromas. Usually, vascular embolization and surgical resection are used. Moderate doses of radiation (such as 3000 cGy) can control relapses.[12] Undifferentiated nasopharyngeal carcinomas can occur and require high-dose radiation, as they do in adults. Recently, chemotherapy has been used to reduce radiation fields and resultant long-term side effects.

Benign and malignant thyroid tumors can arise in adolescents (more often in females). These tumors are surgically approached, and even lymph node metastases do not imply a bad prognosis. External radiation is rarely used, but iodine 131 can be helpful for thyroid ablation or treatment of metastatic lesions.

Keloids and fibromas can be bothersome and cosmetically disfiguring for young people. If repeated resections and steroid injections are not successful, the best control is obtained via resection, followed immediately by low-dose radiation (900 to 1200 cGy in 3 fractions).[49] Unfortunately, the human immunodeficiency virus (HIV) infection epidemic has led to the occurrence of Kaposi's sarcoma in children. Focal painful or disfiguring lesions can be palliated with single doses of 700 cGy, although more lasting results are obtained by a short course to a total dose of over 2000 cGy.[11]

PALLIATIVE RADIATION

Despite the obvious goal of cure for pediatric malignancies, **palliation** or symptom-relieving treatments are sometimes necessary. In a recent forum the Children's Hospital of Philadelphia reported 13% of their patients from 1988 to 1994 were referred for emergency radiation.[47] Mediastinal malignancies may cause airway or vascular compromise. Low doses of radiation or treatment of only a portion of the mass may relieve symptoms without compromising the histological diagnosis. Spinal cord compression at the time of presentation or late in the course of the illness demands immediate treatment to avoid paralysis.

The palliative needs of children in the final stages of cancer must be addressed carefully and compassionately. The goal of such treatments is much different than the usual curative protocols. The attempt must be made to relieve symptoms quickly with a minimum number of treatments to limit the hospital personnel's invasion of the family's remaining time together. The successful treatment of painful or disfiguring masses can reduce the need for narcotics or hospitalization and improve cosmetics and quality of life during precious final days or weeks. In these instances immobilization and simulation techniques are altered in deference to the comfort of the child. Frequently, high daily doses are used for rapid palliation when long-term effects are not of concern.[55] Although this is a difficult time for radiation staff members, such palliative efforts in times of great need are of immeasurable importance to the children and their families.

ROLE OF RADIATION THERAPIST

Almost all patients in radiation oncology centers are adults. In addition to the diseases and their treatment, the personal needs of pediatric patients pose a challenge. As outlined in this chapter, techniques such as CSI are technically demanding. In some patients sedation (even to the point of general anesthesia) is required. This produces unique demands because treatment techniques may need to be altered for anesthetic safety. Close cooperation between radiation therapists, nurses, and anesthesia staff members is necessary for patient positioning and visibility of monitors. This takes much longer than a normal treatment time, so blocking out the schedule sufficiently is important. Usually, this is done early in the morning to reduce disruption of the child's feeding patterns and avoid emergency anesthesia conflicts. Radiation oncologists must plan ahead for such instances and should not perform significant sedations alone. Therapists often must juggle an already crowded schedule of adults, but most patients are willing to change in deference to children and their families.

Most pediatric patients are on an investigational protocol, requiring careful documentation of treatment setups, daily doses, and quality assurance. Clear instructions between the simulator and treatment machine therapists are essential. Polaroid pictures of patient positioning, verification of initial portal films, and dose calculations are usually sent for immediate review by national clinical research groups. Careful adherence to protocol guidelines reflects positively on the quality of a radiation oncology department.

The psychosocial elements of pediatric oncology can be immense. Families who are constantly at the hospital have an extremely difficult time maintaining jobs and homes. In addition, children evoke sympathy and compassion from everyone involved. However, behavorial limits may need to be placed on patients or families to ensure quality treatments. If children are less cooperative when parents are in the treatment room, it is best to have the parents watch the monitors outside. Rewards such as stickers or toys should not be used daily, but therapists are the best judges of when a difficult or sick child needs an uplifting gift. When terminal cancer children come for palliation, it is an especially difficult time. However, the value of the radiation therapist's technical expertise and heartfelt compassion cannot be overstated.

The uniformly multidisciplinary approach to pediatric oncology is always a learning experience. This strategy has led to dramatic increases in cure rates for childhood cancers over the past 30 years (Table 14-9) to reach an overall survival rate of nearly 70%. However, numerous late sequelae must be considered. In addition to organ toxicities, childhood cancer survivors have psychological scars. Social, employment, and insurance discrimination may exist throughout adulthood. For the radiation therapist, the treatment of children can truly be the most joyous or sorrowful portion of the job.

Table 14-9 5-year survival trends for cancers in children ages 0 to 14 years

Diagnosis	Survival rate (%) for 1960-1963	Survival rate (%) for 1974-1976	Survival rate (%) for 1986-1991
Acute lymphocytic leukemia	4.0	52.4	78.0
Brain tumor	35.0	53.7	60.0
Neuroblastoma	25.0	51.9	61.0
Wilms' tumor	33.0	74.3	92.0
Hodgkin's disease	52.0	78.7	92.0
All sites	28.0	55.2	70.0

Modified from Parker SL et al: Cancer statistics, 1996, *CA Cancer J Clin* 46:5-27, 1996.

Review Questions

Multiple Choice

1. Which of the following tumors does *not* spread through the entire central nervous system?
   a. Medulloblastoma
   b. Craniopharyngioma
   c. Ependymoma
   d. Dysgerminoma
2. What is the approximate survival rate of Stage IV Wilms' tumor?
   a. 10%
   b. 30%
   c. 50%
   d. 70%
3. To what is survival in neuroblastoma related?
   a. Age
   b. Stage
   c. n-myc amplification
   d. All of the above

True or False

4. The retinoblastoma gene is a tumor promoter.
   True ___________ False ___________
5. Successful treatment of histiocytosis X lesions requires at least 2000 cGy.
   True ___________ False ___________

Fill in the Blank

6. The usual dose for occult Wilms' tumor is approximately ________ cGy.
7. The tolerance of the lung and kidney is about _____ cGy.
8. The most likely second malignant neoplasm after radiation for retinoblastoma is __________.

Questions to Ponder

1. Why is shifting the junction between the brain and spinal fields important during craniospinal irradiation?
2. Discuss some characteristics of Stage IV-S neuroblastoma.
3. Detail some technical considerations for the simulation of craniospinal irradiation.
4. List examples of chromosome and gene abnormalities associated with pediatric cancer.
5. What types of counseling and advice are needed for long-term survivors of childhood cancer?
6. Note possible long-term effects of high-dose brain radiation, and discuss remedies.
7. What organ-sparing techniques are possible by combining chemotherapy, radiation, and surgery?

REFERENCES

1. Abramson DH: Retinoblastoma: diagnosis and management, *CA Cancer J Clini*32:130-140. 1982.
2. Abramson DH et al: Second nonocular tumors in retinoblastoma survivors: are they radiation induced? *Ophthalmology* 91:1351-1355, 1984.
3. Allen JC, Kim JH, Packer RJ: Neoadjuvant chemotherapy for newly diagnosed germ cell tumors of the central nervous system, *J Neurosurg* 67:65-70, 1987.
4. Bouchard J: *Radiation therapy of tumors and diseases of the nervous system,* Philadelphia, 1988, Lea & Febiger.
5. Breslow N et al: Prognosis for Wilms' tumor patients with non-metastatic disease at diagnosis—results of the Second National Wilms' Tumor Study, *J Clin Oncol* 3:521-531, 1985.
7. Brodeur GM et al: Gene amplification in human neuroblastomas: basic mechanisms and clinical implications, *Cancer Genet Cytogenet* 19:101-111, 1986.
6. Brodeur GM, Sekhon GS, Goldstein MN: Chromosomal aberrations in human neuroblastomas, *Cancer* 40:2256-2263,1977.
8. Chang CH, Housepian EM, Herbert C: An operative staging system and a megavoltage radiotherapeutic technique for cerebellar medulloblastoma, *Radiology* 93:1351-1359, 1969.
9. Chun MS, Masko GD, Hetelekidis S: Radiation therapy in the treatment of pituitary adenomas, *Int J Rad Oncol Bio Phys* 15:305-309, 1988.
10. Cohen ME, Duffner PK: Brain tumors in children: principles of diagnosis and treatment, New York, 1984, Raven Press.
11. Cooper JS, Fried PR: Defining the role of radiotherapy for epidemic Kaposi's sarcoma, *Int J Rad Oncol Biol Phys* 13:35-39, 1987.
12. Cummings BJ, Blend R: Primary radiation therapy for juvenile nasopharyngeal angiofibroma, *Laryngoscope* 94:1599-1605, 1984.
13. D'Angio GJ, Evans A, Koop CE: Special pattern of widespread neuroblastoma with a favorable prognosis, *Lancet* 1:1046, 1971.
14. Deutsch M: The impact of myelography on the treatment results of medulloblastoma, *nt J Radiat Oncol Biol Phys* 10:999-1003, 1989.
15. Douglas EC et al: Abnormalities of chromosome 1 and 11 in Wilms' tumor, *Cancer Genet Cytogenet* 14:331-338, 1985.
16. Druja TP et al: Homozygosity of chromosome 13 in retinoblastoma, *N Engl J Med* 310:550-553, 1984.
17. Duffner PK, Cohen ME: Treatment of brain tumors in babies and very young infants, *Pediatr Neurosci* 12:304-310, 1986.
18. Farber S: Chemotherapy in the treatment of leukemia and Wilms' tumor, JAMA 138:826,1966.
19. Finley JL, Uteg R, Giese WL: Brain tumors in children. II. Advances in neurosurgery and radiation oncology, *Am J Pediatric Hem Oncol* 9:256-263, 1987.
20. Flickinger JC, Kondziolka D, Lunsford LD: Radiosurgery of benign lesions, *Semin Radiat Oncol* 5:220-224, 1995.
21. Fraumeni JF, Miller RW, Hill JA: Primary carcinoma of the liver in childhood: an epidemiologic study, *J Natl Cancer Inst* 40:1087-1099, 1968.
22. Freeman CR et al: Hyperfractionated radiation therapy of brainstem tumors, *Cancer* 68:474-481,1991.
23. Friedman HS, Schold SC: Rational approaches to the chemotherapy of medulloblastoma, *Neurol Clin* 3:843-854, 1985.
24. Gerbaulet A, et al: Iridium afterloading curietherapy in the treatment of pediatric malignancies, *Cancer* 56:1274-1279, 1985.
25. Giacomantonio M et al: 30 years of experience with pediatric primary malignant liver tumors, *J Pediatr Surg* 19:523-526, 1984.
26. Hernandez JC, et al: Conservative treatment of retinoblastoma: the use of plaque brachytherapy, *Am J Clin Oncol* 16:397-401, 1993.
27. Heyn RM, et al: The role of combined chemotherapy in the treatment of rhabdomyosarcoma, *Cancer* 34:2128-2142,1974.
28. Hirsch JE, et al: Medulloblastoma in childhood: survival and functional results, *Acta Neurochir* 48:1-15, 1979.
29. Hoffman HJ, Becker I, Craven MA: A clinically and pathologically distinct group of benign brainstem gliomas, *Neurosurgery* 7:243-248, 1980.
30. Hughes EN, et al: Medulloblastoma at the Joint Center for Radiation Therapy between 1968 and 1984, *Cancer* 61:1992-1998, 1988.
31. Israel MA: Molecular and cellular biology of pediatric malignancies. In Pizzo PA, Poplack DG, editors: *Principles and practice of pediatric oncology,* Philadelphia,1989,JB Lippincott.
32. Kissane JM, Smith MG: Pathology of infancy and childhood, St Louis, 1967, Mosby.
33. Kun LE: Patterns of failure in tumors of the central nervous system, *Cancer Treat Symp* 2:285-294, 1983.
34. Lawson AP, Adler GF: Radiotherapy in the treatment of ovarian dysgerminoma, *Int J Rad Oncol Biol Phys* 14:431-434. 1988.
35. Lemere J et al: Effectiveness of preoperative chemotherapy in Wilms' tumor: results of SIOP clinical trials, *J Clin Oncol* 1:604-610,1983.
36. Lingley JF et al: Neuroblastoma: management and survival, *N Engl J Med* 277:1227-1230, 1967.
37. Mathey KK et al: Patterns of relapse after ABMT for neuroblastoma, *Proc ASCO* 10:312, 1991.

38. Maurer HM et al: The Intergroup Rhabdomyosarcoma Study-I: a final report, *Cancer* 61:209-220, 1988.
39. Newton WA Jr et al: Histopathology of childhood sarcomas, IRS I and II: Clinicopathologic correlation, *J Clin Oncol* 6:67-75,1988.
40. Nishi M et al: Effects of the mass screening of neuroblastoma in Sapporo city, *Cancer* 60:433-436, 1987.
41. Oberfield SE et al: Thyroid and gonadal function and growth of long term survivors of medulloblastoma/PNET. In Green DM, D'Angio GJ, editors: *Late effects of treatment for childhood cancer,*New York,1992, Wiley-Liss.
42. Palma L, Guidetti B: Cystic pilocytic astrocytomas of the cerebral hemispheres: surgical experience with 51 cases and long term results, *J Neurosurg* 62:811-815, 1985.
43. Patterson E, Farr RF: Cerebellar medulloblastoma: treatment by irradiation of the whole central nervous system, *Acta Radiol* 39:323-336, 1953.
44. Raney B: Soft tissue sarcoma in adolescents. In Tebbi CK, editor: *Adolescent oncology,* Mt Kisco, New York, 1987, Futura Publishing.
45. Reese A: *Tumors of the eye,* Hagerstown, Maryland, 1976, Harper & Row.
46. Rorke L: The cerebellar medulloblastoma and its relationship to primitive neuroectodermal tumors, *J Neuropathol Exp Neurol* 42:2-15, 1983.
47. Rudoler S, et al: Patterns of presentation, treatment, and outcome of children referred for emergent/urgent therapeutic irradiation. Presented at The Evolving Role of Radiation in Pediatric Oncology Conference, Philadelphia, 1995.
48. Silverman CL, Simpson JR: Cerebellar medulloblastoma: the importance of posterior fossa dose to survival and patterns of failure, *Int J Radiat Oncol Biol Phys* 8:1869-1876, 1982.
49. Stevens KR Jr: The soft tissue. In Moss WT, Cox JD: *Radiation oncology: rationale, techniques, results,* ed 6, St Louis, 1989, Mosby.
50. Tarbell NJ, Buck BA: *Postgraduate advances in radiation oncology: the treatment of medulloblastoma,* Berryville, Virginia, 1990, Forum Medicum.
51. Tefft M, Wharam M, and Gehan E: Local and regional control of rhabdomyosarcoma by radiation in IRS II, *Int J Rad Oncol Biol Phys* 15(suppl 1):159, 1988.
52. Thomas PRM: Personal communication, 1994.
53. Thomas PRM et al: Validation of radiation dose reductions used in the Third National Wilms' Tumor Study, Proc ASCO 29:227, 1988 .
54. Van den Berge JH et al: Intracavitary brachytherapy of cystic craniopharyngiomas, *J Neurosurg* 77:545-550, 1992.
55. Young JA, Eslinger P, Galloway M: Radiation treatment for the child with cancer, *Issues Comp Pediatri Nurs* 12:159-169, 1989.

BIBLIOGRAPHY

D'Angio GJ et al" *Practical pediatric oncology:* New York, 1989, Raven.

Green DM, D'Angio GJ, editors: *Late effects of treatment for childhood cancer,* New York, 1992, Wiley-Liss.

Halperin EC et al: *Pediatric radiation oncology,* New York, 1989, Raven.

Kun LE: Childhood cancers. In Moss WT, Cox JD, editors: *Radiation oncology: rationale, techniques, results,* St Louis, 1989, Mosby.

Matus-Ridley M et al: Histiocytosis X in children: patterns of disease and results of treatment, *Med Pediatr Oncol* 11:99-105, 1983.

Pizzo PA et al: *Principles and practice of pediatric oncology,* Philadelphia, 1993, JB Lippincott.

Schwartz CL et al: Survivors of childhood cancer: assessment and management,

Weiss DR, Cassady JR, Peterson R: Retinoblastoma: a modification in radiation therapy technique, Radiology 114:705-708, 1975.

APPENDIX

A

Glossary

abdominoperineal resection An anterior incision into the abdominal wall, with the construction of a colostomy followed by a perineal incision to remove the rectum and anus and draining lymphatics.

accelerated fractionation The technique in which the overall treatment time is shortened through the use of doses per fraction less than conventional doses two to three times per day.

accelerated hyperfractionation Treatment more than once a day, with fraction sizes and the number of treatment days equivalent to accelerated fractionation but with a higher total dose.

actinic keratosis A warty lesion with areas of red, scaly patches occurring on the sun-exposed skin of the face or hands of older, light-skinned individuals.

achalasia The loss of the normal peristaltic activity of the lower two thirds of the esophagus, resulting in dilation of the esophagus. The risk factor for the development of esophageal cancer.

adenohypophysis The anterior lobe of the pituitary.

adjuvant therapy The use of one form of treatment in addition to another.

akimbo The position in which the arms are bent by the side.

alopecia Hair loss.

American Joint Committee on Cancer (AJCC) A classification and anatomical staging system.

anaplastic A pathological description of cells, describing a loss of differentiation and more primitive appearance.

aneuploid A condition in which the cells have an abnormal number of chromosomes.

Ann Arbor staging system A classification system used for non-Hodgkin's lymphomas and Hodgkin's disease.

anterior resection An abdominal incision to remove an affected portion of the bowel with the margin plus the adjacent lymphatics. An end-to-end anastomosis is constructed, maintaining the continuity of the gastrointestinal tract (no colostomy).

astrocytoma A central nervous system tumor originating from the nonneuronal-supportiong cells. It can be low grade or anaplastic.

asymmetric collimation A process using collimators in which the blade pairs are capable of independent movement.

atypical hyperplasia The proliferation of unusual-appearing cells in a normal tissue arrangement.

auer rods Structures in the cytoplasm of myeloblasts, myelocytes, and monoblasts.

autologous bone marrow transplant (ABMT) A technique of using a patient's own previously removed bone marrow to rescue the patient from the potentially fatal hematological toxicity of extremely high-dose chemotherapy and radiation.

B symptoms A group of symptoms (fevers, night sweats, weight loss) associated with lymphomas.

Barrett's esophagus A condition in which the distal esophagus is lined with a columnar epithelium rather than a stratified squamous epithelium. It usually occurs with gastroesophogeal reflux. This condition is associated with an increased risk in the development of adenocarcinomas of the distal esophagus.

basal cell carcinoma A slow-growing, locally invasive, but rarely metastasizing neoplasm derived from basal cells of the epidermis or hair follicles.

benign prostatic hypertrophy (BPH) An enlargement of the prostate gland common in men over 50 years old. It generally causes a narrowing of the urethra.

bitemporal-hemianopsia The loss of peripheral vision.

blood-brain barrier The barrier system that hinders penetration of some substances into the brain and cerebrospinal fluid. The blood-brain barrier exists between the vascular system and brain. Its purpose is to protect the brain from potentially toxic substances.

Bowen's disease A precancerous dermatosis or form of intraepidermal carcinoma characterized by the development of pink or brown papules covered with a thickened, horny layer.

bronchogenic carcinoma Cancer of the lung that arises in the anatomy of the bronchial tree.

carcinoma in situ Malignant changes at the cellular level in epithelial tissues without extension beyond the basement membrane.

carina Bifurcation of the trachea at the level of T4.

cervix The part of the uterus that protrudes into the cavity of the vagina.

childhood cancer The incidence of malignancies in people less than 18 years old.

chromophobe adenomas Nonfunctioning pituitary tumors.

chronic ulcerative colitis Extensive inflammation and ulceration of the bowel wall resulting in bloody mucoid diarrhea several times a day. It is associated with an increased risk of the development of colorectal cancer.

cold thyroid nodule A nodule having no uptake.

concomitant The situation in which two types of treatment take place at the same time.

conformal radiation therapy Therapy that, with the use of three-dimensional treatment planning, allows the delivery of higher tumor doses to selected target volumes without increasing treatment morbidity.

contiguous Systematic and predictable, as in the spread of Hodgkin's disease.

conventional fractionation Fractionation in which the total dose of radiation is typically divided into 180 or 200 cGy increments and delivered once a day, 5 days a week.

coplanar A geometrical principle describing two radiation fields configured in such a way that the beam edges lie in the same plane. (The central ray is not parallel opposed.)

craniospinal irradiation (CSI) Complex irradiation of all central nervous system and cerebrospinal fluid regions from behind the eye down to the midsacrum for treatment of medulloblastoma and other cerebrospinal fluid seeding tumors.

cryotherapy The use of cold temperatures to treat a disease.

cryptorchidism Undescended testes.

cerebrospinal fluid (CSF) A clear, colorless fluid resembling water composed of proteins, glucose, urea, and salts. CSF performs several functional roles, including buoyancy to protect the brain, an aid in controlling the chemical environment of the central nervous system, a means of exchanging nutrients and waste products with the central nervous system, and a channel for intracerebral transport.

cystectomy Surgical removal of the bladder.

debulking surgery Surgery for reducing a large, unresectable tumor.

de novo A Latin term that means "anew".

dermis The deeper layer of the skin composed of connective tissue that contains blood and lymphatic vessels, nerves and nerve endings, sweat glands, and hair follicles.

desquamation An acute effect of irradiation characterized by shedding of the epidermis.

diaphysis The shaft or long axis of the bone.

diffuse adenomas Pituitary tumors that usually fill the entire sella turcica and can erode its wall.

drop metastases Secondary tumors that occur via the cerebrospinal fluid.

dysphagia Difficulty in swallowing. The sensation of food sticking in the throat.

EAM External auditory meatus.

ecchymoses The escape of blood into the tissues, causing large, blotchy areas of discoloration.

electrocautery An instrument for directing a high-frequency current through a local tissue area.

endocavitary radiation therapy A sphincter-sparing procedure in which the radiation treatment is delivered by a 50-kVp contact unit inserted into the rectum. Only a select group of low-middle-third rectal lesions that have small exophytic tumors confined to the bowel wall are eligible candidates for this treatment.

endophytic pattern A growth pattern that invades within the lamina propria and submucosa.

ependymoma Tumors arising from the ependymal cells lining the brain ventricles and central spinal canal. They may be low or high grade.

epidemiology The study of disease frequency and distribution.

epidermis The extremely thin outer layer of the skin composed of four to five distinct layers of cells.

epiphyseal line Cartilage at the junction of the diaphysis and epiphysis in young bones that serves as a growth area for long-bone lengthening.

epiphysis The knoblike part of a long bone made up of spongy bone. It is located at either end of a long bone.

epistaxis A nosebleed.

erythema This acute radiation effect, manifested by redness and inflammation of the skin or mucous membranes, is due to capillary congestion, caused by dilatation of the superficial capillaries.

erythroplasia Reddened, velvetlike patches on the mucous membranes.

esophagitis Inflammation of the esophagus. Patients complain of substernal pain and food sticking. Esophagitis begins after 2 weeks of radiation therapy and continues for 2 to 4 weeks after treatment.

exophytic A noninvasive neoplasm that projects out from an epithelial surface.

familial adenomatous polyps (FAP) A hereditary disease in which the entire large bowel is studded with polyps. If left untreated, the patient develops a cancer of the large bowel.

fibrosis The abnormal formation of fibrous tissue caused by alterations in the structure and function of blood vessels.

friable tumors Tumors that are easily broken or pulverized.

Gardner's syndrome An inherited disorder (similar to familial adenomatous polyps) consisting of adenomatous polyposis of the large bowel, upper gastrointestinal polyps, periampullary tumors, lipomas, fibromas, and other tumors. This condition is associated with an increased risk in the development of colorectal cancer.

gadolinium A noniodine-based intravenous contrast agent used for computed tomography and magnetic resonance imaging scans. Gadolinium helps differentiate between edema and a tumor.

germ cell tumors Tumors developing from embryological nests of tissue located throughout the body, from the brain down to the ovaries and testes.

hematuria A common symptom of bladder and kidney tumors with an abnormal presence of blood in the urine.

hemiglossectomy The surgical removal of half the tongue.

hereditary nonpolyposis colorectal syndrome The frequent occurrence of colorectal cancer in families *without* adenomatous polyposis. This syndrome is associated with an increased risk of developing a second malignancy of the colon and adenocarcinomas of the breast, ovary, endometrium, and pancreas.

hilum The area of an organ where blood, lymphatic vessels, and nerves enter and exit.

histiocyte A phagocytic cell found in loose connective tissue.

histiocytosis X A spectrum of diseases caused by abnormal proliferaton of a variety of immune cells affecting single or multiple organs.

Horner's syndrome A condition caused by paralysis of the cervical sympathetic nerves. It may cause sinking in of the eyeball, ptosis of the upper eyelid, slight elevation of the lower lid, constriction of the pupil,and flushing of the affected side of the face.

hot thyroid nodule A nodule having a radionuclide uptake much higher than the rest of the thyroid gland.

hyperfractionation Fractional doses smaller than conventional, delivered two or three times daily to achieve an increase in the total dose in the same overall time.

hyperparathyroidism A condition caused by a tumor in the parathyroid, where calcium is leaked from the bones, resulting in softening and deformity as the mineral salts are replaced by fibrous connective tissue.

hyperthyroidism Hyperactivity of the thyroid gland.

hypophysis The pituitary gland.

hypothyroidism Underactivity of the thyroid gland.

impotence A significant side effect associated with the treatment of prostate cancer in which the adult male is unable to obtain an erection or ejaculate after achieving an erection.

induration The process of becoming hard and firm in soft tissues.

infundibulum Stalklike structures that attach the pituitary to the hypothalamus.

interstitial implant The application of a brachytherapy implant directly into the tissues via devices such as needles, ribbons, or seeds placed in the at-risk tissues.

intrauterine tandem A brachytherapy device placed through the cervical os into the uterus and subsequently afterloaded to give the dose application directly to the cervix, uterus, and upper vagina.

intraoperative radiation therapy (IORT) A boost technique in which a single dose of 10 to 20 Gy is delivered directly to the tumor bed with electrons or photons. The tumor bed has been surgically exposed, allowing critical normal structures to be shielded or displaced out of the radiation beam.

isthmus Connects the lobes of the thyroid gland.

intravenous pyelogram (IVP) A radiographic procedure using contrast media to outline the kidneys, ureters, and bladder.

jugulo-digastric The group of high neck nodes below the mastoid tip.

Kaposi's sarcoma A slow-growing, temperate tumor thought to arise from vascular tissue and associated with nodular purple lesions that are often multifocal.

Karnofsky performance scale (KPS) A scale that measures the neurological and functional status. KPS allows measuring of the quantity and quality of neurological defects. The scale ranges from 1 to 100 and is measured in decades.

keratin An extremely tough, waterproof, protein substance in hair, nails, and horny tissue.

keratinocyte Any one of the cells in the skin that synthesizes keratin.

keratoacanthoma A papular lesion filled with a keratin plug that can resemble squamous cell carcinoma. It is benign and usually subsides spontaneously within 6 months.

keratosis A lesion on the epidermis marked by the presence of a circumsized overgrowth of the horny layer.

latent period The time between the exposure and incidence of an abnormality.

leukoencephalopathy Widespread demyelinating lesions of the brain, brain stem, and cerebellum.

leukopenia An abnormal decrease in the white blood cell count, usually below 5000 per cu mm.

leukoplakia Small, white, raised patches on the mucous membrane.

Lhermitte's syndrome Pain resembling sudden electric shock throughout the body. It is produced by flexing of the neck or some cervical trauma.

limb salvage surgery (LSS) Radical or wide en bloc resection for soft tissue sarcoma that requires a 1- to 3-cm normal tissue margin that allows the limb and extremity to remain intact (avoids amputation).

lytic Pertaining to the destruction of cells.

malignant melanoma The most lethal form of skin cancer which arises from the melanocytes found in the stratum basale of the epidermis.

mantle field The radiation field that treats the lymph nodes superior to the diaphragm.

mediastinum Tissue and organs separating the lungs. The mediastinum contains the heart and its large vessels, trachea, esophagus, thymus, lymph nodes, and other structures.

medullary The cavity within the bone that contains fats or yellow bone marrow.

medulloblastoma A highly malignant cerebellar tumor usually arising in the midline with the propensity to spread via the cerebrospinal fluid.

melanin The pigment that gives color to the skin and hair and serves as protection from ultraviolet light.

melanocyte The melanin-forming cell found in the stratum basale of the epidermis.

menarche The beginning of a woman's first menstrual period.

menopause The end of a woman's menstrual activity.

menorrhagia Pain during menstruation.

mesothelioma Malignant tumors that develop in the mesothelial lining, the pleura, and possibly the pericardium.

Mohs' surgery A surgical method in which the tumor is removed one layer at a time and examined microscopically. It is used for tumors in high risk sites for recurrence and those with aggressive histological subtypes. Mohs' surgery is known for its high success rate.

multicentric Arising from many foci and having multiple origination.

multidisciplinary Having two or more modalities in a combined effort to treat a disease process.

Musculoskeletal Tumor Society (MTS) A surgical staging system—classification and anatomical staging system used for soft tissue sarcomas.

mycosis fungoides A chronic, progressive lymphoma arising in the skin. Initially, the disease stimulates eczema or other inflammatory dermatoses. In advanced cases, ulcerated tumors and infiltrations of lymph nodes may occur.

nadir The lowest point and the time of greatest depression of blood values.

necrosis Death or disintegration of a cell or tissue caused by disease or injury.

neuroblastoma Cancer of neural crest tissues, usually adrenal medulla or spinal ganglia, with frequent metastases.

neurohypophysis The posterior lobe of the pituitary.

nevus A benign, localized cluster of melanocytes arising in the skin, usually early in life.

odontalgia A toothache.

odynophagia Painful swelling.

Ohngren's line The line that connects the medial canthus of the eye with the angle of the mandible. It divides the maxillary antrum into anterior-inferior/superior-posterior halves.

oncogene A gene that regulates the development and growth of cancerous tissues.

oophorectomy The surgical removal of the ovaries.

oophoropexy Fixation of the ovaries behind the uterus.

orthogonal films Two films taken 90 degrees apart. They are required for treatment-planning purposes to define the location and relationship of various anatomical structures relative to the field's isocenter.

orthopnea Difficulty breathing, except in an upright position.

osseous Composed of bone or resembling bone; bony.

osteoblasts Bone-forming cells.

osteomyelitis Infection of bone and marrow caused by the growth of germs in the bone. Infection may reach the bone through the bloodstream or direct injury.

otalgia An earache.

Paget's disease A disease characterized by excessive and abnormal bone reabsorption and formation. It may affect any part of the skeletal system but primarily strikes the spine, pelvis, femur, and skull.

palliation Noncurative treatment to relieve pain and suffering.

pancoast tumor A malignant superior sulcus tumor in the apex of the lung with clinical symptoms that includes (1) pain around the shoulder and down the arm (2) atrophy of the muscles of the hand (3) Horner's syndrome caused by involvement of the brachial plexus, and (4) bone erosion of the ribs and sometimes vertebrae.

papilledema Swelling of the optic disk, usually associated with increased intracranial pressure.

paraaortic field The radiation field that treats the subdiaphragmatic nodes.

parametrium Tissues lateral to and around the uterus.

paraneoplastic syndrome A collective term for disorders arising from metabolic effects of cancer on tissues remote from the tumor. Such disorders may appear as endocrine, hematological, or neuromuscular disorders.

parity Viable pregnancy (500 gm birth weight or 20-week gestation), regardless of the outcome.

pelvic inlet The upper entrance into the pelvis, bordered by the sacral promontory, medial pelvic sidewalls, and pubic bones.

perineum The part of the body dorsal to the pubic arch, ventral to the tip of the coccyx, and lateral to the inferior rami of the pubis, ischium, and sacrotuberous ligaments. These are the tissues surrounding the genitals and anal opening.

periosteum The glistening-white, double-layered membrane covering the outer surface of the diaphysis.

peritoneal cytology Pathological examination of cells obtained from the fluid surrounding the abdominal wall and its contained viscera.

peritoneal seeding The shedding or sloughing of tumor cells into the abdominal (peritoneal) cavity.

petechiae Minute red spots caused by the escape of small amounts of blood.

pigmentation Coloration of the skin caused by the presence or absence of melanin.

ploidy The number of chromosome sets in a cell. (Haploid cells have one set, and diploid cells have two sets.)

Plummer-Vinson syndrome Iron-deficiency anemia characterized by esophageal webs and atrophic glossitis. It predisposes an individual to the development of esophageal cancer.

pluripotent Pertaining to an embryonic cell that can form different kinds of cells.

polyurethane mold An immobilization-repositioning device in which polyurethane (a synthetic rubber polymer) foam hardens and shapes to the patient's body build.

primary site compartment Natural anatomical boundaries surrounding the soft tissue sarcoma primary. It is composed of common fascia plane(s) of muscles, bone, joint, skin, subcutaneous tissues, and major neurovascular structures.

progenitor Originator or precursor.

prostate A walnut-shaped organ that surrounds the male urethra, located between the base of the bladder and urogenital diaphragm.

pruritis Itching.

prostate-specific antigen (PSA) Testing that involves an evaluation of plasma levels. Prostatic antigen is found not only in prostate tissue and seminal fluid, but also in the sera of patients with benign prostatic hypertrophy or cancer.

pseudocapsule Soft tissue sarcomas that are surrounded by compressed normal tissue, reactive inflammation, and fibrosis to give the gross anatomical appearance of a capsule.

purpura Blotchyness and red spots caused by pectechiae and ecchymoses.
radiation necrosis Tissue death resulting from the effects of radiation.
radiosensitizers Chemicals that help enhance the lethal effects of radiation.
Reed-Sternberg cell A giant connective tissue cell with one or two large nuclei that is characteristic of Hodgkin's disease.
regeneration The repair, regrowth, or restoration of a part (as tissue).
retinoblastoma A primitive neuroectodermal tumor of the retina that may be inherited. It usually occurs in children under 4 years old.
rhabdomyosarcoma (RMS) A malignancy of skeletal-muscle origin that can occur in many areas of the body and disseminates early.
Rouvièr's node A node located just inferior to the base of the skull and medial to the internal carotid artery.
second malignant neoplasm (SMN) Cancer developing years after the treatment of an initial tumor related to genetics and previous carcinogenic chemotherapy and radiation.
seminoma The most common malignant testicular tumor.
shelling A surgical procedure that removes the primary tumor and its pseudocapsule, giving it the gross appearance of having removed all viable tumor.
shine over The falloff of the radiation beam over a surface that misses tissue and projects in the air; also known as *fall off.*
shrinking fields A technique that reduces the treated field area one or more times during the course of treatment in response to a tumor that reduces in size and/or the need to limit doses to normal structures.
smegma A white secretion located under the prepuce of the foreskin in the adult male. It is carcinogenic in animals.
soft tissue sarcoma (STS) A malignant tumor arising primarily, but not exclusively, from mesenchymal connective tissues. The following are types of sarcomas:

- **liposarcoma**—STS arising from fat
- **leiomyosarcoma**—STS arising from smooth muscle
- **rhabdomyosarcoma**—STS arising from striated muscle
- **fibrosarcoma**—STS derived from collagen-producing fibroblasts
- **malignant fibrous histiocytoma (MFH)**—Deep STS tumor showing partial fibroblastic and histiocytic differentiation with a variable pattern and giant cells
- **neurofibromatosis (von Recklinghausen's disease)**—Small, discrete, pigmented skin lesions (cafe au lait spots and/or pigmented nevi) that develop into multiple neurofibromas along the course of peripheral nerves; may undergo malignant transformation.
- **schwannoma**—Nonencapsulated tumor resulting from disorderly proliferation of Schwann cells that includes portions of nerve fibers; typically undergoes formation to malignant Schwannomas

staging laparotomy A surgical procedure that includes a splenectomy, lymph node biopsy, and bone marrow biopsy; used in staging lymphomas
stereotactic radiosurgery The use of a high-energy photon beam with multiple ports of entry convergent on the target volume.
stomatitis Inflammation of the mouth.
striae Lines or bands elevated above or depressed below surrounding tissue.
stridor Harsh, rasping breath.
subcutaneous layer A layer of areolar connective tissue and adipose tissue that lies beneath the dermis and contains nerves and blood vessels.
superior vena cava syndrome Edema of the face, neck, or upper arms due to increased venous pressures caused by compression of the superior vena cava. It is most commonly caused by a metastatic, mediastinal lymph node tumor in lung cancer.
synergistic A body organ, medicine, or substance that cooperates with another or others to produce a total effect greater than the sum of the individual elements.
$TD_{5/5}$ The dose of radiation that is expected to produce a 5% complication rate within 5 years.
$TD_{5/50}$ The dose of radiation that is expected to produce a 50% complication rate within 5 years.
telangiectasia Dilation of the surface blood vessels caused by the loss of capillary tone, resulting in a fine spider-vein appearance on the skin surface.
tenesmus Ineffective and painful straining during a bowel movement.
three-point setup Three marks placed on a patient to define the isocenter. It is used to position and level the patient daily to ensure reproducibility and consistency of the setup and treatment.
thrombocytopenia An abnormal decrease in the number of platelets.
total nodal irradiation A system of radiating all the major lymph nodes.
trigone The portion of the bladder (shaped like a triangle) formed by the openings of the two ureters and orifice of the urethra.
transurethral resection (TURP) A surgical procedure of the prostate performed through the urethra.
ulceration A rare, late radiation reaction exhibited by an open sore on the skin or mucous membrane. It is caused by the shedding of dead tissue.
vaginal colpostats Paired brachytherapy devices that allow insertion into the lateral vaginal fornices or apex of the vagina for intracavitary treatment. These are usually shielded anteriorly and posteriorly for greater lateral throw of the dose and often look like small golf clubs.
vaginal cuff The small rim of vaginal tissue at the apex of the vagina around the cervix. Some of this is removed during a hysterectomy, and some remains as the new apex of the vagina with surgical scarring.
vaginal cylinder A domed-ended tubular brachytherapy device used to give even dose distribution to the apex or entire vaginal surface. This resembles a candle with a central hollow canal for later afterloading.
vulva Female external genitalia composed of the mons veneris, labia majora, labia minora, vestibule of the vagina, and vestibular glands.

Waldeyer's ring The ring of tonsillar tissue that encircles the nasopharynx and oropharynx: two palatine tonsils, lingual and pharyngeal tonsils.

warm thyroid nodule A nodule having a slightly higher concentration than the rest of the thyroid gland.

wide resection A surgical procedure for soft tissue carcinoma. The procedure involves a wide en bloc excision for limb salvage and/or wide through-bone amputation.

Wilms' tumor Childhood embryonal kidney cancer.

xeroderma pigmentosum A rare disease of the skin starting in childhood and marked by disseminated pigment discolorations, ulcers, cutaneous and muscluar atrophy, and death.

APPENDIX

B

Answers to Review Questions

CHAPTER 1

1. a
2. c
3. b
4. b
5. a
6. b
7. c
8. d
9. b
10. a

CHAPTER 2

1. b
2. a,b,c,d
3. c
4. c
5. b
6. d
7. a
8. d
9. d
10. c

CHAPTER 3

1. c
2. d
3. c
4. b
5. a
6. d
7. c
8. a
9. c
10. c

CHAPTER 4

1. Submandibular, occipital, cervical, supraclavicular, infraclavicular, axillary, hilar, and mediastinal.
2. Fever (above 38° C), night sweats, and weight loss. About 33% of Hodgkin's disease patients experience B symptoms, but only 10% to 15% of lymphoma patients experience them.
3. Lymphocyte predominant (most favorable), nodular sclerosing, mixed cellularity, and lymphocyte depletion (least favorable)
4. Borders of a mantle field: anterior—superior border (inferior portion of mandible) inferior border (insertion of the diaphragm [T-10]), laterally (to include axilla); posterior—superior border (includes the occipital nodes), other borders are the same.
   Daily dose: 150 to 200 cGy; total dose: 3500 to 4400 cGy for mantle *and* paraaortic fields.
5.

Common side effects	**Management**
Fatigue	Rest, change in daily routines
Occipital hair loss	Nothing
Erythemia	Application of aloe vera or skin creams, protection from sun
Sore throat	Throat lozenges, altered diet (soft foods, no alcohol)
Nausea	Antinauseant, perhaps altered diet

6. Rappaport system: categorized by survival differences, did not account for lymphomas which commonly progress from low to high grade during the-course of the disease, contained some inaccuracies. Working Formulation: bases subtypes (10) according to morphology, clinical features, and prognosis.
7. Nodular lymphomas
8. CHOP, C-MOPP, BACOP, COMLA (most common)
9. Interferon alpha and bone marrow transplants
10. 4000 to 5000 cGy.

CHAPTER 5

1. a
2. b
3. c
4. b
5. Testes, central nervous system
6. ALL, AML, CLL, CML
7. Chemotherapy
8. Ionizing radiation
9. CNS treatment, total body irradiation, control of hepatomegaly or splenomegaly

CHAPTER 6

1. False
2. False
3. False
4. a and c
5. d
6. c
7. Stereotactic radiosurgery
8. Microadenomas
9. Left
10. Stage

CHAPTER 7

1. Increased duration of smoking, increased use of unfiltered cigarettes, increased number of cigarettes consumed
2. Stage, performance (Karnofsky) status, weight loss
3. Mediastinal and intrapulmonic
4. 6000 to 7500 cGy
5. Dermatitis, erythema, esophagitis
6. d
7. c
8. d
9. b
10. c

CHAPTER 8

1. a. Swelling, ulcer fails to heal
   b. Stridor, hoarseness
   c. Bloody discharge, difficulty hearing
2. Lateral borders, anterior two thirds surface
3. T_1 Confined to true cords, normal mobility
   T_2 Supra or subglottic extension, slightly impaired mobility
   T_3 Cord fixation or extension into epiglottis or hypopharynx
4. Anterior: Posterior third of the orbit
   Posterior: 2 cm posterior to spinous process
   Superior: Base of brain
   Inferior: Below angle of the jaw
5. Nasopharyngeal cancer
6. C-3
7. Dry mouth, loss of taste and smell, dysphagia, sore throat, mucositis
8. Leukoplakia and erythroplasia
9. Spinal accessory, supraclavicular, jugular, juglo-digastric (receives nearly all lymph nodes draining the neck)
10.

Cranial Nerve	Function
Olfactory	Smell
Optic	Sight
Oculomotor	Eye (up-down movement)
Trochlear	Eye (rotation)
Trigeminal	Sensory for jaw and face
Abducens	Eye (lateral movement)
Facial	Muscle contractions
Acoustic	Hearing
Glossopharyngeal	Tongue, throat movement
Vagus	Talking, sounds
Spinal accessory	Head, shoulders movement
Hypoglossal	Chewing, tongue

CHAPTER 9

1. c (Gliomas comprise 50% of all primary brain tumors)
2. c
3. e
4. a
5. d
6. c (Although primary brain tumors are relatively uncommon, metastases occur in approximately 30% of all patients with cancer and are the most common brain lesions.)
7. True
8. True (However, children under the age of 4 present a problem with respect to the treatment regimen. Therapy must be modified because of the developing brain. Because the developing brain is more sensitive to radiation, treatment in children under 4 years old must be avoided.)
9. True
10. True

CHAPTER 10

1. Colorectal cancer spreads by direct extension, lymphatic spread, and hematogenous (blood borne) spread.
2. Patients should be on a low-residue diet, avoiding fresh fruits and vegetables, whole-grain breads and cereals, and milk products. Recommended foods include white bread, baked or broiled meats, bananas, macaroni, and cooked vegetables. Antidiarrheal agents (Lomotil) are prescribed to assist in the medical management of diarrhea.
3. d
4. c
5. d
6. a
7. c
8. d
9. c
10. a

CHAPTER 11

1. False
2. False
3. True
4. False
5. True
6. b
7. a
8. d
9. c
10. e

CHAPTER 12

1. b
2. d
3. a
4. d
5. a
6. c

CHAPTER 13

1. d
2. c
3. d
4. a
5. c
6. a
7. a
8. c
9. b
10. b
11. a
12. c

CHAPTER 14

1. b
2. d
3. d
4. False
5. False
6. 1000
7. 1500
8. Osteosarcoma

Index

R

W

X

Y

Z